Primary Care Rheumatology

Primary Care Rheumatology

Edward D. Harris, Jr., MD
George DeForest Barnett Professor
Department of Medicine
Division of Rheumatology and Immunology
Stanford University School of Medicine
Palo Alto, California

Mark C. Genovese, MD
Assistant Professor
Department of Medicine
Division of Rheumatology and Immunology
Stanford University School of Medicine
Palo Alto, California

W.B. SAUNDERS COMPANY
A Division of Harcourt Brace & Company
Philadelphia   London   Toronto   Sydney

W.B. SAUNDERS COMPANY
A Division of Harcourt Brace & Company

The Curtis Center
Independence Square West
Philadelphia, Pennsylvania 19106

Library of Congress Cataloging-in-Publication Data

Primary care rheumatology / [edited by] Edward D. Harris, Jr., Mark C. Genovese.—1st ed.

p. cm.

ISBN 0–7216–7172–1

1. Musculoskeletal system—Diseases. 2. Rheumatology. 3. Primary care (Medicine) I. Harris, Edward D. Jr., 1937- . II. Genovese, Mark C. [DNLM: 1. Musculoskeletal Diseases. 2. Primary Health Care. We 140 P952 2000]

RC925.P6865 2000 616.7—dc21

DNLM/DLC   99–17269

PRIMARY CARE RHEUMATOLOGY   ISBN   0–7216–7172–1

Printed in the United States of America.

Last digit is the print number: 9 8 7 6 5 4 3 2 1

To *Ned, Edie, Andrew, Eliza, Tom, Kate, Maeve, Chandler,* and *Waldo*   —**EDH**

To *Nancy, Alexandra,* and *Danielle for your patience, and to* **Ted** *for your direction*   —**MCG**

Christopher F. Beaulieu, MD, PhD
Assistant Professor, Department of Radiology,
Stanford University School of Medicine, Palo Alto,
California
Musculoskeletal Imaging in Rheumatologic Disorders

Ann Gabrielle Bergman, MD
Associate Professor, Department of Radiology,
Stanford University School of Medicine, Palo Alto,
California
Musculoskeletal Imaging in Rheumatologic Disorders

Alan P. Bocko, MD
Podiatric Fellow, Department of Functional
Restoration, Division of Orthopaedic Surgery,
Stanford University School of Medicine, Palo Alto,
California
Management of Common Foot Problems

Peter Brukner, MBBS, FACSP
Clinic Director, Olympic Park Sports Medicine Centre,
Melbourne, Australia
Overuse Injuries

Eugene J. Carragee, MD, FACS
Associate Professor, Department of Functional
Restoration, Division of Orthopaedic Surgery,
Stanford University School of Medicine; Director,
Orthopaedic Spine Surgery, Stanford University
Medical Center, Palo Alto, California
*Neck Pain; Musculoskeletal Pain and Emotional
Disorders; Infections of the Spine*

Loretta B. Chou, MD
Assistant Professor, Department of Functional
Restoration, Division of Orthopaedic Surgery,
Stanford University School of Medicine, Palo Alto,
California
Foot and Ankle Pain

Edward Damore, MD
Private Practice, Los Gatos, California
Hand and Wrist Pain

Elaine S. Date, MD
Associate Professor, Department of Functional
Restoration; Chief, Division of Physical Medicine
and Rehabilitation, Stanford University School of
Medicine, Palo Alto, California
Low Back Pain

Michael F. Dillingham, MD
Clinical Professor, Department of Functional
Restoration, Stanford University School of Medicine;
Executive Director, UCSF/Stanford Health Center,
Sports Medicine Program, Palo Alto, California
*Trauma—Management by the Primary Care Physician
and the Orthopaedic Surgeon*

Maurice L. Druzin, MD
Professor, Department of Gynecology and Obstetrics;
Chief, Section of Maternal Fetal Medicine, Stanford
University School of Medicine; Chief of Obstetrics,
Lucile Salter Packard Children's Hospital at Stanford,
Stanford University Medical Center, Palo Alto,
California
Rheumatic Diseases and the Pregnant Woman

Gary S. Fanton, MD
Clinical Assistant Professor, Department of Functional
Restoration, Division of Orthopaedic Surgery,
Stanford University School of Medicine, Palo Alto,
California
*Trauma—Management by the Primary Care Physician
and the Orthopaedic Surgeon*

James F. Fries, MD
Professor of Medicine, Department of Medicine,
Division of Immunology and Rheumatology, Stanford
University School of Medicine, Palo Alto, California
Drugs that Relieve Pain and Inflammation

Raymond R. Gaeta, MD
Associate Professor, Department of Anesthesiology,
Stanford University School of Medicine; Director,
Stanford Pain Management Service UCSF/Stanford
Health Care, Palo Alto, California
Pain—Its Origin, Consequences, and Management

Mark C. Genovese, MD
Assistant Professor, Department of Medicine, Division
of Rheumatology and Immunology, Stanford
University School of Medicine, Palo Alto, California
*Aspiration and Injection of Joints and Soft Tissue;
Rheumatic Diseases and the Pregnant Woman;
Differential Diagnosis of Soft Tissue and Joint Pain;
Systemic Lupus Erythematosus and Systemic Vasculitis;
ICD-9 Codes for Diagnosis in Rheumatic Diseases;
Representative Case Studies*

Stuart B. Goodman, MD, PhD, FRCSC, FACS
Professor, Department of Functional Restoration, Division of Orthopaedic Surgery, Stanford University School of Medicine; Chief, Orthopaedic Clinics, Stanford University Medical Center, Palo Alto, California
The Primary Care Physician and the Specialist: Guidelines for Referral

Edward D. Harris, Jr., MD
George DeForest Barnett Professor, Department of Medicine, Division of Rheumatology and Immunology, Stanford University School of Medicine, Palo Alto, California
The Primary Care Physician and the Specialist: Guideline for Referral; The Initial Evaluation: An Approach to Rapid Diagnosis; A Guide to Efficient Examination and Diagnosis of the Musculoskeletal System; Differential Diagnosis of Soft Tissue and Joint Pain; Rheumatoid Arthritis and Lyme Disease; Scleroderma; Heritable Diseases Affecting the Immune and Musculoskeletal Systems

Halsted R. Holman, MD
Berthold and Belle N. Guggenhime Professor, Department of Medicine, Division of Rheumatology and Immunology, Stanford University School of Medicine, Palo Alto, California
Systemic Lupus Erythematosus and Systemic Vasculitis

Elizabeth C. W. Hughes, MD
Clinical Instructor, Department of Dermatology, Stanford University School of Medicine, Palo Alto, California
The Skin and Musculoskeletal Diseases

Amy L. Ladd, MD
Associate Professor of Surgery, Department of Functional Restoration, Stanford University School of Medicine, Palo Alto, California
Hand and Wrist Pain

Nancy E. Lane, MD
Associate Professor of Medicine, Department of Medicine, Division of Rheumatology, University of California, San Francisco, California
Osteoarthritis of the Extremities

Philipp K. Lang, MD
Assistant Professor, Department of Radiology, Stanford University School of Medicine, Palo Alto, California
Musculoskeletal Imaging in Rheumatologic Disorders

Todd L. Lincoln, MD
Assistant Professor, Department of Functional Restoration, Division of Orthopaedic Surgery, Stanford University School of Medicine, Palo Alto, California
The Child with Joint, Limb, or Back Pain

Kate Lorig, RN, DrPH
Associate Professor, Department of Medicine, Division of Rheumatology and Immunology, Stanford University School of Medicine, Palo Alto, California
Helping Patients to Learn to Live With Arthritis

Nisha J. Manek, MD
Senior Fellow, Division of Rheumatology and Immunology, Stanford University School of Medicine, Palo Alto, California
Inflammation and Noninflammatory Myopathies: Clinicopathologic Features and Treatment

Robert Marcus, MD
Professor, Department of Medicine, Division of Endocrinology, Gerontology, and Metabolism, Stanford University School of Medicine, Palo Alto, California
Osteoporosis

Gordon O. Matheson, MD
Associate Professor, Department of Functional Restoration and Chief, Division of Sports Medicine, Stanford University School of Medicine, Palo Alto, California
Overuse Injuries

Lawrence M. Oloff, MD
Department of Functional Restoration, Chief of Podiatry, Stanford University School of Medicine, Palo Alto, California
Management of Common Foot Problems

Glen S. O'Sullivan, MD
Assistant Professor, Division of Orthopaedic Surgery, Stanford University School of Medicine, Palo Alto, California
Osteoarthritis of the Spine

James Posever, MD
Fellow in Immunology and Rheumatology, Stanford University Medical Center, Palo Alto, California
Infections of Peripheral Joints

Boris Ratiner, MD
Rheumatology Fellow, Department of Medicine, Division of Rheumatology, University of California, San Francisco, San Francisco, California
Osteoarthritis of the Extremities

Marc A. Samson, MD
Fellow in Orthopaedics, Department of Functional Restoration, Stanford University School of Medicine, Palo Alto, California
Trauma—Management by the Primary Care Physician and the Orthopaedic Surgeon

Stephen A. Schendel, MD
Professor and Chair, Department of Functional Restoration, Stanford University School of Medicine, Palo Alto, California
Pain in the Jaw Joint: Diagnosis and Treatment

David J. Schurman, MD
Professor, Department of Functional Restoration,
Division of Orthopaedic Surgery, Stanford University
School of Medicine, Palo Alto, California
*A Guide to Efficient Examination and Diagnosis of the
Musculoskeletal System; Differential Diagnosis of Soft
Tissue and Joint Pain*

Christopher F. Snow, MD
Clinical Professor, Department of Medicine, Stanford
University School of Medicine, Palo Alto; Associate
Director, Primary Care, Santa Clara Valley Medical
Center, San Jose, California
Laboratory Testing for Musculoskeletal Diseases

Susan M. Swetter, MD
Assistant Professor, Department of Dermatology,
Stanford University School of Medicine, Palo Alto,
California
The Skin and Musculoskeletal Diseases

Jeffrey Ken Teraoka, MD
Assistant Professor, Department of Functional
Restoration, Division of Physical Medicine and
Rehabilitation, Stanford University School of
Medicine, Palo Alto, California
*Physical Modalities in Management of Pain and
Inflammation*

Andrew E. Turk, MD
Assistant Professor, Department of Functional
Restoration, Plastic and Reconstructive Surgery,
Stanford University School of Medicine, Palo Alto,
California
Pain in the Jaw Joint: Diagnosis and Treatment

Ronald F. van Vollenhoven, MD, PhD
Assistant Professor, Division of Rheumatology and
Immunology, Stanford University School of Medicine,
Palo Alto, California
*Aspiration and Injection of Joints and Soft Tissue;
Recordkeeping for Rheumatic Diseases; Inflammatory
and Noninflammatory Myopathies: Clinicopathologic
Features and Treatment*

Michael M. Ward, MD, MPH
Assistant Professor, Division of Rheumatology and
Immunology, Stanford University School of Medicine,
Palo Alto, California
*Special Problems of Musculoskeletal Disease in the
Elderly Patient; Seronegative Spondyloarthropathies;
Crystal Arthritis*

Peter B. J. Wu, MD, MPH
Clinical Assistant Professor, Department of Physical
Medicine and Rehabilitation, Stanford University
School of Medicine, Palo Alto Medical Foundation,
Palo Alto, California
*Physical Modalities in Management of Pain and
Inflammation; Differential Diagnosis of Soft Tissue and
Joint Pain*

Preface

One of the fascinating, yet bewildering, aspects of musculoskeletal diseases is that there are so many different disciplines of medicine and surgery that have an interest (and yes, a stake) in them. This reality is brought home each day as we triage patients referred to the Center for Musculoskeletal Diseases at Stanford University Medical Center. Who would be the best physician for the patient with a sore shoulder? The rheumatologist? The orthopaedic surgeon? The physiatrist? Although it is accepted that the patient with scleroderma should be referred to the rheumatologist, no one can ignore that the dermatologist can help with treatment. In addition, our colleagues in laboratory medicine and in radiology have broad arrays of diagnostic tests and imaging that help all of us. However, for the practicing internist or family practitioner, the potential menu for obtaining help for a patient can be confusing.

Our objective in developing *Primary Care Rheumatology* has been to help our colleagues in primary care diagnose and treat patients with multiple syndromes and diseases that affect the musculoskeletal and immune systems. It is exciting and rewarding for a practitioner to use successfully a new medication in a patient with an illness that he or she rarely sees. On the other hand, it is useful to know how and when to refer a patient for consultation; and it is equally important to know what kind of help is available from which specialist.

In *Primary Care Rheumatology* we have not arbitrarily said ". . . refer a patient with disease X to specialist Z." Rather, we have presented views of syndromes and diseases from multiple perspectives. For example, two analyses of foot pain are presented, one by an orthopaedic surgeon who subspecializes in diseases of the foot, and another by a podiatrist. A physiatrist and rheumatologist have combined to help give direction in assessment and treatment of soft tissue pain and inflammation. Compared with the usual "disease-oriented" text of rheumatology or orthopaedic surgery, many more pages are used in evaluating symptoms with an eye towards helping the primary care physician effectively manage patients, thereby avoiding expensive referrals.

The chapter that details musculoskeletal diseases in children is complete and very useful. Any family practitioner or pediatrician will find help in differential diagnosis of pain and apparent discomfort in those too young to talk, as well as help with the syndromes affecting uncommunicative adolescents. Similarly, we have not ignored the somatic response to life's stresses that can be expressed as pain and can manifest as back pain, diffuse body pain, or generalized misery that spills over into muscles, bones, and joints.

At the end of many chapters, we have included algorithms and tables from Peter Lipsky's painstakingly prepared system for diagnosis and therapy published in the American Journal of Medicine in 1997. These are complementary to, but independent of, the contributors' presentations.

The vignettes that are included as appendices to the text chapters should be considered a "graduate course." Those who have read the book will have an easier time with these cases and appreciate many of the subtleties of diagnosis and treatment presented.

Finally, we have included an appendix of commonly used ICD-9 codes for connective tissue diseases and soft tissue injury. This can provide a helpful reference in the office.

We have been helped extensively by our editorial assistant, Jean Doran Matua, and by our experienced editor at W.B. Saunders, Richard Zorab.

If this book can in some way help primary care physicians build their confidence in diagnosis and treatment of musculoskeletal complaints, realize when referral is needed, and know to whom to refer, we will have succeeded in our objective.

EDWARD D. HARRIS, JR.
MARK C. GENOVESE

Guide to the Organization of the Algorithms for the Diagnosis and Management of Musculoskeletal Complaints

This organizational guide provides a simplified overview of the algorithms for the diagnosis and management of musculoskeletal complaints. The individual algorithms are indicated by the black-boxed letter; for example, the approach to nonarticular disorders is defined more completely in Algorithm B. A double border indicates a critical-decision point, where choosing the next step may be particularly important and/or difficult.

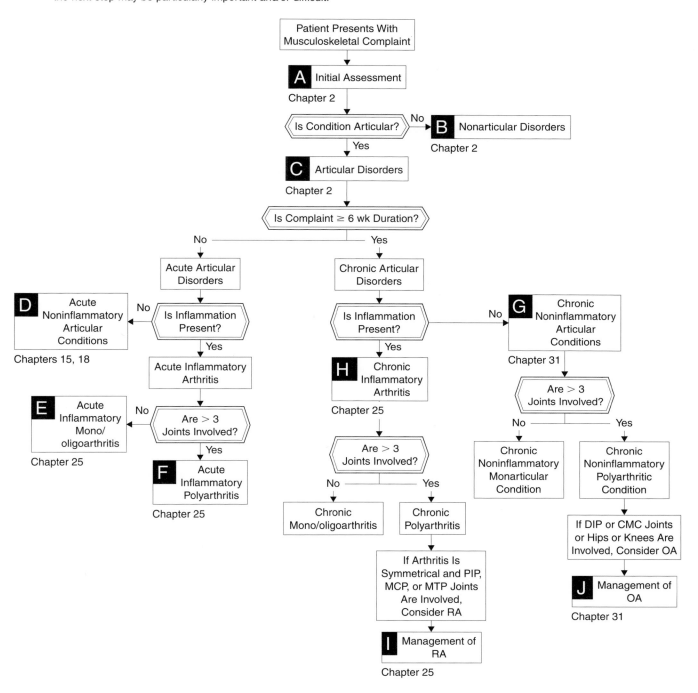

From Lipsky PE: Algorithms for the diagnosis and management of musculoskeletal complaints. Am J Med 103(6A):51S, 1997.

Contents

Part III

RECOGNITION AND MANAGEMENT OF PATIENTS WITH SPECIFIC RHEUMATOLOGIC PROBLEMS

APPENDIX

Part 1

GENERAL APPROACH TO MUSCULOSKELETAL DISORDERS

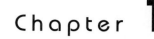

Chapter **1**

The Primary Care Physician and the Specialist: Guidelines for Referral

Edward D. Harris, Jr. ■ Stuart B. Goodman

For the primary care physician in a managed care environment, the challenge of cost-effective care of patients often involves judicious use of specialists. In patients with connective tissue disease, arthralgias, or musculoskeletal pain, this use of specialists involves consultation with rheumatologists, orthopaedic surgeons, hand surgeons, neurologists, physiatrists, and clinical immunologists. The etiquette of consultation and referral is, in general, poorly understood, and these misunderstandings lead to zigzags on the route to ideal care. The issues surrounding consultation and referral can be classified as follows:

- When to refer a patient
- To whom to refer a patient
- How to refer a patient
- What to expect from a referral

WHEN TO REFER A PATIENT

A referral should be made only after a primary care physician has used each of his or her capacities for acquiring a complete history and doing a complete physical examination but before complex laboratory or imaging tests not often used by the physician are ordered. Premature referral can generate unnecessary cost and can place both the consultant and the referring physician in a difficult position.

Consider the following scenario: *A patient is referred to the rheumatology clinic from a general internist with the following note: "Please see, diagnose, and initiate therapy. (signed) Dr. Smith."*

On initial review of this 58-year-old woman, her principal complaint is pain under both patellae and a history of lateral dislocation of the patella bilaterally (once on each side). There are no other symptoms of arthritis or arthralgia. On examination, she was obese and had high and lateral riding patellae with signs of symptomatic chondromalacia. Because no information about her general examination was provided, a relatively full physical examination was performed, which led to the findings that her blood pressure was 168/

110 mm Hg, her heart was enlarged, and her lungs were congested. She later said that she had not mentioned dyspnea to her new internist, just the pain in her knees, and that he had performed only a cursory examination. In addition, her referring physician had sent off the following laboratory tests: fluorescent antinuclear antibody, extractable nuclear antigen, anti-DNA, anti-Sm, anti-RNP, rheumatoid factor, and antimitochondrial antibody.

This type of scenario puts the consultant and patient in a difficult position. The quick referral had saved time for the primary care physician and had guaranteed billing for complete services for the consultant, but it exemplified poor medical care. The patient had to be sent back to her primary care physician for acute management of her hypertension. The immunologic panel was of little use in this woman with obesity and high-riding lateral patellar syndrome and was expensive for her and her insurance company. In addition, the primary care physician had little enjoyment in doing what a primary care physician should enjoy: encountering new symptoms and signs and defining the abnormalities.

The contrast, equally harmful, is the patient who is referred too late to the specialist for appropriate therapy. A case in point is a hard-working mechanic who developed tingling and night pain in his thumb and first two fingers of the right hand. His primary care physician pointed out that because he was left-handed the problem was of little significance. Aspirin and diclofenac (a popular nonsteroidal anti-inflammatory drug) were of little help. No other abnormalities were found on physical examination; radiographs of the cervical spine; and laboratory tests, including a complete blood count, comprehensive survey panel, and erythrocyte sedimentation rate. A diagnosis of carpal tunnel syndrome was made, but by the time the patient presented independently without referral to a hand surgeon there was irreversible loss of muscle mass and function in the thenar muscles.

Similarly, when a patient has an illness that the primary care physician recognizes to be progressive and

3

predictably will need intervention by an orthopaedic surgeon, one should be consulted early rather than later. The surgeon appreciates getting to know the patient with severe degenerative joint disease of the knees long before a total knee joint replacement or osteotomy is necessary.

The keys of *when* to refer patients are as follows:

- Spend substantial time analyzing patients who have poorly defined diagnoses or who are resistant to therapy. Refer those for consultation who are at an impasse in the course of their disease.
- Avoid ordering laboratory tests or imaging tests without a clear rationale for how therapy or diagnosis will change as a result of the tests. Most specialists have strong feelings about the benefit of certain laboratory tests; they usually prefer to order the ones they want after seeing the patient.
- Refer patients when they face a significant progression of functional loss or escalation of pain or anti-inflammatory medicine.

TO WHOM TO REFER A PATIENT

One of the most common problems in dealing with patients with connective tissue disease is determining which subspecialty or consultants to use for which patient. Acute problems are the easiest, and the orthopaedic surgeon is the logical consultant for injury on the playing field or ski slope. More complicated are the regional problems that are associated with chronic pain. Consider the following patient.

A new patient, a 62-year-old woman, arrives in your office complaining of low back pain that is debilitating and chronic. She wants you to refer her to an orthopaedic surgeon. The back pain has resulted in addiction to propoxyphene (Darvon Compound-65) and alprazolam (Xanax). You determine that (1) the pain has not changed significantly over 10 years; (2) it is not related to any specific activity; (3) it has not affected bladder or bowel function; and (4) on physical examination there are intact (but diminished) deep tendon reflexes, straight leg raising to 75 degrees bilaterally, down-going Babinski response, and no localizing tenderness in the lumbar/sacral spine to a light blow of the fist. You review the most recent radiographs of the spine (taken 2 months previously) and read the interpretations of computed tomography scans and magnetic resonance imaging examinations done within the last 6 months; this review reveals evidence for mild lumbar scoliosis with new bone proliferation on the concave side of vertebral bodies and facet joints. You obtain some baseline laboratory tests: complete blood count, erythrocyte sedimentation rate, alkaline phosphatase, serum protein electrophoresis, and renal function tests are all normal. At this point (her third visit), you have decided that this is not an acute process that deserves more imaging studies, that control and management of pain is the principal problem, and that giving her pain a name may be counterproductive.

How do you as the primary care physician manage this patient? The important first step, arriving at a diagnosis of a chronic pain syndrome rather than an acute, surgically or medically reversible process, is the most important one. The next step is reviewing the data with the patient, pointing out that although no *cure* is likely or probable, help in *management* is available. A major challenge for the primary care physician in the care of these types of patients is to convince them that there is no fancy and reversible diagnosis that has been missed all these years. You emphasize that you know that the pain is not imagined, but that mind and body are closely linked in problems such as these. Most crucial, you convince the patient that referral to yet another orthopaedic surgeon would have minimal yield and that pain specialists and physiatrists are the appropriate route of referral.

Several months later, the patient returns to your office. The pain is still present but is manageable with a *pain cocktail* devised by the pain service and a transcutaneous electrical nerve stimulation unit positioned by the physiatrists. Physical therapists have worked with her to strengthen muscle groups in her abdomen. This has relieved some of her late afternoon back pain. She is even back at part-time work as the accountant for her husband's plumbing business.

The points to focus on in this case are as follows:

- Down-regulation of diagnostic and therapeutic alternatives may be better than escalation to more specialized consultants and complex testing in cases in which musculoskeletal pain is chronic and only slowly progressive.
- Appropriate use of selected health professionals (e.g., physical therapists, occupational therapists, speech therapists) may be more effective than multiple medicines and consultations by superspecialists.

Another, often overlooked or ignored component of good referral is the art (or skill) of referring to the specialist who is most likely to do what the primary care physician and patient want accomplished. For example, consider the primary care physician who invariably uses Dr. X for his patients with osteoarthritis of the knee. Dr. X is extremely effective in performing total knee replacements and recommends no other procedure for this disease. The primary care physician, however, has a patient with isolated right and left medial compartment osteoarthritis secondary to marked genu varum (i.e., bow-legs). Only the right knee is symptomatic. The patient's older brother had the same deformity and had effective relief of symptoms after a tibial osteotomy. The patient wants relief of pain but will agree only to an osteotomy, not total knee replacement. Dr. X would be the wrong choice for referral, whereas Dr. Y, with much experience in performing tibial osteotomy, is the preferred consultant. The obvious prerequisite for this form of targeted referral is that the primary care physician learn the preferences as well as skill levels of potential consultants and refer patients accordingly.

HOW TO REFER A PATIENT AND WHAT TO EXPECT FROM A REFERRAL

It is important that referral and consultation be managed at the peer level. No matter how busy the primary care physician is, he or she should make personal contact with the specialist or send signed written requests. Having a nurse call in the referral is not sufficient. If the patient is asked to make his or her own appointment, a letter should be prepared that is attached to relevant data sheets outlining exactly why the referral is being made and stating the questions that the referring physician wants answered. The phrase *relevant data sheets* is important. Having an administrative assistant photocopy every piece of paper in the chart is wasteful of both time and paper. A request for consultation is not like a legal deposition. Only important data are worth inclusion. Chronologic sequencing of events and laboratory tests and careful listing of all drugs that the patient has received should be included in the referral letter. As mentioned previously, the referring physician should detail exact questions that need to be answered. When one is 90% sure of a diagnosis or preferred treatment option, it should be stated in the referral. Consultant specialists actually enjoy corroboration of the current therapy when they know the pressure is off to make a new diagnosis or radically change therapy.

SUMMARY

Precision is perhaps the best noun to describe the most effective consultation. The referring physician must know precisely when it is appropriate to refer a patient and precisely what help that a specific specialist can provide. He or she must provide a clear road map to the consultant about the problem, the data already gathered, and the unambiguous outline of expectations of both the patient and the primary care physician. Referrals generated in this manner have a good chance of providing the opinions and therapies that patients need. The American College of Rheumatology[1] has rec-

ommended that referral to a specialist be done in the following situations:

- Suspected septic arthritis
- Undiagnosed multisystem or systemic rheumatic disease
- Acute myelopathy or mononeuritis multiplex
- Undiagnosed synovitis, in which arthrocentesis or synovial biopsy may be needed
- Musculoskeletal pain undiagnosed after 6 weeks
- Unexplained immunochemical test abnormalities suggestive of an underlying rheumatic disease
- Musculoskeletal pain not adequately controlled with therapy
- Musculoskeletal pain associated with severe or progressive loss of function or work productivity
- Conditions for which treatment with steroids or immunosuppressive drugs is considered
- Systemic rheumatic disease in a pregnant or postpartum patient
- Dysfunction out of proportion to objective findings
- Suspected acute tendon or muscle rupture
- Acute internal derangement with severe pain, poor function, or instability
- End-stage joint disease

Many primary care physicians feel comfortable with diagnosis and treatment of some or many of the above-listed situations and need not refer patients with those entities. The American College of Rheumatology Guidelines for Rheumatology Referral, revised in 1996 and still appropriate, are reprinted in the chapter Appendix.

Appendix

American College of Rheumatology Guidelines for Rheumatology Referral*

Robin K. Dore ▪ Phillip J. Clements ▪ Robert I. Fox ▪
Daniel E. Furst ▪ Herbert Kaplan ▪ Rodanthi C. Kitridou

GUIDELINES

1. Patients with Uncertain Diagnosis

- Normal laboratory findings but local or generalized pain and swelling.
- Abnormal laboratory findings but symptoms and/or examination do not fit criteria for any specific rheumatic disease.
- Patient's complaints are out of proportion to findings on laboratory or physical examination.
- Unexplained symptoms/physical findings such as rash, fever, arthritis, anemia, weakness, weight loss, fatigue or anorexia.

2. Patients with a Presumed or Confirmed Diagnosis

A. INFLAMMATORY ARTHRITIS

714.0	Rheumatoid arthritis
714.3	Juvenile rheumatoid arthritis (adults with hx of)
99.3	Reactive arthritis (including Reiter's syndrome)
696.0	Psoriatic arthritis
718.	Arthritis assoc with inflammatory bowel disease
720.0	Ankylosing spondylitis
88.81	Lyme disease
711.	Infectious arthritis

Diagnosis

Establish or confirm diagnosis; e.g., differentiate erosive osteoarthritis and inflammatory arthritis, differ-entiate crystal induced arthropathy and seronegative spondyloarthropathy.

Uncontrolled Disease

- Disease onset with significant pain, stiffness or swelling requiring immediate/aggressive therapy.
- Pain, stiffness or swelling which **does not respond** to NSAID therapy **within 3-4 months** after disease onset.
- Previously stable disease becomes active.
- **Erosions** appear or progress on x-ray at any time in the course of the disease.
- **Functional** deterioration affecting quality of life.
- **Rapid disease progression** (physical signs of) e.g., nodules, new onset of deformities, subluxation or loss of motion in one or more joints.

Disease Complications

- **Cardiac** involvement causing chest pain and/or pericardial effusions.
- **Eye** involvement presenting as dry, red and/or painful eyes, especially if unilateral.
- **Renal** disease presenting as pedal edema, proteinuria.
- **Pulmonary** involvement causing SOB, cough, nodules on chest x-ray or pleural effusions/infiltrates.
- **Vasculitis, cutaneous or systemic,** causing rash, skin ulcerations, neuropathy.

Medication Complications

Treatment is effective but drug toxicity or intolerance occurs; e.g., steroid myopathy, osteoporosis, multiple recurrent infections, pneumonitis, bone marrow suppression.

*From Lipsky PE (ed): Algorithms for the diagnosis and management of musculoskeletal complaints. Am J Med 103(6A), 1997.

Management

- **Corticosteroid** therapy (chronic) is required to control disease.
- **Immunosuppressive** drug therapy is considered to control disease or to taper corticosteroids.
- **Joint injections,** particularly when prior joint injections have not provided sufficient relief or an injection of a small or difficult to access joint is involved, e.g., finger, wrist, elbow, ankle.
- **Long-term treatment** plan/goals for patients with chronic, long-standing disease must be established.
- **Physical/occupational therapy** recommendations, including appropriate use and duration of PT/OT.
- **Pre/Post surgery medication** modifications/coordination.
- **Surgical opinion** opinion/second opinion regarding the timing of and need for surgical intervention.

B. CONNECTIVE TISSUE DISEASE

710.0	Lupus
710.1	Scleroderma
710.2	Sjögren's syndrome
710.3	Dermatomyositis
710.4	Polymyositis
710.8	Mixed connective tissue disease (MCTD)
710.9	Unspecified connective tissue disease (UCTD)
725.	Polymyalgia rheumatica
279.8.	Antiphospholipid antibody syndrome

Diagnosis

- Establish or confirm diagnosis.
- Differentiate **sicca** syndrome and **Sjögren's** syndrome.
- Evaluate recurrent **fetal losses** or unexplained **thromboses.**
- Interpret serologic laboratory tests.

Uncontrolled Disease

- Previously stable disease becomes active.
- **Elevated CPK, ESR** on corticosteroid therapy.
- **Normal ESR** but symptoms persist.
- **Pleurisy or arthritis** not controlled by NSAIDs.
- **Skin** tightening, rash, not controlled by topical therapy.
- **Signs/symptoms** (other) persist despite therapy, e.g., Raynaud's, digital ulcers, muscle weakness, dry eyes and/or mouth.

Disease Complications

- **Ankylosis** causing loss of motion.
- **Cardiac** involvement causing pericarditis/myocarditis, pericardial effusion.
- **Hematologic** involvement causing anemia, neutropenia, thrombocytopenia, ITP.
- **Eye** disease with recurrent corneal ulcerations or change in vision.
- **Fetal** losses or thromboses occur while on therapy such as ASA or anticoagulation.
- **GI** involvement causing motility disorders or abdominal pain.
- **Lung** involvement causing shortness of breath, cough.
- **Lymph** node involvement causing lymphadenopathy, lymphoma or pseudolymphoma.
- **Malignant hypertension** (scleroderma and others).
- **Peripheral/central nervous system** disease; e.g., confusion, disorientation, neuropathy, paresthesias, seizures, TIAs, CVAs.
- **Renal** insufficiency/nephrotic syndrome/glomerulonephritis/renal tubular acidosis causing fluid retention, decreased urine output.
- **Vasculitis,** cutaneous or systemic.

Medication Complications

Treatment is effective but drug toxicity or intolerance occurs; e.g., steroid myopathy, osteoporosis, multiple recurrent infections.

Management

- Establish a treatment plan.
- **Anticoagulation** therapy, e.g., ASA, heparin or Coumadin in presence of antiphospholipid antibodies.
- **Corticosteroid therapy** (chronic) is required to control disease.
- **Immunosuppressive** drug therapy is considered to control disease or to taper corticosteroids.
- Apheresis, IV immunoglobulin or other non-DMARD therapy is considered.
- **Physical/occupational therapy** recommendations, including appropriate use and duration of PT/OT.
- **Pre/Post surgery medication** modifications/coordination.

C. SYSTEMIC VASCULITIS

287.0	Henoch Schonlein purpura
446.0	Polyarteritis nodosa (PAN)
446.4	Wegener's granulomatosis
446.5	Giant cell arteritis
446.7	Takayasu arteritis
287.0	Churg-Strauss syndrome
273.2	Cryoglobulinemia
711.2	Behcet's syndrome
446.20	Hypersensitivity vasculitis

Diagnosis

Establish or confirm diagnosis; presenting symptoms may include fever, weight loss, malaise, rash, arthritis, renal insufficiency, chronic sinusitis, unilateral headache, cough and/or SOB.

Uncontrolled Disease

Progressive systemic involvement despite therapy.

Disease Complications

- **Eye** involvement, e.g., iritis, uveitis.
- **Lung** involvement causing shortness of breath, cough, pulmonary hemorrhage, infiltrates, nodules or cavities.
- **Mesenteric** infarction/perforation causing abdominal pain, distention.
- **Renal** insufficiency/glomerulonephritis.
- **Peripheral/central nervous system** disease; e.g., confusion, disorientation, paresthesias, seizures, TIAs, CVAs.

Medication Complications

Treatment is effective but drug toxicity or intolerance occurs; e.g., bone marrow suppression, opportunistic infections, hemorrhagic cystitis (cyclophosphamide induced), steroid myopathy, osteoporosis.

Management

- Establish a treatment plan.
- Apheresis, IV immunoglobulin or other non-DMARD therapy is considered.
- **Corticosteroid** therapy (chronic) is required to control disease.
- **Immunosuppressive** drug therapy is considered to control disease or to taper corticosteroids.
- These diseases should in almost all instances be managed by subspecialists (e.g., rheumatologists, nephrologists, pulmonologists); concurrent care may be provided by other physicians.

D. UNCOMMON RHEUMATIC DISEASES

277.3	Amyloidosis
275.0	Hemochromatosis
733.99	Relapsing polychondritis
713.7	Sarcoidosis

Diagnosis

- Establish or confirm diagnosis; e.g., differentiate between infectious arthritis and sarcoidosis.
- Interpret laboratory tests; e.g., angiotensin converting enzyme.
- Determine need for tissue biopsy.

Uncontrolled Disease

- Previously stable disease becomes active.
- Signs/symptoms persist despite therapy; e.g., dry eyes and/or mouth, rash, arthritis.

Disease Complications

- **Cardiac** involvement causing cardiomyopathy, pericarditis.
- **Eye** involvement with uveitis.
- **Hematologic** involvement causing hyperviscosity, bone marrow suppression.
- **Lung** involvement causing shortness of breath, cough, nodules, cavities or infiltrates.
- **Lymph node** involvement causing lymphadenopathy.
- **Peripheral/central nervous system disease;** e.g., entrapment neuropathy, paresthesias, vasomotor instability.
- **Renal** insufficiency/nephrotic syndrome causing peripheral edema, decreased urine output.
- **Vasculitis,** cutaneous or systemic.

Medication Complications

Treatment is effective but drug toxicity or intolerance occurs; e.g., steroid myopathy, osteoporosis, opportunistic infections.

Management

- Establish a treatment plan.
- Apheresis, IV immunoglobulin or other non-DMARD therapy is considered.
- **Corticosteroid** therapy (chronic) is required to control disease.
- **Immunosuppressive** drug therapy is considered to control disease or to taper corticosteroids.

E. OSTEOARTHRITIS

Diagnosis

Establish or confirm diagnosis; e.g., differentiate erosive osteoarthritis and inflammatory arthritis, differentiate osteoarthritis and crystal induced arthropathy.

Uncontrolled Disease

Single or multiple joint involvement which does not respond to NSAID therapy.

Medication Complications

NSAID treatment is effective but drug toxicity or intolerance occurs.

Management

- **Joint injections,** particularly when prior joint injections have not provided sufficient relief or an injection of a small or difficult to access joint is involved, e.g., finger, wrist, elbow, ankle.
- **Physical/occupational therapy** recommendations, including appropriate use and duration of PT/OT.
- **Pre/Post surgery medication** modifications/coordination.
- **Surgical opinion** opinion/second opinion regarding the timing of and need for surgical intervention.

F. REGIONAL MUSCULOSKELETAL DISORDERS

722.xx	Degenerative disk disease
	Radiculopathy
	Spinal stenosis
726.xx	Bursitis/tendinitis
727.xx	Tenosynovitis
728.5	Hypermobility syndrome
	Regional pain syndromes
	Repetitive use syndromes

Diagnosis

Differentiate between a regional musculoskeletal problem and a generalized systemic disorder.

Uncontrolled Disease

Functionally compromising or unresponsive to primary treatment.

Medication Complications

NSAID treatment is effective but drug toxicity or intolerance occurs.

Management

- **Periarticular injections,** particularly when prior joint injections have not provided sufficient relief.
- **Physical/occupational therapy** recommendations, including appropriate use and duration of PT/OT.
- **Surgical opinion** opinion/second opinion regarding the timing of and need for surgical intervention.

G. FIBROMYALGIA/MYOFASCIAL PAIN

Diagnosis

Differentiate articular disease, soft tissue rheumatism and systemic inflammatory disease (e.g., rule out lupus in patients with positive ANA and lacking other diagnostic criteria).

Uncontrolled Disease

Persistent rheumatic symptoms, sleep disturbance, fatigue, pain, despite therapy including anti-depressants and exercise.

Medication Complications

Treatment is effective but drug toxicity or intolerance occurs.

Management

- Establish a treatment plan.
- **Family/patient counseling,** including reassurance that condition is not life-threatening.
- **Pain management program** recommendations.
- **Physical/occupational therapy** recommendations, including appropriate use and duration of PT/OT.

H. METABOLIC BONE DISEASE

733.xx	Osteoporosis
731.0	Paget's disease
713.0	Endocrine arthropathy
733.7	Reflex sympathetic dystrophy (RSDS)
588.0	Renal osteodystrophy
268.2	Osteomalacia

Diagnosis

- Establish or confirm diagnosis.
- Interpret metabolic laboratory tests.
- Evaluate bone density studies and nuclear medicine bone scans.
- Determine need for bone biopsy.

Uncontrolled Disease

- Corticosteroid therapy (chronic) is necessary to control life threatening or disabling primary disease.
- Elevated alkaline phosphatase in Paget's disease despite therapy.
- Functional deterioration affects quality of life.
- Osteopenia despite hormone replacement therapy (HRT) or other therapy.
- Osteopenia when HRT contraindicated or not desired.
- Persistent pain and/or swelling despite therapy in RSDS.

Disease Complications

- Chronic pain.
- Fractures.

Medication Complications

Treatment is effective but drug toxicity or intolerance occurs.

Management

- Establish a treatment plan.
- Evaluate and treat fractures caused by these diseases.

I. CRYSTAL INDUCED ARTHROPATHY

274.9 Gout
712.2 CPPD disease
712.8 Hydroxyapatite deposition disease
271.8 Calcium oxalate deposition disease

Diagnosis

- Differentiate polyarticular crystal disease and inflammatory arthritis.
- Establish diagnosis by joint aspiration and crystal identification.
- Interpretation of abnormal laboratory values (calcium, uric acid, phosphorus).

Uncontrolled Disease

- Recurrent episodes despite appropriate therapy.
- Pain, stiffness and swelling which does not respond to NSAID therapy.

Disease Complications

- Polyarticular gout.
- Tophaceous gout.

Medication Complications

Treatment is effective but drug toxicity or intolerance occurs.

Management

Hypouricemic drug therapy is considered.

J. CHILDREN WITH RHEUMATIC DISEASES

Diagnosis, treatment recommendations and concurrent care with pediatrician or family practitioner.

K. PREGNANT WOMEN WITH RHEUMATIC DISEASES

Diagnosis, treatment recommendations and concurrent care with obstetrician or family practitioner during pregnancy and three months post partum.

Chapter 2

The Initial Evaluation: An Approach to Rapid Diagnosis

Edward D. Harris, Jr.

In a busy primary care practice, there is only a small amount of time for the physician to provide effective, accurate triage of a new patient with a complaint of symptoms involving bones, joints, or muscles. Twenty minutes may be the upper limit of time allocated for a first visit of a new patient who has called for an appointment because of joint pain.

The most efficient use of the 20-minute office visit is as follows:

- *10 minutes*—a focused history, including the chief complaint, past medical history, and medications and allergies
- *7 minutes*—physical examination of relevant systems
- *3 minutes*—impressions and advice to the patient; interim diagnostic testing; institution of empirical therapy, if indicated

Focused History

When the primary care physician encounters a new patient with pain in and around joints, determining whether the discomfort involves one or many joints is extremely important. When multiple areas are involved, it is much less likely that the patient has an acute process (infection, crystal synovitis, structural damage [e.g., fracture]) than if only one joint is involved.

ONE JOINT

If only *one* area is involved, the possibility of trauma or infection must be ranked higher in the differential diagnosis, with crystal-associated synovitis a possibility as well. Questions to the patient must focus on these possibilities.

SEXUAL ACTIVITY? A younger age is directly proportional to the likelihood of developing a sexually transmitted disease. Gonorrhea is still a common cause of acute synovitis in one or few joints. Middle-aged and elderly individuals, however, can also contract gonorrhea.

MEDICATIONS? Oligoarticular synovitis from gout may be associated with the following medications or families of medications that cause hyperuricemia:

Diuretics. Gout in women is more associated with diuretic use than any other causative factor, particularly if the patient is obese or a heavy user of alcohol.

Salicylates, low dose (>500 mg/day, <1500 mg/day).

Antituberculous drugs. Pyrazinamide and ethambutol both retard urinary excretion of uric acid.

Others. Nicotinic acid is used in hypercholesterolemia, and cyclosporine is used in patients with rheumatoid arthritis and in organ transplantation.

TRAUMA? The individual who engages in athletic activity on the weekend may deny trauma to joints or be relatively unaware of a sprain that, by Monday morning, becomes acutely swollen and painful (see Chapters 15 and 16).

MORE THAN ONE JOINT COMPLEX

If multiple areas are involved, the interview of the patient must extend to many topics (see Chapter 18).

ARE THE INVOLVED JOINTS STIFF IN THE MORNING? This question is useful for differentiating inflammatory from noninflammatory sources of pain. In inflamed tissues at relative rest during sleep, edema and products of inflammation gather in extracellular tissues; the result is a joint or set of joints that are stiff but not necessarily painful on wakening in the morning.

ARE THERE SYSTEMIC SYMPTOMS? A rash, Raynaud's syndrome, alopecia, sicca syndrome, uveitis, or cramping bowel symptoms can be the key associated symptoms that lead to diagnosis of diseases such as systemic lupus erythematosus (SLE), rheumatoid arthritis, scleroderma, or spondyloarthropathies. Weight loss, fever, fatigue, and muscle aching can be associated with all diffuse connective tissue diseases as well as with more complex systemic diseases, including endocarditis and malignancies. At a 20-minute office visit, there is a limited number of questions permissible. During this interview, however, the physician must begin the process of data integration and must be formulating hypotheses to test during the physical examination.

Targeted Physical Examination

A short, focused examination must be done with full view of the involved as well as uninvolved joints and muscles. The following are reasonable questions that should be answered during the examination.

IS THE PATHOLOGY WITHIN THE SYNO-VIUM OR IN PERIARTICULAR TISSUES? The answer to this question is a crucial one. Remembering anatomy is useful. Any process that begins as a synovitis works from the inside to the outside of the joint. A moderate inflammation of the joint lining may not produce erythema and only slight warmth of skin overlying the joint, whereas a subcutaneous process may produce moderate-to-severe swelling along with warmth and erythema over a joint but not be associated with any synovial inflammation.

A helpful guide to determine whether a synovitis is present may be found in the difference, if any, in pain on moving the joint passively compared with symptoms when the patient moves the joint actively. In general, synovitis is associated with pain both on passive and on active motion of the joint. In contrast, a subcutaneous process that happens to occur over a joint may often produce intense pain when the patient moves the joint actively but be only slightly painful when the examiner slowly moves the joint through its range of motion.

An example of this is erythema nodosum when it occurs in cutaneous structures over a joint such as the ankle. Although the skin is red and tender, resembling cellulitis or acute, severe gout, it may be possible for the examiner, holding the calf and the foot well distal to the inflammation, to move the ankle in extension and flexion while causing only minimal discomfort. An acutely inflamed gouty ankle or septic joint is virtually impossible to move passively without inducing severe pain.

It is also important to differentiate pain and tenderness in a joint from tenderness in the long bones on either side of a joint. An example of the latter problem is hypertrophic osteoarthropathy. This problem is associated with lung cancer or long-standing hypoxia (e.g., cystic fibrosis, congenital heart disease) and is caused by periostitis, sometimes with concentric layers of new bone being laid down, particularly on the distal ends of long bones.

IF THERE IS JOINT SWELLING, IS IT CAUSED BY BONY ENLARGEMENT, SYNOVITIS, OR BOTH? Joint swelling is the principal finding that differentiates synovitis such as that found in rheumatoid arthritis from osteoarthritis. Palpation gives the answer. Fluid in a joint such as a metacarpophalangeal joint produces a rubbery, elastic sensation to the palpating fingers. Soft tissue (e.g., synovitis) without much fluid in the joint space produces a softer, nonelastic sensation, whereas the bony proliferation that accompanies osteoarthritis is hard and unyielding. At the same examination, the range of motion of the involved joints can be noted quickly.

The two situations in which this finding is most useful are in differentiating osteoarthritis from rheumatoid arthritis when only the fingers or knees are involved. In erosive osteoarthritis, for example, the fingers can be deformed with striking limitation of motion of proximal interphalangeal joints but with virtually no soft tis-

sue proliferation, only bony thickening and ankylosis. In osteoarthritis involving the hands, the first carpometacarpal is often involved with pain, tenderness, and a progressive inability to abduct the thumb; the thumb lies fairly flat against the second finger. Therefore, to generate a more functional grip, the distal phalanx of the thumb hyperextends and may become fixed in that position.

In the knee, even small amounts of joint fluid, in the absence of detectable synovial proliferation or bony thickening, can be detected. One should look for the *bulge* sign (Fig. 2–1): With the leg in full extension and relaxed, pressure with the back of the examiner's hand sweeps from the middle of the joint across the quadriceps to an area approximately 3 inches above the patella and lateral to it. This maneuver pushes fluid, if it is present, into the superior recesses of the suprapatellar pouch. Then, without hesitation, the fingers are used to tap against the suprapatellar area; a slow, rolling bulge seen at the normally concave region medial and inferior to the middle of the patella border indicates that there is probably 4 to 8 mL of fluid in that knee. When more fluid than this is present, the bulge sign cannot be demonstrated.

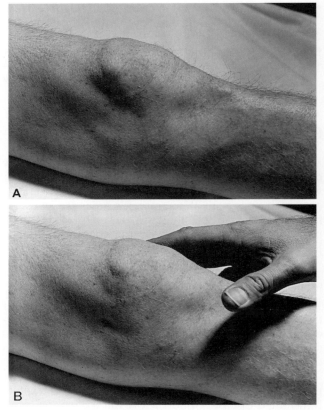

Figure 2–1. Demonstration of the *bulge sign* for a small synovial effusion in the knee. A, The synovial fluid is to be moved from the shaded, depressed area on the medial aspect of the knee. B, Bulge appears in previously shaded area after lateral aspect of the knee is tapped. (From Polley HF, Hunder GG: Rheumatologic Interviewing and Physical Examination of the Joints, 2nd ed. Philadelphia, WB Saunders, 1978.)

HOW MANY JOINTS ARE INVOLVED? It is important to determine whether the process involves a single joint or is a polyarticular disease. All joints should be examined. One begins with the opposite joint or joint complex; if the involved metacarpophalangeal joint is on the right hand, the left hand is examined first. Symmetric involvement implies diffuse connective tissue diseases, especially rheumatoid arthritis and possibly SLE, scleroderma, or dermatomyositis (see Chapters 25, 27, 28, and 29).

If there is asymmetric involvement, it is then appropriate to examine the spine for flexibility. Ankylosing spondylitis and reactive arthritis associated with HLA-B27 frequently involve peripheral joints (particularly those in the lower extremity) in an asymmetric fashion (see Chapter 26). Diminished flexion of the lumbar spine may be present even before there are any radiographic changes. In the *Schober* test, a mark is made on the midline skin of the back at the level of the dimples of Venus (S1) or close to them; another mark is made 10 cm up from there. When the normal person then is asked to bend over as far as possible with the knees straight, these two marks on the skin spread to 14 to 16 cm from each other as the lumbar vertebrae move posteriorly away from their neighbors. In spondylitis, ligamentous thickening fixes the spine, and the distance between the skin spots moves less than 2 cm during spine flexion (see Chapter 3 and Fig. 3–4 and Chapter 25).

The hands should always be examined, even if the patient complains little about them. In addition to the fact that there are 15 joints distal to the wrist that may be involved with arthritis, there is much cutaneous pathology that may be found, including nail pitting associated with psoriasis, the flat plaques (Gottron's papules) found over proximal interphalangeal joints in dermatomyositis, clubbing of the fingers (hypertrophic osteoarthropathy), sclerodactyly (scleroderma), and Dupytren's contractures (see Chapters 17, 23, 28, 29).

PLAN FOR THE NEXT VISIT

In the last 3 minutes of the office visit, the physician must communicate his or her preliminary findings to the patient, order appropriate laboratory tests and radiographs, initiate some therapy, and arrange the next appointment.

Tempo of the Evaluation

The intensity of subsequent evaluation should be directly proportional to the acuity of the suspected diagnosis. If the physician suspects that a patient has acute gout, pseudogout, or a septic joint, the work-up must proceed quickly. The joint must be tapped and fluid examined for crystals and sent for cell count, Gram stain, and culture. Primary care physicians generally should feel comfortable in doing an arthrocentesis of the knee, the great toe, and perhaps the wrist and shoulder (see

Chapter 6). A rheumatologist or orthopaedic surgeon, however, should be consulted for other joints less easy to aspirate or for any joint that the physician is uncomfortable about tapping.

Another major diagnosis that, once suspected, demands quick action is temporal arteritis in a patient who has presented with transient loss of vision (usually in one eye); tenderness along the temporal artery on that side; and other symptoms suggestive of this process, including fever, weight loss, and jaw claudication. Glucocorticoid therapy (usually, prednisone 40 to 60 mg/24 hours) should be given immediately to these patients (even before baseline laboratory tests have been completed and a biopsy requested) to help prevent permanent blindness from thrombosis within the ophthalmic artery. As pointed out in Chapter 27, a close relative of temporal arteritis is polymyalgia rheumatica; this latter process need not be so aggressively treated and may even be managed by non-steroidal anti-inflammatory drugs (NSAIDs).

Laboratory Tests and Radiographic Images

It is rare that a specific laboratory test provides a diagnosis of connective tissue disease. There are obvious exceptions to this (e.g., serum iron or iron-binding capacity could indicate that degenerative arthritis of the second and third metacarpophalangeal joint is related to hemochromatosis, or a platelet count could confirm that palpable purpura is not secondary to thrombocytopenia). Clinical impressions gained from history and physical examination, however, are the most important diagnostic aids.

At the end of a 20-minute visit, it is often appropriate to order some basic laboratory tests. Chapter 5 provides guidance in the use of laboratory studies; however, evaluation should start with complete blood count (hemoglobin, hematocrit, white blood cell count, and platelet count) and an erythrocyte sedimentation rate (which gives an index of inflammation). In addition, if rheumatoid arthritis, SLE, or another of the diffuse connective tissue diseases is suspected, tests for rheumatoid factor, a fluorescent anti-nuclear antibody test, serum creatinine, and a urinalysis are appropriate. It is rare that any additional tests should be ordered at that first visit, unless there is a high probability of a specific diagnosis that can be confirmed by one or two laboratory tests.

Similarly, it is rare that radiographic images help in diagnosis unless the pathologic process has been present for many months. Chapter 4 provides guidance in the use of imaging studies. In patients with inflammatory joint disease, for example, periarticular osteopenia develops only after several months of active synovitis, and this finding tells the clinician little more than he or she could ascertain from a good joint examination. There are exceptions; for example, if hypertrophic osteoarthropathy is suspected, periosteal new bone formation would be visible shortly after the time that symptoms develop. Stress fractures may be seen in metatarsal bones if careful radiographic studies are completed, and calcium salt deposits in areas of bursitis can often be observed. A solid fund of knowledge helps the physician in knowing what tests or images to order. The asthmatic patient, for example, who has been treated with high doses of glucocorticoids for several years then develops progressive hip pain may well have avascular necrosis of the femoral head; for this problem, magnetic resonance imaging is more sensitive and specific than normal plain films of the hip.

Diagnosis

Rarely can a diagnosis can be made during the first short visit. A diagnosis should not be forced and the patient should be reassured that except for possible sepsis, gout, or vasculitis the longer one goes along before his or her symptom complex meets criteria sufficient to make a specific diagnosis, the better the prognosis. This is a concept difficult for a patient to grasp, but it is crucial for optimal management. Aches and pains are not on a parallel with, for example, finding a lump in one's breast; although the latter situation demands mammography and perhaps fine-needle aspiration or lumpectomy, watchful waiting and empirical therapy over time before committing to a diagnosis of connective tissue disease is a useful plan.

Therapy

During the first 20-minute visit, it is likely that a firm diagnosis cannot be made. The physician arranges for blood to be drawn for basic tests (see earlier) and perhaps orders some radiographic images. Initial treatment in a patient without a diagnosis can be started with NSAIDs or acetaminophen. The latter is useful for pain if associated inflammation is not present; NSAIDs are indicated if a noninfectious inflammatory illness seems likely.

CONCLUSION

At the end of the first office visit, the patient should feel confident that the physician has been thorough, has listened, has touched and palpated sore or tender areas, has listed some alternative diagnoses, and has indicated the path for both relief of symptoms and the approach to a final diagnosis. The next visit to the office should follow closely on completion of the laboratory tests or after several weeks of a therapeutic trial. At this next visit, scheduled for 30 minutes, if possible, the physician should ask for details of the history not obtained during the first visit because of the press of time, determine the response to the empirical therapy if any was prescribed, and correlate laboratory tests and images with the clinical presentation. The appendix contains several algorithms and tables relevant to the initial evaluation.

Algorithms and Tables for the Diagnosis and Management of Musculoskeletal Complaints*

Algorithm A: Initial Assessment

From the initial physical examination and rheumatologic history of the patient, the provider should determine whether there is a musculoskeletal condition and, if so, whether it is articular.

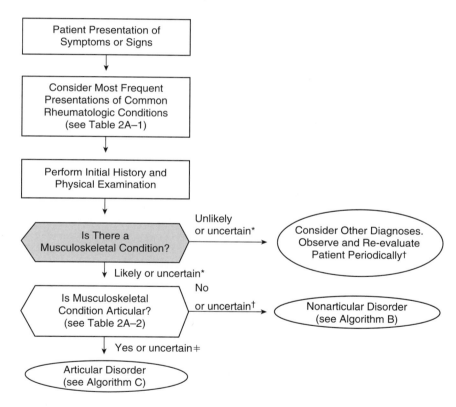

* It is uncertain if condition is musculoskeletal in nature if history and physical findings are inconsistent, atypical, or both. If the provider still believes that the patient's report of symptoms may be explained by a musculoskeletal disorder, further evaluation as though a rheumatologic condition were present is warranted.

† As many rheumatologic conditions cannot be accurately diagnosed at onset, patients should be re-evaluated periodically for development of a known rheumatologic disorder or resolution of the complaint.

‡ If provider is uncertain whether the condition is articular or nonarticular, the patient should be evaluated for both.

---

*All algorithms and tables in Appendix are reprinted with permission from Lipsky PE (ed): Algorithms for the diagnosis and management of musculoskeletal complaints. Am J Med 103(6A): 52S–54S, 62S–64S, 1997.

B Algorithm B: Nonarticular Disorders

If the musculoskeletal complaint is not or probably is not articular, the provider should determine whether fibromyalgia or polymyalgia rheumatica is present or further investigation is necessary.

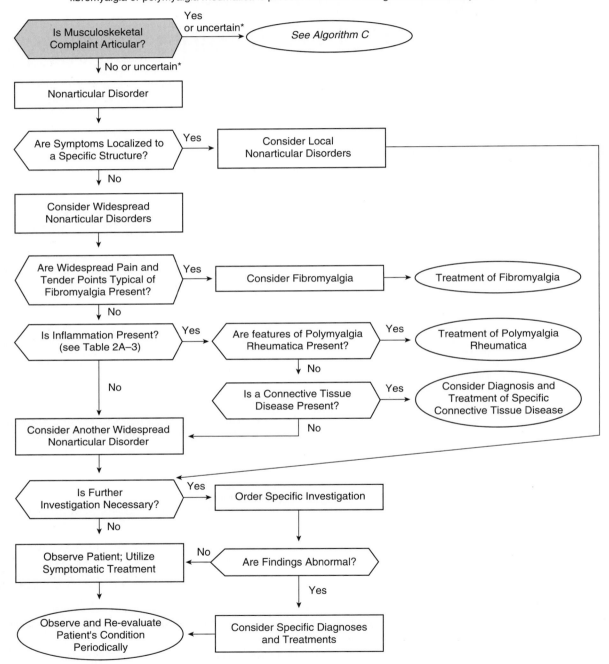

* If provider is uncertain whether the condition is articular or nonarticular, the patient should be evaluated for both.

Algorithm C: Articular Disorders

If the musculoskeletal complaint is or probably is articular, the provider should determine whether the complaint is chronic or acute and, if acute, whether an inflammatory or noninflammatory condition is present.

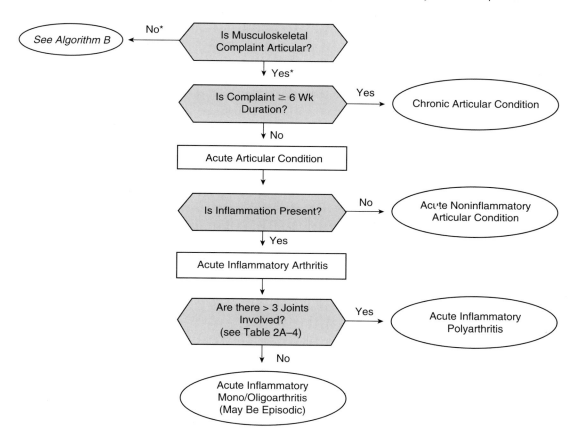

* If provider is uncertain whether the condition is articular or nonarticular, the patient should be evaluated for both.

Table 2A–1. COMMON RHEUMATOLOGIC CONDITIONS, CONDITIONS ARE LISTED IN APPROXIMATE ORDER OF PREVALENCE.

Age (yr)	Men		Women	
	Noninflammatory	Inflammatory	Noninflammatory	Inflammatory
18–34	• Injury/overuse[*] • Low back pain	• Spondyloarthropathies[‡] • Gonococcal arthritis • Gout	• Injury/overuse[*] • Low back pain	• Gonococcal arthritis • RA • Systemic lupus erythematosus
35–65	• Low back pain • Injury/overuse[*] • OA • Entrapment syndromes[†]	• Bursitis • Gout • Spondyloarthropathies[‡] • USP[§]	• Osteoporosis (postmenopausal) • Low back pain • Inury/overuse[*] • Fibromyalgia • Entrapment syndromes • OA • Raynaud's phenomenon	• Bursitis • RA • USP[§]
>65	• OA • Low back pain • Osteoporosis • Fracture	• Bursitis • Gout • USP[§] • RA • Pseudogout • Polymyalgia rheumatica • Septic arthritis	• Osteoporosis • OA • Fibromyalgia • Low back pain • Fracture	• Bursitis • USP[§] • RA • Gout • Pseudogout • Polymyalgia rheumatica • Septic arthritis

*Injury/overuse includes fracture, soft-tissue injuries, tendinitis, and "nonarticular rheumatism"; †entrapment syndrome includes carpal tunnel and tarsal tunnel syndromes: ‡spondyloarthropathies include ankylosing spondylitis, psoriatic arthritis, and Reiter's syndrome §USP = undifferentiated seronegative (self-limited or persistent) polyarthritis, usually inflammatory, that is not associated with increased titers of rheumatoid factor and is atypical of RA or fails to meet ACR criteria for the classification of RA.

Table 2A–2 MUSCULOSKELETAL CONDITIONS: FEATURES THAT DISTINGUISH ARTICULAR FROM NONARTICULAR DISORDERS

		Articular	Nonarticular

Anatomic Structures		• Juxtaarticular bone • Synovial fluid
		• Articular cartilage • Synovium
		• Intraarticular • Joint capsule
		  ligaments
		• Menisci (knee)
			• Tendons • Fascia
			• Bursae • Bone
			• Extraarticular • Nerve
			  ligaments
			• Muscle • Skin

Symptoms and Signs	Pain/tenderness	• Localized to joint • Deep and poorly localized • Specific referral patterns	• Localized to extraarticular structure • "Point" tenderness, superficial
	Pain on movement	• With active and passive movement • With movement in many planes • Localized to joint	• With active movement • With movement in specific planes • Rarely localized to joint

	Swelling	• Common, related to articular structure
		  1. Synovial effusion
		  2. Synovial thickening
		  3. Bony enlargement
			• May be present
			• Not limited to articular structure

	Limitation of motion	• Frequent on both passive and active range of movement • Related to mechanical derangement or joint pain	• May be present but usually limited to active range of movement • Related to extraarticular mechanical abnormality, diffuse pain, or weakness
	Crepitation	• May be present	• Absent/unrelated
	Instability	• May be present	• Absent/unrelated
	Locking of joint	• May be present	• Absent/unrelated
	Deformity	• May be present • Localized to joint • Secondary to joint damage	• Rare, except with antecedent trauma • Associated with extraarticular abnormality
Radiographic changes		• Common in chronic conditions • Uncommon in acute conditions except trauma	• Uncommon/unrelated • Soft tissue calcification

Table 2A–3 SPECIFIC FEATURES THAT ARE USEFUL IN DISTINGUISHING INFLAMMATORY FROM NONINFLAMMATORY CONDITIONS

Feature	Characteristics of the Condition	
	Inflammatory	Noninflammatory
Joint pain	Yes (with activity and rest)	Yes (with activity)
Joint swelling	Soft tissue	Bony (if present)
Local erythema	Sometimes	Absent
Local warmth	Sometimes	Absent
Morning stiffness*	Prolonged (>60 min)	Variable (<60 min)
Systemic symptoms	Common	Rare
ESR, CRP	Increased	Normal for age
Hemoglobin	Normal or low	Normal
Serum albumin	Normal or low	Normal
Synovial fluid WBC/mm^3	≥2000	<2000
Synovial fluid % PMN	≥75%	<75%

*Presence, duration, and functional impact of morning stiffness have been suggested to be poor discriminators of RA and chronic noninflammatory joint pain (Hazes, JMW, et al. *J Rheumatol.* 1993;20:1138–1142.) However, 87% of 489 practicing rheumatologists reported that prolonged (>60 min) morning stiffness was useful in differentiating inflammatory from noninflammatory arthritis.

Table 2A–4 DISCRIMINATING FEATURES OF COMMON CHRONIC POLYARTICULAR DISORDERS

Clinical/Laboratory Finding	OA	RA	Spondyloarthropathy
Morning stiffness >60 min*	−	+	+
Back pain	+	−	+
Distribution of articular involvement	Asymmetric	Symmetric	Asymmetric
Joints commonly involved	DIP, PIP, 1st CMC, hip, knee, spine	PIP, MCP, MTP, wrist, knee, hip	Hip, knee, SI joints
Nature of joint involvement	Bony enlargement, intermittent effusion	Synovial swelling and effusion	Synovial swelling and effusion
Enthesitis	−	−	+
Extraarticular features	−	+	+
Increased ESR, CRP	−	+	+
Increased rheumatoid factor	−	+	−
Synovial fluid analysis	WBC < 2000/mm^3 PMN < 75%	WBC ≥ 2000/mm^3 PMN ≥ 75%	WBC ≤ 2000/mm^3 PMN ≥ 75%
Radiographic findings	Joint space narrowing, osteophytes, subchondral sclerosis	Periarticular demineralization, erosions	Sacroiliitis

+ = highly characteristic
− = uncommon
*Presence, duration, and functional impact of morning stiffness have been suggested to be poor discriminators of RA and chronic noninflammatory joint pain (Hazes JMW, et al. *J Rheumatol.* 1993;20:1138–1142.) However, 87% of 489 practicing rheumatologists reported that prolonged (>60 min) morning stiffness was useful in differentiating inflammatory from noninflammatory arthritis.

Chapter **3**

A Guide to Efficient Examination and Diagnosis of the Musculoskeletal System

David J. Schurman ■ Edward D. Harris, Jr.

The primary care physician refers more adult patients to the rheumatologist and orthopaedic surgeon for consultation than any other physician. This is, in part, due to the general interest of the public in fitness and exercise and the fact that musculoskeletal complaints become more common as the body ages. *Staying fit* implies not only exercising the cardiorespiratory system, but also often involves repetitive stresses to musculoskeletal units, including bones, joints, muscles, tendons, and ligaments. Musculoskeletal *catastrophes,* such as fracture of a long bone, are easily diagnosed by the primary care physician; these are case scenarios that most physicians learn about in medical school and begin treating during their internship. Some of the more acute conditions that are not as catastrophic, but are painful and disabling, (e.g., a bad ankle sprain) and subacute and chronic conditions (e.g., rotator cuff tendinitis) often pose a dilemma for the primary care physician, who may have had little experience in the diagnosis and treatment of these musculoskeletal conditions. This chapter gives broad guidelines for efficient examination and diagnosis of different anatomic disorders in the musculoskeletal system as well as to aid in the timely referral to a specialist. Indepth discussions of most of these conditions are found in later chapters. The key with musculoskeletal complaints is to take a detailed but focused history because many active patients experience a myriad of musculoskeletal aches and pains over the years. With some persistence and judicious direction by the physician, the details of the injury (e.g., how and when did it happen, where does it hurt, what are the quality and frequency of pains or other symptoms, where does the pain radiate to, and what treatments have been instituted) can be obtained.

The physical examination is an extension of the history, in which the primary care physician concentrates on the affected body part and adjacent and related parts and performs a neurologic and vascular examination. For example, a shoulder complaint usually prompts an examination of the neck, elbow, and hand. The contralateral side is usually a good benchmark for compar-

ison. This chapter includes references to therapy of various abnormalities (e.g., patellofemoral syndromes) that are found on physical examination.

Many patients have no complaints referable to bones and joints, even after specific questioning during the review of systems. For that reason, during the general physical examination, time should not be taken for a complete examination of the musculoskeletal system. Instead, different functions of more than one group of muscles and joints can be evaluated quickly, yielding a relatively complete assessment for the physician of full locomotor function. All of this examination should take less than 5 minutes (see Chapter 2 for a description of a 20-minute work-up of patients with new musculoskeletal complaints).

OBSERVATION OF GAIT

When a patient enters the office, takes off his or her coat or puts down her purse, sits in a chair, and gets up to change into an examining gown, these are excellent opportunities for an observant physician to identify areas worth more intensive examination. Most important, observing gait during these activities takes no extra time. A *limp* is always abnormal and may indicate unrecognized pathology, an old injury, a congenital abnormality, acute inflammation, or one manifestation of systemic problems. In the dynamics of limping, the individual bears weight on the painful leg for a shorter part of the walk cycle than on the normal pain-free leg. Whether the discomfort is in the foot, ankle, knee, or hip is more difficult to determine by a brief glance at gait. A *coxalgic* gait is caused as the patient leans over the diseased hip during the phase of weight bearing on that hip. A *Trendelenburg* gait[1] is caused most often by a relative weakness of abductors of the leg at the hip, a problem that forces the patient to lean to the right, for example, as the pelvis droops to unweight the left leg, and vice versa. Obese individuals may waddle, yet have no intrinsic hip disease. A test is positive when a patient stands on one leg and the pelvis droops toward

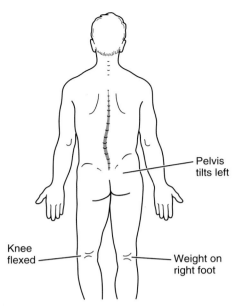

Figure 3–1. Weakness in pelvis abductors is demonstrated by having the patient stand on one foot. Normally the *unweighted* side of the pelvis rises above the weighted side. With abductor weakness, the unweighted side falls. During gait, there is a noticeable oscillation of the pelvic brims from left to right and back again.

the others (unweighted) side because abductors on the weighted side lack strength (Fig. 3–1).

Heel pain forces toe walking. In contrast, a person with a painful ankle walks with a flat-footed gait because he or she cannot spring off the toes. A patient with a painful knee and a large effusion does not straighten the knee when walking because full extension diminishes the intra-articular volume, intensifying pain as the pressure within the joint increases.

SCREENING EXAMINATION

It is impossible to examine a patient's muscles and joints when he or she is draped in a gown. The patient should wear underwear without stockings. At any point during the screening examination that an abnormality is found, it must be followed up at that time.

Shoulder Girdle

The physician faces the patient and says, "Hold your arms as I do and move them along with mine," then puts his or her upper arm in a neutral position (the shoulders in 0 degrees of rotation) with the hands held out in front. Then the physician (and the patient) brings up the arms in flexion to 90 degrees; this is the easiest shoulder motion. The next motion is to swing the arms out so that the shoulders are in position of 90 degrees of abduction (with forearms in the "I surrender" position). Next the physician (and the patient) rotates the forearms down so that they are pointed toward the floor.[2] This latter motion puts the shoulder into internal rotation, by far the most difficult motion for this joint. (Fig. 3–2). Additional tips in examination of the shoulder are included in Chapters 15 and 18.

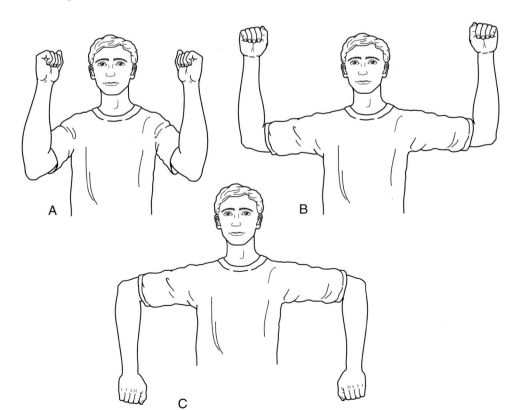

Figure 3–2. *A*, The 10-second test for shoulder function. The patient is asked to simulate movement of the physician. This motion is forward flexion, easiest for most to perform. *B*, From flexion of the humerus, the patient copies the examiner and moves into abduction. *C*, From abduction, the patient is asked to roll down into internal rotation in abduction. This is a difficult maneuver for patients with rotator cuff problems or bursitis.

Neck

A patient with a normal neck should be able to touch the chin to the chest, look up at the ceiling, and rotate the neck to at least 80 degrees both right and left.[3]

Hands, Wrists, and Elbows

Adequate elbow function can be documented simply by having the patient move the palms from supination to pronation while beginning the hand examination. This motion is caused by the radius rotating over the ulnar head. The ulnar head stays in the same position. Loss of full extension at the elbow can be asymptomatic in diseases that cause inflammation here, such as rheumatoid arthritis.

Rather than assess finger joint function one by one in a screening examination, it is sufficient to ask the patient to squeeze several fingers of the examiner's hands, both hands at the same time. Equal pressure should be exerted by the squeeze of both hands. Any asymmetry or obvious symmetric weakness should be investigated further. If the patient winces in discomfort, the symptom can be followed up by specific examination.

Hips

The physician should ascertain that the hip extends fully and rotates completely in extension. Frequently, patients complain of pain generally localized to the pelvis. If passive rotation in full extension is normal, it is unlikely that there is serious intrinsic hip disease. Every person with normal musculature and no inflammation of the hip or knee should be able to hold the leg off the bed (with knee extended) for at least 45 seconds. This can be tested while other parts of the physical examination are being carried out.[4]

Knees

So long as the patient can fully extend the knee, it is unlikely that there is significant inflammation in that joint. In a screening examination, there is little return from thorough evaluation of range of motion unless the knee had been focused on by complaint or gait abnormalities.[4]

Ankle

The ankle is the most stable joint in the body. It is one of the few that can be fused and yet function sufficiently well to enable the individual to function well. There is no indication for routine screening of motion of the ankle.[5]

Foot

Feet bear the brunt of full body weight and impact loads. Ranging from calluses to stress fracture, the feet are at risk for trauma and inflammation. Patients generally complain about painful feet.[5] Therefore, without complaints, it is unlikely that more than rotation of the ankle and squeezing of the metatarsophalangeal joints during screening examinations is worthwhile (see Chapter 21).

EVALUATION OF SPECIFIC COMPLAINTS

Aching

"I ache all over" may be one of the most common complaints relating to the musculoskeletal system and certainly is the most difficult to label with a specific diagnosis or to treat effectively. Fibromyalgia and the chronic fatigue syndrome, diagnoses frequently given to such patients, are discussed in Chapter 18. Many practitioners find it too easy to dispense these diagnoses and frequently label patients with them who have not truly met diagnostic criteria.

Many patients who *ache all over* have symptoms that begin in the joints but are severe enough so that the muscles surrounding joints generate pain as well. This situation can be determined by careful palpation of the involved joint and determination of range of motion. The majority of patients who have significant inflammation of the joints do *not* have muscles that are tender to palpation, even though they have pain in these tissues. In contrast, patients with primary fibromyalgia rarely have swelling or tenderness in the joints themselves. The fibromyalgia patient has characteristic *tender points* that are demonstrated in Figure 18-1, but these patients should *not* have tenderness all over the body (see Chapter 18).

The patient with *pain all over* generally can perform the motions outlined in the screening examination, but he or she does so slowly while letting the examiner know that it is difficult. These patients rarely have cutaneous findings, muscle atrophy, or symmetric deformity. Women with severe osteopenia secondary to osteomalacia with superimposed osteoporosis may be exceptions to this; they are often slight of build with marked kyphosis and generally weak and tender muscles. Another exception is hypothyroidism. These patients may have thick brawny edema in the lower legs that histologically is a mixture of extracellular fluid and glycosaminoglycans.

Pain Defined by Exotic Adjectives

"It feels like there are little men with track shoes inside my knee."
"It feels like there is a screwdriver reaming out the veins in my legs."

All physicians can add descriptors that their patients have used that come across as either bizarre or incredibly creative. Sometimes true organic problems bring forth original adjectives, but these also make it likely that there is substantial emotional overlay to the symptoms. Symptoms that appear to be generated or enhanced by an active mind, however, are nevertheless symptoms and as such need to be managed, no matter how they are generated. The primary care physician as well as the rheumatologist should remember that a patient with symptoms in an extremity characterized as *burning* or *tingling* are at higher risk of having a neuropathy than the patient who complains of an *aching* joint, a common term used by those who have arthritis.

Weakness

"*I'm weak as a kitten, Doctor!*", a direct enough complaint, is often one of the most difficult for the physician to decipher and to treat.[6] Every organ system and most psychogenic disorders lay claim to producing weakness. The lack of specificity of the complaint is high. Almost everyone recovering from a winter's bout of influenza complains of weakness. Depression and cancer are associated with phlegmatic weakness and, without other signs, are impossible to differentiate from one another.

A complete history is extremely important for providing a guide for focus in the physical examination. *Pain or claudication* in muscles that are weak suggests a more acute process, possibly ischemic or inflammatory, than does painless weakness. *Double vision, drooping eyelids, or slurring of speech* should direct focus on specific tests for myasthenia gravis. *Painless progressive proximal weakness* suggests inflammatory myopathy (e.g., polymyositis). *Ascending weakness* can indicate the early stages of an inflammatory neuropathy (e.g., Guillain-Barré syndrome). *Asymmetric intermittent weakness* can be a presenting symptom of multiple sclerosis, as can abnormalities of speech.

To ensure record keeping that is effective in these patients, the physician must do a screening examination that allows comparison of findings at different time points. A five-point system is useful (Table 3–1). It is not essential at this first examination of the patient with weakness to examine every muscle in detail. An adequate screening examination includes the following:[7]

1. Effective swallowing; bulbar weakness or myositis may lead to aspiration of food or fluid into the lungs.

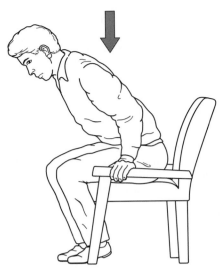

Figure 3–3. This patient has weak hip and knee extensor muscles. To rise from a chair, he must rock forward and backward, putting his weight over his arms. The arrow indicates his center of gravity as he finally stands.

2. Ability to stand (without using arms for help) from a chair; this tests both hip and knee extensor function (Fig. 3–3).

3. Squeezing the examiner's index and second fingers; a normal squeeze should produce mild pain for the examiner.

4. Downward pressure on arms held in abduction; the physician cannot break this position in normal persons.

5. Resistance to:
   • Neck flexion with head in extension
   • Neck extension with head in flexion
   • Depression of shoulder girdle in shrugging position
   • Extension of elbow with flexed forearm
   • Flexion of hand with wrist held in extension
   • Flexion of lower leg with knee in extension
   • Flexion of forefoot with ankle-foot in dorsiflexion.

Each of these short muscle tests begins with the muscle group to be tested held in a position of contraction, not relaxation. This position provides the patient with maximal and reproducible resistance.

Back Pain

Everyone has back or neck pain at some time during his or her lifetime. Back and neck pain can be due to a local musculoskeletal cause or to referred pain from other organ systems.

HISTORY

The complaint, "I've got terrible pain in my back," is common, accounting for as many as one third of complaints referable to the musculoskeletal system, and in primary care practices, it is a problem that represents

Table 3–1. FIVE-POINT SYSTEM		
Grade	**Strength**	**Criteria**
5	Normal	Can resist the physician
4	Mild weakness	Physician can break patient's contraction
3	Moderate weakness	Patient cannot use muscle group in functional effort; discoordinated and slow motion
2	Severe weakness	Minimal voluntary motion; no movement against gravity
1	Paralysis	No significant voluntary motion

approximately 5% of reasons for physician visits.[8] Over the years, it has become recognized that true herniation of the nucleus pulposus accounts for only 5% of back disorders, and this knowledge has accelerated the need for better evaluation and treatment of these patients. Common causes of pain include low back strain, lumbar disc disease, neurogenic pain from encroachment of a lumbar nerve root (lumbar radiculopathy), and narrowing of the spinal canal secondary to degenerative changes (lumbar spinal stenosis) (see Chapters 19 and 32). Two anatomic points are worth emphasizing before analyzing a proper back examination.

- Adjacent vertebrae are connected by the anterior intervertebral discs and by posterior zygoapophyseal joints. Anterior and posterior ligaments strengthen the alignment (see Chapters 19 and 32). Other posterior ligaments that have some distensibility and elasticity link the vertebral arches and spinous processes.
- The posterior muscle supports of the lower back are the sacrospinalis (connecting the posterior surface of the sacrum and iliac crest with the lower ribs) and multifidus muscles (that run from transverse processes to the spinous processes several vertebrae higher). The latter muscles act to rotate the spine.

The characteristics of low back pain from different origins sometimes help in diagnosis.

- *Spinal pain* from a pathologic process that stimulates sensory nerve endings often increases with spine motion, can be dull or sharp, and is localized to a specific place in the back, initially.
- *Radicular pain* is accentuated by motion that stretches the nerve root; it improves with rest and can have associated motor weakness, paresthesias, and numbness.
- *Discogenic pain* is exacerbated by motion or position that increases intradisc pressure (e.g., sitting, Valsalva maneuver, bending, or lifting). It rarely has associated neurologic findings.
- *Spinal stenosis pain,* in contrast to discogenic pain, often presents as claudication that is accentuated by walking and relieved by sitting. It is more diffuse and is alleviated when the spine is flexed. The compression of spinal cord and cauda equina by intrusion of internal osteophytes can be diagnosed more readily by computed tomography and magnetic resonance imaging.
- *Referred back pain* from pelvic or abdominal viscera has a deep aching quality in a dermatomal distribution.

EXAMINATION

The spine must be visible. First, with the patient standing, the physician looks for the extent of lumbar lordosis, thoracic kyphosis, and scoliosis with and without paravertebral muscle spasm. The physician should be aware of posturing that borders on histrionic activity. The patient should be asked to bend forward with the knees as straight as possible. Forward bending accentuates idiopathic dorsal scoliosis found in young people;

such scoliosis is usually convex to the right. The Schober test (make a pen mark at S1 and 10 cm cephalad from there, and measure the distance that the marks move apart on maximal lumbar flexion) should be used in any patient in whom ankylosing spondylitis may be a possible diagnosis (Fig. 3–4). Specific diagnostic tips can be as follows:

- *Schober measurements less than 12 cm in flexion:* ankylosing spondylitis. A positive Schober test demands measurement of chest expansion.
- *Exquisite localized tenderness on one spinous process:* localized pathology (i.e., infection, vertebral compression, or tumor).
- *A step on palpation at L4 through S1:* spondylolisthesis (Table 3–2).
- *Midline nevi or localized hair growth:* spina bifida.
- *Tender sciatic notch and calf tenderness:* sciatic nerve compression.
- *Uneven pelvis/iliac crest:* leg length discrepancy.

Neurologic examination related to back pain is best carried out initially on a supine patient. At the same time, peripheral pulses can be examined as well as skin and hair of the lower legs and feet.

Weakness of the lower leg muscles (e.g., calf) can often be found only by having the patient stand and do toe lifts and heel lifts as well as toe-toe/heel-heel gait. Malingering as a cause or contributor to back pain can be brought out by certain maneuvers. For example, in the patient *unable* to lift the heel off of the bed, there should be a downward push during true effort underneath the contralateral heel.

The history and physical examination, including

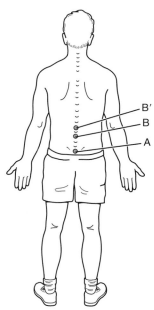

Figure 3–4. The Schober test. A mark is made at *A,* parallel with the dimples of Venus. A second mark is made at *B,* 10 cm above *A.* When the patient bends forward with knees extended, points *A* and *B* should move apart by more than 3 cm, indicating normal flexibility of the lumbar spine. Point *B′,* at 15 cm from *A,* is the distance that *A* and *B* separate in healthy young people.

Table 3-2. NERVE ROOT FINDINGS

Nerve Root	Pain/ Dysesthesia	Weakness/ Atrophy	Decreased Reflexes
L4	Posterior thigh across the knee	Quadriceps	Knee jerk
L5	Anteromedial thigh Anterolateral leg Medial foot and hallux	Extensor hallucis longus atrophy	None
S1	Posterior thigh Posterior leg Posterolateral foot Lateral toes	Gastrosoleus	Ankle jerk
Sacral roots S2–S4	Buttocks and perineum Posterior thigh Posterior leg Plantar foot	Gluteus maximus Hamstrings Gastrosoleus Anal/bladder sphincters	Ankle jerk Absent Plantar toe response

From Lipson SJ: Low back pain. In Kelly WN, Harris ED, Ruddy S, Sledge CB, eds: Textbook of Rheumatology, 5th ed. Philadelphia, WB Saunders, 1997, p 439.

neurologic examination, are important to the diagnosis, and a special questioning of changes in bowel and bladder habits recognizes the special sacral nerve root innervation of these organ systems. Radiographs may not be immediately indicated in the younger patient before treatment. In the elderly patient, however, metastatic disease, osteoporosis-associated vertebral collapse, and degenerative conditions as sources of ongoing pain can be appreciated with radiographic examination. Orthopaedic referral should be initiated for most traumatic injuries, cases with deformity, neurologic deficit, change in bowel or bladder habit not attributable to other causes, progressive pain especially associated with night pain, and repeated occurrences of disabling pain or functional deficits.

Cervical Spine

The most common musculoskeletal causes of neck pain include an acute cervical strain, cervical disc disease, neurogenic pain from encroachment of a cervical nerve root (cervical radiculopathy), and narrowing of the spinal canal secondary to degenerative changes (cervical spondylosis).[3] These are sometimes interrelated; for example, the patient with neck pain secondary to cervical disc disease may also have a radiculopathy. The key to diagnosis is the history and physical examination, including a thorough neurologic examination to detect motor and sensory deficits in the upper and lower extremities.

The cervical spine can be assessed by palpation and by active flexion, extension, and rotation. In patients with rheumatoid arthritis, anterior dislocation of C1 on C2 can sometimes be found by noting a particularly prominent spinous process at C2.[3] Rarely, posterior

pressure on the forehead combined with anterior pressure on C2 can detect a small amount of motion and even a *click* as the subluxed odontoid process falls back on the anterior portion of C1 (Fig. 3–5). In such patients, the opposite motion (i.e., anterior pressure on the occiput) should *never* be done for fear of causing cervical spinal cord compression.

Cervical radiographs and more sophisticated radiologic studies are important in instances of trauma, persistent pain, neurologic deficit, systemic symptoms, and deformity. If none of these are present, and the symptoms are mild to moderate, treatment may be commenced with counseling of the patient about the condition, physical means to keep the neck mobile and alleviate pain (referral for physical therapy), control of pain and spasm as indicated, and alteration of lifestyle (e.g., sleeping practices). Orthopaedic referral should be made for most traumatic injuries; for cases with neurologic deficit, deformity, or persistent pain; and when the primary care physician is in doubt about the cause.

SPECIFIC JOINT EXAMINATION—THE KEY TO SPECIFIC DISEASE DIAGNOSIS

There is no substitute for careful observation and palpation of joints involved in a patient's complaints or suggested by the history. This section focuses on specific joints, with the assumption that these examinations will be used in patients with pain or limitation of motion in those areas that have been defined during the screening examination. There are certain generalities about joint examination that are useful to consider:

- If an involved joint lacks full range of motion, that loss should be expressed in degrees lost (e.g., *the right hip lacks 20 degrees full extension*) or in degrees achieved (e.g., *the right wrist extends only 30 degrees*).
- Any swelling in or around a joint is abnormal.

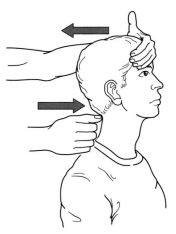

Figure 3–5. Test for C1–C2 instability at the atlanto-occipital joint. The left hand pulls the forehead toward the examiner, while the thumb of the examiner presses the spinous process of C2. In patients with rheumatoid arthritis who have posterior subluxation of the odontoid process, the patient and examiner may feel a click as it hits the arch of the atlas.

Swelling can be subtle. The concavities of normal anatomy (e.g., medioinferior and lateroinferior to the edge of the patellae, medial to the olecranon processes, posterior to the malleoli of the ankle, between metacarpophalangeal joints, and the volar surface of the wrist) should be kept in mind. When they are obliterated in a non-obese patient, there is either excess soft tissue or fluid present.

- Crepitus found on passive motion of a joint may represent relatively normal vibrations produced when one layer of soft tissue glides over another. Crepitus is not necessarily pathologic.
- If a joint has diminished motion, the reason why usually can be determined on physical examination. For example, if a proximal interphalangeal joint cannot extend fully, this could be related to an extensor tendon nodule, extensor tendon rupture, bound-down skin (in scleroderma), a tense synovial effusion, or bone/cartilage destruction (see Chapter 23). If none of these appear to be a problem, a neurologic cause must be considered.

Temporomandibular Joint

Both degenerative and inflammatory processes can affect the temporomandibular joint, which is crucial for maintaining adequate nutrition. Details of examination are included in Chapter 22. Temporomandibular joint dysfunction is likely to be the cause of an inability fully to open the mouth. The exception to this is the patient with scleroderma in whom skin contracture around the mouth limits mandibular motion.

Cricoarytenoid Joints

The cricoarytenoid joints are often overlooked as being true joints. In rheumatoid arthritis, their synovial linings may become inflamed and proliferative, resulting in hoarseness and, exceedingly rarely, stridor.

Sternoclavicular, Manubriosternal, and Costochondral Joints

Of the sternoclavicular, manubriosternal, and costochondral joints, the sternoclavicular joint is the only one that has substantial motion and therefore is a true diarthrodial joint with articular cartilage on both sides of the joint and substantial synovial lining. Tenderness and swelling of the sternoclavicular joint can be associated with inflammatory synovitis (particularly rheumatoid arthritis) and can be a focus of septic arthritis, especially in patients who use intravenous drugs (Fig. 3–6).

Costochondral joints can be painful (and inflamed) in polychondritis (a primary disease of articular and fibrocartilage) but rarely are involved in rheumatoid arthritis or other inflammatory arthritis. Patients with chest pain presenting at emergency departments with a diagnosis of *rule out myocardial infarction* should al-

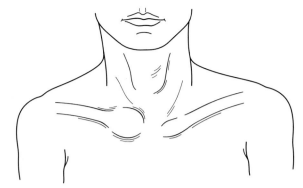

Figure 3–6. This sketch of a swollen, painful, red sternoclavicular joint is from an intravenous drug user who usually injected veins in his right arm. Rheumatoid arthritis is another cause of sternoclavicular inflammation.

ways have costochondral joints palpated; focused tenderness there may indicate costochondritis (Tietze's syndrome).

Shoulder

The basic motion of shoulders during the screening test was described earlier. When pain or limitation of motion is present, it is likely that the pathology is related to one of three categories (Table 3–3). There is a more extensive discussion of the shoulder examination in Chapter 18 and evaluation and management of rotator cuff impingment syndrome in Chapter 15.

One shoulder can have both periarticular and glenohumeral pathology. An example of this is the patient with a rotator cuff tear and a glenoid labrum tear. The labrum complex serves to enlarge the net surface area of contact for the humeral head. Tenderness at the glenohumeral joint may reflect a tear of this complex that functionally may behave similarly to a tear in the

Table 3–3. SHOULDER SYNDROMES	
Periarticular disorders	Rotator cuff tendinitis and tear
	Impingement disorders
	Calcific tendinitis
	Rotator cuff tear
	Bicipital tendinitis
	Subscapular neuropathy
	Thoracic outlet syndrome
Glenohumeral Disorders	Inflammatory arthritis
	Osteoarthritis
	Septic arthritis
	Osteonecrosis
	Adhesive capsulitis
	Glenohumeral instability
	Glenoid labrum tears
Regional Disorders	Cervical radiculopathy
	Nerve entrapment syndromes
	Reflex sympathetic dystrophy
	Fibromyalgia
	Polymyalgia rheumatica.

From Thornhill TS: Shoulder pain. In Kelly WN, Harris ED, Ruddy S, Sledge CB, ed: Textbook of Rheumatology, 5th ed. Philadelphia, WB Saunders, 1997, p 413.

meniscal cartilage in the knee. Diagnosis may depend on arthrography or MRI.

Palpation of the subacromial area produces pain early in impingement syndromes when there is mild inflammation of the supraspinatus tendon, a major component of the rotator cuff and the component most at risk from inflammation and tears. It is believed that *rotator cuff* tendinitis is the most common cause of shoulder pain. The principal finding on physical examination is the severe pain produced when the patient is asked to abduct the arm. The complexity and variety of imaging techniques and arthroscopy have made referral to a skilled orthopaedic surgeon essential for patients with persistent shoulder pain and loss of function.

A subset of people (generally young) have a predilection to develop *calcific tendinitis* in response to repetitive mild shoulder trauma. This is outlined in greater detail in Chapters 18 and 30. The intensity of pain and inflammation may resemble gout (Fig. 3–7). The deposits of calcium hydroxyapatite are often visible on simple radiographs, and injection of the local area with 20 mg triamcinolone hexacetonide is an appropriate therapeutic option for the primary care physician.

The following points may help the primary care physician in assessment of disability or pain in the shoulder (see Chapters 15 and 18).

- Long-standing tears of the rotator cuff are often associated with atrophy of the supraspinatus and infraspinatus muscles.
- *Bicipital tendinitis* may mimic rotator cuff pathology; the diagnosis of the former may be indicated if pain in the bicipital groove occurs when the examiner resists supination of the pronated forearm with the elbow flexed at 90 degrees (Yergason's supination sign).
- Rupture of the long head of the biceps tendon pro-

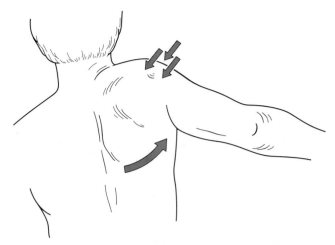

Figure 3–8. This patient is attempting to abduct his shoulder. He has severe rotator cuff disease, and this motion produces pain in the area of the small arrows. The glenohumeral joint is almost motionless. Partial abduction (pseudo-abduction) is possible as he wings out his scapula (large curved arrow).

duces a bulbous enlargement in the muscle bundle just proximal to the elbow.

- *Osteonecrosis* may produce dull aching pain with an essentially negative physical examination.
- *Adhesive capsulitis* is often the end stage of rotator cuff tendinitis, calcific tendinitis, bicipital tendinitis, and glenohumeral arthritis and generally occurs in persons older than 40.
- When testing for ability to abduct the shoulder, care must be taken by the examiner to hold the scapula in place to prevent *pseudoabduction* by winging of the scapula (Fig. 3–8).

Elbow

The skin over the olecranon (nodules in rheumatoid arthritis, plaques in psoriatic arthritis) should be examined closely (Fig. 3–9). The ulnar/humeral joint can be palpated on either side of the olecranon during flexion. The elbow can develop completely asymptomatic flexion contractures in response to only minimal inflammation. This tendency is accentuated in preadolescents with juvenile polyarthritis. Examination of the epicondyles is covered in the discussion of ailments linked to activity or sports (see Chapter 15).

Wrist

The true wrist joint is formed proximally by the radius and distally by the scaphoid (navicular), lunate, and triquetrum (triangular) carpal bones, and it is this joint—not carpometacarpal joints—that permits wrist flexion and extension. There is a distal radioulnar joint, but no true ulnocarpal joint. The first carpometacarpal joint is the only one of these that has substantial movement. This joint is symptomatic in *deQuervain's stenosing tenosynovitis* (see Chapter 23). Caused by irritation

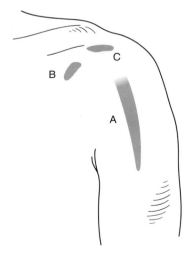

Figure 3–7. Common sites of shoulder pain. *A* represents the course of the long head of the biceps that can be both acutely and chronically inflamed. *B* marks the medial/anterior border of the glenohumeral joint that is tender or swollen when synovitis of this joint is present. *C* represents tenderness and pain in impingement syndromes. Pain associated with rotator cuff tears may be found throughout the upper surfaces of the shoulder.

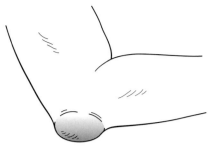

Figure 3–9. Classic location of nodules in patients with seropositive rheumatoid arthritis. Nodules can be firm and rubbery or soft and fluctuant. The fibroblasts and macrophages in these nodules produce large amounts of proteolytic enzymes.

of the extensor tendons and long abductor tendon of the thumb, pain in the area between the radial styloid and metacarpophalangeal joint can be reproduced by having the patient grasp the thumb in the palm by making a fist, then forcing the wrist into ulnar deviation. (Fig. 3–10).

The carpal tunnel is formed by the carpal bones and the flexor retinaculum. This tunnel contains tendons and their sheaths as well as the median nerve, the reason that when inflammation occurs in tendon sheaths the nerve may be compressed causing the *carpal tunnel syndrome* (see Chapter 23). Tinel's sign (paresthesias elicited in the fingers by gentle tapping over the carpal tunnel) and Phalen's maneuver (increasing paresthesias after maximal wrist flexion for 1 minute) are present in less than 55% of patients with carpal tunnel syndrome (Fig. 3–11). In every patient in whom the diagnosis of carpal tunnel syndrome seems possible, careful search for weakness of thumb abductors and flexors of the second finger is essential; if found, immediate referral to a hand surgeon after ob-

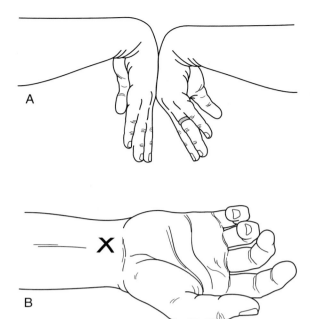

Figure 3–11. *A,* Phalen's maneuver (i.e., holding the wrists in maximal flexion for 1 minute) often produces paresthesias in distribution of the median nerve in patients with carpal tunnel syndrome. *B,* Tinel's sign. By tapping the area marked *X* with a strong finger or percussion hammer, a patient who has carpal tunnel syndrome often experiences tingling in the distribution of the medial nerve.

taining electromyography is indicated. More extensive discussion of the evaluation and management of disease in the wrist is found in Chapter 23.

Hand

The following aspects of examination of the hands have relevance for primary care physicians (see Chapter 23).

- Cutaneous abnormalities include tight skin with loss of wrinkles over the knuckles, which is characteristic of *scleroderma*. The loss of capillaries or presence of dilated capillary loops at the base of fingernails can be seen by use of the +40 lens of an ophthalmoscope. *Dupytren's contracture* is caused by fibrosis of the palmar aponeurosis, and this can draw fingers into progressive flexion contracture at the metacarpophalangeal joint or proximal interphalangeal joint.
- Nail abnormalities, such as punctate pitting or onycholysis, may be the only sign on hands of psoriatic arthritis. Fine, linear subungual hemorrhage may be seen in systemic vasculitis. True clubbing can be associated with pain in distal long bones found in *hypertrophic osteoarthropathy*.
- Bony thickening at the distal interphalangeal joints is known as *Heberden's nodes* and represents localized osteoarthritis with loss of cartilage and chaotic new bone growth without substantial synovitis. Similar changes at the proximal interphalangeal joints are known as *Bouchard's nodes.*
- Loss of abduction of the first carpometacarpal joint is

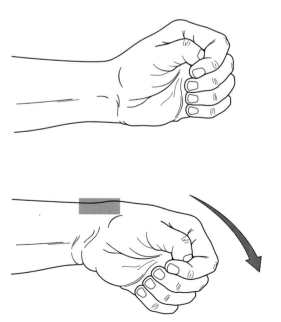

Figure 3–10. Test for de Quervain's stenosing tenosynovitis. Pain is induced in the track of the long extensor and abductor tendons (dark rectangle) as the wrist is forced into ulnar deviation (arrow).

characteristic of osteoarthritis as well as rheumatoid arthritis. It results in a reactive hyperextension of the distal interphalangeal joint so that pinch still is functional.

- Strength of grasp can be gauged roughly by having the patient squeeze a wound sphygmomanometer cuff inflated to 20 mmHg. Intrinsic hand muscle strength can be estimated by having the patient squeeze a 3 × 5 card between outstretched fingers against the examiner squeezing the other end of the card in the same way.
- A *swan-neck* deformity is flexion of the metacarpophalangeal joint, hyperextension of the proximal interphalangeal joint, and flexion of the distal interphalangeal joint. The *boutonnière deformity* is a flexion contracture of the proximal interphalangeal joint and hyperextension of the distal interphalangeal joint. Both are the result of inflammation in rheumatoid arthritis or other inflammatory synovitis (see Fig. 25–5 in Chapter 25).
- Fluid in small joints of the hand can be demonstrated by the examiner using fingers of both hands to press from three sides of the joint while reserving one finger to test for fluid by pressure on the fourth side.
- Inflammation of proximal interphalangeal and metacarphophalangeal joints can be determined most efficiently by simple squeezing of all four at once, as in a handshake; even minimal inflammation results in pain.

Hip

The hip joint is the weight-bearing articulation that connects the lower extremity with the axial skeleton. The hip is subjected to extremely large forces (sometimes as large as seven times body weight) during stair climbing, getting up from a chair, running, and jumping. Conditions such as inflammatory and degenerative arthritis of the hip, avascular necrosis of the femoral head, and trochanteric bursitis are common disorders that often are treated in their earlier stages by the primary care physician.

Tenderness to palpation directly laterally over the hip area is more likely to represent *trochanteric bursitis* than hip disease. Conversely, pain or limitation of gentle rotation of the leg relaxed in extension of the hip is a reliable sign of hip pathology, either inflammatory or degenerative. A painful hip can be appreciated best by pressure on the capsule at the hip in the groin or by pressure from the buttocks. As individuals age, external rotation of the hip in flexion becomes progressively difficult and does not necessarily connote osteoarthritis. If the supine patient holds the contralateral knee in flexion, a position that holds the pelvis in a neutral position, a flexion contracture in the other hip is demonstrated by an inability to make contact of the popliteal space with the examining table.

For arthritis of the hip, treatment of the inciting condition (e.g., by anti-inflammatory medication in rheumatoid arthritis), weight reduction, activity modification, the use of canes and other aids, analgesics and anti-inflammatory medication, and, in some cases, phys-

ical therapy are the mainstay of conservative treatment. Occasionally, a hip joint injection performed under radiographic control, using local anesthetic and glucocorticoid, may be both diagnostic and therapeutic. For unresponsive cases, total joint replacement is usually performed.

Avascular necrosis of the hip joint is usually idiopathic in origin but may be associated with the use of glucocorticoids, excessive alcohol intake, seropositive or seronegative arthritis, trauma, hemoglobinopathies, Caisson's disease, and other causes. Early referral to an orthopaedic surgeon assists in the staging of the disease (which affects prognosis and treatment options) and the determination of the status of the index hip, the contralateral hip, and other susceptible bones.

Trochanteric bursitis is a type of overuse syndrome causing pain at the insertion of the hip abductors into the greater trochanter. The pain may radiate distally and often is confused with hip arthritis and sciatica. Trochanteric bursitis may be treated by analgesics and anti-inflammatory medication, stretching exercises, or local injection of local anesthetic and glucocorticoid.

Knee

Problems around the knee joint are perhaps the most common reason for referral of a patient for orthopaedic consultation. Conditions associated with recurrent effusions, diffuse or localized subacute or chronic pain, locking, giving way, maltracking of the quadriceps-patellar mechanism, and arthritis with or without deformity usually are seen initially in the general physician's office.

Descriptions of examination for meniscal and ligamentous tears and patellofemoral syndromes are discussed in Chapter 16, and the bulge sign for fluid is described in Chapter 2 (see Fig. 2–7). Much information about knee function is gained by observing the standing patient. *Genu varum* (medial deviation of the lower leg) or *genu valgum* (lateral deviation of the lower leg) can be well tolerated by young individuals but may result in extra stress on medial or lateral compartments of the knee joint producing symptoms and signs of osteoarthritis at a later age.

Atrophy of the quadriceps muscles begins shortly after pain or inflammation develops in the knee and is a sign that the patient, for one reason or another, is not effectively using these muscles. Synovial effusion or difficulty in fully exending the knee often accompanies or is a cause of quadriceps atrophy.

High-riding or laterally displaced patellae often accompany pain localized in the patellofemoral articulations. If lifting the patella away from contact with the femur during passive flexion relieves pain, this indicates that patellofemoral contact is the source of the pain.

The popliteal region of the knee should be palpated for an arterial pulse and to define a popliteal (Baker's) cyst, if present. A popliteal cyst or ruptured popliteal cyst into the gastrocnemius/soleus muscles can mimic thrombophlebitis of the lower leg, causing swelling and pain in the calf.

The suprapatellar pouch or recess of the joint may extend as much as 5 to 7 cm proximal to the superior border of the patella.

Although acute traumatic injuries to one or two knee ligaments (most commonly the medial collateral ligament and anterior cruciate ligament) can initially be assessed clinically and radiographically by the primary care physician, immediate orthopaedic consultation often hastens diagnosis so that a treatment plan can be quickly decided on. For subacute injuries, timely orthopaedic consultation, usually within 1 week, usually suffices.

Minor recurrent effusions are indicative of intraarticular pathology, such as a meniscal tear, arthritis, or other cause. If not associated with locking, severe pain, or disability, and radiographs do not show loose bodies or end-stage arthritis, treatment may be initially commenced with analgesics and anti-inflammatory medication and a knee-strengthening program. More advanced knee signs and symptoms or failure of conservative management should prompt an orthopaedic referral. If knee radiographs are negative and a ligament injury or meniscal tear is suspected, a magnetic resonance imaging scan of the knee is often helpful before referral. Anterior knee pain from the patellofemoral joint, which is common in young women, may also be treated conservatively at first (Fig. 3–12). Persistent pain associated with maltracking of the patellofemoral joint with subluxation/dislocation, however, should be referred to the orthopaedic surgeon for consultation and treatment.

The Ankle and Foot

The ankle and foot are complex anatomic sites for diagnosis and treatment by the clinician (see Chapter 21). Similar to the wrist and hand, this area is comprised of numerous articulating bones and joints. In contrast to the upper extremity, multiples of the patient's body weight pass through the small joints of the foot and ankle during simple walking and stair climbing. Furthermore, the social aspects associated with modern footwear are complex. Shoes seem to emphasize style over comfort and often thwart the attempt to treat common foot disorders with shoe modifications.

Displaced fractures and dislocations in the ankles and feet should be seen by the orthopaedic surgeon immediately. Minor fractures of the toes and most sprains may be seen within 48 hours. These injuries often swell enormously. Splinting, elevation, icing, and analgesics are the cornerstones of treatment.

For less acute foot and ankle complaints, the history and physical examination are important starting points. Changes in weight, physical and social activities, and shoe wear can often herald the beginning of ankle and foot pain. Systemic illnesses should always be considered; for example, a diabetic foot sore may lead to an amputation if not aggressively diagnosed and treated. The patient as well as his or her stockings and shoes should be examined. The physician should look for associated deformity in the lower extremities. An attempt should be made to localize the pain primarily to the ankle, hindfoot, midfoot, or forefoot for diagnosis and treatment. Associated signs and symptoms, such as deformity, bunions, calluses and corns, and sores, should be noted. A neurovascular examination is extremely important. As noted early in this chapter, the physician should watch the patient walk. The patient's shoes should be at least as wide as the patient's foot, comfortable, and supportive. General foot care should be discussed with the patient. It is prudent to refer more complex issues to the orthopaedic surgeon with a special interest in the ankle and foot.

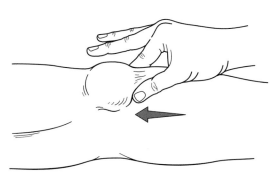

Figure 3–12. The patellar compression test. In patients complaining of pain around or under the patella, noted particularly when descending stairs or hills, sharp and intense pain is felt in that area when the examiner applies pressure at the upper border of the patella in the direction of the feet (arrow). The pain subsides immediately on release of pressure. This test lacks specificity but when positive suggests the diagnosis of chondromalacia, a softening and mild fissuring of patellar cartilage. There is no evidence that chondromalacia leads directly to osteoarthritis.

REFERENCES

1. Moder KG, Hunder GG: Examination of the joints. In Kelly WN, Harris ED, Ruddy S, Sledge CB, eds: Textbook of Rheumatology, 5th ed. Philadelphia, WB Saunders, 1997, p 363.
2. Thornhill TS: Shoulder pain. In Kelly WN, Harris ED, Ruddy S, Sledge CB, eds: Textbook of Rheumatology, 5th ed. Philadelphia, WB Saunders, 1997, p 413.
3. Nakano KK: Neck pain. In Kelly WN, Harris ED, Ruddy S, Sledge CB, eds: Textbook of Rheumatology, 5th ed. Philadelphia, WB Saunders, 1997, p 394.
4. Dillingham MF, Barry NN, Lannin JV: Hip and knee pain. In Kelly WN, Harris ED, Ruddy S, Sledge CB, eds: Textbook of Rheumatology, 5th ed. Philadelphia, WB Saunders, 1997, p 457.
5. Scardina RJ, Wood BT: Ankle and foot pain. In Kelly WN, Harris ED, Ruddy S, Sledge CB, eds: Textbook of Rheumatology, 5th ed. Philadelphia, WB Saunders, 1997, p 479.
6. Felsovanyi AS: Weakness. In Kelly WN, Harris ED, Ruddy S, Sledge CB, eds: Textbook of Rheumatology, 5th ed. Philadelphia, WB Saunders, 1997, p 388.
7. Wortmann RL: Inflammatory diseases of muscle and other myopathies. In Kelly WN, Harris ED, Ruddy S, Sledge CB, eds: Textbook of Rheumatology, 5th ed. Philadelphia, WB Saunders, 1997, p 1177.
8. Lipson SJ: Low back pain. In Kelly WN, Harris ED, Ruddy S, Sledge CB, eds: Textbook of Rheumatology, 5th ed. Philadelphia, WB Saunders, 1997, p 439.

Chapter **4**

Musculoskeletal Imaging in Rheumatologic Disorders

Ann Gabrielle Bergman ▪ Philipp K. Lang ▪ Christopher F. Beaulieu

Radiologic imaging techniques allow noninvasive detection, evaluation, and serial assessment of structural or gross-pathologic abnormalities in rheumatologic disorders. A broad array of imaging techniques, each modality having its own strengths and weaknesses, is currently available. The specific tools and areas of imaging expertise available to a primary physician depend on the practice setting. With increasing capability and sophistication of medical imaging of the musculoskeletal system, it has become increasingly important to choose carefully the modalities employed for imaging, so that a diagnosis can be reached as efficiently as possible without overuse of expensive technology.[1] This chapter discusses the role of the radiologist as consultant, the different imaging techniques available for assessment of rheumatologic conditions (Table 4–1), and imaging approach to the most frequent rheumatic disorders (Table 4–2).

RADIOLOGIST AS A CONSULTANT

The importance of providing a concise and specific clinical history when ordering an imaging examination, whether in writing as on a request form or verbally in direct consultation with a radiologist, cannot be overemphasized. Although the images themselves do portray the central, objective product of diagnostic radiology studies, the clinical history helps direct and refine a radiologist's search pattern in viewing the images and in arriving at the best diagnosis or differential diagnosis for a particular patient. Because the imaging appearances of many disorders overlap, having a relevant history often makes a major difference in the final radiologic impression. With increasing complexity and expense of imaging examinations, the role of the radiologist as a consultant to ordering clinicians is becoming more important. As a consultant, the radiologist takes on a more active and guiding role in patient care, not only by interpreting the results of completed examinations, but also by helping to select a specific imaging study for a particular clinical condition and in tailoring that study to answer the pertinent clinical questions. Additionally the radiologist may perform subsequent diagnostic or therapeutic procedures based on the consensus of clinical and imaging diagnoses.

Because the technology of imaging has advanced rapidly, literature on which test is optimal for a given circumstance is not always readily available, and often the best source of practical, up-to-date information is the consulting radiologist. Whenever in doubt as to which imaging examination to order for a patient the physician should consider contacting a radiologist directly for advice. Spending time on these interactions is ultimately beneficial to the quality of patient care and helps keep overall costs at a minimum.

OVERVIEW OF IMAGING TECHNIQUES

The imaging techniques available for evaluation of rheumatologic disorders include conventional radiography, computed tomography (CT), magnetic resonance imaging (MRI), scintigraphy (radionuclide bone imaging), arthrography, and ultrasound. Each modality has strengths and weaknesses that determine the diagnostic sensitivity and specificity for disorders involving different anatomic components of the musculoskeletal system. The modalities also vary as to overall cost and availability. Table 4–1 lists commonly available imaging modalities and indicates their relative strengths and weaknesses in providing image information on bony structures versus soft tissues. In the sections that follow, more specific information regarding applications of these modalities is given. Detailed texts are available for readers who want to review more images.[1, 2]

Conventional Radiography

Conventional x-rays (plain radiographs) remain the primary initial imaging study for virtually all rheumatologic disorders. Radiography is relatively inexpensive, is widely available, and often allows either a specific diagnosis or reassurance that a serious condition is not being overlooked. The interactions of x-irradiation with tissues, such as scattering and absorption, create a differential density on the exposed film. Regardless of the physical interactions involved, different classes of tissues result in a predictable hierarchy of decreasing film density, so that the film goes from being

Table 4–1. STRENGTHS AND WEAKNESSES OF IMAGING TESTS				
Modality	Bone	Soft Tissues	Cost
Conventional radiography	+++	+	+
Computed tomography	+++	++	+++
Magnetic resonance imaging	++*	+++	++++
Ultrasound	+†	+++ (superficial)	++
Scintigraphy	+++‡	−	++

*Magnetic resonance imaging is primarily sensitive to evaluation of bone marrow abnormalities as opposed to trabecular bone architecture and cortical integrity.

†Ultrasound does not penetrate bone, but reflectance off of cortical surfaces can allow detection of cortical step-off or discontinuity in fractures.

‡Scintigraphy is highly sensitive to bone turnover and metabolic activity but is primarily a functional rather than an anatomic technique.

relatively black (exposed) to relatively white (less exposed) as one encounters objects with density ranging from gas to fat, water, calcium, and metal. Because radiography is a projection technique, density information from a three-dimensional structure is represented on a two-dimensional plane. This summation of density results in relatively lower contrast resolution than that obtained with tomographic techniques, such as CT or MRI.

The chief value of conventional radiographs is in their depiction of bone. Information obtained includes qualitative global assessment of bone mineral content as well as highly detailed anatomy of the osseous structures, including periosteal, endosteal, and subchondral surfaces. In addition, some information is available related to cancellous bone structure and pathologic processes affecting this compartment, such as resorptive, reparative, or destructive processes. Soft tissue information is relatively limited. Because the bulk of periarticular and articular soft tissues has a density near that of water, little or no image contrast is available. Even so, useful insights into regional soft tissue swelling, joint capsular distention and effusions, and sharpness of soft tissue interfaces can be obtained with appropriate techniques and interpretive skills. Soft tissue masses, such as ganglion cysts, bursal distention, and nodules in rheumatoid arthritis and gout, may be depicted with appropriate soft tissue radiographic technique. Another valuable attribute of conventional radiography is in the depiction of pathologic calcifications occurring in soft tissues, which often provide useful diagnostic clues as described later.

Routine evaluation of most joints includes at least two different radiographic projections. Although specific projections are tailored to each anatomic region, in general, a combination of anteroposterior and lateral projections is obtained. An important consideration in designing radiographic protocols relates to patient position, such as whether or not the patient is weight bearing during the examination. For example, an anteroposterior radiograph of the knee in the supine position may show a normal tibiofemoral cartilage space, whereas the same exposure done with the patient standing upright during weight bearing may show narrowing indicating loss of articular cartilage.

Computed Tomography

CT can be viewed as a sophisticated extension of conventional radiography, in which irradiation is used to produce thin-section tomograms that depict bony anatomy with high detail and provide for much higher soft tissue contrast than does conventional radiography. CT images are generated in a plane that is parallel to the donut-shaped scanner gantry (i.e., in the transverse or [axial] plane when the patient lies supine on the scanner table). Thin-section axial CT sections can be reformatted into images in the sagittal or coronal planes, thereby aiding in evaluation of complex anatomic structures. In general, CT plays a relatively limited diagnostic role as a routine procedure in rheumatologic disorders but can be used effectively in certain body areas, such as the spine and sacroiliac joints. In these areas, transverse CT sections provide a unique and valuable depiction of the vertebral column and related soft tissues. For evaluation of degenerative disc disease, CT is sometimes combined with injection of iodinated contrast material into the spinal subarachnoid space (CT-myelography) to depict nerve roots and the spinal cord; however, this procedure has largely been replaced by MRI. In the sacroiliac joints and pelvis, CT is useful because it overcomes the frequent limitation of conventional radiographs in which superimposition of soft tissue and gas-containing bowel loops degrades bony visualization. Finally, CT is used commonly to guide biopsy procedures in the musculoskeletal and other systems.

Magnetic Resonance Imaging

MRI is based on the behavior of the hydrogen nuclei of water and fat molecules in a strong, external magnetic field. Hydrogen is used for MRI because of its abundance in biologic tissue and its high sensitivity to the magnetic resonance phenomenon. Behaving as miniature magnets themselves, the hydrogen nuclei (protons) undergo a process of precession or rotation about the external magnetic field. MRI signals are obtained from the precessing protons by probing the body with radiofrequency energy. Once a specific radiofrequency pulse is turned on, then off, the protons themselves produce a radiofrequency signal that is mapped into an image. The intensity of the emitted signal from a given point in the patient depends on several factors, including hydrogen density and magnetic properties of protons in a specific chemical environment called the *T1* and *T2* relaxation times. The assessment of these parameters provides the potential for physiologic and biochemical information about the imaged tissue.

A key feature of MRI, as compared with conventional radiography and CT, is its superior soft tissue contrast. Muscle, cartilage, ligaments, tendons, nerves, and blood vessels each produce different MRI because the water protons within them have differing T1 and T2 relaxation times. In addition to the excellent soft tissue contrast, MRI has the capability of providing direct images in any plane.

Although relatively expensive, MRI is an excellent tool for work-up of traumatic, degenerative, and inflammatory conditions affecting joints because of its ability to depict soft tissues directly. Moreover, direct depiction of articular cartilage is afforded by high-resolution MRI, information that is unavailable with any other imaging technique. Because little MRI signal is generated directly from the protons in the crystalline matrix of mature bone, it is commonly thought that MRI is not useful for imaging bone. This statement is far from correct, as long as the appropriate context is appreciated.[3] Although it is true that obtaining the same bone surface and trabecular detail with MRI as with high-resolution CT is difficult, MRI provides unique information about the bone marrow space and edema or inflammatory processes affecting the bone marrow. In addition, surface reactions of bone, such as periostitis, often are associated with tissue edema that is well depicted by MRI.

In orthopaedics and sports medicine, MRI of the knee, shoulder, ankle, and hip is commonly performed for comprehensive evaluations of osseous and soft tissue structures. Because of its diagnostic accuracy, MRI has replaced diagnostic arthrography in most patients and has markedly decreased the amount of exploratory or diagnostic arthroscopy. In the detection and characterization of stress injury to bone, MRI compares well with radionuclide bone scanning and often provides a more specific diagnosis.

With adequate equipment and technique, MRI is uniquely capable of imaging articular cartilage. The overall thickness, smoothness, and internal signal characteristics of articular hyaline cartilage can be assessed at a single time point or followed serially to assess the efficacy of cartilage repair and regrowth procedures under development. Currently, imaging of naturally thicker areas of cartilage, such as that in the knee, is more successful than imaging of joints with thinner cartilage, such as the hip or in small joints such as the wrist. Finally, inflamed or infected synovial tissue undergoes enhancement on MRI after intravenous injection of gadolinium chelates, a phenomenon that has been taken advantage of in characterization and follow-up of inflamed joints.

Radionuclide Bone Imaging

Radionuclide bone imaging or scintigraphy can be viewed as a highly sensitive but nonspecific imaging modality for detection of increased bone turnover occurring in trauma, inflammation, infection, or neoplasia. The technique involves intravenous injection of technetium-99m-radiolabeled phosphate compounds, followed by imaging of radiopharmaceutical activity with a gamma camera. Immediate imaging after injection can give some information on alterations in regional blood flow and blood pool activity, whereas *delayed* imaging at 2 to 4 hours after injection depicts activity

resulting from radiotracer interactions with bone, as the isotope is localized by chemoabsorption onto the hydroxyapatite crystals at bone surfaces. Activity is usually greatest in regions with high ratios of bone surface to blood flow, such as the cancellous bone around joints. In arthritis, localization of these agents results primarily from the increase in blood flow to juxta-articular bone in regions of active synovitis. Another important application of joint scintigraphy is the evaluation of joint prostheses. Mechanical loosening and pyogenic infection are infrequent but important complications of joint replacement and may be detected by use of radionuclide scintigraphy.

Arthrography and Tenography

Injection of contrast material into the joint cavities (arthrography) or tendon sheaths (tenography) has been employed less frequently as MRI is used more. These procedures, however, still have important clinical applications. Arthrography may be applied to the evaluation of many different joints and is usually performed using x-ray fluoroscopy. After contrast opacification of the joint, CT or MRI may be performed. For magnetic resonance arthrography, intra-articular injection of gadolinium-containing compounds is performed, whereas for conventional arthrography, iodinated contrast material, air, or a combination of these two is employed. Although such procedures usually now assume a secondary role to noninvasive imaging in rheumatologic disorders, the functional information obtained can be unique. Opacification of the joint cavity allows assessment of synovium and detection of communications between joints and surrounding bursae or in situations such as rupture of a popliteal cyst. In addition, imaging-guided injection of the joint of interest can be combined with injection of local anesthetic or glucocorticoids for therapeutic purposes.

Tenography is a specialized technique in which opacification of a tendon sheath is used to evaluate for irregularities resulting from synovitis or inflammation, most commonly performed for ankle tendons. A selective injection of a combination of radiographic contrast material, local anesthetic, and glucocorticoid helps target the patient's symptoms to a specific tendon sheath and provides therapy.

In sports medicine, magnetic resonance arthrography is currently the imaging gold standard for evaluation of partial-thickness rotator cuff tears and glenoid labral injury of the glenohumeral joint. The technique excels over that of conventional MRI because the high signal material injected into the joint produces high-quality anatomic delineation of the structures of interest and provides distention of the joint capsule, thereby separating normally neighboring anatomic structures.

Ultrasound

Ultrasound (or sonography) of the musculoskeletal system is widely used outside the United States, owing in part to lesser availability of MRI. The technique involves placement of a transducer on the skin overlying the structure of interest and imaging using high-frequency sound waves. The procedure is harmless and painless for the patient and has the benefits of being relatively inexpensive as well as mobile.[4] A significant disadvantage of ultrasound is that it requires a skilled operator with a detailed knowledge of the regional anatomy. In some centers, ultrasound plays a primary role in detection of rotator cuff degeneration and tears, with diagnostic accuracy comparable to MRI. Other superficial structures, such as the Achilles and patellar tendons, are also accessible by ultrasound. In the wrist and hand, ultrasound can be useful for detection of and characterization of ganglion cysts and in evaluating tenosynovitis and tendinitis. Some centers also have excellent experience using ultrasound to evaluate tendons in the ankle and foot, such as the peroneal and posterior tibial tendons.

RADIOGRAPHIC FEATURES OF RHEUMATOLOGIC DISORDERS

Rheumatoid Arthritis

Radiologic manifestations that reflect the gross pathologic changes of rheumatoid arthritis (RA) are seen in the periarticular soft tissues, the articular cartilage and synovium, and the subchondral bone. Most frequent joint involvement is seen in the small joints of the hands, wrists, knees, and feet (Fig. 4–1). The process can begin with a monoarticular or asymmetric, pauciarticular distribution, which, in time, becomes polyarticular and symmetric. Occasionally, advanced disease is asymmetric and nonuniform. Axial skeletal involvement in adult RA usually occurs later, is less striking than peripheral involvement, and is generally limited to the cervical spine.

CONVENTIONAL RADIOGRAPHIC FEATURES

SOFT TISSUES. Swelling of the periarticular soft tissues is a hallmark of RA involvement. Swelling results from periarticular edema, synovial proliferation, and accumulation of joint fluid. Radiographically, symmetric uniform swelling around the joints is most easily detected in the small joints of the hands and wrists.

CARTILAGE. Radiographic narrowing of the interosseous space, reflecting cartilage loss, presents later than does periarticular soft tissue swelling. Occasionally, widening of the joint may reflect capsular distention by hypertrophied synovium and excessive fluid. In late disease, the interosseous space may be asymmetrically narrowed or widened as a result of advanced destruction and fragmentation of subchondral bone and damage to supporting capsular and ligamentous structures.

OSTEOPENIA. Regional osteopenia characteristically accompanies soft tissue swelling in RA. Initially, it is most apparent in the periarticular regions. This re-

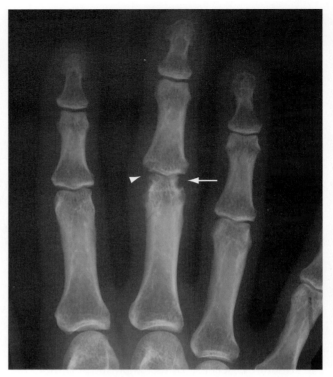

Figure 4–1. Posteroanterior view of the hand in a 68-year-old woman shows characteristic changes of rheumatoid arthritis in the proximal interphalangeal joint of the third finger: soft tissue fullness; a large erosion on the ulnar aspect (*arrow*); and a small erosion in the bare area on the radial aspect (*arrowhead*), seen only as absence of the subchondral cortical white line.

sorption of cancellous bone produces periarticular demineralization. It is seen radiographically as radiolucency and sometimes a relative accentuation of primary trabeculae, as secondary trabeculae are resorbed. In late disease, the regional, irregular, patchy osteopenia is superseded by a more uniform demineralization.

EROSIONS. Articular erosions represent destruction of subchondral cortical bone. Their radiographic appearance provides an important parameter for serial assessment of activity of disease and response to therapy, with the preceding soft tissue swelling and focal osteopenia being more sensitive but less specific radiographic features. Erosions generally begin intraarticularly at the periphery of the joint, in the *bare area* where the cartilage ends and the capsule inserts (see Fig 4–1). As pannus develops, the underlying cortical and cancellous bone becomes rarefied and indistinct, and as it is focally destroyed, bony erosions are produced.

ALIGNMENT. As disease progresses and capsular, ligamentous, and tendinous structures become weakened or destroyed, joint malalignment, such as subluxation or dislocation, may take place. These changes are most common in the small peripheral joints of the hands and feet and in the cervical spine (Figs. 4–2 and 4–3).

ANKYLOSIS. Bony ankylosis, although not prominent in adult RA, has been reported in approximately 10% of patients with advanced disease and involves predominantly the carpal and tarsal joints.

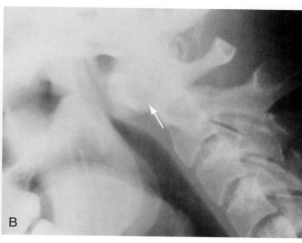

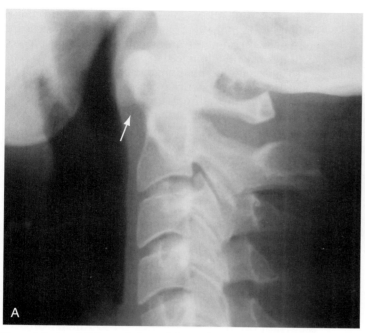

Figure 4–2. *A* and *B,* Lateral views of the cervical spine in a 21-year-old woman with rheumatoid arthritis were obtained during extension and flexion and show normal alignment in extension but atlantoaxial (C1–C2) instability (*arrows*) in flexion. Laxity or erosions of the transverse ligament allows the odontoid process to subluxate posteriorly in flexion of the head, resulting in a more than a 3 mm space between the posterior margin of the anterior arch of the atlas and the anterior surface of the odontoid process (shown faintly in part *B*).

IMAGING FEATURES WITH MAGNETIC RESONANCE IMAGING

MRI has a greater sensitivity in detecting carpal erosions when compared to conventional radiography and may become a useful tool for evaluating and quan-

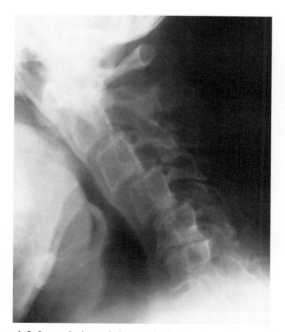

Figure 4–3. Lateral view of the cervical spine in a 63-year-old man with rheumatoid arthritis was obtained during flexion and shows a *stepladder* appearance with mild anterior shift of C2 on C3 and more pronounced anterior subluxation at C3–C4 and C4–C5.

titating response to anti-inflammatory therapy. MRI provides excellent delineation of the soft tissue changes, cartilaginous defects, and osseous erosions associated with RA. The signal intensity of inflamed synovium or pannus varies markedly on T1-weighted and T2-weighted MRI, reflecting different degrees of inflammation and fibrosis in the proliferative tissue. In evaluating inflammatory soft tissue changes in RA, MRI may be supplemented by the use of paramagnetic contrast agents, such as gadolinium–diethylenetriaminepenta-acetic acid (Gd-DTPA). The contrast enhancement at bony erosions after administration of Gd-DTPA indicates the presence of perfused, actively enhancing granulation tissue in the erosion. MRI is unique in that it provides a direct delineation of the pathologic tissue at the site of the erosive process. In imaging the craniocervical junction in RA patients, MRI affords superior delineation of brain stem or spinal cord compression resulting from atlantoaxial subluxation or pannus.

Systemic Lupus Erythematosus

Systemic lupus erythematosus (SLE) is a chronic disease with many manifestations, of which polyarthritis and polyarthralgia are the most common. Exclusive of soft tissue swelling, radiographic changes occur in only 5% to 30% of these patients. As in RA, involvement is frequently polyarticular and symmetric with an identical pattern of joint involvement, whereas severe progressive joint destruction is rare.

In the hands, the most common finding is soft tissue swelling at the proximal interphalangeal, metacarpophalangeal, and wrist articulations. Periarticular osteoporosis is sometimes seen, whereas more generalized osteoporosis is frequent in late disease and often accentuated by glucocorticoid therapy. The most characteristic radiographic change is pronounced joint deformity without presence of bony erosions. The synovitis of SLE is generally less pronounced than that of RA, without pannus formation. Rather the periarticular, capsular, and ligamentous supporting structures are involved and account for the characteristic joint malalignments. Most commonly, ulnar deviation and volar subluxation of the metacarpophalangeal joints, hyperextension at the proximal interphalangeal joints, flexion of the distal interphalangeal joints, and carpal subluxation in ulnar direction take place.

Avascular osteonecrosis, most commonly involving the femoral heads, is seen in approximately 5% of patients with SLE, usually associated with glucocorticoid medication.

Scleroderma

Progressive systemic sclerosis or scleroderma is a generalized disorder of connective tissue characterized by inflammation, fibrosis, and degeneration. Raynaud's phenomenon and arthralgia are frequent and associated with characteristic radiographic changes in about two thirds of patients. During the early phase, soft tissue swelling in the hands is seen diffusely. Tapering of the soft tissues of the fingertips is a characteristic radiographic feature. Soft tissue calcification is generally a late manifestation. Resorption of distal phalanges in severe disease is defined well by radiographs.

Seronegative Spondyloarthropathies

The seronegative spondyloarthropathies, including ankylosing spondylitis, enteropathic arthritis, psoriatic arthritis, and Reiter's syndrome, share many common features. They are characterized clinically and radiographically by prominent involvement of the spine, proliferative new bone formation, and bony ankylosis. Enthesopathy or inflammation and degeneration at sites of ligamentous or tendinous insertion in bone, which are called *entheses*, as well as prominent synovitis and, occasionally, severe destruction of phalangeal joints, are characteristic.

ANKYLOSING SPONDYLITIS

In ankylosing spondylitis, the axial skeleton is most frequently and most severely involved. In addition to synovitis of the diarthrodial joints, these patients have prominent inflammation at ligamentous, tendinous, and capsular attachments to bone.

SACROILIAC JOINTS. Abnormal sacroiliac joints can be seen radiographically even before the onset of focal symptoms. Almost all patients have radiographic changes at this site within 12 months of clinical onset of the disorder. Conventional radiography is frequently difficult because of the curved and angled configuration of the sacroiliac joint, and therefore a special view consisting of an angled anteroposterior projection is usually obtained.

Early radiographic change in the sacroiliac joint consists of loss of the discrete subchondral cortical line resulting from focal bony erosion, accompanied by reactive sclerosis in the subjacent cancellous bone (Fig. 4–4). Early on, the process may be unilateral or asymmetric, but it soon becomes bilateral and eventually symmetric. The process characteristically progresses to intra-articular bony ankylosis.

SPINAL INVOLVEMENT. In the spine, radiographic changes consist of anterior vertebral squaring, syndesmophytosis (Fig. 4–5A), apophyseal joint ankylosis, and ligamentous ossification and usually first appear at the region of the thoracolumbar junction. Vertebral squaring, seen on a lateral radiography of the spine, results from subtle bone resorption at the anterior longitudinal ligament insertion, which leads to a loss of the normal concavity of the anterior surface of the vertebral body. This focal inflammation can also be associated with osteitis and sclerosis, the so-called shiny corner appearance.

Syndesmophytes are linear paravertebral ossifications that appear in the outer fibers of the anulus fibrosus and the adjacent connective tissues, along the anterior and lateral aspects of the spine at the level of the disc interspace. They differ from osteophytes or new bone formation in diffuse idiopathic skeletal hyperostosis (DISH) (Fig. 4–5B, C), which orginate from the cartilaginous end-plate in response to degeneration of the disc and are oriented parallel to the end-plates.

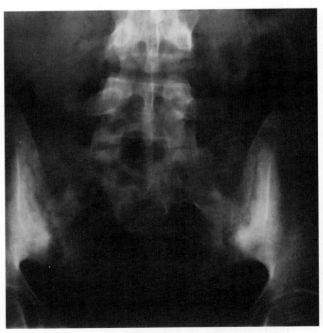

Figure 4–4. Tilted anteroposterior view of the sacroiliac joints in a young man with ankylosing spondylitis, showing advanced changes of sacroiliitis, including absence of the subchondral cortex with indistinct joint margins resulting from bony erosions and extensive sclerosis.

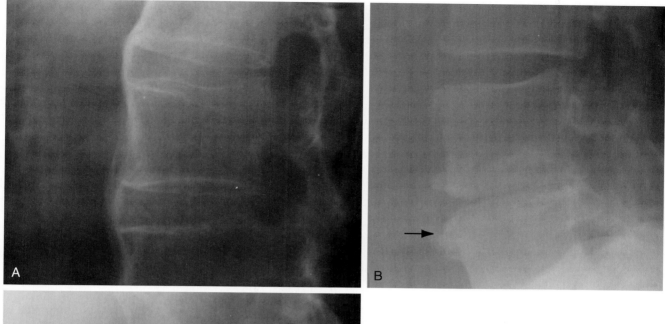

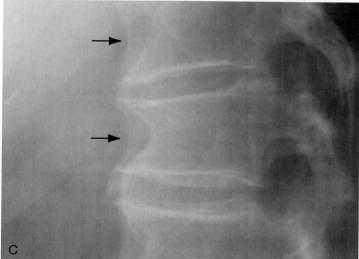

Figure 4–5. Lateral view of the upper lumbar spine in a man with long-standing ankylosing spondylitis (*A*), demonstrating the characteristic appearance of syndesmophytes as smooth linear densities along the distribution of the anterior longitudinal ligament. For comparison, a lateral view of the midlumbar spine in a middle-aged man with degenerative spine disease (*B*), showing osteophyles (*arrow*) and the upper lumbar spine in an older man with diffuse idiopathic skeletal hyperostosis (DISH) (*C*) showing bone formation also along the anterior cortex of the vertebral bodies (*arrows*).

Syndesmophytes differentiate ankylosing spondylitis from other spondylitic disorders. In ankylosing spondylitis, syndesmophytes are typically marginal and symmetric and eventually result in the classic radiographic finding of a *bamboo spine*.

Involvement of the apophyseal joints in ankylosing spondylitis can result in erosion, narrowing, and sclerosis. Later the apophyseal joints become fused.

In patients with advanced disease, linear densities can be seen posteriorly resulting from ossification of the interspinous ligaments in the midline plane and, less commonly, of the capsules and ligaments that span the apophyseal joints in the parasagittal plane. Thus, anteroposterior lumbar radiographs may have a distinct double-track or triple-track appearance.

PERIPHERAL JOINTS. Involvement of the appendicular skeleton is usually transient in the peripheral joints. In the proximal joints, however, advanced destructive arthropathy is common. The hips often are

involved in ankylosing spondylitis, with a ridge of bone formation surrounding the perimeter of the femoral head similar to a collar. Total arthroplasty of the hip is often required but is associated with an increased risk of extensive postoperative heterotopic ossification.

PSORIATIC ARTHROPATHY

The radiographic changes of psoriatic arthropathy in the axial skeleton result from enthesopathy and synovitis and resemble ankylosing spondylitis in many respects, whereas the peripheral manifestations may simulate aggressive RA. Manifestations of axial joints are nearly indistinguishable radiographically from those of Reiter's syndrome.

Sacroiliitis is an early, frequent feature but differs from that of ankylosing spondylitis in that asymmetry is seen in about 50% of patients. The spondylitis of psoriasis is characterized by broad, nonmarginal syndesmophytes and sometimes also the more subtle syndesmophytes seen with ankylosing spondylitis. Skip areas are frequent, and advanced cervical spine changes may be seen in the absence of involvement of the thoracic, lumbar, or even sacroiliac joints. Atlantoaxial subluxation is common but is generally less dramatic than in RA.

Peripheral psoriatic arthritis affects predominantly the small joints of the hands and feet, whereas destructive changes are less common in the larger joints. Radiographic changes range from those characteristic of psoriatic arthropathy to those indistinguishable from RA. Typically an asymmetric arthropathy affects the distal interphalangeal joints and, less severely, the proximal interphalangeal, metacarpophalangeal, metatarsophalangeal, carpal, or tarsal joints. In about one fourth of patients, diffuse swelling of an entire digit (*sausage finger*) may be present. Characteristic findings at articular margins and at capsular attachments consist of a combination of focal bone resorption and linear periosteal new bone formation.

REITER'S SYNDROME

In Reiter's syndrome, early diagnosis when the syndrome is incomplete may be aided by careful radiographic assessment. Radiographic features of Reiter's syndrome consist of asymmetric, pauciarticular involvement of the feet, ankles, knees, and lower spine. The upper extremity is usually spared except for soft tissue swelling and, rarely, periostitis. One or several joints of the feet, most commonly the first interphalangeal or other proximal interphalangeal joints, are sites of pronounced soft tissue swelling, moderate periarticular osteoporosis, proliferative erosion, and periosteal new bone formation. The peripheral manifestations simulate psoriatic arthropathy closely and may be indistinguishable clinically and radiographically (Fig. 4–6). Features that may distinguish Reiter's syndrome from psoriatic arthritis include predominant distribution in the lower extremity, involvement of fewer joints, sparing of the distal interphalangeal joints, and greater periarticular osteoporosis. Sacroiliitis, often asymmetric, is common in patients with Reiter's syndrome, whereas spinal involvement is less common than in psoriasis.

DEGENERATIVE AND ISCHEMIC ARTHROPATHIES

Osteoarthritis

Osteoarthritis, also known as *osteoarthrosis* or *degenerative joint disease*, is a common joint disorder characterized predominantly by noninflammatory deterioration of articular cartilage accompanied by formation of new bone at joint margins. Osteoarthritis occurs in two major forms: primary and secondary. Primary osteoarthritis develops in joints without antecedent history of insult and affects predominantly the distal and proximal interphalangeal joints (Fig. 4–7); first carpometacarpal joints in the hands; spine; and larger weight-bearing joints, such as the hips and knees. Primary generalized osteoarthritis predominantly affects the hands in middle-aged women but frequently involves the knees, hips, and spine as well.

Secondary osteoarthritis results from alterations in metabolism or mechanics of the joint subsequent to other conditions. These conditions include traumatic injury; inflammatory arthritis; infection; osteonecrosis; developmental abnormality; neurologic deficit; and disorders such as ochronosis, Wilson's disease, pseudogout, and acromegaly. Secondary osteoarthritis may be the end stage of other common primary arthritides, such as RA, juvenile RA, and gout.

The radiographic manifestations of osteoarthritis consist of irregular narrowing of the joint, subchondral sclerosis and cyst formation, and marginal osteophytes. Often there also is mild soft tissue swelling and some joint malalignment, whereas the mineralization remains normal. The variable expression of these components depends on many factors, such as the stage of disese, underlying disorder, and local joint anatomy.

COMPUTED TOMOGRAPHY AND MAGNETIC RESONANCE IMAGING

MRI is unique in that it affords direct visualization of cartilage. Focal thinning of cartilage, irregularity of the cartilage surface, and inhomogeneity of signal intensity are MRI signs of cartilage loss in osteoarthritis. MRI can demonstrate cartilage loss before joint space narrowing is evidenced radiographi-

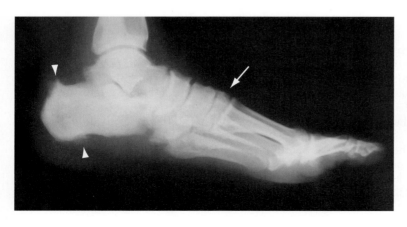

Figure 4–6. Lateral view of the foot in a young man with Reiter's syndrome, showing the characteristic combination of bony erosions (*arrow*) and enthesopathy with bone formation (*arrowheads*). The involvement is most pronounced in the hindfoot.

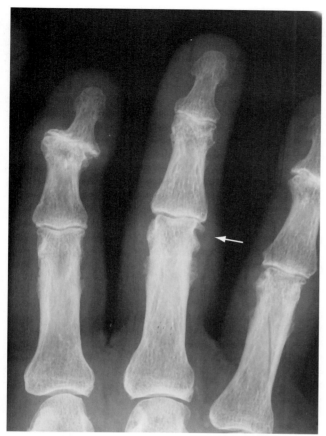

Figure 4–7. Posteroanterior view of the hand in a 74-year-old man shows features of osteoarthritis, including narrowing or obliteration of the cartilage space at the joints and marginal osteophyte formation. Prominent osteophytes can sometimes lead to an appearance mimicking erosions (*arrow*) in adjacent bone, but there is normal continuity of the cortex and no bony lysis.

cally and may also demonstrate osseous as well as cartilaginous intra-articular bodies. Subchondral sclerosis causes low signal intensity within the high signal intensity marrow space on all sequences. Subchondral cysts produce low signal intensity on T1-weighted images and high signal intensity on T2-weighted images. MRI may be used as a noninvasive tool for monitoring progression of early osteoarthrities and may be particularly useful for longitudinal studies that assess the influence of different therapies on the long-term course of this disease.

Neuroarthropathy

Sometimes called *Charcot joint*, neuroarthropathy describes painless, unstable, and frequently deformed joints associated with a neurologic deficit (Fig. 4–8). Most common among the diseases causing neuroarthropathy are diabetes mellitus, syringomyelia, and spinal cord injury or anomaly. The radiographic features depend on the underlying disease and the stage and rate of evolution. In established neuroarthropathy, these features consist of joint effusion, subluxation, subarticu-

lar sclerosis, fracture and fragmentation, marginal osteophytosis, and heterotopic calcification and ossification. Any of these features may exist separately, or they may be combined, as is common in advanced disease. The common sites of neuropathic involvement are the midfoot, ankle, and knee, and less commonly the hip, spine, shoulder, and wrist, although other joints may be affected. Both in rapidly and in slowly evolving forms of neuroarthropathy, one sees similar radiographic features of extensive subarticular bone resorption, the atrophic phase, with joint deformity and instability. This resorption is followed by intense sclerosis, prominent osteophytosis, and periarticular ossification, the hypertrophic phase. The late changes are similar to those of advanced degenerative joint disease.

Osteonecrosis

Osteonecrosis or avascular necrosis may affect the epiphyseal region of bones. The most common site of involvement is the femoral head (Fig 4–9). Other commonly involved sites are the humeral head, distal femoral condyles, carpal scaphoid bone, and talar dome. Several different clinical and radiographic staging systems have been reported for osteonecrosis of the hip. The most frequently used classification has been introduced by Ficat and Arlet.[5] This system denotes five successive stages of osteonecrosis: Stage 0 is preradi-

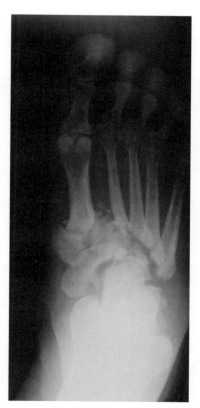

Figure 4–8. Anteroposterior view of the foot in a middle-aged woman with diabetes mellitus and neuroarthropathy, also called *Charcot joint changes*. These include bony lysis, sclerosis, fragmentation, and malalignment.

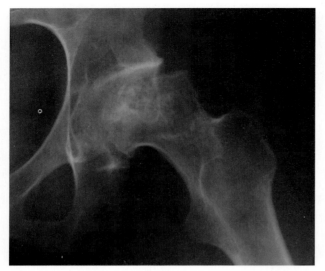

Figure 4–9. Frogleg lateral view of the hip in a young man with advanced changes of avascular necrosis, showing marked flattening of the femoral head with sclerosis and osteophyte formation indicating the presence of secondary osteoarthritis.

ographic and preclinical. In stage 1, the patient has hip pain but no radiographically detectable disease in one hip. In stage 2, the patient has pain, and radiographs demonstrate diffuse or localized areas of sclerosis or cysts. Stage 3 is characterized by the appearance of a bony sequestrum on the radiograph. A transition between stages 2 and 3 is evidenced by a crescentic line resulting from subchondral fracture and segmental flattening (Fig 4–10). In stage 4, progressive loss of articular

cartilage and the development of acetabular osteophytes are observed. Nontraumatic osteonecrosis is most frequently observed between the 20s and 40s. The incidence of osteonecrosis is fourfold greater in men than in women. Bilateral involvement, often asynchronous, is found in up to 70% of patients.

MRI is the most sensitive imaging technique for detecting osteonecrosis and is sometimes positive for osteonecrosis when conventional radiography, scintigraphy, and CT are still negative. In contrast to scintigraphy, MRI also demonstrates the exact location and extent of the necrotic zone and is characterized by a high specificity in differentiating osteonecrosis from other hip disorders.

CRYSTAL DEPOSITION DISEASES

Gout

Gout, a form of crystal-induced disease caused by monosodium urate monohydrate crystal deposition, affects predominantly the small joints in the feet, hands, wrists, ankles, and elbows. During the early acute episodes of gout, the only radiographic manifestation is soft tissue swelling over the painful joint and sometimes mild focal demineralization. Even with chronic gout, radiographic evaluation may not show any abnormalities, but after several years of recurrent disease, radiographic changes consisting of periarticular soft tissue swelling with erosions usually appear. Characteristically, erosions are sharply marginated with a sclerotic border, as opposed to the ill-defined and focally de-

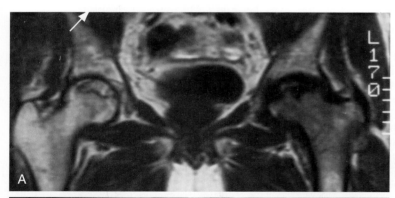

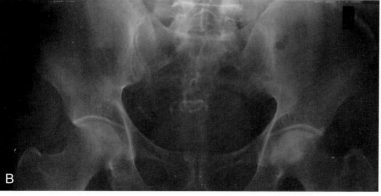

Figure 4–10. Magnetic resonance imaging (*A*) of the hips in a middle-aged man with known avascular necrosis of the left hip shows involvement also of the right hip, with a characteristic irregular demarcation line in the upper aspect of the femoral head. A plain radiograph taken 2 weeks earlier (*B*) does not show diagnostic changes of the avascular necrosis of the right hip, but the sclerosis and subtle flattening of the left femoral head can be seen.

mineralized erosions of RA. In about 40% of patients with gouty erosions, a characteristic overhanging edge is seen, resulting from adjacent new periosteal bone formation. This appearance is uncommon in other erosive articular disorders. Usually, there is maintenance of normal cartilage thickness and normal or mildly decreased bony mineralization. Tophi characteristic of gout appear radiographically as a soft tissue density, usually calcified, in a periarticular location. Tophi are particularly common at the first metatarsophalangeal joint of the foot.

Pseudogout

Abnormal deposition of a type of calcium salts in the hyaline and fibrocartilage of joints, often accompanied by acute or chronic synovitis, is called *pseudogout* or *calcium pyrophosphate dihydrate* crystal deposition disease. The radiographic features of pseudogout consist of linear and punctate calcifications of fibrocartilage and hyaline cartilage of multiple joints, frequently bilateral and symmetric. Characteristically, this calcification is often seen at the knees, the wrist, and the symphysis pubis. The synovial lining and capsule of joints and less commonly extra-articular structures such as tendons and bursae may also sometimes calcify.

Articular chondrocalcinosis in pseudogout is frequently accompanied by degenerative arthropathy. The arthropathy consists of narrowing of the cartilage, subchondral sclerosis, osteophytosis, and presence of sub-

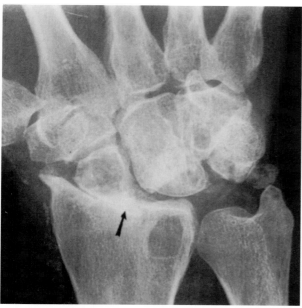

Figure 4–11. Calcium pyrophosphate crystal deposition disease (CPPD). In this patient, the changes of pyrophosphate arthropathy include narrowing of the radiocarpal joint with collapse of the scaphoid into the radial articular surface (*arrow*) as well as the presence of numerous subchondral cystic lesions. Calcification of the triangular fibrocartilage can also be noted. (From Resnick D, Yu JS, Sartoris D: Imaging. In Kelley WN, Harris ED Jr, Ruddy S, Sledge CB [eds]: Textbook of Rheumatology, 5th ed. Philadelphia, WB Saunders, 1997, p 675.)

chondral cysts (Fig. 4–11). These are all features of osteoarthritis but differing in that cysts are more prominent and the joints involved differ from that of conventional osteoarthritis. Also, the pronounced and often isolated involvement of the patellofemoral compartment, the radiocarpal joint, and the metacarpophalangeal joints is characteristic of pseudogout.

Hydroxyapatite Deposition Disease

Calcific periarthritis or peritendinitis is a crystal deposition disease affecting tendons and bursae. Characteristically the supraspinatus tendon and the subacromial bursa of the shoulder are involved, but other regions may be affected, such as the hips, elbows, and wrists. Generally the calcification is seen radiographically as a periarticular homogeneous deposit with well-defined margins. Absence of involvement of the articular cartilage distinguishes hydroxyapatite deposition disease from calcium pyrophosphate dihydrate crystal deposition disease.

JOINT INFECTION

Septic Arthritis

Joint infection is generally diagnosed clinically. In the early phase, radiography may remain normal, whereas MRI or a radionuclide bone scan may be helpful for early diagnosis. Joint aspiration for microscopy and culture is essential for early diagnosis and treatment. The radiographic appearance depends on the age of the patient, the mechanism of inoculation, the virulence of the organism, the stage of disease, the influence of therapy, the local anatomic features, and the presence of underlying articular disorders. Any joint may be involved, but the spine, hips, and knees are the most common, followed by wrists, ankles, shoulders, and sacroiliac joints.

Infectious arthritis may result from direct hematogenous spread to the synovium, from osteomyelitis adjacent to a joint, or from direct extent by cellulitis. Articular destruction complicating metaphyseal osteomyelitis can occur in adults and infants in whom the subarticular blood supply is continuous with the major nutrient supply to the metaphysis and diaphysis. In children, however, the cartilaginous epiphyseal growth plate acts as an effective barrier to the spread of pyogenic infection from its common site of origin in the metaphysis. An exception is when the metaphysis is located within the joint capsule, such as in the hip, where metaphyseal osteomyelitis frequently leads to septic arthritis. Another exception is osteomyelitis caused by tuberculous or fungal infection, which readily destroys and crosses the epiphyseal plate and leads to septic arthritis.

Pyogenic infection generally involves a single joint except in instances of underlying systemic disease, immunosuppressive therapy, or drug abuse. Pyogenic infection is characterized radiographically by capsular

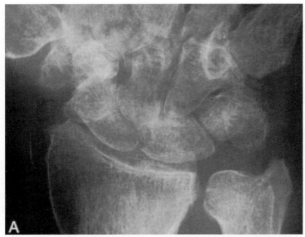

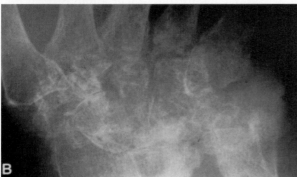

Figure 4–12. Tuberculosis. Note the gradual progression of destructive changes in radiographs obtained 18 months apart. *A,* There is prominent soft tissue swelling and osteoporosis with marginal osseous erosions at multiple sites. *B,* The process has progressed to virtually complete destruction of the carpus. A large erosion of the distal radius is also present. (From Resnick D, Yu JS, Sartoris D: Imaging. In Kelley WN, Harris ED Jr, Ruddy S, Sledge CB [eds]: Textbook of Rheumatology, 5th ed. Philadelphia, WB Saunders, 1997, p 677.)

distention recognizable several days after the onset of symptoms and soon followed by patchy osteoporosis related to hyperemia, cytokine production, and disuse. Initially the joint space may be widened because of effusion, but uniform loss of articular cartilage soon appears from rapid destruction of cartilage by polymorphonuclear leukocyte and synovial cell enzymes. Within a few weeks, diffuse lysis of the subchondral cortex is seen, resulting in an appearance distinct from that of tuberculous arthritis or RA, in which articular erosions are focal and marginal. Later, complete destruction of cartilage and subchondral bone causes fragmentation, reactive sclerosis, and pronounced deformity.

The most common cause of nonpyogenic joint infection is tuberculosis, whereas fungal infections, such as coccidioidomycosis, blastomycosis, actinomycosis, sporotrichosis, and brucellosis, are relatively rare. Tuberculous involvement of joints is characterized radiographically by mild-to-moderate soft-tissue swelling, marginal erosions, and preservation of cartilage. Mixed demineralization and patchy sclerosis are common (Fig. 4–12).

Tuberculosis of the spine is characterized by narrowing of the disc space, end-plate destruction, and large, occasionally calcified paraspinal abscesses. Moderate reactive sclerosis may be seen. The posterior elements are generally spread, whereas adjacent vertebral bodies are frequently involved at several levels. Striking anterior collapse and wedging may result in a characteristic kyphosis. Occasionally, in both tuberculosis and coccidioidomycosis, isolated focal destruction of the anterior surface of the vertebral body may cause a scalloped erosion deep to the anterior longitudinal ligament.

In evaluating septic arthritis, MRI provides more accurate and detailed information regarding the extent of involvement than conventional radiography, CT, and radionuclide studies. It may permit the differentiation

Table 4–2. COST-EFFECTIVE STRTEGIES FOR THE COMMON GENERAL COMPLAINTS AND DISEASE PROCESSES

Hands
  Rule out inflammatory joint disease: *radiography,* posteroanterior and oblique (ballcatcher's view) of both hands
Wrist pain
  Rule out inflammatory disease and ligament or tendon injury: *radiography,* posteroanterior, lateral, and oblique; *MRI,* consider intra-articular contrast injection (MR arthrogram)
Neck pain
  Rule out inflammatory or degenerative disease: *radiography,* anteroposterior and lateral (lateral in flexion and extension); cervical-spine *MRI* without contrast administration
Shoulder pain
  Rule out inflammatory disease: *radiography,* anteroposterior in internal rotation, Grashey view in external rotation, axillary view; *MRI* of the shoulder without contrast administration
Lumbar-spine pain
  Rule out osteoporotic fractures, degenerative changes or disc herniation: *radiography,* anteroposterior and lateral; *MRI* of the lumbar spine without contrast administration. Use intravenous contrast material if question is reherniation versus fibrosis.
Sacroiliac-joint pain
  Rule out sacroiliitis: *radiography,* angled anteroposterior (replacing oblique views)
Hip pain
  Rule out inflammatory or degenerative disease, avascular necrosis, *radiography,* anteroposterior or stress fracture: and frog-leg lateral; hip *MRI,* unilaterally (bilaterally if to rule out avascular necrosis), no contrast administration
Knee pain
  Rule out inflammatory or degenerative disease: *radiography,* anteroposterior, lateral, tunnel, and skyline views (with patient weight bearing); knee *MRI* to rule out meniscal tear and other soft tissue pathology
Foot and ankle pain
  Rule out inflammatory or degenerative disease, stress fracture: *radiography,* anteroposterior, lateral oblique (with patient weight bearing); *MRI* of the foot or ankle without contrast administration
Acute joint pain and signs of infection
  Rule out infection: *radiography* or *bone scintigraphy* to evaluate bony structures; *MRI* to evaluate bone and soft tissue structures; if joint may be infected, aspirate as soon as possible for Gram stain and culture

MRI, magnetic resonance imaging.

of septic arthritis from osteomyelitis and demonstrate joint effusion, abscess formation, loss of cartilage, and lysis of subchondral bone.

Summary

The variety and cost of imaging for musculoskeletal diseases are great. For that reason, it must be re-emphasized that the radiologist should be used as a consultant for the primary care physician to suggest the modality that is appropriate for the specific bone, joint, or extra-articular symptoms and signs. Table 4–2 provides some useful strategies for these issues. Although the primary care physician will often want to work with subspecialists (e.g., rheumatologists or orthopaedic surgeons) in choosing a specific image for a given patient, these strategies can be used as guidelines.

REFERENCES

1. Resnick D (ed): Diagnosis of Bone and Joint Disorders, 3rd ed. Philadelphia, WB Saunders, 1994.
2. Brower A: Arthritis in Black and White, 2nd ed. Philadelphia, WB Saunders, 1996.
3. Atlas S: MR of the Brain and Spine. Philadelphia, Lippincott-Raven, 1998.
4. Jacobson JA, van Holsbeeck MT: Musculoskeletal ultrasonography. Orthop Clin North Am. 29: 135–167, 1998.
5. Ficat RP, Arlet J: Imaging in avascular necrosis of bone. In Hungerford DS (ed): Ischemia and Necrosis of Bone. Baltimore, Williams & Wilkins, 1989, pp 85–91.

Chapter **5**

Laboratory Testing for Musculoskeletal Diseases

Christopher F. Snow

Musculoskeletal disorders are among the most common conditions encountered by the primary physician. In most instances, the use of laboratory testing in the evaluation of these complaints is unnecessary. Testing is most helpful when the physician has a working diagnosis and wishes to test a specific hypothesis. The type of testing chosen depends on the hypothesis. When gout is suspected, synovial fluid analysis is important. If ankylosing spondylitis is a diagnostic consideration, radiologic evaluation is especially useful. The appropriate and cost-effective use of blood tests in the evaluation of rheumatologic complaints is the primary focus of this chapter.

GENERAL PRINCIPLES OF LABORATORY TEST INTERPRETATION

Test Characteristics

Each laboratory test has *performance characteristics. Sensitivity* refers to the percentage of patients with the disease in whom the test is positive. The *false-negative rate* is 100% minus the sensitivity. Using rheumatoid arthritis (RA) as an example, about 80% of patients are positive for rheumatoid factor (RF). Therefore, the sensitivity of RF for the diagnosis of RA is 80%, and the false-negative rate is 20%. *Specificity* refers to the percentage of patients without the disease in whom the test is negative. The *false-positive rate* is 100% minus the specificity. The specificity of RF for the diagnosis of RA in patients with polyarthritis is greater than 90% (10% false-positive rate).

Sensitivity and specificity, although thought of as intrinsic characteristics of a laboratory test, are affected by the clinical setting in which the test is performed. For example, only about one third of RA patients seroconvert in the first 3 months of illness. Therefore, for the primary care physician, who is likely to see an RA patient early in the course of the disease, the sensitivity of RF is lower than for a rheumatologist, who is likely to encounter the patient at a later stage of illness. Similarly the specificity of RF is lower in the hospital setting than among outpatients because hospitalized patients are more likely to have other conditions associated with a false-positive RF. Sensitivity and specificity also vary depending on the definition of the normal range. A wider normal range increases specificity at the cost of sensitivity (i.e., increases false-negative rates and reduces false-positive rates).

Pretest and Post-Test Probabilities, Predictive Value, Bayes' Theorem

The *pretest probability* refers to the likelihood based on clinical and demographic criteria that the person being tested has the disease in question. For the general population, the pretest probability (or prevalence) of RA is about 1%. The *positive predictive value* is the probability that, given a positive test result, the patient has the disease. The *negative predictive value* is the probability that, given a negative test result, the patient does not have the disease. The *post-test probability* is the probability of the disease after the results of the test are known. *Bayes' theorem* is an algebraic formulation of the principle that the post-test probability of a disease depends on both the pretest probability and the performance characteristics of the test. The results of Table 5–1 were calculated using Bayes' theorem and illustrate how the post-test probability of a diagnosis of RA is affected by varying pretest probabilities.

Guidelines for Appropriate Laboratory Testing

Before ordering laboratory tests, the clinician should keep in mind the following guidelines:

1. Laboratory tests should not be ordered in lieu of an appropriate history and physical examination.

2. Laboratory tests should be ordered only if the result is likely to affect patient management in some way.

3. Diagnostic testing is most likely to be useful in situations in which the pretest probability of disease is in the intermediate range (see Table 5–1).

4. Unless the time element is crucial, physicians should avoid ordering multiple laboratory tests at one

Table 5–1. EFFECT OF RHEUMATOID FACTOR TESTING ON THE PROBABILITY OF RHEUMATOID ARTHRITIS*

Pretest Probability of RA (%)	RF Test Result	Post-Test Probability of RA (%)
1	(−)	0.3
	(+)	33.1
30	(−)	9.7
	(+)	95.5
60	(−)	27.3
	(+)	98.7
90	(−)	69.2
	(+)	99.7

*Assumes test sensitivity of 80% and specificity of 98%. RA, rheumatoid arthritis; RF, rheumatoid factor.

time because this practice increases the likelihood of false-positive results (Table 5–2).

LABORATORY TESTING IN RHEUMATOLOGY

Several factors are of particular importance in reference to laboratory testing for rheumatologic disorders.

Importance of Titer

Many rheumatologic tests are reported in a quantitative fashion using a serum dilution titer. In general, the higher the titer, the lower the false-positive rate of the test. For example, one study in which RA patients were compared to patients with other inflammatory rheumatic disorders found the RF to have a false-positive rate of 6% at a titer of 1:160 but only 1% at a titer of 1:1280.[1]

"Cross-Reacting" of Laboratory Tests

A particular problem in the evaluation of rheumatologic disorders is that a laboratory test ordered to evaluate the possibility of one disease is often positive in distinct diseases that may present with similar

Table 5–2. RELATIONSHIP OF FALSE-POSITIVE TESTS TO NUMBER OF TESTS ORDERED*

No. of Tests	Probability of at Least One False-Positive Result (%)
1	5
3	14
5	23
7	30

*Assumes 5% false-positive rate for a single test and that test results are independent of one another.

symptoms. For example, both RA and systemic lupus erythematosus (SLE) may present with a symmetric polyarthritis. Antinuclear antibody (ANA) testing, ostensibly ordered to evaluate a possible diagnosis of SLE, is positive in 30% or more of RA patients, resulting in a lowering of the positive predictive value of ANA testing for the diagnosis of SLE.

Measurement Error

Rheumatologic tests are often technically difficult to perform, increasing the chance of interlaboratory variability in test accuracy. In one study, two university immunology laboratories differed in their classification of duplicate serum samples as normal or abnormal in 11% of cases for ANA testing, in 15% of cases for DNA binding testing, and in 27% of cases for serum complement (C3) testing.[2]

USE OF LABORATORY TESTING IN THE EVALUATION OF COMMON CLINICAL SYNDROMES

Nonarticular Pain and Muscle Weakness

A variety of disorders may present with nonarticular musculoskeletal pain with or without weakness (Table 5–3). For anatomically localized symptoms, blood tests usually are not helpful; an exception may be in the investigation of unexplained neuropathies. Patients with more generalized nonarticular musculoskeletal complaints inevitably require a comprehensive clinical evaluation. Some patients, such as those meeting clinical criteria for fibromyalgia, may need no further testing. Often, however, laboratory testing may be indicated. Ideally, specific clinical symptoms and signs should prompt specific laboratory testing (Table 5–4). More detailed information regarding selected laboratory tests used in the diagnosis of nonarticular rheumatologic disorders is summarized in Table 5–5.

When specific diagnostic clues are lacking, further direction may be obtained from commonly ordered laboratory tests, including the complete blood count and blood chemistries. For example, in the patient with muscle pain, the presence of eosinophilia may suggest the possibility of trichinosis. Because many patients with polymyalgia rheumatica and thyroid dysfunction have subtle or nonspecific symptoms, it is not unreasonable to order an erythrocyte sedimentation rate (ESR) and thyroid-stimulating hormone test even when classic symptoms and signs are lacking (see Table 5–4).

Noninflammatory Articular Disorders

Usually the common noninflammatory articular disorders (Table 5–6) are diagnosed clinically and by

Table 5–3. DISORDERS THAT OFTEN PRESENT WITH NONARTICULAR PAIN, MUSCLE WEAKNESS, OR BOTH*

Localized Symptoms

Fracture, soft tissue injury
Tendinitis, bursitis
Regional myofascial pain syndromes
Entrapment syndromes and radiculopathies
Reflex sympathetic dystrophy
Other neuropathic syndromes

More Generalized Symptoms

Fibromyalgia
Somatization disorder
Polymyalgia rheumatica
Endocrine disorders
 Hypothyroidism and hyperthyroidism
 Adrenal insufficiency
 Cushing's disease
 Hyperparathyroidism
Chronic fatigue syndrome
Myositis and other muscle disorders
 Polymyositis
 Dermatomyositis
 Drug-induced myositis
 Myasthenia gravis
 Toxic myopathies
 Alcohol
 Glucocorticoids
 Others
Inherited disorders of muscle
Infections

 HIV
 Trichinosis
 Others

*For suspicion of disorders listed in italic type, laboratory testing may be useful. HIV, human immunodeficiency virus.

Table 5–4. EXAMPLES OF LABORATORY TESTING BASED ON CLINICAL CLUES IN PATIENTS WITH NONARTICULAR MUSCULOSKELETAL DISORDERS

Symptoms and Signs	Possible Diagnosis	Tests to Consider
Shoulder girdle pain, headache onset after age 50	PMR/temporal arteritis	ESR
Cold or heat intolerance, menorrhagia, delayed relaxation of deep tendon reflexes, tremor, goiter	Hypothyroidism or hyperthyroidism	TSH
Proximal muscle weakness	Myositis, hyperthyroidism, PMR	Creatine kinase, aldolase, TSH, ESR
Thrush, multiple sexual partners, intravenous drug use	HIV infection	HIV antibody
Recent steroid use, nausea, hyperpigmentation, hypotension	Adrenal insufficiency	ACTH stimulation test
Cushingoid body habitus, striae, hypertension	Cushing's syndrome	Overnight dexamethasone suppression test

PMR, polymyalgia rheumatica; ESR, erythrocyte sedimentation rate; TSH, thyroid-stimulating hormone; HIV, human immunodeficiency virus; ACTH, adrenocorticotropic hormone.

Table 5–5. SELECTED LABORATORY TESTS USED IN THE DIAGNOSIS OF NONARTICULAR DISORDERS

Possible Diagnosis	Test	Performance Characteristics	Comments
PMR/ temporal arteritis	ESR	Sensitivity for PMR approximately 80%.[3] Rarely normal in temporal arteritis unless prior steroid therapy	Use of Westergren method is preferred. Formula for upper limit of normal = age/2 (males), (age + 10)/2 (females)[4]
Myositis	CK	Relatively specific for cardiac or skeletal muscle source. Elevated in 95% of polymyositis/dermatomyositis patients at some point but less sensitive at onset of symptoms.[5] Elevated in up to 90% of hypothyroid patients	Typically the first test ordered in cases of suspected myositis. An algorithm using CK, CK-MB, and AST levels to distinguish among chronic myopathies has been proposed[6]
Myositis	Aldolase	Present not only in muscle cells, but also in hepatocytes and erythrocytes. Comparably sensitive to CK and more sensitive than transaminases in inflammatory myopathies[5]	Less specific than CK for myositis; no need to order this test if CK elevated. May occasionally be elevated in inflammatory myopathies when CK is normal
Myositis	Anti Jo-1	An antibody directed against tRNA histydyl synthetase. Occurs in up to 30%–40% of patients with inflammatory myopathies. Highly specific for inflammatory myositis	Presence correlates with subgroup of inflammatory myopathies associated with interstitial lung disease and aggressive course.[7] More appropriately used by rheumatologists than by primary care physicians

PMR, polymyalgia rheumatica; ESR, erythrocyte sedimentation rate; CK, creatine kinase; AST, aspartate aminotransferase.

Table 5–6. DISORDERS THAT OFTEN PRESENT WITH NONINFLAMMATORY ARTICULAR PAIN*

Common

Osteoarthritis
Mechanical back pain
Joint injury
Osteonecrosis

Uncommon

Hemarthrosis
Charcot (neuropathic) arthropathy
Metabolic arthropathies
   Hemochromatosis
   Acromegaly
   Hypothyroidism
   Hyperparathyroidism
Tumors

*For suspicion of disorders listed in italic type, laboratory testing may be useful.

Table 5–8. DISORDERS THAT OFTEN PRESENT WITH INFLAMMATORY MONOARTHRITIS OR OLIGOARTHRITIS*

Bacterial arthritis (including gonococcal arthritis)
Crystalline arthritis
   Gout
   Pseudogout
   Hydroxyapatite arthritis and periarthritis
Lyme arthritis
Viral arthritis
   HIV
   Herpesviruses
   Others
Tuberculous arthritis
Fungal arthritis
Spondyloarthropathies
   Psoriatic arthritis
   Reiter's syndrome
   Other reactive arthritides
   Inflammatory bowel disease
   Ankylosing spondylitis
   Palindromic rheumatism

*Synovial fluid analysis is often required for accurate diagnosis. Joint fluid white blood cell counts >50,000/mm³ are found essentially only in bacterial arthritis, gout, or severe rheumatoid arthritis. For disorders listed in italic type, other laboratory testing may also be useful. HIV, human immunodeficiency virus.

radiographic techniques rather than by the use of laboratory testing. However, it may not always be easy to distinguish noninflammatory articular disorders from mild inflammatory articular disorders. The findings on the joint examination and the presence of historical clues, such as prolonged morning stiffness, are important in this regard. If an effusion is present, the presence of less than 2000 white blood cells/mm³ (<75% polymorphonuclear forms) in synovial fluid suggests a noninflammatory disorder. In the absence of other evidence, it is questionable whether the common practice of ordering an ESR to rule out inflammation is worthwhile because there is a considerable overlap in ESR values between inflammatory and noninflammatory disorders. For example, about 15% of women with osteoarthritis have an ESR of at least 30 mm/hour,[8] whereas subjects with mild RA may have a

Table 5–7. C-REACTIVE PROTEIN MEASUREMENT COMPARED TO ERYTHROCYTE SEDIMENTATION RATE MEASUREMENT

	CRP	ESR
Measurement of the acute-phase response	Direct indicator	Indirect indicator
Affected by blood parameters* unrelated to inflammation	No	Yes
Affected by age, sex	No	Yes
Rate of rise and fall as related to changes in clinical evidence of inflammation	Rapid	Slow
Accurate quantitation in the higher range	Yes	No
Cost	Moderate	Low

*Hemoglobin level, erythrocyte shape, presence of monoclonal immunoglobulins or elevated lipoproteins. CRP, C-reactive protein; ESR, erythrocyte sedimentation rate.

Table 5–9. EXAMPLES OF TESTING (OTHER THAN SYNOVIAL FLUID ANALYSIS) BASED ON CLINICAL CLUES IN PATIENTS WITH MONOARTHRITIS AND OLIGOARTHRITIS

Clinical Clues	Diagnosis	Tests
Tenosynovitis, pustular skin lesions, history of sexually transmitted diseases	Gonococcal arthritis	Cultures of extra-articular sites
Erythema chronicum migrans, history of tick bite	Lyme disease	Serology* for antibodies to *Borrelia burgdorferi*. Western blot (if ELISA indeterminate)
Conjunctivitis, urethritis, balanitis, heel pain	Reiter's syndrome	Urethral culture and/or serologies for *Chlamydia* species
Indolent arthritis, primary focus elsewhere	Tuberculous arthritis	PPD, synovial biopsy
Diarrhea, rectal bleeding, systemic symptoms	Inflammatory bowel disease	Colonoscopy/biopsy
History of intravenous drug use or high-risk sexual activity	HIV infection, hepatitis, gonococcal arthritis	HIV antibody, hepatitis B, C, cultures of extra-articular sites

*Enzyme-linked immunosorbent assay (ELISA). PPD, purified protein derivative; HIV, human immunodeficiency virus.

normal ESR. Although C-reactive protein (CRP) has several advantages when compared to the ESR as an indicator of inflammation (Table 5–7), its use in the detection of subclinical inflammatory arthritis has not been validated. Among RA patients, the finding of an elevated CRP and a normal ESR is a more likely finding than the converse.[9] In contrast, patients with chronic liver disease or the nephrotic syndrome who have little systemic inflammation but abnormal serum proteins are likely to have an elevated ESR and a normal CRP.

Inflammatory Monoarthritis and Oligoarthritis (Fewer than Three Joints Involved)

In patients presenting with inflammatory arthritis involving one or a few joints, the principal diagnostic considerations are the crystalline and infective arthritides (Table 5–8). Consequently a strong argument can be made for performing arthrocentesis in all patients as the initial diagnostic maneuver.[10] In acute cases, joint fluid analysis must always include a cell count, Gram stain, and bacterial culture. This is true even if crystals are present because septic arthritis and gout can co-exist.

As a practical matter, some primary care physicians and rheumatologists may forego arthrocentesis when there is a strong clinical suspicion of gout.[11] This approach is supported by data suggesting that certain clinical criteria (a history of attacks that begin abruptly and remit within 2 weeks, a single episode of podagra, presence of a suspected tophus) have high specificity for the diagnosis of gout.[12] Arthrocentesis is required in cases of possible infection and when consideration is given to committing patients to long-term therapy with allopurinol or probenecid.

Radiologic testing is rarely helpful in the evaluation of acute inflammatory monoarthritis and oligoarthritis. When arthrocentesis is nondiagnostic or other specific clinical clues are present, other testing may be appropriate (Table 5–9). Specific information regarding selected tests used in the laboratory evaluation of monoarthritis and oligoarthritis is summarized in Table 5–10.

Inflammatory Polyarthritis (More than Three Joints Involved)

Among disorders usually considered as likely causes of inflammatory polyarthritis, blood testing is often of value as an adjunct to a careful clinical evaluation

Table 5–10. SELECTED LABORATORY TESTS USED IN THE DIAGNOSIS OF MONOARTHRITIS AND OLIGOARTHRITIS

Possible Diagnosis	Test	Performance Characteristics	Comments
Gout	Serum uric acid	Among a group of patients with various arthritides, serum uric acid of >7% (male) and >6% (female) was 55% sensitive and 93% specific for gout[12]	Of little value in diagnosis because of high false-positive and false-negative rates. May be used in monitoring response to therapy
Gout	24-hour urine for uric acid		May be indicated if use of probenecid is considered
Nongonococcal bacterial arthritis	Blood cultures	Positive in about 50% of cases. If positive, may confer worse prognosis[13]	Although the standard of practice is to obtain blood cultures, the results rarely affect management because the causative organism should be recoverable from joint fluid
Tuberculous arthritis	PPD	Sensitivity 50%–75%	Should not be used to rule out tuberculous arthritis. Synovial biopsy may be needed to confirm diagnosis
Lyme arthritis	ELISA for antibodies to *B. burgdorferi*	Low sensitivity during early stages of disease, but highly sensitive when frank arthritis is present.[14] A positive serology may reflect past or asymptomatic infection with *B. burgdorferi* or may relate to cross-reactive antibodies associated with autoimmune diseases or from infection with other agents[15]	Test is poorly standardized and often leads to overdiagnosis in patients with vague and nonspecific symptoms. Most useful if pretest probability of disease between 20% and 80%.[15] Western blot recommended if ELISA is indeterminate[15]
Gonococcal arthritis	Culture of extra-articular sites for gonorrhea	Sensitivities:[16, 17] Endocervical, 57%–90%; urethral (men), 50%–75%; blood, 10%–30%; skin lesions, 28%; pharynx, 5%	These cultures are important because in gonococcal arthritis genitourinary culture yield is higher than synovial fluid Gram stain or culture yield
Reiter's syndrome	Urethral culture or serologies for *Chlamydia* species	More than half of patients have serologic evidence of chlamydial infection, and 16% have a positive urethral chlamydial culture.[18] Antibiotic therapy may be indicated if evidence of recent infection exists	It is reasonable in suspected cases to test for IGM and IgA antibodies (only high titers are relevant)[19] to chlamydial species and to culture patients with current or recent symptoms of urethritis

PPD, purified protein derivative; ELISA, enzyme-linked immunosorbent assay.

Table 5–11. DISORDERS THAT MAY PRESENT WITH INFLAMMATORY POLYARTHRITIS*

Rheumatoid arthritis
Systemic lupus erythematosus
   Idiopathic
   Drug-induced
Arthritis associated with other collagen vascular diseases
   Progressive systemic sclerosis
   Polymyositis/dermatomyositis (see Tables 5–4, 5–5)
   Mixed connective tissue disease
   Polyarteritis nodosa
   Others, including the seronegative spondyloarthropathies
     (psoriatic arthritis, Reiter's syndrome, ankylosing spondylitis)
Acute rheumatic fever
Viral arthritis
   Parvovirus B-19
   Hepatitis B, C
   Rubella
   Others

*For suspicion of diagnoses in italic type, laboratory testing may be useful.

(Table 5–11). Synovial fluid analysis is less important in this setting than in the evaluation of the patient with monoarthritis, but it must be recognized that both crystalline and infective arthritides may present with polyarticular involvement. Joint aspiration is mandatory in suspected polyarticular septic arthritis; clinical clues include the presence of known RA or immunosuppression, fever, leukocytosis, or infected skin lesions.[20] As always, it is best to order laboratory tests only after specific clinical clues have increased the pretest probability of disease (Table 5–12).

In the evaluation of systemic inflammatory disorders, primary physicians find the use of ANA testing to be especially confusing. Although the ANA is highly sensitive for the diagnosis of SLE, its specificity is poor (see Table 5–14). In one retrospective review from a large teaching hospital, the positive predictive value of the ANA test was only 11% for SLE and 11% for other rheumatic diseases.[21] Adding to the confusion caused by the poor specificity of ANA testing is the issue of fluorescence pattern interpretation. More than 30 antigenic specificities for ANA have been identified; depending on the antigens involved, the fluorescence pattern varies. The patterns (eg., speckled, nucleolar diffuse/homogeneous, peripheral/rim, anticentromere) are not so sensitive or specific that the presence of a given autoantibody can be ruled in or ruled out according to the pattern reported. The most that can be said is that the finding of a positive ANA in a homogeneous (diffuse) pattern at low titer is less likely to denote significant disease than a positive ANA at high titer or with an inho-

Table 5–12. CLINICAL CLUES IN PATIENTS WITH INFLAMMATORY POLYARTHRITIS THAT MAY INDICATE THE USE OF SPECIFIC LABORATORY TESTING

Clues	Possible Diagnosis	Tests to Be Considered*
Symmetric involvement, often including hands, wrists, knees, feet. Onset age 35–50	Rheumatoid arthritis	Rheumatoid factor

Multisystem disorder (90% of cases in women) involving joints, skin, serosal surfaces, kidney, central nervous system	Idiopathic SLE	ANA
		If ANA positive:
		  Antibodies to double-stranded DNA (anti-ds DNA)
		  Antibodies to extractable nuclear antigens (anti-ENA)

Fever and joint pain in a patient taking procainamide, hydralazine, isoniazid, or certain other drugs	Drug-induced SLE	ANA If ANA positive: Antihistone antibodies; anti-ds DNA

Sclerodactyly, Raynaud's phenomenon, esophageal dysmotility	Progressive systemic sclerosis or mixed connective tissue disease	ANA
		If ANA positive:
		  Antiribonucleoprotein (anti-U1 RNP)
		  Anti–topoisomerase 1; Anticentromere

Asymmetric involvement, often of large joints. Evidence of carditis, chorea, erythema marginatum, subcutaneous nodules	Acute rheumatic fever	Throat culture ASO
		  If ASO titer low or borderline:
		  Anti–deoxyribonuclease B (anti-DNAase-B)

Symmetric large and small joint involvement. Lymphadenopathy	Arthritis due to parvovirus B-19 or adult-onset Still's disease	IgM antibody to B-19 Serum ferritin
Abnormal liver function tests, anorexia, malaise	Hepatitis B, hepatitis C	Hepatitis B surface antigen; Antibody to hepatitis C virus
Urticarial or maculopapular rash	Hepatitis B, rubella	Hepatitis B surface antigen; rubella titers

*In many of these clinical scenarios, other less specific laboratory tests are often ordered, including an erythrocyte sedimentation rate (ESR) or C-reactive protein (CRP), a complete blood count, and blood chemistries. The role of the ESR or CRP in ruling out or in following the course of these disorders has not been well-defined. SLE, systemic lupus erythematosus; ANA, antinuclear antibodies; ASO, antistreptolysin O.

Table 5–13. IMPORTANT AUTOANTIBODIES IN RHEUMATOLOGIC DISEASES

Autoantibodies	Clinical Associations	Comments
Antibodies to double-stranded DNA (anti-DS DNA)	Present in about 60%–70% of active SLE patients and in about 20% of inactive SLE patients. Highly specific for idiopathic SLE. Absent in drug-induced SLE	Presence and titer can correlate with renal disease activity in SLE. Tests for single-stranded DNA are nonspecific and should not be ordered
Antibodies to extractable nuclear antigens (anti-ENA) Antiribonucleoprotein (Anti-U1 RNP)	Present in 35%–40% of SLE patients, usually, in conjunction with anti-Sm. Mixed connective tissue disease defined in part by presence of high-titer anti-U1 RNP and absence of anti-Sm	In SLE patients, presence is associated with relatively mild disease and low prevalence of nephritis[22]
Anti-Sm (Smith)	Present in about 25% of SLE patients, with wide racial disparity (more common in African-Americans and Asians than in whites)[23] Highly specific for SLE	Should not be confused with test for antibodies to smooth muscle
Anti-histone	Present in 95% of drug-induced SLE and in 50% of idiopathic SLE. May be present in RA or juvenile RA.	Can be used to help rule out drug-induced SLE, if absent
Anti-Ro (SSA)	Present in about 40% of SLE patients, in one third of antinuclear antibody–negative SLE patients, in 60% of primary Sjögren's patients, and in 1% of healthy controls	Because of association with neonatal lupus and congenital complete heart block, healthy pregnant women with a prior history of these problems and all pregnant SLE patients should be tested
Anti-La (SSB)	Present in 50% of primary Sjögren's patients and in 15% of SLE patients	Generally of little diagnostic value, although anti-Ro and anti-La can have adjunctive utility in the diagnosis of Sjögren's syndrome
Antiphospholipid antibodies Elevated aPTT Anticardiolipin antibody Dilute Russel Viper Venom Time	Associated with coagulopathy, thrombocytopenia, recurrent fetal loss, livedo reticularis	Appropriate to order in patients with unexplained cerebrovascular events and in women with recurrent miscarriages
Anti-topoisomerase 1 (Anti-ScL-70)	Present in 30% of patients with PSS. Highly specific for PSS	Can be predictive of worse outcome in patients with PSS
Anticentromere	Present in 80%–90% of patients with CREST variant of PSS, in 30% of patients with PSS, and in 25% of patients with idiopathic Raynaud's syndrome	Whether presence in patients with Raynaud's syndrome suggests that CREST will develop is unclear

SLE, systemic lupus erythematosus; RA, rheumatoid arthritis; PSS, progressive systemic sclerosis.

Table 5–14. SELECTED LABORATORY TESTS USED IN THE DIAGNOSIS OF INFLAMMATORY POLYARTHRITIS

Possible Diagnosis	Test	Performance Characteristics	Comments
RA	Rheumatoid factor	Sensitivity about 80%; sensitivity at presentation 50%; positive predictive value 24%.[24] High titers correlate with more erosive disease and extra-articular features. Often positive in other collagen vascular diseases (especially Sjögren's syndrome, MCTD, cryoglobulinemia) and in other disorders (pulmonary fibrosis, biliary cirrhosis). Positive in 1% of normal adults, although this figure rises with age	Presence neither sufficient nor necessary for diagnosis. Most useful in cases in which suspicion of RA is neither very low nor very high (see Table 5–1). Not useful to reorder in patients known to be seropositive. No established diagnostic utility for disorders other than RA[24]
SLE	ANA	Sensitivity >95% (idiopathic SLE). By definition, sensitivity is 100% for drug-induced SLE. Positive in 75% of Sjögren's, 50% of PSS, and 15%–35% of RA patients. Positive in 1%–45% of healthy blood donors, depending on age and titer.[25] Active SLE likely to be associated with high titer	Should not be used to screen for collagen vascular disease when diagnostic suspicion low or to monitor disease activity in patients with a known collagen vascular disease. Because of autoantibody specificities (see Table 5–13), it is useful to order an ANA in suspected cases of PSS, CREST, and MCTD
SLE	LE preparation	Present in 50%–75% of patients with SLE. Nonspecific	Tedious to perform. Of historical interest only
SLE Other disorders	Serum complement (CH$_{50}$, C3, C4)	Poor sensitivity and specificity for any rheumatic disease. Low values may be caused by malnutrition or hepatic dysfunction. May increase as an acute-phase reactant in inflammatory conditions	In general, of no use to the primary care physician in the evaluation of rheumatologic disease. May be useful to the rheumatologist in monitoring SLE nephritis activity or in diagnosis of certain types of vasculitis
Acute rheumatic fever	Throat culture	Sensitivity <25%.[26] Positive culture may indicate coincidental pharyngeal carriage of streptococci	Inexpensive. Reasonable to order in suspected cases despite insensitivity
Acute rheumatic fever	ASO titer	Sensitivity 80%. Elevated titer may reflect coincidental streptococcal infection	Titer rises and falls more rapidly than anti-DNAase B
Acute rheumatic fever	Anti-DNAase B	If titer is low in conjunction with low ASO titers, diagnosis of acute rheumatic fever is unlikely	Should be ordered if strong clinical suspicion and ASO titer borderline or low[27]
Parvovirus B19–associated arthritis	IgM antibody to B19	Usually present by the time arthritis develops. Undetectable by 2–3 mo after onset of illness[28]	When clinically suspected testing can be useful

RA, rheumatoid arthritis; MCTD, mixed connective tissue disease; SLE, systemic lupus erythematosus; PSS, progressive systemic sclerosis; ANA, antinuclear antibody; ASO, antistreptolysin O.

mogeneous fluorescence pattern. Specific autoantibodies of interest to the primary physician are listed in Table 5–13. In general, there is no point in ordering these expensive tests unless the initial ANA test is positive. Exceptions are anti-Ro antibodies, which are present in about one third of ANA-negative patients with SLE, and antiphospholipid antibodies. Further information about the ANA test and other tests used in the evaluation of inflammatory polyarthritis is given in Table 5–14.

Table 5–15. OTHER LABORATORY TESTS USED IN THE EVALUATION OF RHEUMATOLOGIC DISORDERS

Disorder	Test	Performance Characteristics	Comments
Mixed cryoglobulinemia	Serum cryoglobulins	Titer (cryocrit) correlates poorly with symptoms and prognosis	Reasonable to order in patients with palpable purpura (histologic leukocytoclastic vasculitis), unexplained digital gangrene, nephritis or nephrosis of unknown cause. Presence often associated with hepatitis C infection
Ankylosing spondylitis	HLA-B27	Sensitivity 90%. Positive in 50%–80% of Reiter's patients. Positive in 6%–10% of normal whites in North America	Use should be avoided because of poor specificity and use of clinical and radiographic criteria for the diagnosis of AS
Wegener's granulomatosis	c-ANCA	Sensitivity in active generalized disease >90%. If disease localized or inactive, sensitivity lower. Specificity about 95%	Because of risks associated with therapy, use as a substitute for a tissue diagnosis should be avoided. Possibly useful in monitoring disease activity
Other vasculitides	p-ANCA	Sensitivity and specificity generally poor. Present in other collagen vascular diseases, nephritis, inflammatory bowel disease, some infections	Of little diagnostic utility

OTHER LABORATORY TESTS

Other laboratory tests used in the diagnosis of rheumatologic disorders with which the primary care physician should be familiar are listed in Table 5–15.

REFERENCES

1. Wolfe F, Cathey MA, Roberts FK: The latex test revisited: Rheumatoid factor testing in 8,287 rheumatic disease patients. Arthritis Rheum 34:951, 1991.
2. Feigenbaum PA, Medsger TA, Kraines RG, et al: The variability of immunologic laboratory tests. J Rheumatol 9:408, 1982.
3. Helfgott SM, Kieval RI: Polymyalgia rheumatica in patients with a normal erythrocyte sedimentation rate. Arthritis Rheum 39:304, 1996.
4. Miller A, Green M, Robinson D: Simple rule for calculating normal erythrocyte sedimentation rate. BMJ 286:266, 1983.
5. Tymms KE, Webb J: Dermatopolymyositis and other connective tissue diseases: A review of 105 cases. J Rheumatol 12:1140, 1985.
6. Hood D, Van Lente F, Estes M: Serum enzyme alterations in chronic muscle disease: A biopsy-based diagnostic assessment. Am J Clin Pathol 95:402, 1991.
7. Love LA, Leff RL, Fraser DD, et al: A new approach to the classification of idiopathic inflammatory myopathy: Myositis-specific autoantibodies define useful homogenous patient groups. Medicine 70:360, 1991.
8. Rafnsson V, Bengtsson C, Lurie M: Erythrocyte sedimentation rate in women with different manifestations of joint disease. Scand J Rheumatol 11:87, 1982.
9. Amos RS, Constable TJ, Crockson RA, et al: Rheumatoid arthritis: Relation of serum C-reactive protein and erythrocyte sedimentation rates to radiographic changes. BMJ 1:195, 1977.
10. Baker DG, Schumacher HR: Acute monoarthritis. N Engl J Med 329:1013, 1993.
11. Wallace SL, Robinson H, Masi AT, et al: Preliminary criteria for the classification of the acute arthritis of primary gout. Arthritis Rheum 20:895, 1977.
12. Rigby AS, Wood PHN: Serum uric acid levels and gout: What does this herald for the population? Clin Exp Rheumatol 12:395, 1994.
13. Kelly PJ, Martin WJ, Coventry MB: Bacterial (suppurative) arthritis in the adult. J Bone Joint Surg 52:1595, 1970.
14. Craft JE, Grodzicki RL, Steere AC: Antibody response in Lyme disease: Evaluation of diagnostic tests. J Infect Dis 149:789, 1984.
15. Tugwell P, Dennis DT, Weinstein A: Laboratory evaluation in the diagnosis of Lyme disease. Ann Intern Med 127:1109, 1997.
16. Scopelitis E, Pindaro MO: Gonococcal arthritis. Rheum Dis Clin North Am 19:363, 1993.
17. Eisenstein BI, Masi AT: Disseminated gonococcal infection and gonococcal arthritis: I. Bacteriology, epidemiology, host factors, pathogen factors, and pathology. Semin Arthritis Rheum 10:155, 1981.
18. Vilppula AH, Granfors KM, Yli-Kerttula UI: Infectious involvements in males with Reiter's syndrome. Clin Rheumatol 3:443, 1984.
19. Bas S, Cunningham T, Kvien TK, et al: The value of isotope determination of serum antibodies against chlamydia for the diagnosis of chlamydia reactive arthritis. Br J Rheumatol 35:542, 1996.
20. Dubost JJ, Fis I, Denis P, et al: Polyarticular septic arthritis. Medicine 72:296, 1993.
21. Slater CA, Davis RB, Shmerling RH: Antinuclear antibody testing: A study of clinical utility. Arch Intern Med 156:1421, 1996.
22. Reichlin M, Mattioli M: Correlation of a precipitin reaction to an RNA protein antigen and a low prevalence of nephritis in patients with systemic lupus erythematosus. N Engl J Med 286:908, 1972.
23. Field M, Williams DG, Charles P, et al: Specificity of anti-Sm antibodies by ELISA for systemic lupus erythematosus: Increased sensitivity of detection using purified peptide antigens. Ann Rheum Dis 47:820, 1988.
24. Shmerling RH, Delbanco TL: The rheumatoid factor: An analysis of clinical utility. Am J Med 91:529, 1991.
25. Fritzler MJ, Pauls JD, Kinsella D, et al: Antinuclear, anticytoplasmic, and anti-Sjogren's syndrome antigen A (SS-A/RO) antibodies in female blood donors. Clin Immunol Immunopathol 36:120, 1985.
26. Dajani AS, Ayoub EM, Bierman FZ, et al: Guidelines for the diagnosis of rheumatic fever: Jones criteria, updated 1992. JAMA 268:2069, 1992.
27. Dajani AS: Rheumatic fever. In Braunwald E (ed): Heart Disease. Philadelphia, WB Saunders, 1997, p 1769.
28. Ytterberg SR: Viral arthritis. In Koopman WJ (ed): Arthritis and Allied Conditions. Baltimore, Williams & Wilkins, 1997, p 2341.

Chapter **6**

Aspiration and Injection of Joints and Soft Tissue

Mark C. Genovese ■ Ronald F. van Vollenhoven

The *aspiration* of synovial fluid from joints and (rarely) inflamed tendons or bursae fulfills an important role in the diagnosis of rheumatic diseases. Similarly, joint and soft tissue *injections* are important as therapeutic modalities employed to treat a wide range of musculoskeletal diseases. The proper role of these procedures, including the medical situation in which they are properly employed; the choice of the most appropriate instruments, medications, or both; and the potential risks and side effects are sufficiently well defined so that the primary care physician can be equipped to perform these procedures in a wide range of clinical situations and in a time-efficient manner. Although injections are not without potential risks, in the hands of an experienced operator, they can provide needed short-term and long-term benefit for the appropriate condition.

INDICATIONS FOR JOINT ASPIRATION

The evaluation of synovial fluid can be invaluable in arriving at the correct diagnosis in the setting of monoarticular or polyarticular inflammation. In the work-up of acute monoarticular arthritis, in which infection and crystal-induced causes are the leading diagnostic concerns, arthrocentesis is a mandatory diagnostic procedure. Even in the setting of chronic, polyarticular disease, joint fluid analysis can help distinguish between inflammatory diseases (rheumatoid arthritis, Reiter's syndrome), degenerative arthritis, and crystalline arthritis (gout and pseudogout). Synovial fluid should in almost every occasion be sent for cell count with differential, Gram stain and culture, and crystal analysis. The last-mentioned can conveniently be done in the office. Synovial fluid should be sent to the laboratory for a cell count using a tube that prevents clotting. Individual laboratories may express preferences; usually a purple-top tube containing ethylene diaminetetraacetic acid is preferred, but a green-top tube containing heparin should also be acceptable. Testing of synovial fluid for protein, glucose, lactate dehydrogenases, and complement and other chemistry tests have not proven useful in clinical practice. In some difficult cases of polyarthritis with negative serum rheumatoid

factor, a positive synovial fluid rheumatoid factor titer has been diagnostically helpful, but this should not be ordered routinely. Synovial fluid characteristics are listed in Table 6–1.

Occasionally a practitioner may encounter a situation in which no fluid can be aspirated from the joint in question; this is typically known as a *dry tap*. If this situation occurs, it usually necessitates removal of the needle, reorientation of landmarks, repeat antiseptic procedures, and a second arthrocentesis using a larger-gauge needle (sometimes as large as a 16-gauge needle). Failing this, the joint under examination can be lavaged with sterile saline, and the fluid thus obtained can be analyzed for crystals or sent to the laboratory for Gram stain and culture.

INDICATIONS FOR INTRA-ARTICULAR INJECTION

Intra-articular injections are most commonly given for the treatment of inflammatory arthritis, crystalline arthritis, and osteoarthritis. Although systemic inflammatory disorders, such as rheumatoid arthritis, seronegative spondyloarthropathies (Reiter's syndrome, psoriatic arthritis, ankylosing spondylitis), and systemic lupus erythematosus, are treated with systemic agents, it also may be of use to provide local intra-articular injections. Thus, injections are seldom used as a primary treatment modality but rather considered more of an adjuvant therapy to both systemic treatment, such as disease-modifying antirheumatic drugs and nonsteroidal anti-inflammatory drugs, and local treatments, such as hot and cold compresses, rest, splints, exercise, and physical and occupational therapy. In addition to their local effects, injections with glucocorticoids often provide generalized benefits, presumably related to systemic absorption. They are a highly effective means of bridging therapy (temporary use of glucocorticoids while awaiting disease-modifying antirheumatic drugs to take effect) and occasionally are used as solitary therapy in a noninfectious monoarthritis. Injections are commonly used when the systemic disease appears generally controlled, but monoarticular or oligoarticular inflammation remains.

Table 6–1. ANALYSIS OF SYNOVIAL FLUID

	Normal	Noninflammatory	Inflammatory	Septic
Color	Clear	Straw/yellow	Yellow	Variable
Clarity	Transparent	Transparent	Hazy-opaque	Opaque
Viscosity	High	High	Low	Low-high
White blood cells	0–200	200–2000	2000–75,000	>50,000
Neutrophils	Low	Low	Medium-high	High

Injection is also considered for particularly refractory joints that do not appear to be responding to appropriate therapy or when escalation of systemic therapy is contraindicated. In the setting of crystalline arthritis (gout and pseudogout), glucocorticoid injection after aspiration often provides prompt and significant resolution of symptoms while longer-term therapies are implemented. Use of intra-articular glucocorticoids in the setting of osteoarthritis is somewhat more contentious. However, if the joint is stable, without substantial cartilage loss, and there is evidence of inflammation, intra-articular injection may provide substantial relief of pain and swelling. To understand better the landmarks and needle placement, some of the more frequently injected joints (knee, shoulder, wrist, elbow, ankle) are pictured in Figures 6–1 to 6–4.

INDICATIONS FOR EXTRA-ARTICULAR INJECTION

Depot-glucocorticoids (e.g., depot-methylprednisolone) can be injected intramuscularly in an attempt to relieve polyarticular inflammation without resorting to oral preparations or to multiple intra-articular injections. Intramuscular injection can provide benefit for periods lasting days to weeks. More importantly, extra-articular injections can be administered for a number of localized musculoskeletal disorders. The local injection of glucocorticoids into periarticular structures can be especially beneficial when used with other local therapies. Inflammation of tendons, tendon sheaths, or tendon insertions can warrant injection. Sites commonly injected include the rotator cuff, bicipital tendon, and extensor pollicis brevis and abductor pollicis longus of the thumb (for DeQuervain's tenosynovitis). Bursitis is a relatively common affliction, and injections of the subacromial (shoulder) (Fig. 6–5), greater trochanteric (hip), olecranon (elbow), anserine (knee), and prepatellar (knee) bursae are relatively easily performed and frequently produce excellent results. Injection of the epicondyles, medial (golfer's elbow) and lateral (tennis elbow) (Fig. 6–6), can have good results, especially when done in concert with conservative therapy. Injections can also be considered for adhesive capsulitis (frozen shoulder) (see Fig. 6–5), synovial cysts, flexor tenosynovitis (trigger finger), entrapment neuropathies (carpal tunnel syndrome), plantar fasciitis, and myofascial pain syndromes.

PREPARATION FOR INJECTION

Before inserting a needle for arthrocentesis or injection, proper informed consent should be obtained. The site should then be selected and prepared in an appropriate fashion. Although the site need not be draped, the injection itself should be performed using both universal precautions and sterile technique. The site should be cleaned using a povidone-iodine solution,

Figure 6–1. Knee injection, medial approach. The needle is inserted under the patella parallel with the floor and aimed slightly proximally. (From Genovese MC: Joint and soft-tissue injection. A useful adjuvant to systemic and local treatment. Postgrad Med 103:125–134, 1998.)

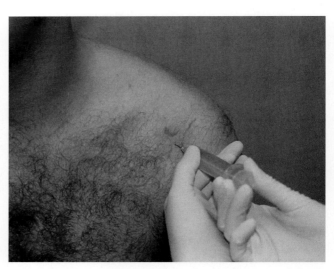

Figure 6–2. Shoulder injection, anterior approach. The arm is externally rotated, and the needle is inserted below and lateral to coracoid process but medial to the head of the humerus. (From Genovese MC: Joint and soft-tissue injection. A useful adjuvant to systemic and local treatment. Postgrad Med 103:125–134, 1998.)

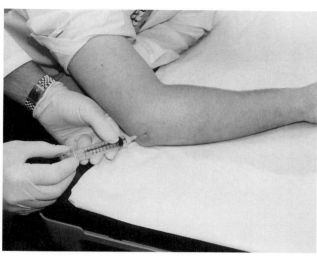

Figure 6–3. Elbow injection. With the elbow bent at 90 degrees, the needle is inserted on the lateral side of the elbow and is directed toward the base of the thumb. (From Genovese MC: Joint and soft-tissue injection. A useful adjuvant to systemic and local treatment. Postgrad Med 103:125–134, 1998.)

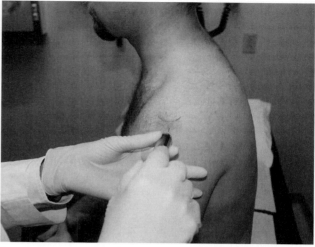

Figure 6–5. Injection of the subacromial bursa. The needle is inserted below the distal tip of the acromion and inserted horizontally. (From Genovese MC: Joint and soft-tissue injection. A useful adjuvant to systemic and local treatment. Postgrad Med 103:125–134, 1998.)

and the antiseptic solution should be allowed to dry. A topical anesthetic, such as ethyl chloride, may be applied if the operator perceives it will lessen the discomfort of the injection or the anxiety of the patient. Commonly, a small quantity of a 1% to 2% lidocaine hydrochloride preparation is injected subcutaneously with a 25- to 27-gauge needle before an intra-articular or extra-articular injection to provide a local anesthetic. Often the glucocorticoid preparation is mixed with a small quantity of 1% to 2% lidocaine. This approach helps to provide temporary analgesia at the time of injection and to dilute the crystalline suspension so that it might better diffuse in the injected structure. Although this is a common practice and we have never encoun-

tered a problem at our institution, many manufacturers recommend against this because of a theoretical risk of clumping and precipitation of steroid crystals.[1]

GLUCOCORTICOID PREPARATIONS FOR INJECTION

Many agents are available for intra-articular and extra-articular injection. The drugs differ based on their potency, solubility, and crystalline structure. Although cortisone was the first agent injected intra-articularly, more potent and less soluble agents are more com-

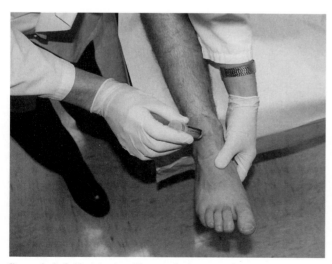

Figure 6–4. Ankle injection. The needle is inserted approximately 2 cm distal to the line connecting the medial and lateral malleoli and just medial to the tendon of the extensor hallucis longus (the patient is asked to raise the big toe); the needle is directed straight posteriorly. (From Genovese MC: Joint and soft-tissue injection. A useful adjuvant to systemic and local treatment. Postgrad Med 103:125–134, 1998.)

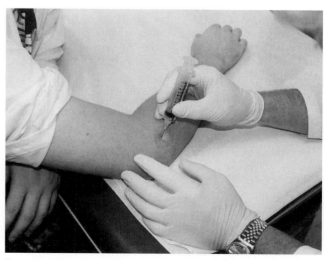

Figure 6–6. Injection of the lateral epicondyle. The needle is inserted into the area of maximal tenderness at the lateral epicondyle. The clinician should not inject directly into the tendon. (From Genovese MC: Joint and soft-tissue injection. A useful adjuvant to systemic and local treatment. Postgrad Med 103:125–134, 1998.)

Table 6–2. GLUCOCORTICOIDS USED FOR JOINT AND SOFT TISSUE INJECTIONS

Glucocorticoid Preparations	Hydrocortisone Equivalents per mg	Concentrations (mg/mL)
Betamethasone sodium phosphate and acetate suspension*	25	6
Dexamethasone sodium phosphate*	25	4
Dexamethasone acetate*	25	8
Triamcinolone acetonide*	5	10, 40
Triamcinolone hexacetonide*	5	20
Methylprednisolone acetate	5	20, 40, 80
Prednisolone tebutate	4	20
Hydrocortisone acetate	1	25

*Fluorinated compounds.

Table 6–4. DOSAGE OF TRIAMCINOLONE HEXACETONIDE TYPICALLY USED PER JOINT

Structure	Dose (mg)	Joint Size	Volume of Injection (mL)
Knee	40	Large	1.0–4.0
Shoulder	30		
Elbow	20–30		
Ankle	20–30	Medium	0.5–1.0
Wrist	20		
Interphalangeal	5–10	Small	0.25–0.5
Metacarpophalangeal	5–10		
Metatarsophalangeal	5–10		
Bursa*	20		0.5–1.5
Tendon sheath*	5–20		0.25–1.0

*Dose of methylprednisolone typically used for soft tissue injection.

monly used today. A list of potential compounds and their relative potencies are compared in Table 6–2. Although few studies have been performed comparing relative efficacies of different agents, the duration of effect is thought to correlate inversely with the solubility of the preparation.[2] The less soluble an agent, the longer it is believed to remain within the joint and, therefore, the more prolonged the effect. Table 6–3 lists relative solubilities. Triamcinolone hexacetonide is believed to be the least soluble and longest acting of the available glucocorticoid preparations.[3] It subsequently has become a favored agent for intra-articular injection. Some practitioners favor other agents, including combination agents that contain short-acting compounds with long-acting suspensions, such as betamethasone sodium phosphate and acetate suspension. Shorter-acting solutions are less likely to precipitate postinjection flare (to be discussed later), whereas longer-acting suspensions have a greater duration of effect.[1] As can be seen based on the agents listed in Table 6–2, preparations are available in different concentrations depending on the dose and volume of suspension the physician wishes to inject. The dose of glucocorticoid used is based on the size of the joint or soft tissue structure; general guidelines for intra-articular injections are given in Table 6–4.

The same properties that make fluorinated, low-solubility agents favored for intra-articular injection make them unacceptable for extra-articular injection. Less soluble agents, such as triamcinolone hexace-tonide, should not be used for soft tissue injection because they are more likely to result in atrophy of surrounding tissues, such as tendons, ligaments, and fascia.[3] Methylprednisolone acetate is a commonly used agent for extra-articular injection.

CONTRAINDICATIONS TO INJECTION

As crucial as arthrocentesis and injection can be in diagnosis and treatment of localized and systemic illness, it is just as crucial to know when not to inject an articular or extra-articular structure. The contraindications to injection are listed in Table 6–5. Should the patient report prior idiosyncratic reaction to the use of lidocaine, it should be avoided during the procedure. In addition to these contraindications, there are also a number of locations in which injection should not be attempted. Injections of the hip and spine should be attempted only by experienced individuals and usually only under fluoroscopic guidance. When performing soft tissue injection, care must be taken never to inject directly into a tendon or ligament. In addition, the area surrounding the Achilles tendon is also rarely injected because of the potential risk of rupture.

EFFICACY OF INJECTIONS

One overriding question prevails when it comes to the use of injections. How well do they work? Efficacy is difficult to establish because it depends

Table 6–3. SOLUBILITY OF GLUCOCORTICOID PREPARATIONS

Intra-Articular Glucocorticoid Preparation	Solubility (% wt/vol)
Dexamethasone sodium phosphate	0.01
Triamcinolone acetonide	0.004
Hydrocortisone acetate	0.002
Methylprednisolone acetate	0.001
Prednisolone tebutate	0.001
Triamcinolone hexacetonide	0.0002

Table 6–5. CONTRAINDICATIONS TO GLUCOCORTICOID INJECTION

Absolute Contraindications
  Infection suspected
  Bacteremia
  Prosthetic joint
  After acute injury/fracture
Relative Contraindications
  Joint instability
  Coagulopathy
  Overlying cellulitis or infection
  Lack of prior efficacy

on many factors, including the structure being injected, the agent being injected, and disease for which it is being used. Intra-articular glucocorticoid injections in rheumatoid arthritis have been shown to be efficacious in a number of studies, and synovitis can be suppressed for periods lasting days to months.[2, 4] Other forms of inflammatory and crystalline arthritis also have been found to respond well to injection. There are no conclusive data, however, on whether glucocorticoids injected intra-articularly retard erosions and ultimately influence progression of disease. The data on efficacy in osteoarthritis have been conflicting. Despite numerous anecdotal and case series reports of benefit, there are only a limited number of controlled studies suggesting either modest or no benefit.[2] It has been suggested that among patients with osteoarthritis, those with greatest benefit are those with clear evidence of effusion and those in whom synovial fluid is aspirated before injection.[5] The majority of studies have shown substantial benefit from soft tissue injections in the treatment of tendinitis and bursitis.[2] To obtain maximal efficacy, glucocorticoid injections should be followed by rest of the affected structure for 24 hours.[6] Given lack of sufficient data, expert opinion and consensus recommend not injecting the same joint or extra-articular structure more frequently than every third or fourth month.[1–3] As well, injection should not be repeated if a patient should fail to achieve a benefit or have only a short-lasting benefit after one or two injections.

MECHANISM OF ACTION OF INJECTED GLUCOCORTICOIDS

Through the years, many potential mechanisms have been suggested to account for the apparent benefits of intra-articularly injected steroids. These mechanisms have included alterations in neutrophil chemotaxis and function, increases in viscosity, inhibition of metalloproteases, alterations in hyaluronic acid synthesis, transient decreases in synovial fluid complement, alterations in synovial permeability, and changes in synovial fluid leukocyte counts.[1] Although it is known that glucocorticoids suppress inflammation, the mechanism of action is not fully understood. These compounds are known to enter cells and bind to cytoplasmic receptors. The steroid receptor complex then moves into the nucleus of the cell, where it acts as a transcription factor. The complex may either activate or suppress genes after binding to them. Through this process, glucocorticoids are believed to increase the expression of an inhibitory protein $I\kappa Ba$. This protein, in turn, prevents the access of another transcription factor nuclear factor-κB (NF-κB) into the nucleus of a cell where it normally functions as an activator of the immune system and cytokine secretion.[7, 8] Alterations in this system ultimately are believed to lead to decreased neutrophil aggregation at sites of inflammation and reduction of protease and cytokine release by various cell types.[9] In higher doses, there is increasing evidence that nongenomic, receptor-mediated or physicochemical mechanisms are involved in the action of glucocorticoids.

COMPLICATIONS OF INJECTIONS

Although glucocorticoid injections have clear benefits in the appropriate setting, they are not entirely without potential complications. As with the use of any glucocorticoid, a risk of adrenal suppression exists. Systemic absorption is known to take place from both articular and extra-articular injections, albeit at a slower rate than orally administered agents.[2] The rate of absorption is believed to correlate with the solubility of the suspension. The degree of absorption is increased when multiple structures are injected, which may be secondary to the greater surface area of synovial membrane exposed to drug when more than one joint is injected. As well, when glucocorticoids are injected intra-articularly in more than one joint, the hypothalamic-pituitary-adrenal axis may be suppressed 2 to 7 days.[2]

Although it is exceedingly difficult to predict to what extent an individual patient may be affected, it is probably prudent to avoid injecting multiple large joints simultaneously. Similarly, steroids in any form may worsen the hyperglycemia of diabetes, although a study suggests that diabetics can be given soft tissue steroid injections of up to 40 mg of methylprednisolone without raising blood glucose.[10] Occasionally, patients may also manifest diaphoresis, erythema, and warmth after glucocorticoid injections. In addition, abnormal uterine bleeding in both premenopausal and postmenopausal women has been reported.[1]

Intra-articular injection has been associated with the introduction of infection into a sterile space, the development of hemarthroses, postinjection exacerbation of inflammation, and, probably most concerning, steroid arthropathy. With the introduction of a foreign body into a sterile space comes the risk of introducing an iatrogenic infection. The frequency of this occurrence is operator-dependent but reported in the range of 1 in 7000 to 50,000 injections.[2, 11] Besides the risk of introducing an infection during the procedure, there is also the risk that transient damage to joint integrity might lead to septic arthritis in a bacteremic patient secondary to hematogenous seeding.

Any instrumentation of an articular structure carries with it the risk of hemarthrosis. Coagulopathy is not surprisingly a relative contraindication to both aspiration and injection. Although there is no absolute cut-off as to when injection or aspiration can no longer be safely carried out in the setting of coagulopathy, there needs to be an analysis of the goals and urgency of the procedure as well as the proficiency of the operator.

The term *postinjection flare* has been coined to describe the occasional increase in local inflammation that may follow a glucocorticoid injection and potentially last from hours to days. Postinjection flare may be difficult to distinguish from infection. The cause of inflammation occasionally following joint injection is not known but has been associated with the preservative in the steroid suspension as well as with formulations that have larger or more needle-shaped crystalline structures.[1]

The development of *steroid arthropathy* (destruction of cartilage and articular surfaces) has been associated with the use of intra-articular glucocorticoids. Initially, it was thought that the pain relief provided by the glucocorticoid injection would lead to overuse of the affected joint. It was impossible, however, to differentiate possible steroid-related effects from the natural progression of disease.[2, 3] In 1966, Mankin and Conger[12] reported decreased glycine incorporation into rabbit articular cartilage compared with controls 6 hours after intra-articular hydrocortisone injection. Subsequently, Behrens, *et al*[13] published work suggesting increased numbers of fissures in cartilage after intra-articular hydrocortisone injection in rabbits. They found a decrease in hexosamine incorporation, synthesis of proteoglycans, and collagen production in cartilage. Researchers studying subprimate animal models have postulated that steroids decrease synthesis of cartilage matrix components which, in turn, leads to decreased resiliency of cartilage and, ultimately, to cartilage damage with repetitive weight bearing.[1]

Researchers have challenged this notion with data from primate models, which suggest possible protective effects of intra-articular steroids, particularly against fibrillation and osteophyte formation in the setting of experimentally induced articular damage.[14, 15] Monkeys that underwent repeated intra-articular injection with methylprednisolone showed only minor degenerative changes, and those changes were no different than those found after repetitive injections of a control solution.[16] In the setting of chemically induced cartilage damage in guinea pigs, the injection of triamcinolone hexacetonide produced a dose-dependent protective effect.[14] In the Pond-Nuki dog model of osteoarthritis, dogs who received intra-articular injection with triamcinolone hexacetonide had reduced severity of osteoarthritis and structural changes in cartilage.[15] Research suggests that intra-articular use of glucocorticoids has no net effects on bone resorption and only transient effects on bone formation, suggesting intra-articular use may prove to be safer on bone metabolism than oral use of glucocorticoids.[17] Most studies have shown no long-term adverse effects on cartilage from repeated intra-articular injections.[2] Additionally, glucocorticoid injection in rheumatoid arthritis does not appear to increase the need for total joint arthroplasty.[18] Despite the limited evidence of steroid arthropathy, the frequency with which intra-articular glucocorticoids may be given safely remains unclear. In the lack of clear evidence, consensus recommends not injecting the same joint more frequently than every third or fourth month.[1–3]

EXTRA-ARTICULAR COMPLICATIONS

In addition to the articular complications listed previously, there are a number of complications associated with extra-articular injections. Injection of glucocorticoids may lead to the development of soft tissue atrophy as well as thinning and pigmentation changes in the overlying skin. Although uncommon, rupture of tendons has been reported secondary to glucocorticoid injection. Particular attention should be paid to avoid direct injection of a tendon. Examples of tendon ruptures include the Achilles tendon and bicipital tendon. Although uncommon, care must be taken to avoid surrounding nerves for fear of potential damage. Examples include the median nerve when injecting the carpal tunnel or the ulnar nerve when injecting for medial epicondylitis.[1, 2]

INTRA-ARTICULAR USE OF VISCOSUPPLEMENTATION

Alternatives to glucocorticoids are available for intra-articular injection in patients who suffer from osteoarthritis (detailed to a greater extent in Chapter 30). Synthetic hyaluronic acid can be administered intra-articularly in the knee. There are currently two agents available in the United States. These agents are administered through a series of either three or five weekly injections. The agents themselves are believed to be slow-acting and may modify symptoms, but do not modify the course of osteoarthritis. The mechanism of action of these agents is not fully understood, but the following mechanisms have been postulated: short-term lubrication, anti-inflammatory effects through binding of inflammatory mediators and destructive enzymes, and the stimulation of synovial cells to produce a more "normal" hyaluronic acid. In clinical studies these agents appear to reduce pain and improve mobility. When compared to intra-articular glucocorticoid injection, the hyaluronic acid agents appear to have longer-lasting benefits. These agents appear to have analgesic and anti-inflammatory benefits comparable to those seen with the use of NSAIDs. This type of therapy remains expensive; however, these agents may have utility in individuals with osteoarthritis limited to the knee, those at risk for side effects from the use of NSAIDs, or those who are not candidates for surgical correction with osteotomy or knee replacement surgery.

ALGORITHM FOR GUIDE TO SYNOVIAL FLUID ANALYSIS AND GLUCOCORTICOID INJECTIONS

Joint and soft-tissue injection can augment systemic and local conservative treatment and have long-lasting benefits. Inflammatory and crystalline arthritis, synovitis, tendinitis, bursitis, and many other conditions respond well to injection. Corticosteroid preparations should be chosen on the basis of solubility and potency desired and the size of structure to be injected. Injections should not be made directly into a ligament

Guide to synovial fluid analysis

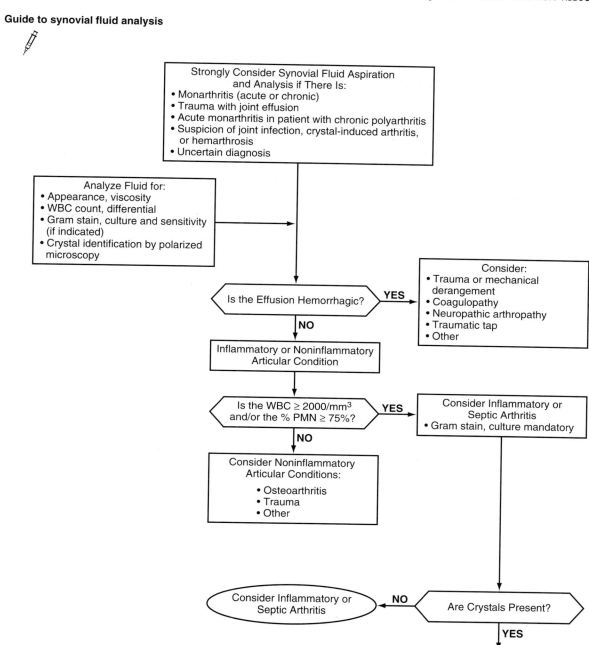

Strongly Consider Synovial Fluid Aspiration
and Analysis if There Is:
• Monarthritis (acute or chronic)
• Trauma with joint effusion
• Acute monarthritis in patient with chronic polyarthritis
• Suspicion of joint infection, crystal-induced arthritis,
  or hemarthrosis
• Uncertain diagnosis

Analyze Fluid for:
• Appearance, viscosity
• WBC count, differential
• Gram stain, culture and sensitivity
  (if indicated)
• Crystal identification by polarized
  microscopy

Is the Effusion Hemorrhagic? — **YES** →

Consider:
• Trauma or mechanical
  derangement
• Coagulopathy
• Neuropathic arthropathy
• Traumatic tap
• Other

NO

Inflammatory or Noninflammatory
Articular Condition

Is the WBC ≥ 2000/mm³
and/or the % PMN ≥ 75%? — **YES** →

Consider Inflammatory or
Septic Arthritis
• Gram stain, culture mandatory

NO

Consider Noninflammatory
Articular Conditions:
• Osteoarthritis
• Trauma
• Other

Consider Inflammatory or
Septic Arthritis ← **NO** — Are Crystals Present?

YES

Identification of Crystal and
Definitive Diagnosis of
Crystal induced Arthritis*

*Presence of crystals does not rule out the possibility of concurrent infection.

Reprinted with permission from Lipsky PE (ed): Algorithms for the diagnosis and management of musculoskeletal complaints. Am J Med 103(6A):
67S, 1997.

or tendon and should be limited to every third or fourth month. With attention to the usual cautions required with corticosteroid use and avoidance of contraindications (e.g., bacteremia, fracture), injection is usually safe and effective, particularly as a bridging technique to long-term therapy.

REFERENCES

1. Owens DS: Aspiration and injection of joints and soft tissues. In Kelly WN, Harris ED, Ruddy S, Sledge CB, eds: Textbook of Rheumatology, 5th ed. Philadelphia, WB Saunders, 1997, pp 591–608.

2. Gray RG, Gottlieb NL: Intra-articular corticosteroids: An updated assessment. Clin Orthop 177:235–263, 1983.

3. McCarthy GM, McCarty DJ: Intrasynovial corticosteroid therapy. Bull Rheum Dis 43:2–4, 1994.

4. McCarty DJ: Treatment of rheumatoid joint inflammation with triamcinolone hexacetonide. Arthritis Rheum 15:157–173, 1972.

5. Gaffney K, Ledingham J, Perry JD: Intra-articular triamcinolone hexacetonide in knee osteoarthritis: Factors influencing the clinical response. Ann Rheum Dis 54:379–381, 1995.

6. Chakravarty K, Pharoah PDP, Scott DGI: A randomized controlled study of post-injection rest following intra-articular steroid therapy for knee synovitis. Br J Rheumatol 33:464–468, 1994.

7. Scheinman RI, Cogswell PC, Lofquist AK, Baldwin AS Jr: Role of transcriptional activation of IκBa in mediation of immunosuppression by glucocorticoids. Science 270:283–286, 1995.

8. Auphan N, DiDonato JA, Rosette C, et al: Immunosuppression by glucocorticoids: Inhibition of NF-κB activity through induction of IκB synthesis. Science 270:286–290, 1995.

9. Harris ED Jr: The role of glucocorticoids. In Harris ED Jr, ed: Rheumatoid Arthritis. Philadelphia, WB Saunders, 1997, pp 350–363.

10. Slotkoff AT, Clauw DJ, Nashel DJ: Effect of soft tissue corticosteroid injection on glucose control in diabetics. Arthritis Rheum 37(suppl 6): S347, 1994.

11. Hollander JL, Jessar RA, Brown EM: Intra-synovial corticosteroid therapy: A decade of use. Bull Rheum Dis 11:239–240, 1961.

12. Mankin HJ, Conger KA: The acute effects of intraarticular hydrocortisone on articular cartilage in rabbits. J Bone Joint Surg 48:1383–1388, 1966.

13. Behrens F, Shepard N, Mitchell N: Alteration of rabbit articular cartilage by intraarticular injections of glucocorticoids. J Bone Joint Surg 57:70–76, 1975.

14. Williams JM, Brandt KD: Triamcinolone hexacetonide protects against fibrillation and osteophyte formation following chemically induced articular cartilage damage. Arthritis Rheum 28: 1267–1274, 1985.

15. Pelletier JP, Martell-Pelletier J: Protective effects of corticosteroids on cartilage lesions and osteophyte formation in the Pond-Nuki dog model of osteoarthritis. Arthritis Rheum 32:181–193, 1989.

16. Gibson T, Burry HC, Poswillo D, Glass J: Effect of intraarticular corticosteroid injections on primate cartilage. Ann Rheum Dis 36:74–79, 1977.

17. Emkey RD, Lindsay R, Lyssy J, et al: The systemic effect of intraarticular administration of corticosteroid on markers of bone formation and bone resorption on patients with rheumatoid arthritis. Arthritis Rheum 39:277–282, 1996.

18. Roberts WN, Babcock EA, Breitbach SA, et al: Corticosteroid injection in rheumatoid arthritis does not increase rate of total joint arthroplasty. J Rheumatol 23:1001–1004, 1996.

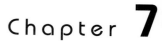

Chapter **7**

Pain—Its Origins, Consequences, and Management

Raymond R. Gaeta

The experience of pain is a necessary part of human survival. Consider Fabry's disease, a condition in which patients are congenitally insensate to pain; it leads to tremendous injury because of the loss of the protective mechanism of pain. Affected individuals usually succumb at an early age because of cumulative and devastating trauma. Rather than the absolute elimination of pain, a more laudable goal for physicians is to seek a better understanding of the nature of pain and the means by which it can be managed in a manner that optimizes functionality and preserves a quality way of life.

Pain has been defined by the International Association for the Study of Pain as both a sensory and an emotional experience associated with real or potential tissue damage.[1] This definition encompasses the key elements in the field of pain and recognizes the complex interplay of the physical world with the neurochemical signals of the nervous system and finally the integration with the affective components of the higher cortical centers. The chapter discusses pain from this perspective in an attempt to define and explain its consequences better. From this basis of understanding, rational treatment plans are formulated that deal with the entire patient.

BASIC NEUROPHYSIOLOGY

An understanding of the basic pain pathways is an important aspect in the diagnosis and management of pain.[2] Neuroanatomic examination can localize lesions within the body and even discern when pain is likely referred from another site in the body. Interruption of the neurochemical signals that carry the pain impulses anywhere along the pathway can lead to effective therapeutic intervention. Opioids, local anesthetics, and nonsteroidal anti-inflammatory drugs (NSAIDs) all interact along portions of this pain pathway to achieve pain relief with different side-effect profiles. Despite the numerous agents available, the complete control of pain in every circumstance remains an elusive goal. Future research efforts will focus on specific and novel modalities to achieve such an effect.

Transduction

The interface to the outside world occurs at specialized nerve fibers that transduce physical phenomena and convert them to the electrochemical signals of the nervous system (Fig. 7–1). The pain fibers, A-delta and C fibers, are termed *nociceptors* and are capable of sensing potentially injurious temperature, mechanical, and chemical stimuli. Some nerve types, termed *unimodal nociceptors,* respond only to one type of stimuli, whereas polymodal fibers are capable of sensing, as the name implies, multiple types of stimuli.[3] Various algesic substances, such as bradykinin, histamine, and potassium, are capable of directly stimulating nociceptors and setting up a complex and cascading interaction at the site of stimulus (Fig. 7–2). When tissue injury occurs, prostaglandins are elaborated locally by the enzyme cyclooxygenase. Prostaglandins are sensitizing agents for nociceptors causing them to fire with a weaker stimulus, thus causing surrounding tissue to become sensitive to otherwise subthreshold stimuli. Some nociceptors have large receptive fields and have a less well-localized spatial discrimination, whereas others, as on the fingertips, have small, discrete fields capable of exquisite localization.

Conduction

As the influx of sodium occurs along the membrane, a signal is conducted along the nerve toward the central nervous system. These fibers conduct at various speeds depending on their state of myelination. Myelinated A-delta pain fibers conduct much faster than unmyelinated C pain fibers. This differential rate of conduction leads to the phenomenon of *fast* and *slow* pain experienced by many after injury (Fig. 7–3). The faster-conduction A-delta fibers are responsible for the fast, well-localized pain sensation that is followed by the slow-onset, poorly localized gnawing pain initiated by the same injury. Despite the terms *slow* and *fast,* these nociceptive fibers conduct at roughly 1 and 10 m/sec. This is in contrast to motor fibers, which conduct an order of magnitude faster.

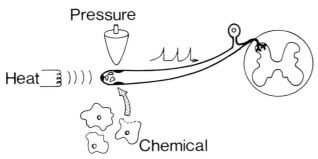

Figure 7–1. Sensitivity range of the C-polymodal nociceptor. Available evidence suggests that the terminals are sensitive to direct heat or mechanical distortion. Thus, transduction can occur at the terminal. The terminals are also sensitive to chemicals released from damaged cells. In this manner, any tissue cell can serve as an intermediate in the transduction process. In a sense, all tissue cells are *receptors* for injury. (From Fields HL: Pain. New York, McGraw-Hill, 1987, p 27.)

Central Integration

Afferent fibers from the periphery have their cell bodies in the dorsal root ganglion. Projections of these cell bodies continue into the spinal cord entering via the dorsal root. Fibers enter this area from a dermatomal distribution. This concept leads to the phenomenon of referral patterns of pain. The diaphragm and the shoulder are innervated by the fourth cervical dermatome. In the case of cholecystitis with inflammation of the diaphragm, the pain can be felt in the shoulder. In the same way, angina pectoris can be felt not only in the chest, but also in the neck and arms owing to the same principle of referred pain (Fig. 7–4).

The spinal cord has an internal organization known as the *rexed laminae I through X* (Fig. 7–5). These laminae contain the cell bodies and synapse responsible for the transmission of information to the higher centers of the central nervous system. In the dorsal horn region of the spinal cord, the afferent fibers synapse with cell bodies in lamina I, also known as the *marginal zone*. The marginal zone cells can then send further projections to interact with other important sites within the central nervous system. Some fibers interact with cell bodies of the anterior motor horn leading to reflex arcs that allow painful stimuli to cause retraction of a limb without the involvement of higher cortical centers. Other fibers in the pain pathway interact with specialized cells in laminae II through IV. Of particular interest is lamina II, also known as the *substantia gelatinosa,* which is the site of numerous opioid receptors and is thought to be responsible for spinally mediated analgesia. Deeper, in laminae III to IV, wide dynamic range neurons serve to integrate pain signals from the periphery before its presentation to higher centers of the spinal cord and cerebral cortex. The cell bodies of the sympathetic nervous system reside in the lateral aspect of the spinal cord in the thoracolumbar region and are subject to projections from the pain pathways. Interaction with this system is responsible for the sympathetic response to injury and may even play a role in the development of the sympathetically mediated pain syndromes, such as those known as *complex regional pain syndromes,* formally known as *reflex sympathetic dystrophy* and *causalgia.*

Ascending Pathways

The pain signals ascend to the cerebral cortex passing through various discrete sites, including the nucleus raphe magnus and the nucleus reticularis gigantocellularis (Fig. 7–6). These nuclei have projections into the thalamus and the periaqueductal gray, where elaboration of endogenous enkephalins along with input from the nucleus reticularis gigantocellularis interact with descending pathways of the nucleus raphe magnus. This intimate relationship between the ascending and descending tracts in the nuclei is a fascinating area of future research. The ascending signals that do reach the thalamus synapse in the venteroposterolateral (VPL) and centromedian (CM) nuclei. Projections from the VPL are directed to the somatosensory cortex in the somatotopic arrangement of the homunculus. This VPL projection allows for the localization of the pain to a specific site of the body and face. The other nucleus projects signals to the hypothalamus and other centers responsible for the affective components of pain. The fear, loathing, and suffering associated with the experience of pain are derived from this portion of the central nervous system. Lesions in one particular area of the frontal cortex, the cingulate gyrus, can be especially effective in managing this affective component and lessen the suffering associated with some chronically painful conditions.

Descending Pathways

In a parallel construct, the descending pathways follow the ascending pathways, passing through many of the same nuclear centers (see Fig. 7–6). This proximity allows for interaction between the two systems and even modulation of the ascending signals by descending inhibitory control. This pathway is thought to play a major role in the body's ability to control or self-modulate painful events. The soldier who is able to continue in battle despite tremendous wounds and the athlete who competes with a seemingly disabling injury are two examples of this descending control. The pathway has far-reaching consequences as projections of this system extend all the way to the level of the dorsal horn, where pain signals make their entry into the central nervous system. At this level, these descending pathways may exert some of their more potent effects as the multiple neural cell types and the multitudinous receptors provide many sites for modification of the pain signals.

Neurotransmitters and Receptors

The propagation of pain signals within the nervous system uses specific chemicals called neurotransmitters. Norepinephrine and acetylcholine are common agents that transmit signals in the nervous system. Serotonin is

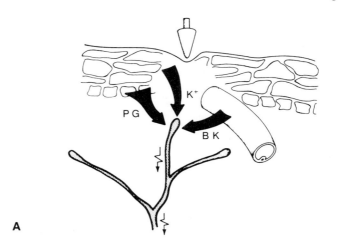

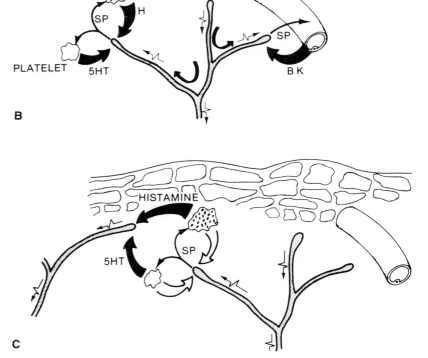

Figure 7–2. Events leading to activation, sensitization, and spread of sensitization of primary afferent nociceptor terminals. *A,* Direct activation by intense pressure and consequent cell damage. Cell damage leads to release of potassium (K^+) and to synthesis of prostaglandins (PG) and bradykinin (BK). Prostaglandins increase the sensitivity of the terminal to bradykinin and other pain-producing substances. *B,* Secondary activation. Impulses generated in the stimulated terminal propagate not only to the spinal cord, but also into other terminal branches, where they induce the release of peptides, including substance P (SP). Substance P causes vasodilation and neurogenic edema with further accumulation of bradykinin. Substance P also causes the release of histamine (H) from mast cells and serotonin (5HT) from platelets. *C,* Histamine and serotonin levels rise in the extracellular space, secondarily sensitizing nearby nociceptors. This leads to a gradual spread of hyperalgesia, tenderness, or both. (From Fields HL: Pain. New York, McGraw-Hill, 1987, p 36.)

also recognized as a ubiquitous neurotransmitter involved in many different aspects in both the perception and the regulation of pain. Migraine headaches, in particular, are heavily influenced by serotonin and its effects on vascular stability and inflammation. In the dorsal horn of the spinal cord, new transmitters are now recognized as playing important roles in the pain pathways. Receptors for substance P, α_2 agonists, γ-aminobutyric acid, *N*-methyl-D-aspartate, glycine, and aspartate have all been identified in addition to the well-described opioid receptors (Table 7–1). Intracellular mechanisms involving

cyclic adenosine monophosphate (AMP) and G-proteins are then responsible for the action of these transmitters. Nitric oxide has been shown to participate in some of the final common pathways of these receptors. Depending on the site of the receptor, either presynaptic or postsynaptic, these agents can serve either to facilitate or to block the transmission of pain by altering the transmembrane potentials or changing the permeability to various ions (Fig. 7–7). Specialized channels termed *N-type calcium channels* regulate the influx of calcium and have also been localized in the

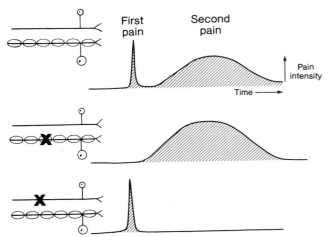

Figure 7–3. *Top,* First and second pain are carried by two different primary afferent axons. First pain is abolished by selective blockade of myelinated axons (*middle*) and second pain by blocking C fibers (*bottom*). (From Fields HL: Pain. New York, McGraw-Hill, 1987, p 26.)

dorsal horn in the same region as the opioid receptors. Blockade by a compound known as ziconotide produces strong analgesia.

CLINICAL PAIN CONCEPTS

Although pain is such a common human experience, words often fail to describe it in clinical settings. In the midst of an emergency department visit for a compression fracture, the patient may not be able to discern whether the horrible pain in the back and chest is related solely to the fracture or perhaps even to some dynamic nerve root compression. It is important for the practitioner not only to diagnose the cause of the pain, but also to tease out the various components of pain that may lead to significant differences in therapy. The area of pain taxonomy is unsettled as various categorizations vie for predominance. No system is encompassing enough to describe adequately the myriad of pain symptoms and syndromes. The *visceral versus somatic* system does not yield valuable information when dealing with the patient in whom the pain in a limb may be related to a tenosynovitis or a mononeuropathy.

A simple and descriptive taxonomy uses the historical features and the physical examination to categorize pain as either *nociceptive* or *neuropathic.* Nociceptive pain is pain related to a noxious stimulus or source. Fractures and incisions are easily identifiable examples of nociceptive pain. Generally, nociceptive pain is described as sharp or dull or stabbing or boring. Neuropathic pain is pain related to the abnormal function of the nervous system with no ongoing noxious stimulus required. Postherpetic neuralgia and diabetic neuropathy represent two classic types of neuropathic pain. Although the initiating cause of the injury may have waned, the incredibly descriptive reports of shooting, electrical, and burning pain are unmistakable as those of neuropathic pain. Although this categorization may be far too simplistic for some, this categorization can help guide therapy because the two areas generally respond to different classes of therapeutic agents. Although they are not mutually exclusive, the nociceptive and neuropathic categorization does stratify patients into groups and give reasonable attention to the class of nerve injury–type pains that many times are not diagnosed in a proper and timely fashion. From this broad categorization, more specific diagnoses can be

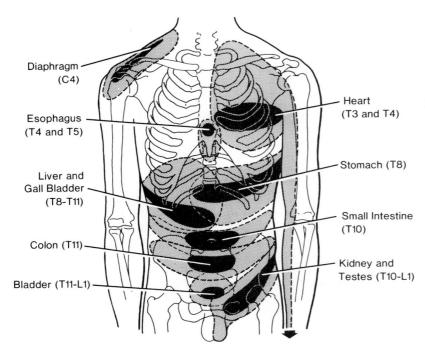

Diaphragm (C4)

Esophagus (T4 and T5)

Liver and Gall Bladder (T8-T11)

Colon (T11)

Bladder (T11-L1)

Heart (T3 and T4)

Stomach (T8)

Small Intestine (T10)

Kidney and Testes (T10-L1)

Figure 7–4. Viscerotomes. Approximate superficial areas to which visceral pain is referred, with related dermatomes in brackets. The dark areas are those most commonly associated with pain in each viscus. The gray areas indicate approximately the larger area that may be associated with pain in that viscus. (From Cousins M: Visceral pain. In Andersson S, Bond M, Mehta M, Swerdlow M, eds: Chronic Non-Cancer Pain: Assessment and Practical Management. Lancaster, MTP Press, 1987.)

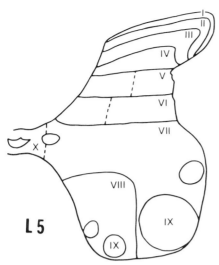

Figure 7–5. Rexed's scheme for lamination of the spinal gray matter. Outlines of fifth lumbar (L5) segments of the adult cat. (From Rexed B: A cytoarchitectonic atlas of the spinal cord in the cat. J Comp Neurol 96:415–495, 1952.)

made to direct specific therapies. The classification does have some difficulty in categorizing some situations, such as headaches, for example; however, headache is such a well-defined syndrome that it has its own appropriate classification.

The clinical encounter, particularly related to chronic painful conditions, is directed not only to the diagnosis, but also to the overall state of the patient.[4] The historical features should include aspects of the patient's functional capacity. Attention to function in the social and recreational areas also discloses limitations that have a tremendous impact on the well-being of the patient. Depression occurs to a high degree in patients with chronic debilitating pain. Patients with depression experience their pain as more severe, and they see little hope for relief from the interventions of health care providers. The effects of the depression can be far reaching and can sabotage what would otherwise be considered effective medical therapies.

Evaluation of the more severely depressed and debilitated patient may sometimes require a multidisciplinary approach, so that the medical, physical, and emotional components of the patient's pain experience are given their proper weight as diagnostic and treatment plans are elaborated. From a psychological standpoint, depression is not the only factor that affects pain evaluation and treatment. Other Diagnostic and Statistical Manual of Mental Disorders (DSM-IV)[5] axis I states, such as bipolar disorders and anxiety disorders, can disrupt any treatment plan that does not offer attention to these states. More subtle than the axis I disorders are the axis II personality disorders, which are equally disruptive. The personality disorders are long-standing patterns of behavior that affect the manner in which patients react to their environment. Many patients have personality disorders that are unrecognized until such time as they become stressed, such as during the course of an acute or chronic illness. Avoidant and dependent

personality types are managed differently than borderline or histrionic personalities. It is with patients within this axis II category of disorders that many practitioners have the most difficulty, yet do not seek the assistance of a clinical psychologist. The information obtained from a clinical psychologist, especially one trained in pain management, can make the management of these patients appropriate and reasonable.

Despite the emphasis on the psychological state of the patient, the goals of pain management are to return the patient to the premorbid state, including optimal physical and social function. The input of a physical or occupational therapist can be invaluable

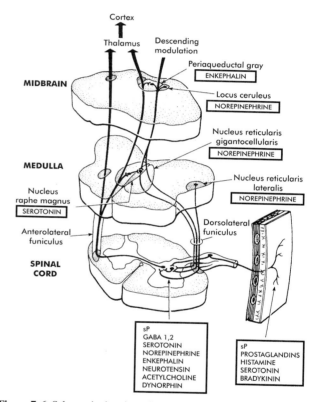

Figure 7–6. Schematic drawing of nociceptive processing, outlining ascending (*left side of diagram*) and descending (*right side of diagram*) pathways. Stimulation of nociceptors in the skin surface leads to impulse generation in the primary afferent. Concomitant with this impulse generation, increased levels of various endogenous algesic agents (substance P [sP], prostaglandins, histamine, serotonin, and bradykinin) are detected near the area of stimulation in the periphery. The noxious impulse is conducted to the dorsal horn of the spinal cord, where it is subjected to local factors and descending modulation. The endogenous neurochemical mediators of this interaction at the dorsal horn that have been characterized are listed in the figure. Primary nociceptive afferents relay to projection neurons in the dorsal horn that ascend in the anterolateral funiculus to end in the thalamus. En route, collaterals of the projection neurons activate the nucleus reticularis gigantocellularis, whose neurons project to the thalamus and activate the periaqueductal gray of the midbrain. Enkephalinergic neurons from the periaqueductal gray and noradrenergic neurons from the nucleus reticularis gigantocellularis activate descending serotoninergic neurons of the nucleus raphe magnus. These fibers join with noradrenergic fibers from the locus coeruleus reticularis lateralis to project descending modulatory impulses to the dorsal horn via the dorsolateral funiculus. GABA, γ-aminobutyric acid. (From Brose WG, Cousins MJ: Gynecologic pain. In Coppelson M, ed: Gynecologic Oncology. Edinburgh, Churchill Livingstone, 1992, pp 1439–1479.)

Table 7–1. SPINAL NEUROTRANSMITTERS, RECEPTORS, AND LIGANDS

Neurotransmitter System	Proposed Receptor	Endogenous Ligand	Exogenous Ligand
Opioid	μ	β-Endorphin; Met/Leu-enkephalin	Morphine
	δ	Met/Leu-enkephalin	DADL
	κ	Dynorphin	U50488H
Adrenergic	α_1	Norepinephrine	Methoxamine
	α_2	Norepinephrine	Clonidine
	β	Epinephrine	Isoproterenol
Serotoninergic	5-HT	Serotonin	Serotonin
GABAergic	A	GABA	Baclofen
	B	GABA	Muscimol
Neurotensin	—	Neurotensin	Neurotensin
Cholinergic	Muscarinic	Acetylcholine	Oxotremorine

GABA, γ-aminobutyric acid; 5-HT, 5-hydroxytryptamine (serotonin).
Modified from Taksh TL: Neurologic mechanisms of pain. In Cousins MJ, Bridenbaugh PO, 2ed: Neural Blockade in Clinical Anesthesia and Management Of Pain. 2nd ed. Philadelphia, JB Lippincott, 1988, p 820.

in designing a treatment plan that has a patient as physically fit and independent as possible. The use of assisted devices when appropriate can make a tremendous difference for the patient. For other patients, a general conditioning program is the key to better levels of function.

PAIN MANAGEMENT MODALITIES

One of the most important features in the management of chronic painful conditions is an approach that strives to return patients to a productive and happy lifestyle with a great degree of independence.[6] The

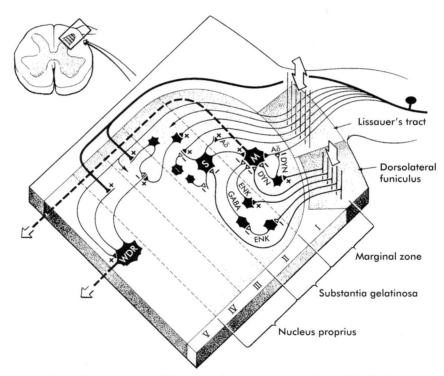

Figure 7–7. Dorsal horn processing. Large-diameter and small-diameter primary neurons have their cell bodies in the dorsal root ganglia. These fibers segregate as they approach the spinal cord. Large-diamter afferents (*thick solid lines*) travel in the medial portion, whereas small-diameter afferents (*thin solid lines: C and Aδ*) segregate to the lateral portions of the entry zone. The spinal terminals of the small fibers enter the cord, where they may ascend or descend for several segments in the dorsolateral tract (Lissauer's tract) and subsequently terminate throughout the dorsal horn of the spinal cord. Aδ fiber afferents terminate primarily in lamina I (marginal zone), whereas C fiber afferents terminate in lamina II (substantia gelatinosa). In lamina I, nociceptive fibers synapse on dendrites of the large marginal (M) neurons. Smaller neurons in lamina I may exert presynapse inhibition of the marginal neuron. Other nociceptive fibers (Aδ) synapse with stalked (S) neurons in lamina II. These S neurons stimulate M neurons in lamina I. The relay between primary afferent fibers and S neurons is also subject to modulation by inhibitory islet (I) neurons in lamina II. Central transmission is accomplished by M neurons directly, wide dynamic range neurons (WDR) directly, or S neurons indirectly. M neurons are subject to inhibition by neurons in lamina II. Descending serotoninergic neurons from the nucleus raphe magnus, which travel in the dorsolateral funiculus, are also shown. These neurons terminate throughout the spinal cord on interneurons (γ-aminobutyric acid [GABA] and enkephalins [ENK]) to provide inhibition of nociceptive transmission. DYN, dynorphin. (From Yudofsky SC, Hales RE: Neuropsychiatry. Washington, DC, American Psychiatric Press, 1997, p 360.)

blueprint for such a construct must be discussed before initiation of treatment, although obviously modifications are made along the way based on progress of the patient. Once the plan is described, the multiple tools available, including medical, interventional, and nonmedical, can be properly employed. Each of these interventions can be tested against the plan to determine whether it is an essential component. Medications or other interventions that do not contribute can be changed or even eliminated. The use of goal sheets, which track specific behaviors on a daily basis, is an essential component of the management style. The ability to identify prospectively progressively more strenuous and productive activities gives the patient specific targets to be achieved. When analyzed at intervals, these goal sheets can document improvements or perhaps lack of progress in response to specific interventions. The type of intervention can be in any of the domains, such as medical, interventional, rehabilitative, or psychological. At the end of treatment, the goal sheets can be compared from beginning to end to demonstrate the tremendous improvements that are sometimes difficult to appreciate on a day-to-day basis.

Analgesics

Most of the medications available to patients are considered palliative and provide symptom management rather than a cure for pain.[7] An exception to this is the class of NSAIDs, which are able to modify the inflammatory response as well as provide analgesia.

NONSTEROIDAL ANTI-INFLAMMATORY DRUGS

NSAIDs are invaluable in the management of mild-to-moderate pain. Their analgesic properties as well as their anti-inflammatory profile make them a well-suited choice for many clinical scenarios, including acute sprains, strains, and even fractures. Muscular aches and pains associated with chronic pain syndromes also respond favorably to this class of medications. Used in conjunction with opioids, the NSAIDs provide the mainstay of most analgesic regimens. As with many medications, the side-effect profile may limit clinical effectiveness. Both have renal and gastrointestinal side effects, particularly in the elderly and medically complicated patients. The release of cyclooxygenase type 2 inhibitors that inhibit new prostaglandin synthesis at the site of injury should help improve the safety profile of these drugs.

OPIOIDS

No other class of analgesic agent has so much history yet so much misconception. Although it is clear that opioids are potent analgesics that interact with specific receptor sites in the body and are concentrated in the central nervous system, the debate concerning the appropriate use of opioids rages to this day. Throughout history, opioids have been used to relieve pain, such as

in an acute fracture and in surgical trauma.[8] The response is dose dependent and generally complete, and the patient is considered to have *opioid-responsive pain.* In cancer patients in the United States, the use of opioids is recognized as both appropriate and humane. Most physicians would not hesitate to provide an opioid, such as morphine, to alleviate a cancer patient's pain and suffering. Contrast this, however, with patients with nonmalignant pain, in whom the bias and concern about liability for addiction often limits access to medications even when the pain is opioid responsive, such as vertebral compression fracture.

The concerns surrounding the use of opioids are valid but must be better understood when the use of a valuable palliative agent is in question. The most significant concern is about addiction or psychological dependence. *Psychological dependence* is manifest when there is evidence of abnormal behaviors directed toward the acquisition of the drug, evidence of harm associated with its use, and continued use and abuse despite the knowledge that harm exists. True addiction is a real concern and medical problem that requires specific treatment when it does occur; however, this fear of addiction should not prevent the prescription and monitoring of opioids in appropriate patient populations. Adding to the confusion are two physiologic phenomena that occur normally and are not to be confused with true psychological dependence. The first is *physical dependence,* which refers to the complex of symptoms that can be seen when opioid medications are discontinued. Just as the abrupt withdrawal of clonidine can lead to rebound hypertension, the cessation of opioids can cause symptoms of sympathetic overdrive with sweating, tachycardia, abdominal cramping, and diarrhea. The other concept is *tolerance,* which is described as the requirement for increased dosage over time to achieve the same effect. Tolerance is not a universal effect, but when it occurs in an opioid-responsive patient, analgesia is generally recaptured with reasonable increases in the dosage. The final misconception about opioids is called *pseudoaddiction.* This situation occurs primarily when the patient has opioid-responsive pain but is undermedicated. With each increase of medication, improved analgesia is achieved, so that the patient requests further increases in dose. This behavior pattern mimics the drug-seeking pattern of the addict, but it is motivated by the appropriate dose-response relationship of opioid-responsive pain. A good patient-physician relationship is key in the prescription of these medications so as to avoid confusion with these concepts.

Fundamental to the use of opioid medications is the establishment of a unique benefit for the patient with an acceptable side-effect profile. It is incumbent on the practitioner to establish prospective goals with the patients and to assess critically whether the medication helps achieve the goals. A *blinded pain cocktail* is exceedingly useful in this regard. The patient is told of the contents of the cocktail but not the dosage of the medications, which usually are opioids, and a blinding agent with some anticholinergic side effect. The dose of opioid is varied with each refill while the blinding agent remains the same, thus giving a similar experience to the patient with each administration. Over several weeks, the optimal function is determined based on objective criteria, then matched to the dosage contained in the cocktail at that point in time. Patients can then be *unblinded* and given the optimal dose in tablet form. Other times, no matter how high the medication is raised, no substantial increase in function is seen. Similarly, sometimes reductions in the dosage cause no decrement in function, so that the opioid can be weaned entirely. Because these changes occur in a blinded fashion, withdrawal of the medication can be achieved in a safe and less abrupt manner, avoiding withdrawal symptoms.

Specific Opioids

The class of opioids must be considered to be a family of medications with similar efficacy and side-effect profiles. Although individual differences are noteworthy, they relate more to idiosyncratic effects rather than to efficacy. The opioids should be considered as *weak* versus *potent* and *short-acting* versus *long-acting*. This classification best allows the prescription of these medications to match the clinical need. It also helps explain why extensive compounding and repackaging of opioids occurs to move from the short-acting potent class to the long-acting potent class (e.g., the fentanyl patch). Table 7–2 describes multiple opioids along with caveats for dosing and conversion between drugs. In general, the knowledge of four different opioids suffices in clinical practice. Morphine is the gold standard potent, short-acting agent. Conversion between opioids is usually based on morphine equivalency. Methadone is a cost-effective, potent, long-acting agent for use when long-term administration is desired. Fentanyl is a potent, fast-onset opioid useful for conscious sedation in painful procedures. Finally, hydrocodone is a weak, short-acting agent for time-limited use in mild-to-moderate pain. Generally, however, hydrocodone is combined with acetaminophen or ibuprofen to improve its overall potency.

Routes of Administration

The oral route is preferred for the administration of opioids. Onset of action is reasonably rapid, and this route avoids the rapid rise in blood levels seen with intermittent parenteral use. When oral intake is restricted, transdermal delivery becomes a viable alternative. Although rectal administration is possible, suppositories have low popularity in the United States, and thus this route is underused. Inhaled opioids and lozenge opioids are available; they are best suited for acute short-term administration. At the other extreme, as in cases of severe pain, long-term subcutaneous or intravenous use via an ambulatory pump becomes practical. This can be a particularly effective method in the terminally ill, for whom home health agencies can offer excellent care and support with this method.

Adjuvant Medications

In practical terms, the class of adjuvant medications are those that supplement or enhance the analge-sia of other medications. Under the broad definition, there are multiple classes of medications used for pain relief in conditions not listed as the primary indication (Table 7–3). A familiar example is the use of antidepressant agents for treatment of neuropathies. In particular, tricyclic antidepressants in subantidepressant doses are effective in various neuropathic pain states, such as diabetic neuropathy and postherpetic neuralgia. These medications—amitriptyline, nortriptyline, imipramine, and desipramine—are usually prescribed as an evening or bedtime dose and provide an appropriate alternative to the use of benzodiazepines. Poor sleep hygiene is a hallmark of chronic pain and depression so that the sedation is an added benefit. The newer selective serotonin reuptake inhibitors have less sedation; their role in pain management is under review with ongoing clinical trials.

Membrane-stabilizing drugs share a common ability to block the frequency-dependent sodium channels of neural tissue. In neuropathic pain states, the injured nerve is relatively hyperactive at baseline. Agents such as lidocaine and mexiletine both share the ability to block this hyperactivity without disturbing the normal transduction or conduction of the nerve. Side effects, such as nausea, may limit the dosage of these medications, but their use has improved painful neuropathies when no other agent was successful.

Anticonvulsants also play a role in pain management and are useful for painful neuropathies. Carbamazepine has a long history in the treatment of trigeminal neuralgia and continues to have indications for use in other neuropathic states. Although it is initially sedating, most patients become accustomed to this side effect and derive benefit from it. Of more concern, however, is the reversible granulocytopenia that can occur idiosyncratically with carbamazepine. It is recommended that a baseline complete blood count be obtained before starting the medication and every 3 to 6 months thereafter. Evidence of decreased white blood cell count requires discontinuance of the medication. Although valproate and phenytoin have also been used, they are much less effective in regular practice. A newer agent, gabapentin, appears to have some role in the treatment of neuropathies and, in particular, reflex sympathetic dystrophy.

Muscle relaxants, such as baclofen, cyclobenzaprine, carisoprodol, and benzodiazepines, are touted as effective agents for muscular pain. In patients with acute muscular strain, they may provide some relief; in chronic myofascial pain states and fibromyalgia, these agents are less effective. They tend to have nonsustainable effects and generally cause sedation that limits patients as they strive to become more functional and productive.

Newer agents include capsaicin, which depletes the neurotransmitter, substance P. When applied to the affected area, it causes a burning sensation followed by analgesia in some cases. Multiple applications are required, and it is not for use on mucous membranes. Patient compliance generally wanes, especially after the first inadvertent application to the eyes or mouth. Ziconotide an *N*-type calcium channel blocker, administered into the spinal fluid exerts a powerful analgesic

Table 7–2. CHARACTERISTICS OF COMMONLY USED OPIATES

	Drug (Trade Name)	Equianalgesic	Dose* (mg)	Peak (min)	Duration (h)	Standard Dosage† (adults >50 kg)	Comments
Agonist	Propoxyphene (Darvon)	Oral	400	60–90	4–6	65 mg q 4 h	Weak analgesic; overdose may lead to convulsions
	Codeine (Tylenol #3)	Oral	200		4–6	15–60 mg q 4–6 h	
		Parenteral	120	45–90	4–6	15–60 mg q 4–6 h	
	Meperidine (Demerol)	Oral	300	60–120	3–6	Not recommended	Limit dose to <600 mg/24 h, as metabolite normeperidine can accumulate (especially in those with renal failure) and lead to CNS excitation (seizures)
		Parenteral	75	30–60	2–4	50–100 mg q 3–4 h	Combination with MAO inhibitors has caused fatalities. Avoid this combination
							Has atropine-like effect and can induce tachycardia
							Small dose can control postoperative shivering (12–25 mg IV)
	Hydrocodone (Vicodin, Lortab)	Oral	40	30–60	4–5	5–10 mg q 3–4 h	Available in combination with acetaminophen, which limits dosing to maximal 4 g acetaminophen per day (adults >50 kg)
	Oxycodone (Percocet, Tylox)	Oral	30	60	4–5	5–10 mg q 3–4 h	See comment for hydrocodone
	Morphine (Roxanol, MS Contin)	Oral	30	90–120	4	5–30 mg q 2–4 h	Oral slow-release formulation MS Contin useful for long-acting therapy (e.g., in cancer patients). This formulation is dosed q 8–12 h
		Parenteral	10	30–60	3–5	5–15 mg q 4 h	
	Methadone (Dolophine)	Oral	10	90–120	4–12	2.5–20 mg q 12 h	Long and variable half-life (12–48 h) renders this agent good for long-acting treatment. Effect may persist for days after drug is discontinued
		Parenteral	10	30–60	4–8	2.5–20 mg q 8 h	Oral bioavailability essentially equal to parenteral
	Hydromorphone (Dilaudid)	Oral	4	90–120	4–6	2–4 mg q 4–6 h	Available in suppository form
		Parenteral	2	30–60	3–4	1–2 mg q 4–6 h	
	Fentanyl (Sublimaze, Duragesic)	Parenteral	0.1	3–20	0.5–1	0.05–0.1 mg q 1–2 h	Available in skin patch for transdermal administration. Achieving therapeutic level is delayed for 12 h as drug passes through skin initially. In addition, removal of patch still leaves drug in skin, thus delaying actual end of dosing
							Excellent agent to titrate intravenously, as high lipid solubility allows for rapid onset of action (within 5 min)
							Associated with less hemodynamic instability than morphine or meperidine secondary to less histamine release and no vagolytic effect
	Sufentanil (Sufenta)	Parenteral	0.02	3–20	0.5–1	0.005–0.02 mg q 1–2 h	Similar to fentanyl except more potent and less accumulation of drug with infusion
Mixed Agonist-Antagonist	Butorphanol (Stadol)	Parenteral	2	30–60	2–4	1–2 mg q 3–4 h	Nasal preparation available (10 mg/mL; one spray in one nostril is equal to 1 mg)
							See pentazocine
	Nalbuphine (Nubain)	Parenteral	10	30–60	3–6	10 mg q 3–6 h	Similar to pentazocine except fewer hallucinations
	Pentazocine (Talwin)	Oral	150	90–120	2–4	50 mg q 3–4 h	When given to patient chronically on pure opiate agonist, may precipitate withdrawal symptoms
		Parenteral	30	30–60	2–4	30 mg q 3–4 h	May cause hallucinations

*Equianalgesic dose refers to the dose of opiate that would produce the same amount of analgesia as 10 mg of parenterally administered morphine. It does not represent dose recommendations.

†Standard dosage may be excessive in patients with certain conditions.

CNS, central nervous system; MAO, monoamine oxidase; IV, intravenous.

From Ariani K, Gaeta RR: The management of preoperative pain and anxiety. In Niederhuber J, ed: Fundamentals of Surgery. Stamford, CT, Appleton Lange, 1998, pp 40–50.

Table 7–3. ADJUVANT MEDICATIONS

Drugs, by Classification	Indications	Comments

Antidepressant
  Amitriptyline
  Imipramine
  Mianserin
  Clomipramine
  Doxepin
	Chronic pain, neuropathic pain associated with neuropathy and headache	Improves sleep, may improve appetite

Anticonvulsant
  Carbamazepine
  Phenytoin
  Valproate
  Clonazepam
	Neuropathic pain with paroxysmal character	Start slowly, increase gradually while observing for side effects

Membrane stabilizer
  Lidocaine
  2-Chloroprocaine
  Tocainide
  Mexiletine
	Neuropathic pain associated with peripheral neuropathy	Efficacy of oral preparations is not established

Modified from Brose WG, Gaeta RR, Spiegel D: Neuropsychiatric aspects of pain management. In Yudofsky SC, Haels RE, eds: Textbook of Neuropsychiatry, 3rd ed. Washington, DC, American Psychiatric Press, 1997, pp 349–380.

effect. It has shown efficacy in cancer and chronic pain states, particularly in neuropathic pain. It is in the category of neuropathic pain that is of most interest because so few alternatives exist for this population of patients.

Interventional Techniques

Injection therapies can be an important component of pain management in both a diagnostic and therapeutic fashion.[9] Local anesthetic injections with and without steroids can aid in the healing process of various musculoskeletal problems. The pain of localized tender points can temporarily be relieved with direct injection of local anesthetic. Specific nerve blocks with local anesthetics, when combined with active physical therapy, can be of tremendous benefit, particularly in cases of sympathetically maintained pain. The temporary relief afforded by these blocks allows aggressive rehabilitation to proceed when other medications and treatments have plateaued. Sympathetic blockade of the stellate ganglion or the lumbar sympathetic chain is a safe and reasonable option in the treatment of reflex sympathetic dystrophy or causalgia of the upper or lower extremities.

Therapies directed to the neuraxis represent the most invasive of the pain management strategies. Opioids can be delivered to the epidural or subarachnoid space to provide excellent analgesia at a fraction of an equivalent parenteral dose. Delivery of opioids directly to the site of action can have an overall beneficial effect by reducing the total dose and thus limiting side effects. This represents an invasive approach to management, but for the properly selected patient, it offers the possibility of relief where other techniques have failed. Besides opioids, electrical current can be applied to the spinal cord via a spinal cord stimulator that is implanted as an entirely self-contained system under the skin. Patients with radicular back pain and even some

with failed back syndrome have derived benefit from this technique. Patients who require this level of intervention are obvious candidates for a multidisciplinary pain center with the demonstrated ability to perform the procedure and to follow up on these patients adequately.

Physical Therapy

Physical therapy is either active or passive. Passive therapies tend to be modality oriented (e.g., ultrasound, muscle stimulation, and massage therapies). Patients favor this form of treatment. If a patient is to return to higher levels of productivity and function, however, an active program that emphasizes stretching, strengthening, and an overall conditioning program is more important. The educational component of physical therapy deserves equal emphasis. The lifelong body and joint protection exercises are key to sustaining physical capacity.

Psychological Therapies

Interventions from behavioral medicine play a key role in the sustained effort required to help a patient recover from debilitating illness. Although traditional individual counseling is appropriate in some cases, other cognitive-behavioral strategies, such as biofeedback, self-hypnosis, and relaxation techniques, are useful approaches toward patient self-management. Many times, these techniques are a less threatening way in which to expose patients to the mind-body connection. After accepting these techniques, many patients find it easier to proceed with more traditional psychological interventions or even group therapy that serves as an educational tool. Patients actually learn to *live with the pain*.

Comorbid depression is a significant impediment to well-being and productivity and when present must be addressed directly. Patients many times protest that they are understandably depressed related to an injury, which, if treated, would allow the depression to resolve. The depression impedes the patient's progress and thus may require medical management. Because many of the antidepressants also have analgesic properties, patients may be more likely to take them when they are introduced in this fashion. For more recalcitrant cases, referral to a psychiatrist for medicine optimization is warranted.

CONCLUSION

The management of patients with pain requires an understanding of the underlying neuroanatomy and physiology. This knowledge base allows the practitioner to apply therapies rationally and even to incorporate new treatments as they become available. More important is an overall approach that recognizes the patient as a whole and complex being and uses various tools to return patients to optimal function and productivity.

Pain management centers that adhere to a multidisciplinary and rehabilitative approach can be a useful resource for both the patient and the referring physician. The Appendix provides specific recommendations for older patients prepared as clinical practice guidelines by the American Geriatrics Society Panel on Chronic Pain in Older Persons, which are useful for all age groups.

REFERENCES

1. Bonica JJ: Definitions and taxonomy of pain. In Bonica JJ, ed: The Management of Pain, Vol 2, Philadelphia, Lea & Febiger, 1988, pp 18–27.

2. Brose WG, Gaeta RR, Spiegel D: Neuropsychiatric aspects of pain management. In Yudofsky SC, Haels RE, eds: Textbook of Neuropsychiatry, 3rd ed. Washington, DC, American Psychiatric Press, 1997, pp 349–380.

3. Howard LF, ed: Pain. New York, McGraw-Hill, 1987.

4. Loeser JD, Egan KJ, eds: Managing the Chronic Pain Patient. New York, Raven Press, 1989.

5. American Psychiatric Association: Diagnostic and Statistical Manual of Mental Disorders, 4th ed. Washington, DC, American Psychiatric Association, 1994.

6. Russo CM, Brose WG: Chronic pain. Ann Rev Med 49:123–133, 1998.

7. The Medical Letter. Drugs for pain. 40:1033, 1998.

8. Ariani K, Gaeta RR: The management of preoperative pain and anxiety. In Niederhuber J, ed: Fundamentals of Surgery. Stamford, CT, Appleton Lange, 1998, pp 40–50.

9. Cousins MJ, Bridenbaugh PO, eds: Neural Blockade, 2nd ed. Philadelphia, Lippincott, 1988.

Specific Recommendations for Management of Chronic Pain[*]

I. All patients with diminished quality of life as a result of chronic pain are candidates for pharmacologic therapy.

II. The least invasive route of administration should be used (this is usually the oral route).

III. Fast-onset, short-acting analgesic drugs should be used for episodic (i.e., chronic recurrent or noncontinuous) pain.

IV. Acetaminophen is the drug of choice for relieving mild to moderate musculoskeletal pain. The maximum dosage of acetaminophen should not exceed 4000 mg per day.

V. NSAIDs should be used with caution.

  A. High-dose, long-term NSAID use should be avoided.

  B. When used chronically, NSAIDs should be used as needed, rather than daily or around the clock.

  C. Short-acting NSAIDs may be preferable to avoid dose accumulation.

  D. NSAIDs should be avoided in patients with abnormal renal function.

  E. NSAIDs should be avoided in patients with a history of peptic ulcer disease.

  F. NSAIDs should be avoided in patients with a bleeding diathesis.

  G. The use of more than one NSAID at a time should be avoided.

  H. Ceiling dose limitations should be anticipated (i.e., maximum dose may be unattainable because of toxicity or may be accompanied by lack of efficacy).

VI. Opioid analgesic drugs may be helpful for relieving moderate to severe pain, especially nociceptive pain.

  A. Opioids for episodic (i.e., chronic recurrent or noncontinuous) pain should be prescribed as needed, rather than around the clock.

  B. Long-acting or sustained-release analgesic preparations should be used only for continuous pain.

    1. Breakthrough pain should be identified and treated by the use of fast-onset, short-acting preparations. Breakthrough pain includes the following three types:

      a. *End-of-dose failure* is the result of decreased blood levels of analgesic with concomitant increase in pain before the next scheduled dose.

      b. *Incident pain* is usually caused by activity that can be anticipated and pretreated.

      c. *Spontaneous pain*, common with neuropathic pain, is often fleeting and difficult to predict.

    2. Titration should be conducted carefully.

      a. Titration should be based on the persistent need for and use of medications for break-through pain.

      b. Titration should be based on the pharmacokinetics and pharmacodynamics of specific drugs in the older person and the propensity for drug accumulation.

      c. The potential adverse effects of opioid analgesic medication should be anticipated and prevented or treated promptly.

    3. Constipation should be prevented.

      a. A prophylactic bowel regimen should be initiated with commencement of analgesic therapy.

      b. Bulking agents should be avoided.

      c. Adequate fluid intake should be encouraged.

      d. Exercise, ambulation, and physical activities should be encouraged.

      e. Bowel function should be evaluated with every follow-up visit.

      f. Rectal examination and disimpaction should occur before use of motility agents.

---

*Reprinted with permission from American Geriatrics Society Panel of Chronic Pain in Older Persons: The management of chronic pain in older persons. J Am Geriatr Soc 46:635–651, 1998.

g. An osmotic, stimulant, or motility agent should be prescribed, if necessary, to provide regular bowel evacuation.

h. Motility agents should not be used if signs or symptoms of obstruction are present.

i. If fecal impaction is present, it should be relieved by enema or manual removal.

4. Mild sedation and impaired cognitive performance should be anticipated when opioid analgesic drugs are initiated. Until tolerance for these effects has developed:

a. Patients should be instructed not to drive.

b. Patients and caregivers should be cautioned about the potential for falls and accidents.

c. Monitoring for profound sedation, unconsciousness, or respiratory depression (defined as a respiratory rate of <8 per minute or oxygen saturation of <90%) should occur during rapid, high-dose escalations. Naloxone should be used carefully to avoid abrupt reversal of pain and autonomic crisis.

5. Severe nausea may need to be treated with antiemetic medications, as needed.

a. Mild nausea usually resolves spontaneously in a few days.

b. If nausea persists, a trial of an alternative opioid may be appropriate.

c. Antiemetic drugs should be chosen from those with the lowest side-effect profiles in older persons.

6. Severe pruritus may be treated with antihistamine medications.

7. Myoclonus may be relieved by the use of an alternate opioid drug or clonazepam in severe cases.

VII. Fixed-dose combinations (e.g., acetaminophen and opioid) may be used for mild to moderate pain.

A. Maximum recommended dose should not be exceeded to minimize toxicity of acetaminophen or NSAID.

B. Ceiling effect should be anticipated (i.e., maximum dose may be reached without full efficacy because of limits imposed by toxicity of acetaminophen or an NSAID).

VIII. Patients taking analgesic medications should be monitored closely.

A. Patients should be re-evaluated frequently for drug efficacy and side effects during initiation, titration, or any change in dose of analgesic medications.

B. Patients should be re-evaluated on a regular basis for drug effectiveness and side effects throughout long-term analgesic drug maintenance.

1. Patients on long-term opioid therapy should be evaluated periodically for inappropriate or even dangerous drug-use patterns.

a. The clinician should watch for indications of the use of medications prescribed for other persons or of illicit drug use (the latter being very rare in this population).

b. The clinician should ask about prescriptions for opioids from other physicians.

c. The clinician should watch for signs of narcotic use for inappropriate indications (e.g., anxiety, depression).

d. Requests for early refills should include evaluation of tolerance, progressive disease, or inappropriate behavioral factors.

e. These evaluations need to take place with the same medical equanimity accompanying similar evaluations for long-term management of other potentially risky medications (i.e., antihypertensive medications) in order not to burden the patient with excessive worry or unnecessary fears, or to promote "opiophobia."

2. Patients on long-term NSAIDs should be periodically monitored for gastrointestinal blood loss, renal insufficiency, and other drug-drug or drug-disease interactions.

IX. Non-opioid analgesic medications may be appropriate for some patients with neuropathic pain and some other chronic pain syndromes.

A. Carbamazepine is the medication of choice for trigeminal neuralgia.

B. Agents with the lowest side-effect profiles should be chosen preferentially.

C. Agents may be used alone but often are more helpful when used in combination and to augment other pain management strategies.

D. Therapy should begin with the lowest possible doses and increased slowly because of the potential for toxicity of many agents.

E. Patients should be monitored closely for side effects.

F. Clinical endpoints should be decreased pain, increased function, improvements in mood and sleep, not decreased drug dose.

Chapter **8**

Helping Patients to Learn to Live with Arthritis

Kate Lorig

The treatment of patients with arthritis can be likened to a three-legged stool. One leg consists of medical treatments, the second surgical interventions, and the third self-management. Most patients with arthritis must live with their disease for the rest of their lives. In fact, they are often told that they "must learn to live with it." Although this statement is true, it is often all the self-management advice that is ever offered. This chapter discusses how the primary care physician can work with arthritis patients to prepare them to take on the necessary self-management tasks.

WHAT IS SELF-MANAGEMENT?

Self-management is all the activities that a patient must do on a day-to-day basis to live with a chronic illness. To a great extent, the quality of a patient's life is determined by how well he or she undertakes these tasks. Some tasks, such as taking medication, are fairly simple. Others, such as maintaining an exercise program, are more difficult. The most difficult tasks involve making daily decisions, problem solving, and working effectively with health care providers. Corbin and Strauss[1] have formulated three sets of tasks for patients with chronic conditions:

- Patients must actively deal with the medical demands of the condition. These include visiting with health professionals, complying with medication schedules, and such other activities as maintaining an exercise program or a special diet.
- Patients must give up or alter important life activities. These can range from retiring, from employment or changing jobs to changing the way the family gathers for festive occasions. Everyone has many roles in life, from worker to grandmother to weekend golfer. Having arthritis often means that these roles change. Because quality of life is often closely tied to these life roles, changes resulting from arthritis can be devastating.
- Patients with arthritis must come to terms with the emotional sequelae of having arthritis. Most patients with arthritis have some disease-related emotions, including anger, fear, depression, and frustration. These

emotions are the result of worries about the future, inability to continue valued activities, or alterations in expectations about life.

The impact of arthritis on a patient's life is only loosely related to the severity of the disease. Some people who begin to get Heberden's nodes find this a devastating experience, whereas others with severe rheumatoid arthritis (RA) can cope with crippling.

EFFICACY OF SELF-MANAGEMENT

To date, there are nearly 150 peer-reviewed articles on the effectiveness of arthritis patient education.[2, 3] In fact, the arthritis patient education literature is among the best for any chronic disease. In the mid-1970s, Congress passed the National Arthritis Act creating multipurpose arthritis centers in academic institutions. This act also mandated that each center was to create and evaluate educational programs. This was the impetus for many of today's self-management programs.

Arthritis patient education programs are usually evaluated according to the changes that occur in health behaviors, such as exercise; health status; pain and disability; psychological status, such as anxiety and depression; and health care utilization. The conclusions from a meta-analysis suggest that "patient education interventions provide additional benefits and are 20% to 30% as great as the effects of NSAID (nonsteroidal anti-inflammatory drug) treatment for pain relief in osteoarthritis (OA) and RA, and 40% as great as NSAID treatment for improvement in functional ability in RA."[4] Although there are many different effective behavioral programs for arthritis, some of the best are presented through voluntary arthritis organizations such as the Arthritis Foundations in the United States and Australia, the Arthritis Society in Canada, and Arthritis Care in Great Britain. To find or start local programs, a physician can contact the nearest voluntary agency, chapter, or branch. Because self-management is such an important part of arthritis treatment, some specific self-management tools are examined in this chapter.

PAIN MANAGEMENT

Pain is the most common presenting complaint of patients with arthritis and the number one reason that arthritis patients seek the help of a physician. There is a common belief that pain and disability are closely correlated. This is not entirely true. In studies of large populations, it has been found that up to a certain point people can have pain with little or no disability.[5] Then a small increase in pain can cause a loss of function. The reverse is also true. Sometimes a small reduction in pain can result in large lessening in disability. For this reason, even a small reduction in pain can have a marked influence on one's quality of life.

It is also often assumed that the pain in RA is greater than that suffered by patients with OA. Many studies, however, have demonstrated that although patients with RA have more disability, the amount of pain reported by OA and RA patients is generally the same. Thus, in all patients with arthritis, pain is a symptom that needs to be taken seriously and should be treated behaviorally as well as with medicine and surgery (see Chapter 7). The first step in behavioral pain management is to help the patient understand the nature of the pain. There are four important messages.

1. *The pain of arthritis has several origins.* The disease causes pain, either because of inflamed joints as in RA or from the loss of cartilage and the resulting bone rubbing against bone as in OA. Pain also comes from deconditioning. When a joint is damaged, the surrounding muscles contract in an attempt to compensate for the lack of joint stability. These contracted muscles, especially in a deconditoned patient, cause pain. It is rather like making a tight fist and holding it for many minutes. Pain is also made worse by worry or depression. If patients think that arthritis pain foretells life-altering disability, the pain is often worse.

2. *Hurt does not necessarily mean harm.* Many people with arthritis are afraid to exercise or take part in normal activities if they have pain. They believe that the pain means they are causing themselves permanent medical harm. Many patients need to be reassured that even if an activity is painful, it does not mean they are causing accelerated joint deterioration.

3. *Treat minor pain before it becomes intense.* Once pain becomes severe, it becomes much more difficult to control. Thus, early use of pain medications and behavioral pain management techniques is most effective. People have a tendency to ignore pain until it is so severe that it interferes with activity. Patients should be advised to use pain management techniques and medication early (see Chapter 7).

4. *Much can be done to lessen pain of arthritis.* Studies provide evidence of the success of behavioral pain management for patients with arthritis. This does not mean that patients should not be given medicine or offered surgery when appropriate. Rather it means that the best arthritis pain management includes behavioral as well as medical interventions.

EXERCISE

The single most important self-management activity for patients with arthritis is exercise (see also Chapter 10). Numerous studies have now documented the importance of endurance exercise for patients with both OA and RA.[6–10] Beyond general fitness, there are many benefits, including the reduction in pain, that comes from strengthening weak muscles to reduction in depression and improved sleep. The following are general exercise instructions, which can be given to all arthritis patients regardless of age, type of arthritis, or severity of disease. The exception is patients with infectious arthritis or those now in the midst of an active flare of inflammatory arthritis.

Ask patients how far or how long they can now walk, swim, or bicycle. Wherever patients are at that point in time is where they must begin. For example, if a patient can walk only 1 minute or walk only across the room, he or she should do this once an hour while awake. If patients can walk 5 minutes, they should walk 5 minutes once or twice a day. In all cases, exercise should be done 4 to 5 days a week. The goal for patients with arthritis is the same as that suggested by the Surgeon General for all Americans—120 minutes of activity a week.[11] Most arthritis patients cannot start at this level. By starting where they are and then adding 10% to 20% a week, most arthritis patients can reach this goal within a few months. The total time exercising is more important than the duration of any one exercise session.

Patients worry that pain when exercising may mean that they are causing irreversible damage to joints. The primary care provider can allay this fear by explaining that exercise will not be pain-free. If, however, patients have more pain after exercising than before starting, they have worked too much and should cut back. It is also important to tell patients that they may make themselves sore and stiff, similar to anyone who exercises too much. They will not, however, cause accelerated permanent damage.

Many patients enjoy water exercise, and this is to be encouraged, although there does not seem to be any special benefit beyond that found with walking.[12] The one caveat is that no matter what the exercise program, it should take place 4 to 5 days a week. Thus, a single water exercise class a week does not offer maximal benefit. For these patients, cross-training should be encouraged: water exercise once or twice a week supplemented by walking or bicycling.

If patients enjoy exercise classes, they should be encouraged to go to fitness classes at senior centers. These do not have to be special arthritis classes. The physician should remind patients of the rule that if they have more pain when they have finished than before they start, they should cut back. It may be that at the beginning, patients can take part only in 10 to 15 minutes of the class. There are several excellent arthritis exercise books and videotapes.[13,14] In addition, arthritis exercise classes are offered by the Arthritis Foundation throughout the United States and by voluntary arthritis organizations in other countries.

Range-of-motion and strengthening exercises are also recommended. Patients may learn these from the aforementioned books and videos, from the Arthritis Self-Help Program, or exercise-specific programs offered by the Arthritis Foundation or from a physical therapist. When making a referral to a physical therapist, it should be with the understanding that the patient will be taught an exercise regimen that can be carried out at home. They should also be taught how to increase or decrease their exercise depending on the trends and tempo of the disease.

FATIGUE MANAGEMENT

After pain, fatigue is the most common complaint of many patients with arthritis. Although some types of arthritis, such as RA, can contribute to fatigue, in many cases, fatigue is due to deconditioning, poor nutrition, poor sleep hygiene, medications, boredom, or depression. All of these should be explored when the patient is experiencing fatigue. Too often, patients are told to rest, or to "take it easy." Although this may sometimes be good advice, at other times it is counterproductive. Patients should be encouraged to seek a variety of means to deal with their fatigue.

Self-management of fatigue may include taking part in an exercise program as discussed previously. Sleep hygiene can be improved by having the patient go to bed and, most important, get up at the same times every day. A second tip is to use the bed only for sleeping and sex, not for other activities, such as reading. For the most part, naps should be avoided. If patients want to rest during the day, the physician should suggest that they watch TV, read, or practice cognitive pain management techniques such as visualization or meditation. If evening pain interferes with sleep, patients can try taking pain medication before going to bed, such as over-the-counter time-released aspirin or acetaminophen. In some cases, patients might benefit from taking a low dose of a tricyclic antidepressant before going to bed. There are also tricks for making the bed more comfortable, such as the use of sheepskin or a feather bed under the bottom sheet or a heated electric mattress pad. Patients with neck problems can purchase small neck support pillows from back or travel stores.

COGNITIVE PAIN MANAGEMENT

Cognitive pain management is a term that covers a whole range of techniques from simple distraction to mindfulness meditation. The common denominator of all these techniques is that they are cognitive rather than physical. For this reason, both patients and health professionals are sometimes skeptical about their effectiveness. Research has shown the effectiveness of cognitive techniques, especially for pain management.[15] There is little literature comparing the relative effectiveness of the various techniques. The following is a brief overview of some of the more common cognitive techniques and some suggestions for their use.

Jacobson Progressive Muscle Relaxation

In the Jacobson progressive muscle relaxation[16] technique, patients are taught to consciously relax tense muscles. This is done by having patients first tense then relax various muscle groups usually starting with the feet and progressing toward the head. In reality, this is a combination of a physical and cognitive modality, but it is usually classified as cognitive. It is especially useful for patients who are skeptical about cognitive techniques; most patients can easily understand the differences they feel when muscles are tense as opposed to relaxed.

Distraction

Because it is difficult to concentrate on more than one thing at a time, mild-to-moderate pain can often be relieved by distraction. This is also a good technique to use for short painful activities and dealing with insomnia. Each individual can use his or her favorite technique. The crucial element is to keep the mind occupied. The following are a few samples of distraction techniques.

- Name all the countries in Europe and their capitols.
- Go through the alphabet naming an animal, a city, or an airline for each letter.
- Think of all the cities, states, or countries that you have visited.
- Name all your relatives.
- Count backward from 100 by 3s.

Guided Imagery

Guided imagery is usually done by having patients listen to an audiotape, which guides them through a series of pleasant, relaxing experience, such as a walk along the beach, a visit to a country garden, or a walk in a cool forest. The tapes are usually 10 to 20 minutes long and help the person listening take a mini-vacation, in the midst of a busy or stressful day. Guided imagery is also useful for helping someone first get to sleep or return to sleep after awakening in the middle of the night. Because guided imagery quiets the mind, patients can also use it when they are resting. Use of guided imagery insures that both the mind and the body get needed rest.

A similar technique is semiguided imagery. With this technique, the patient is cued to imagine a pleasant place or time and to fill in all the details. It differs from guided imagery in that it is much more personal with patients providing their own images. Patients often have a definite preference for the type imagery techniques.

Guided and semiguided imagery are especially good for stress reduction. They can also be used to lower pain levels by making the imagery pain specific. For example, patients are guided to think of their pain as a color (usually red), then to change it to a cooler color, such as pink to violet and then to blue. They might also be guided to think of the pain as another sensation, such as numbness. This pain-specific imagery is more difficult to master but is helpful for many patients.

Mindfulness Meditation

Mindfulness meditation has been studied and disseminated by Kabot-Zin at the University of Massachusetts School of Medicine. This form of meditation, adapted from Theravadin Buddhism, asks patients to concentrate on their breathing. There is a growing research base on the effectiveness of this technique for pain management.[17–19] Mindfulness pain and stress reduction courses are generally taught in 10 weekly sessions and are widely available. Mindfulness meditation may be one of the more powerful cognitive pain management techniques. Its only drawback is that it takes an initial commitment of 45 minutes a day for 10 weeks. In contrast to some of the other techniques, benefits are not immediately apparent. Continued practice, however, appears to produce significant long-term benefits.

DEPRESSION MANAGEMENT

These are the voices of people with arthritis:

"The worst part for me is social isolation."
"I get very sad at times when I can't do what I once did like lift weights twice a week."
"I sometimes feel like the song of the little mermaid, who wishes she was like the people on land."

Depression is an often overlooked aspect of arthritis. From our experience and that of others, many arthritis patients are subclinically depressed.[20] This is true for both OA and RA patients. Most of these patients do not need medication or formal psychological counseling but can benefit from recognition of their depression along with some suggestions on how to make it less burdensome.

Exercise, especially endurance exercise as described earlier, is an excellent antidepressant. It usually gets people out of the house, gives them confidence in their physical ability, improves their sleep, and helps with weight reduction. In addition, it may increase endorphin levels.

Socialization is another antidepressant. This can take a variety of forms from talking with friends and family on the telephone to attending formal arthritis support groups. There is also evidence that people with chronic disease benefit from helping others; patients may be urged to take up a volunteer activity that interests them.

Finally, having patients become conscious of the messages they give themselves can help depression. An example is the patient who wakes up in the morning thinking that she has pain so surely her whole day will be ruined. The result is that she decides to stay in bed. A similar patient wakes ups and has pain but thinks that a warm shower will get her started and then she can get on with the things she wants to do. The difference in these two patients has nothing to do with their arthritis. Rather their activity level is a result of the messages that they give themselves. If patients can be taught to identify negative thinking, they can also be taught consciously to change their thought patterns. This is a successful technique for dealing with mild depression.

WEIGHT MANAGEMENT

Excess weight predisposes patients to osteoarthritis of the lower extremities.[21–23] Thus, weight reduction can often help arthritis pain and disability. Although weight loss is difficult to achieve, there are a few things that the physician can do to help the process. First, the physician can suggest to the patient that he or she begin by losing only a small amount of weight, say 4 to 5 pounds in a month. Having a bathroom scale is essential. Many patients can achieve this weight loss with only moderate changes in diet accompanied with starting an exercise program. The important factor is to set a goal that the patient can easily achieve. Once the first goal is accomplished, patients have more confidence in continuing the program.

SHORT SUGGESTIONS FOR HELPING PATIENTS BEGIN SELF-MANAGEMENT

After suggesting a behavioral intervention, a patient should be asked what he or she wants to do in the next week or two: for example, not eat between meals for 4 days a week or walk 15 minutes 3 days a week. The answer should be behavior specific, not general such as *lose weight* or *exercise*. Then the patient should be asked how certain he or she is that the behavior (on a scale of 0, totally uncertain, to 10, totally certain) will be carried out. If the number is 7 or above, there is a good chance that the behaviors will take place. If it is below 7, the physician can ask what the problems might be and renegotiate until the patient is more sure that the behaviors can be accomplished. Patients can be asked to make small changes, the physician should limit suggestions to the most important changes. When faced with many new activities or big changes, there is a tendency for patients to do nothing. Whenever possible, the physician should help the patient make a firm decision. The physician should present alternatives and let the patient make the choice or at least have the opportunity to say that he or she wants the physician to make the choice.

Patients should be referred to chapters of the Arthritis Foundation and other arthritis-related resources. They should take a self-help course or participate in an exercise program. Self-management interventions take time both to teach and to learn. Often, this teaching cannot be accomplished in the busy office practice. The recommendation of the physician is often the motivation patients need to participate in these programs.

REFERENCES

1. Corbin J, Strauss A: Unending Work and Care: Managing Chronic Illness at Home. San Francisco, Jossey-Bass Publishers, 1988.
2. Lorig K, Konkol L, González V: Arthritis patient education: A review of the literature. Patient Educ. Counsel 10:207–252, 1987.
3. Hirano P, Laurent D, Lorig K: Arthritis patient education studies, 1987–1991: A review of the literature. Patient Educ Counsel 24:9–54, 1994.
4. Superio-Cabuslay E, Ward M, Lorig K: Patient education interventions in osteoarthritis and rheumatoid arthritis: A meta-analytic comparison with non-steroidal anti-inflammatory drug treatment. Arthritis Care Res 9:292–301, 1996.
5. Von Korff M, Ormel J, Keefe F, Dworkin S: Grading the severity of chronic pain. Pain 50:133–149, 1992.
6. Ettinger WJ, Burns R, Messier S, et al: A randomized trial comparing aerobic exercise and resistance exercise with a health education program in older adults with knee osteoarthritis. The Fitness Arthritis and Seniors Trial (FAST). JAMA 277:25–31, 1997.
7. Kovar P, Allegrante J, MacKenzie C, et al: Supervised fitness walking in patients with osteoarthritis of the knee. Ann Rheum Dis 116:535–539, 1992.
8. Minor M, Lane N: Recreational exercise in arthritis. Rheum Dis Clin North Am 22:563–577, 1996.
9. Minor M: Exercise in the management of osteoarthritis of the knee and hip. Arthritis Care Res 7:198–204, 1994.
10. Minor MA, Brown JD: Exercise maintenance on persons with arthritis after participation in a class experience. Health Educ Q 20:83–95, 1993.
11. Centers for Disease Control and Health: Surgeon General's report on physical activity and health. JAMA 276:522, 1996.
12. Minor M, Hewett J, Webel R, et al: Efficacy of physical conditioning exercise in patients with rheumatoid arthritis and osteoarthritis. Arthritis Rheum 23:1396–1405, 1989.
13. Good moves for every body [Exercise videotape, 60 min.]. Columbia, University of Missouri, Arthritis Center, 1993.
14. Sayce V: Exercise can beat arthritis: Getting stronger [video]. New York, View Video, 1997.
15. Fernandez E, Turk D: The utility of cognitive coping strategies for altering pain perception: A meta-analysis. Pain 38:123–135, 1989.
16. Jacobson E: Progressive Relaxation. Chicago, University of Chicago Press, 1938.
17. Roth B, Creaser T: Mindfulness meditation-based stress reduction: Experience with a bilingual inner-city program. Nurse Pract 22:150, 1997.
18. Miller J, Fletcher K, Kabat-Zinn J: Three-year follow up and clinical implications of a mindfulness meditation-based stress reduction intervention in the treatment of anxiety disorders. Gen Hosp Psychiatry 17:192–200, 1995.
19. Astin J: Stress reduction through mindfulness meditation: Effects on psychological symptomatology, sense of control, and spiritual experiences. Psychother Psychosom 66:97–106, 1997.
20. Dexter P, Hayes J: Depression in osteoarthritis. In Brandt K, Doherty M, Lohmander LS, eds: Osteoarthritis. New York, Oxford University Press, 1998 pp 338–349.
21. Felson D: Does excess weight cause osteoarthritis and, if so, why? Ann Rheum Dis 55:668–670, 1996.
22. Felson D, Zhang Y, Anthony J, et al: Weight loss reduced the risk of symptomatic knee osteoarthritis in women: The Framingham Study. Ann Intern Med 116:535–539, 1992.
23. Felson D, Zhang Y, Hannan M, et al: Risk factors for incident radiographic knee osteoarthritis in the elderly: The Framingham Study. Arthritis Rheum 40:728–733, 1997.

Chapter **9**

Drugs That Relieve Pain And Inflammation

James F. Fries

Drug management of chronic arthritis has changed significantly. Data from Arthritis, Rheumatism, and Aging Medical Information System (ARAMIS), the large national arthritis data bank, and other sources have helped to provide evidence-based approaches to management of serious arthritic conditions. The primary care provider should understand the implications of two major revolutions in arthritis patient management, one in rheumatoid arthritis (RA) and one in osteoarthritis (OA). The strategies for selection of medications have changed radically from those promoted only a few years ago.

First, in RA, the old *therapeutic pyramid* has been replaced. This approach initiated treatment with aspirin and nonsteroidal anti-inflammatory drugs (NSAIDs) and later moved gradually, in the most seriously affected patients, toward treatment with agents that had the capability of modifying the disease progression. The new approach is a disease-modifying antirheumatic drug (DMARD)–based strategy,in which treatment with the more effective agents (DMARDs) is initiated as early as possible in the disease, and DMARDs are used consistently throughout the entire course of illness. The new strategy has been termed *inverting the pyramid.*

The old strategy was based on three postulates: (1) that rheumatoid arthritis was a benign disease and hazardous therapies should be used only reluctantly, (2) that NSAIDs were generally nontoxic, and (3) that DMARDs were extraordinarily toxic and should be reserved for only the most seriously affected patients. Each of these premises is wrong. RA is a serious disease that results in severe disability in the majority of patients treated under the old therapeutic pyramid strategy and has a mortality rate double that of the general population. NSAIDs, as illustrated subsequently, are a toxic class of therapeutic agents and need to be used with caution. Finally, DMARDs have toxicities roughly equivalent to NSAIDs and are far less toxic than earlier estimates suggested.

A consequence of this new paradigm is that RA, when managed for optimal long-term outcome, requires monitoring and sequencing of drug therapy by a physician familiar with the use of DMARDs. Usually, this is a rheumatologist, and early referral is essential for optimal long-term patient outcome in all except the most

mild of cases of RA. The primary care physician can work in synchrony with the rheumatologist in the carefully monitored care of patients.

In OA, the management revolution has been perhaps more mundane but no less revolutionary. Here again the movement is away from an NSAID-based treatment regimen toward one that emphasizes exercise and mild analgesia (preferably acetaminophen). If NSAIDs are employed, the strategy is to emphasize their use at analgesic (low) doses rather than at anti-inflammatory (high) doses. This radical management change has resulted from increasing evidence that judiciously employed exercise is a major therapeutic agent; that NSAIDs are toxic, particularly in the elderly, and that many patients get just as much pain relief from mild analgesics as from anti-inflammatory agents. Some data even suggest that anti-inflammatory treatment with NSAIDs may accelerate the process of degeneration of the articular cartilage.

This chapter outlines the repertoire of available and soon to be available medications, indicating the logical sequences of drugs appropriate for the major rheumatic diseases, and provides guidelines for referral of patients to the rheumatologist or orthopaedic surgeon. Drug therapy of arthritis is only one aspect of treatment. In many patients, it may not be even the most important aspect of management. Patient self-management, exercise, increase in personal self-efficacy, use of orthoses and devices, and many other approaches can be extremely important.

REPERTOIRE OF MEDICATIONS

Nonsteroidal Anti-Inflammatory Drugs

Many NSAIDs currently are available. The intense marketing efforts by the pharmaceutical industry sometimes can confuse rather than aid the choice of therapy. A few relatively straightforward considerations can ease this decision process. NSAIDs include aspirin and a number of different chemical categories of anti-inflammatory agents; in some countries, more than 40 agents are available. At last count, 17 NSAIDs were available in the United States.

As a class of medications, NSAIDs have clear toxicity, predominantly related to gastropathy induced by depletion of prostaglandins in the gastric mucosa. The major clinical events are peptic ulcers, perforation, and hemorrhage, most frequently in the stomach. The Food and Drug Administration (FDA) estimates 2% to 4% serious reactions for each year of exposure to these drugs, which cause 10,000 to 20,000 deaths yearly in the United States. ARAMIS estimates are a little lower but nevertheless indicate that in RA 1.6% of NSAID-treated patients are hospitalized each year for gastrointestinal causes, and approximately 10% of that number die.

Table 9–1 summarizes some of these data. In an ARAMIS study of 2747 patients with RA followed for nearly 10,000 patient-years, 116 were hospitalized for gastrointestinal causes, nearly all of these while taking NSAIDs. The relative serious risk of gastrointestinal toxicity for patients taking NSAIDs compared with those not taking NSAIDs is 5.2.[1] Other estimates suggest that more than one third of patients hospitalized for gastrointestinal bleeding have NSAID exposure as the cause.

All patients are not at equal risk for developing serious NSAID complications. Increasing age is the most important risk factor, and serious events are four times more likely to occur in those older than age 75 than in those younger than age 50. Other major risk factors are the dosage, the particular NSAID chosen, the concurrent use of prednisone (even in small doses), previous gastrointestinal symptoms or hemorrhage, and the degree of disability.[2]

All NSAIDs are not equal. Although the FDA and many experts had considered these drugs to be of roughly equivalent toxicity, data from ARAMIS and now many other sources indicate major differences in toxicity among NSAIDs. Table 9–2 lists toxicity levels for both DMARDs and NSAIDs. On the right, 10 NSAIDs are compared using a standardized toxicity index, which includes symptomatic side effects, laboratory abnormalities associated with drug use, and hospitalizations related to the medication.[3] Differences in toxicity

are twofold to threefold between the various NSAIDs. Meclofenamate, ketoprofen, tolmetin sodium, indomethacin, fenoprofen, and piroxicam consistently rank among the most toxic drugs in the various studies.[4] There seems little reason to employ these drugs unless a particularly effective response has been previously reported by the patient.

If aspirin were to be included in this table, it would be among the least toxic of medications because in clinical practice it is used in lower doses than in the earlier clinical trials comparing aspirin with NSAIDs. In contrast, the average prescribed dosage of NSAIDs has slowly increased over the years; this increase has undoubtedly made a major contribution to the frequency of NSAID gastropathy.[5] Data are accumulating slowly on the comparative toxicity of the combined use of an NSAID and misoprostol, a prostaglandin analogue, which is expected to have a relatively low toxicity index value, close to that of ibuprofen, nabumetone (Relafen), etodolac (Lodine), and meloxicam (Mobic).

Antacids and H_2 antagonists have been frequently prescribed in an attempt to reduce the risk of gastrointestinal toxicity from NSAIDs. Studies indicate that these agents can actually *increase* the risk of serious events by a substantial amount, probably by masking early warning symptoms and encouraging continued use, in higher doses, of a potentially toxic agent.[6] Misoprostol, a synthetic prostaglandin, has been shown to be useful in protecting against NSAID-induced gastropathy. If used together with any NSAID, it can reduce the risk of serious complications by one half. Problems with misoprostol include the additional cost of a second medication and sometimes diarrhea or other gastrointestinal symptoms related to the misoprostol itself. The proton pump inhibitor omeprazole was shown to be as efficacious as misoprostol in treating ulcers in patients receiving continuous NSAID therapy. During the 6-month maintenance period after initial treatment, there appeared to be a lower rate of relapse with omeprazole than with misoprostol, and it appeared to be better tolerated. Proton pump inhibitors appear to be useful when combined with NSAIDs to reduce the risks of complications.[9]

Since recognition of NSAID gastropathy, new drugs under development or entering the market have been designed to have lower toxicity. Discovery of two cyclooxygenase isozymes (COX-1 and COX-2) point a way toward designing safer NSAIDs. Inhibition of the COX-1 enzyme increases the risk for NSAID gastropathy and other side effects but does not decrease inflammation. Inhibition of COX-2 does not promote gastrointestinal injury but does reduce inflammation. Thus, development of *selective COX-2–inhibiting drugs* offers the possibility of good therapeutic benefit together with greatly reduced or even absent gastrointestinal side effects. The first drug to have these greatly decreased effects upon COX-1 is celecoxib (Celebrex); the second is rofecoxib (Vioxx). Celecoxib has been approved for OA at 200 mg daily and for RA at 200 or 400 mg daily, divided in two doses. It may have efficacy that approxi-

Table 9–1. ARAMIS DATA ON GASTROINTESTINAL HOSPITALIZATION IN PATIENTS WITH RHEUMATOID ARTHRITIS

No. patients	2747
Years of observation	9525
Years taking NSAID	6741
No. patients with gastrointestinal hospitalizations	116
Rate per year, overall (%)	1.22
No. patients taking NSAID	107
Rate per year while taking NSAID (%)	1.58
Relative risk for patients taking NSAID compared with those not taking NSAID	5.2

ARAMIS, Arthritis, Rheumatism, and Aging Medical Information System; NSAID, nonsteroidal anti-inflammatory drug.

From Fries JF: NSAID gastropathy. The second most deadly rheumatic disease? Epidemiology and risk appraisal. J Rheumatol 18 (suppl 28):6–10, 1991.

Table 9–2. COMPARATIVE TOXICITY OF DMARDS AND NSAIDS

Safety Rank	DMARD	Standardized Toxicity Index	NSAID	Standardized Toxicity Index
1			Salsalate	1.28
2	Hydroxychloroquine	1.38		
3			Ibuprofen	1.94
4			Naproxen	2.17
5			Sulindac	2.24
6	Intramuscular gold	2.27		
7			Piroxicam	2.52
8			Fenoprofen	2.95
9	Penicillamine	3.38		
10			Ketoprofen	3.45
11	Methotrexate	3.82		
12			Meclofenamate	3.86
13	Azathioprine	3.92		
14			Tolmetin	3.96
15			Indomethacin	3.99
16	Auranofin	5.25		

DMARDs, disease-modifying antirheumatic drugs; NSAIDs, nonsteroidal anti-inflammatory drugs.
From Fries JF: ARAMIS and toxicity measurements. J Rheumatol 22:995–997, 1995.

mates that of the other available NSAIDs but has a lower rate of causing serious gastrointestinal side effects (e.g., endoscopic ulcers) and no apparent antiplatelet effects. It is much more expensive than the other drugs; therefore, if a patient has been receiving expected and desired efficacy from other NSAIDs (with or without misoprostol or a proton pump inhibitor) without experiencing significant gastrointestinal symptoms or signs, there are few reasons to switch to the selective COX-2 inhibitors.

Rofecoxib, in doses of 12.5 to 25 mg/day, has been as effective as dicolfenac or ibuprofen in OA of the hip or knee, but further comparative studies of its adverse gastrointestinal effects are needed. Similar to traditional NSAIDs, celecoxib and rofecoxib both reduce renal prostaglandin synthesis and thus have the capacity to produce nephrotoxicity.

The following are some general rules for management of patients with NSAIDs:

1. Do not use NSAIDs if acetaminophen suffices.
2. Choose from among the least toxic NSAIDs.
3. Use the lowest dose that provides adequate relief.
4. Discontinue the agent periodically to determine whether it is actually effective; reinstitute treatment if a flare follows discontinuation.
5. Consider misoprostol or possibly a proton pump inhibitor if NSAID treatment is essential and the patient at high risk.
6. Be particularly wary in the older, sicker, disabled, or prednisone-taking patient.

Monitoring of patients for NSAID gastrointestinal toxicity is seldom emphasized because there is no evidence that monitoring procedures increase safety, and there may be expense and sometimes discomfort associated with the monitoring procedure itself. In contrast, identification of the high-risk patient (older, disabled, with gastrointestinal symptoms, and prednisone use) indicates the need for caution. Periodic endoscopic evaluation, hemoglobin checks, liver function tests, and stool guaiac tests have been occasionally recommended but lack evidence of effective prevention. Some of these tests are likely to be performed periodically in any event in the course of routine clinical practice.

Acetaminophen and Other Analgesics

Acetaminophen has become an increasingly important drug for the management of arthritis. In contrast to the NSAIDs, it has no anti-inflammatory activity. However, its analgesic effectiveness is often of a similar magnitude to that of the NSAIDs. Most importantly, toxicity is seldom a problem with acetaminophen; it is by far the safest drug used in arthritis management.

In OA, particularly of the knee, a number of studies have suggested the approximate equivalence of acetaminophen and NSAIDs for the average patient with OA.[7] OA patients are increasingly divided into two groups, one that responds effectively to acetaminophen and one that requires NSAIDs for symptomatic control. The logical strategy is to begin with acetaminophen, switching to NSAIDs if there is lack of effectiveness. Similarly, in RA, treatment centers on the use of DMARDs for the control of inflammation. Hence, the role for NSAIDs is increasingly that of analgesia only, and acetaminophen may often suffice.

The only serious concern of acetaminophen treatment has to do with overdosage, in which life-threatening hepatic necrosis can occur. Hepatic necrosis does not occur in doses of 4 gm or less per day except in rare instances in which heavy alcohol intake occurs at the same time. Hence, the drug should be used with great caution in those with heavy alcohol intake, but is not likely to be a problem in persons with moderate social drinking.

Stronger narcotic-containing analgesics are used too frequently in patients with arthritis. They should be used rarely and then only when no alternative approaches can be safely employed. In chronic arthritis, tolerance develops to narcotic medications (including codeine), there is frequently accentuation of depression by these drugs, and the symptoms of the disease may be masked while disease progression continues.

Disease-Modifying Antirheumatic Drugs

Table 9–1 compares the toxicity of several DMARDs in the left column using the toxicity index methodology.[3] The toxicity of DMARDs is roughly that of the NSAIDs, and there is a wide range of toxicity among DMARDs, with hydroxychloroquine (Plaquenil) being the safest. Sulfasalazine and minocycline, not listed, also have low toxicity.

DMARDs are the best pain relievers in inflammatory arthritis. This clinical paradox, in which pain is best relieved by drugs with no analgesic action whatsoever, is illustrated in Figure 9–1.[8] The average starting pain level for each drug is represented by the dot, and the point of the arrow represents the pain level 3 months later. The hatched areas represent the standard error of the change scores. Gold, penicillamine, and methotrexate (DMARDs) have the strongest effects on reducing subsequent pain, and the NSAID effects are relatively minor and statistically insignificant. The paradox is explained by the underlying pathophysiology of inflammatory arthritis. Inflammation results in pain and ultimately destruction of joint tissues. The drugs that best suppress inflammation, the DMARDs, therefore give the greatest pain relief.

PAIN BY DRUG

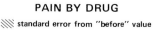

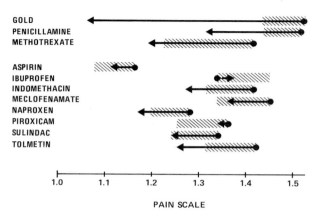

PAIN SCALE

Figure 9–1. Pain by drug: Pain is best relieved by drugs with no analgesic action whatsoever. (From Fries JF, Spitz PW, Mitchell DM, et al: Impact of specific therapy upon rheumatoid arthritis. Arthritis Rheum 29:620–627, 1986.)

HYDROXYCHLOROQUINE

Hydroxychloroquine is relatively safe and moderately effective. Dosage is 200 mg twice daily for most patients. Because of the long drug half-life (4 months), therapeutic effects occur gradually and are not seen before 6 to 12 weeks of treatment. The major side effect of concern is retinal damage, which occurs rarely, occurs gradually, and is reversible in the earlier stages. Hence, ophthalmologic examination with dilated pupils is recommended at baseline and subsequently at 6-month to yearly intervals.

SULFASALAZINE

Sulfasalazine chemically represents a combination of 5-aminosalicylic acid and sulfapyridine. The sulfonamide is poorly absorbed. The therapeutic benefit is due to the sulfonamide component. Dosage is four to six 500-mg tablets daily in divided doses. Effectiveness occurs over several weeks. Hypersensitivity reactions to sulfonamide may occur, and the drug should be avoided in those with a history of such reactions. Gastrointestinal side effects are common and disappear after changes in dose or drug discontinuation. The enteric-coated preparation may be better tolerated. Gastrointestinal hemorrhage and serious gastrointestinal complications are unusual.

MINOCYCLINE

A number of well-performed studies have shown a modest but definite effect of minocycline on RA, and the effect appears to be of the disease-modifying type. The mechanism of action probably involves inhibition of metalloproteases. Dosage is 100 mg twice daily. Side effects include hypersensitivity reactions, gastrointestinal upset, and sometimes thrush or other monilial complications.

AURANOFIN

Auranofin is *oral gold*. It is gradually effective in RA over a number of weeks as the gold is slowly absorbed and stored in the body. Efficacy is moderate but almost entirely limited to patients with early disease, particularly when the drug is used as the first DMARD. Dosage is 3 to 9 mg daily; diarrhea is extremely common and often severe at the 9-mg dose. Auranofin has a poor score on the toxicity rankings principally because of frequent diarrhea and early drug discontinuation. It is tolerated by many for only a short period of time. Few serious toxic reactions are observed, and it is most unusual for hospitalization to be required for a toxic auranofin reaction.

METHOTREXATE

Methotrexate has become the gold standard by which DMARD therapy is judged. It is effective, often dramatically so, over a period of a few weeks, and the effectiveness is often maintained for many years.

Because of the many nuances of treatment with methotrexate, it is recommended that a rheumatologist participate in the treatment decision-making process and subsequent follow-up. Dosage is weekly and ranges from 7.5 to 15 mg weekly in most patients. In some patients the dose must be increased to 20 mg weekly. A mistake in which methotrexate is given daily instead of weekly can have fatal consequences. Folic acid 1 mg/day is recommended to decrease side effects. The most worrisome complication is hepatotoxicity, initially manifested by moderate elevations in hepatic enzymes then slowly by hepatic fibrosis and cirrhosis over many years in a few patients. Hepatic enzyme tests should be checked at 6- to 8-week intervals. Occasional minor liver enzyme elevation is not a problem, but dosage should be lowered or the drug discontinued in patients who demonstrate consistently elevated enzyme levels. Moderation or abstinence from alcohol is recommended. If the drug is pushed despite liver function abnormalities, most clinicians suggest liver biopsy after 2 or 3 years and at similar intervals subsequently. Oral ulcers, gastrointestinal intolerance, pneumonitis, and occasional cytopenias can occur.

LEFLUNOMIDE (ARAVA)

Leflunomide, alone or in combination with methotrexate, is effective in rheumatoid arthritis. Used alone it is similar in both efficacy and toxicity to methotrexate, and it has been shown to reduce the rate of progression of bony erosions in this disease. Leflunomide should be of particular benefit in patients who cannot tolerate methotrexate. A loading dose of leflunomide of 100 mg is taken for three days, followed by 20 mg/day as the maintenance dose. Studies have found it to be effective, without added toxicity, when added to methotrexate in doses up to 15 mg/week in patients with RA who have responded to methotrexate, but without desired control of their synovitis. When taken in combination with methotrexate, the loading dose of leflunomide is 100 mg for two days followed by 10 mg/day and can be increased to the standard dose of 20 mg/day. Liver function tests are recommended at intervals of 6 to 12 weeks, at least for the first year or two of treatment. Its use should be supervised by a physician familiar with the drug.

INTRAMUSCULAR GOLD

Gold shots rival methotrexate in effectiveness but are much less convenient to use. The beneficial effects take 12 to 20 weeks to occur. The usual therapeutic sequence is to give 10 mg as a test dose, 25 mg a week later, then 50 mg weekly to a total of 1000 mg. At this point, granted effectiveness, the frequency of injections is decreased to every 2 weeks or every 3 weeks. Lower doses of *maintenance* therapy are often associated with gradual loss of effectiveness. Although intramuscular gold can cause severe cytopenias, nephrotic syndrome, severe dermatitis, and other major side effects, it is on average a surprisingly well-tolerated drug. This toleration is principally due to the tradition of careful monitoring of urine protein, white blood cell count, hemoglobin, and platelet count as well as questions about rash before each injection. With good monitoring, proteinuria is found quite commonly but disappears after drug discontinuation and seldom results in progression to the nephrotic syndrome. The nuances of treatment with intramuscular gold are such that it is recommended that a rheumatologist supervise this treatment.

D-PENICILLAMINE

Penicillamine is similar to intramuscular gold in effectiveness and in side-effect profile, although the effectiveness is much less predictable. Dosage is generally 250 mg daily for the first month; 500 mg the second month; 750 mg the third month; and, if required, 1000 mg daily for the fourth and subsequent months. Urine protein, hemogram, and chemical screening battery tests are generally performed monthly for 6 months then less frequently if the dose is stable. Effectiveness is generally seen after 3 or 4 months. An unusual side effect is a myasthenia gravis–like syndrome. It is appreciated now that D-penicillamine is one of the more toxic medications available for treatment of RA and is subsequently used much less frequently than other DMARDs.

AZATHIOPRINE (IMURAN)

Azathioprine is effective in some, but not all, patients with RA. Therapeutic effects occur slowly over a period of months. It can be effective treatment even in patients with long-standing disease. It is recommended that a rheumatologist participate in the care of the patients if treatment with azathioprine is undertaken. Major side effects involve reduction in blood elements or gastrointestinal problems, although there is some concern about late development of non-Hodgkin's lymphoma. Dosage is generally 50 to 150 mg/day. Monthly monitoring of hemogram and chemical screening batteries are required for the first several months and less frequently thereafter. Concurrent allopurinol treatment is absolutely contraindicated because it can increase azathioprine blood concentrations to dangerous levels.

CYCLOSPORINE

Cyclosporine, either alone or in combination with methotrexate, has been recommended as a treatment for progressive RA. It should be used only with concurrence of a rheumatologist and by physicians thoroughly skilled in its use. RA patients are particularly susceptible to decreases in renal function as a result of cyclosporine treatment, and doses need to be kept appropriately low (2.5 mg/kg) in most patients. Blood pressure and renal function should be carefully monitored.

PREDNISONE

Low-dose prednisone therapy, 5 to 7.5 mg daily, is used by many patients with RA, although most rheumatologists believe that it should be used sparingly. The paradox is short-term benefit, long-term harm. It acts as a DMARD over periods of up to a year, with slower progression of bony erosions. Clinical benefits, as appreciated by the patients, are immediate and often striking. The side effects are well known; over long periods, there is particular concern about osteopenia, vertebral fractures, cataracts, and acceleration of atherosclerotic development. Over periods of 5 to 10 years, patients on low-dose prednisone have been observed to have twice the frequency of serious NSAID gastrointestinal problems, twice the rate of development of disability, and twice the mortality rate, as contrasted with RA patients not taking prednisone. It is recommended that a rheumatologist participate in the decision to begin prednisone and in the concurrent use of other medications to decrease dosage and the likelihood of side effects.

ETANERCEPT (ENBREL)

This drug is particularly interesting because it is among the first of custom-designed, recombinant products that are targeted at an inflammatory mediator, tumor necrosis factor alpha (TNFα), that has been identified as a cytokine that drives production of other cytokines, such as Interleukin-1 and Interleukin-6 that induce and perpetuate inflammatory synovitis. Etanercept is a fusion protein, formed of a recombinant portion of the TNF receptor found on cells fused with the Fc portion of human IgG. The Fc fragment gives the molecule a sufficient half-life in vivo for it to bind circulating or extracellular TNFα. Its recommended dosage is 25 mg subcutaneously (as one gives insulin) twice weekly. It is recommended as an add-on drug to patients already taking methotrexate in full doses, but who have not, as yet, achieved the desired beneficial effect; it has clear-cut efficacy in these patients. Local injection site reactions have been the only clinical side effect, and most patients with such reactions are willing to continue the drug. Some patients develop antibodies against nuclear antigens, including DNA, but to date these have not been related to any clinical manifestations. As with leflunomide, etanercept can be used in patients to whom methotrexate cannot be given. Its cost is an impediment to wide usage, more than $10,000 per year.

INFLIXIMAB (REMICADE)

This monoclonal antibody to TNFα is approved for use in Crohn's disease, and soon should be approved for patients with RA. It must be given intravenously by a physician or by a closely supervised nurse in separated weekly doses. In Crohn's disease, repeat courses given many months after the first course have produced allergic manifestations, occasionally severe. These reactions are probably caused by the patient's immune reaction against the murine component of the monoclonal antibody.

Newer Approaches

In inflammatory arthritis, a number of biologic agents are under investigation. As noted previously, the most promising are agents directed against tumor necrosis factor-α, but the role of these treatments in the long-term management of RA is far from established. A greater review of these therapies in RA is found in Chapter 25. Hyaluronic acid injections, particularly in osteoarthritis of the knee, show some promise but are cumbersome, are expensive, and appear to be of only moderate benefit. The lay press frequently touts new *cures,* such as glucosamine sulfate, but evidence for effectiveness is scant. Fish oil supplements have been shown to have moderate anti-inflammatory activity but offer little in addition to agents discussed previously.

Because of the chronic nature of many forms of arthritis and the lack of completely satisfactory treatment for many individuals, profiteering from alternative medicine approaches and the use of quack remedies is common. For the most part, these have relatively low toxicity, and the largest problem may be displacement of truly effective therapy at disease stages where it is required to reduce rates of disease progression.

DRUG SEQUENCING IN PROTOTYPIC ARTHRITIC CONDITIONS

In chronic forms of arthritis, outcomes over several decades must be anticipated. Only seldom does a particular drug remain appropriate over the entire course. Each of the major arthritis conditions has its own therapeutic progression sequence. These sequences are always somewhat controversial and are steadily evolving. One can think of each of the disease areas as having several levels of disease ranging from *mild and early* to *late and severe.* The sequences presented in Tables 9–3 through 9–7 are offered as a general framework for considering the appropriate clinical response. Careful clinical judgment is required to decide when treatment at a higher level is required.

Rheumatoid Arthritis

In RA, the necessary progression to higher levels of management usually occurs early in the course. The overall strategy is to employ DMARDs consistently from the onset of disease and to supplement with symptomatic medications, such as NSAIDs, when required. The overall strategy is DMARD based, and the goal is complete or nearly complete suppression of inflammatory activity. Failing a nearly complete response, progression to a more aggressive level of treatment should be rapid.

Table 9–3 shows a scheme for progressive DMARD-based drug therapy for RA. This is sometimes called a *step-up* progression, and there are some who argue, in contrast, for initial use of multiple therapies to establish

Table 9–3. PROGRESSIVE DRUG THERAPY FOR RHEUMATOID ARTHRITIS

Disease Level	Toxicity	Effectiveness
Level 1: Early or mild		
Hydroxychloroquine	Low	Moderate
Auranofin	High (but low less serious toxicity)	Moderate, in early disease only
Sulfasalazine	Low	Moderate
Minocycline	Low	Moderate
Combination of the above agents	Moderate	Moderate
Level 2: Early progressive		
Methotrexate	Moderate	High
Intramuscular gold	Moderate	High
Leflunomide	Moderate	High
Level 3: Continued progressive		
Empirical combinations (e.g., methotrexate and hydroxychloroquine)	Moderate	Moderate
Etanercept	Moderate	High
Infliximab	Moderate	High
Azathioprine	Moderate	Moderate, often best in late disease
D-Penicillamine	Moderate	Moderate
Level 4: Late		
Cyclosporine	High	Moderate
Methotrexate plus cyclosporine	High	High

disease control, then gradual removal of some elements of the combination therapy. The scheme presented here approximates that of the majority of rheumatologists.

Level 1 treatment involves four drugs with low serious toxicity, employed sequentially or in combination. These are not the most effective treatments available but do have favorable toxicity profiles. Each appears to operate through a different mechanism of action, and hence combination treatment with these agents is sensible. The toxicity, even of combination regimens, is at relatively low levels. These drugs are hydroxychloroquine, auranofin, sulfasalazine, and minocycline.

In moderate or severe RA, the transition to level 2 management is likely to be required 3 to 6 months after disease onset. Methotrexate is most commonly used initially at this level and currently is used by more than 40% of patients with RA in the United States. If it is ineffective or poorly tolerated, intramuscular gold is the next choice of most physicians. Methotrexate treatment, appropriately used, is frequently sufficient for manage-

ment for 5 years or more and in some patients seemingly for the duration of the course. With continued progression of disease (level 3), empirical combinations of drugs such as methotrexate and hydroxychloroquine or methotrexate and sulfasalazine may be employed. At level 4, cyclosporine and complex combinations of agents such as methotrexate and cyclosporine may find a role. New disease-modifying drugs are anticipated over the coming years, and they will find their use at one or another level of the therapeutic progression.

Ankylosing Spondylitis and Other Seronegative Spondyloarthropathies

The treatment progressions for ankylosing spondylitis, Reiter's syndrome, psoriatic arthritis, and the arthritis associated with ulcerative colitis or Crohn's disease are approximately similar (Table 9–4). The basic

Table 9–4. PROGRESSIVE DRUG THERAPY FOR ANKYLOSING SPONDYLITIS AND OTHER SERONEGATIVE SPONDYLARTHROPATHIES

Disease Level	Toxicity	Effectiveness
Level 1: Symptomatic		
Exercise and moderate-dose, low-toxicity NSAID	Low to moderate	Moderate
indomethacin or naproxen, dose as required	Moderately high	Moderately high
Level 2: Persistent		
Exercise and NSAID as above, plus sulfasalazine, 2–3 g/d	Moderately high	Moderately high
Level 3: Persistent and progressive		
Exercise and NSAID as above, plus oral methotrexate weekly, 7.5–17.5 mg	Moderately high	Moderately high
Add sulfasalazine as above	Moderately high	Moderately high
Cyclosporine	High	Moderate
Level 4: Disabling		
Level 3 management plus orthopaedic surgery consultation for hip, knee, or shoulder replacement	Moderate	Moderately high

NSAID, nonsteroidal anti-inflammatory drug.

goal is to reduce inflammatory activity such that the patient can exercise vigorously, particularly with flexibility exercises, to prevent the bony fusions that are the late consequences of the spondyloarthritis. At the first level, exercise is combined with relatively low doses of low-toxicity NSAIDs in an attempt to gain control of the disease. If unsuccessful, larger doses of more potent NSAIDs for these conditions, such as indomethacin, are used. Most patients are able to remain at level 1 treatment throughout the course of their disease. When disease persists as symptomatic despite level 1 treatment, addition of sulfasalazine 2 to 3 g daily may be helpful. For more recalcitrant patients, methotrexate, given orally each week, with or without sulfasalazine, can be helpful. In late and disabling disease there may be a role for orthopaedic surgery with regard to hip, knee, or shoulder replacement or procedures on the cervical spine.

Gouty Arthritis

With gout, the goals are to treat acute inflammatory episodes with anti-inflammatory agents and, when required, to reduce the total body pool of monosodium urate by use of allopurinol or probenecid. The scheme for progressive therapy is presented in Table 9–5 (a more thorough discussion of gout is given in Chapter 30.) At first level, the patients with an isolated elevation of serum uric acid has a *nondisease,* which does not require treatment. This patient is, however, at risk for subsequent development of disease at the other levels, although the majority of individuals with mildly elevated serum uric acid never have a gouty consequence.

The second level is acute gouty arthritis with dramatic inflammation of one or several joints, particularly the base of the great toe, the instep, the ankle, or the knee. A short course of NSAIDs, particularly naproxen or indomethacin, is often effective. Some prefer to use oral glucocorticoid with taper over a 5- to 7-day period or adrenocorticotropic hormone (ACTH) injections. The oldest treatment, oral colchicine 0.6 mg hourly until relief, diarrhea, or 12 tablets, is no longer used as frequently because of the frequent occurrence of substantial diarrhea that develops about the time that relief is obtained.

Level 3 is sometimes termed *interval gout* or intercritical gout and represents a patient who has previously had more than one attack of acute gouty arthritis and now has asymptomatic hyperuricemia. This patient is between attacks. Generally a medication to suppress and decrease the frequency of attacks is used at this stage. Oral colchicine at doses of 0.6 to 1.2 mg/day is relatively safe and usually effective. Alternatively, and with greater toxicity, a daily dose of an NSAID may be used. With severe or frequent attacks, most employ, in addition, probenecid or allopurinol to reduce the serum uric acid level and the total body urate pool.

At the fourth level of chronic tophaceous gout, there are large and destructive aggregations of monosodium urate crystals, which can destroy bone and can occupy space in and damage the kidney. If the patient is excreting excessive amounts of uric acid daily, allopurinol is required. Probenecid may be used in those excreting only normal amounts of uric acid daily unless tophi are present. The goal is to reduce the size of the tophi and to remove the excess sodium urate from the body. Allopurinol reduces the production of uric acid, and probenecid increases the rate of its excretion. In difficult cases, the two may be used in combination. Colchicine or an NSAID is required to reduce the frequency of the acute attacks of gout, which are most common during the early months of treatment with either allopurinol or probenecid. Neither probenecid nor allopurinol should be used during an acute attack of gout.

Osteoarthritis

Progressive drug therapy for OA is shown schematically in Table 9–6. In early or mild disease, exercise and acetaminophen may be all that is required.

Table 9–5. PROGRESSIVE DRUG THERAPY FOR GOUTY ARTHRITIS

Disease Level	Toxicity	Effectiveness
Level 1: Asymptomatic hyperuricemia		
No treatment	None	High
Level 2: Acute gouty arthritis		
NSAID course, 1 week	Low	High
ACTH, or steroid burst and taper	Low	High
Oral colchicine	Low	Moderate
Level 3: Interval gout (between attacks)		
Colchicine, oral, 0.6–1.2 mg/d	Low	Moderately high
NSAID, moderate dose	Moderate	Moderately high
Probenecid	Low	Moderately high
Allopurinol	Moderately low	Moderately high
Level 4: Chronic tophaceous gout		
Allopurinol *or*	Moderately low	High
Probenecid *plus*	Low	High
Colchicine, oral, 0.6–1.2 g/d *or*	Low	Moderately high
NSAID, moderate dose	Moderate	Moderately high

NSAID, nonsteroidal anti-inflammatory drug; ACTH, adrenocorticotropic hormone.

Table 9–6. PROGRESSIVE DRUG THERAPY FOR OSTEOARTHRITIS

Disease Level	Toxicity	Effectiveness
Level 1: Early or mild		
Exercise	Very low	Moderate
Add acetaminophen as required	Very low	Moderate
Level 2: Persistent		
Exercise and acetaminophen 2–4 g/d	Low	Moderate
Level 3: Flare		
Decrease exercise and NSAID course, low dose, 7 d	Low	Moderate
NSAID course, high dose, 7 d	Low	Moderate
Glucocorticoid injection	Low	High
Hyaluranate injections	Low	Moderate
Level 4: Continued persistent		
Exercise and NSAIDs, low toxicity, low dose	Moderate	Moderate
NSAIDs, low toxicity, high dose	Moderately high	Moderate
Best NSAID, best dose	High	Moderate
Level 5: Intractable pain and disability		
Orthopaedic surgery consultation for total joint replacement consideration	Moderate	High

NSAIDs, nonsteroidal anti-inflammatory drug.

With persistent symptoms, a regular regimen of acetaminophen may suffice. During flares, episodic treatment with NSAIDs in low or high dose may be helpful, and if the flare is in an accessible joint, such as the knee, a corticosteroid injection or a series of hyaluronate injections may be helpful. With continued persistent disease, regular NSAID treatment may be required. If possible, the dose is kept low and the NSAID chosen to be one of relatively low toxicity. It may, however, be necessary to determine empirically the best NSAID and the best dose for long-term management of severe symptoms. Minocycline may be added for its inhibitory activity on *metalloproteases*. The last level, where joint cartilage has been largely or completely lost, involves surgical salvage. The availability of total joint replacement procedures, particularly for the hip and knee, has revolutionized management of late-stage OA.

REGIONAL SYNDROMES

The majority of all human maladies are probably the regional rheumatic disease syndromes, ranging from low back pain to a variety of sports (or overuse) injuries, strains, and a variety of periarticular pain. These are discussed in detail in Chapters 15, 16, 19, and 24. For the most part, these problems represent minor musculoskeletal injuries, and most heal naturally. Local problems generally suggest local therapy. Treatment is designed to improve comfort levels while awaiting the natural healing process to restore the function of the part. Acutely, in the first 24 to 48 hours, cold packs are helpful, followed by warmth and heat on subsequent days, rest, and use of acetaminophen. The sequence of progressive treatment is shown in Table 9–7. For those whose problem persists into a subacute stage, the therapeutic goals are to continue rest of the injured body part, sometimes with splints or braces, and to use low-dose NSAIDs as required for symptomatic control. The analgesic level of NSAIDs, rather than the anti-inflammatory, is desired. Glucocorticoid injections frequently find a role at this stage and if they are effective for 6 weeks or more may be repeated as often as every 3 months. Chronic problems persistent beyond 6 months may require evaluation by the orthopaedist, neurosurgeon, or rheumatologist.

Table 9–7. PROGRESSIVE DRUG THERAPY FOR REGIONAL RHEUMATIC SYNDROMES (LOW BACK PAIN, PLANTAR FASCIITIS, ACHILLES TENDINITIS, STRAINS, AND PAINS)

Disease Level	Toxicity	Effectiveness
Level 1: Acute		
Cold followed by heat		
Rest of affected body part		
Acetaminophen	Low	Moderately high
Level 2: Subacute (1 wk–6 mo)		
Localized measures		
Rest of affected body part		
Low-dose NSAIDs	Moderately low	Moderately high
Physical therapy	Low	Moderately high
Glucocorticoid injection	Low	Moderately high
Level 3: Chronic (persistent past 6 mo)		
Orthopaedic, neurosurgical, or rheumatologist referral as indicated	Variable	Moderate

NSAIDs, nonsteroidal anti-inflammatory drugs.

WHEN TO REFER THE PATIENT

Many rheumatic disease syndromes may be successfully managed by the primary care provider. The major exceptions are RA and the systemic connective tissue diseases. In these diseases, a rheumatologist's opinion should be sought at the initial suspicion of diagnosis and subsequently at least twice yearly as long as the disease is active. Table 9–8 summarizes minimal indications for referral to the rheumatologist. Diagnostic or therapeutic uncertainty is an obvious indication. Ankylosing spondylitis may be managed alone by the general physician in most cases up to level 3. Additionally, if the generalist is not familiar with or does not have ready access to patient education programs and specific exercise recommendations, referral should be made. Consultation for management of gout is often not required, depending on the confidence of he primary care practitioner, but should be obtained in patients with chronic tophaceous gout at a minimum.

Osteoarthritis usually can be managed well by the general physician. If, as frequently happens, the patient is less than totally satisfied with treatment, referral may be indicated. Referral is needed if pain is intractable or if the patient has significant disability. Regional syndromes may generally be managed by the generalist familiar with effective treatment, but these patients should receive rheumatologic consultation if the condition persists for more than 6 months. Fibromyalgia can require referral because of patient requests, but referral is not medically imperative, as long as the diagnosis is well established and symptoms are adequately controlled. A serious side effect to an antirheumatic medication frequently raises complex questions of minimizing drug toxicity while maintaining therapeutic effectiveness and usually requires rheumatologic referral.

The Appendix contains protocols for medical management of rheumatoid arthritis.

Table 9–8. MINIMAL INDICATIONS FOR REFERRAL TO A RHEUMATOLOGIST

Diagnostic or therapeutic uncertainty
Rheumatoid arthritis
At initial suspicion of diagnosis and at least twice yearly throughout the course
Systemic lupus erythematosus, scleroderma, polymyositis/dermatomyositis, polyarteritis, Wegener's granulomatosis, other suspected vasculitis or systemic connective tissue disease:
At initial suspicion of diagnosis and regularly thereafter
Ankylosing spondylitis
As desired or at level 3, persistent and progressive
Gout
As desired or at level 3, interval gout
Osteoarthritis
As desired, rheumatologist at level 4, continued and persistant pain
Regional syndromes
As desired or at level 3, chronic: persistent at 6 mo
Fibromyalgia
As desired for therapeutic difficulties
Serious side effect (e.g., gastrointestinal hemorrhage, proteinuria, cytopenia) owing to antirheumatic medication

REFERENCES

1. Fries JF: NSAID gastropathy: The second most deadly rheumatic disease? Epidemiology and risk appraisal. J Rheumatol 18(suppl 28): 6–10, 1991.
2. Fries JF, Williams CA, Bloch DA, Michel BA: NSAID-associated gastropathy: Incidence and risk factor models. Am J Med 91: 213–222, 1991.
3. Fries JF, Spitz PW, Williams CA, et al: A toxicity index for comparison of side effects among different drugs. Arthritis Rheum 33:121–130, 1990.
4. Fries JF, Williams CA, Bloch DA: The relative toxicity of nonsteroidal anti-inflammatory drugs (NSAIDs). Arthritis Rheum 34:1353–1360, 1991.
5. Fries JF, Williams CA, Ramey DR, Bloch DA: The relative toxicity of alternative therapies for rheumatoid arthritis: Implications for the therapeutic progression. Semin Arthritis Rheum 23:68–73, 1993.
6. Singh G, Ramey DR, Morfeld D, et al: Gastrointestinal tract complications of nonsteroidal anti-inflammatory drug treatment in rheumatoid arthritis. Arch Intern Med 156:1530–1536, 1996.
7. Bradley JB, Brandt KD, Katz BP, et al: Comparison of an anti-inflammatory dose of ibuprofen, an analgesic dose of ibuprofen, and acetaminophen in the treatment of patients with osteoarthritis of the knee. N Engl J Med 325:87–91, 1991.
8. Fries JF, Spitz PW, Mitchell DM, et al: Impact of specific therapy upon rheumatoid arthritis. Arthritis Rheum 29:620–627, 1986.
9. Hawkey CJ, Karrasch JA, Szczepanski L, et al: Omeprazole compared with misoprostol for ulcers associated with nonsteroidal antiinflammatory drugs: Omeprazole versus misoprostol for NSAID-induced ulcer management (OMNIUM) Study Group. N Engl J Med 338:727–734, 1998.

Appendix

Protocols for the Medical Management of Musculoskeletal Complaints*

Table 9A–1. PROTOCOLS FOR MEDICAL MANAGEMENT OF RHEUMATOID ARTHRITIS

Protocol for Nonsteroidal Antiinflammatory Drugs (NSAIDs)

Toxicity:

GI:	Peptic ulcer, dyspepsia (persons at increased risk of NSAID-induced GI ulceration include those with a history of peptic ulcer disease, history of GI bleed, advancing age, history of serious comorbid disease, and concomitant corticosteroid therapy. In such patients, prophylactic therapy with misoprostol should be considered)
Renal:	Azotemia, interference with antihypertensives
Allergic:	Triad of rhinitis/nasal polyposis/asthma
Heme:	Interference with platelet function, bleeding

Monitoring:

Initial Evaluation:	CBC, creatinine, liver function tests
Follow-up:	CBC, BUN/creatinine q6mo. During the first 6 months, the patient should be evaluated every 4 to 8 weeks. After 6 months, the patient may be seen less frequently (eg, q6mo) depending upon age and comorbid conditions.

Usual Dosing Regimens: Doses vary depending upon the specific agent, however, lower doses often provide analgesia while higher doses are required for antiinflammatory effects

Hold NSAIDs and/or Evaluate if the Following Occur:

1) Evidence of GI bleed
2) Azotemia (increasing creatinine)
3) Worsening hypertension
4) Evidence of bleeding from other organ systems

Protocol for Low-Dose Oral Corticosteroids

Toxicity: (most toxicities are dose-dependent)

Bone:	Osteoporosis (dose-, time-related); risk of osteonecrosis
Endocrine:	Rapid withdrawal of corticosteroids after chronic use, or insufficient supplement of corticosteroids during periods of stress for patients using corticosteroids chronically precipitate adrenal insufficiency
Immune:	Increased risk of infection; may "mask" signs and symptoms of infection by dampening inflammatory response
Metabolic:	May precipitate/exacerbate hyperglycemia and/or diabetes mellitus; dose-related hypercholesterolemia
GI:	May potentiate risk of peptic ulceration in patients concurrently receiving NSAIDs
Muscle:	May be associated with myopathy

---

*Reprinted with permission from Lipsky PE (ed): Algorithms for the diagnosis and management of musculoskeletal complaints. Am J Med 103(6A):81S, 1997.

97

Monitoring:
   Initial Evaluation: Glucose, urinalysis, consider DXA scan
   Follow-up: Glucose, urinalysis, every 3 months
Usual Dosing Regimens: "Low dose" corticosteroids are typically considered by rheumatologists to be ≤7.5 mg/day prednisone. Ensure adequate calcium and vitamin D intake.
Consider Holding or Decreasing Doses of Corticosteroids and/or Evaluate if the Following Occur:
   1) Active infectious problem
   2) Hyperglycemia
   3) GI bleed

Protocol for Sulfasalazine Therapy

Contraindications: Documented allergic reaction to sulfa drugs or aspirin; history of severe hepatic or hematologic disease
Factors Affecting Drug Levels: Acetylator status (may not affect efficacy or outcome, however)
Toxicity: Adverse reaction usually minor and reversible; 75% occur within first 3 mo of treatment
   GI: Nausea, vomiting, anorexia (10–20% d/c Rx), lessened with slow increase in dose, enteric-coated tablets, and dosing with meals ↑ increased liver function tests (0.5–1.5%)
   CNS: Irritability, headache, dizziness (5–10% d/c Rx)
   Skin: Rash, urticaria (4–5% d/c Rx); rarely Stevens-Johnson, TEN
   Heme: Anemia (megaloblastic > hemolytic; <1%), neutropenia (1–1.5%), thrombocytopenia (0–1%)
Usual Dosing Regimens: Maintenance therapy typically 1000 mg bid. In order to minimize GI adverse effects, therapy may be begun at 500 mg/day, and increased at weekly intervals. Maximal dose usually 3–4 g/day

Monitoring:
   Initial Evaluation: CBC, liver function tests, consider analysis for G6PD deficiency
   Follow-up: CBC, liver function tests q4–8wk
Hold Sulfasalazine and/or Evaluate if the Following Occur:
   1) WBC < 3500/mm^3, or absolute PMN count <2000/mm^3
   2) Platelet count < 150,000/mm^3 Hb < 9 g
   3) Severe GI upset
   4) Severe rash
   5) Liver function tests >3× upper limit of normal or >2× on two visits

Protocol for Hydroxychloroquine Therapy

Contraindications: Preexisting retinopathy or other serious ophthalmologic condition
Toxicity: Adverse reactions are infrequent, and (except for ocular toxicity) usually minor and reversible
   GI: Nausea, vomiting, anorexia
   CNS: Irritability, nervousness
   Heme: Anemia (hemolytic; rare)
   Eye: Reversible: blurring of vision, halos around lights (ciliary body and corneal effect); irreversible: retinopathy, macular atrophy (very rare if dosed ≤6.5 mg/kg/day)
Usual Dosing Regimens: Typical therapeutic dose is 400 mg/day. Occasionally higher doses (600 mg/day) or lower doses (200 mg/day) may be utilized.

Monitoring:
   Initial Evaluation: CBC, consider baseline ophthalmologic examination, consider analysis for G6PD deficiency
   Follow-up: Ophthalmologic evaluation Q 6 mo
Hold Hydroxychloroquine and/or Evaluate if the Following Occur:
   1) Altered visual acuity or other ocular complaint
   2) New onset or worsening of anemia
   3) Severe GI upset

Protocol for Methotrexate Therapy

Contraindications: Ethanol abuse; active infection; pregnancy; history of hepatitis; severe hepatic, renal, hematologic, or interstitial pulmonary disease. Increased Risk: Ethanol use, obesity, diabetes mellitus, elderly, impaired renal function.

Factors Affecting Drug Levels: Renal function; use of sulfa antibiotics, dilantin, NSAIDs, probenecid, diuretics; route of administration (po vs IM or SQ).

Toxicity: Folic acid may be prescribed concurrently to try to decrease side effects.

GI: Nausea, vomiting, anorexia, diarrhea (10%); increased liver function tests

Skin: Mucositis, rash (10%), alopecia (1%)

Heme: Leukopenia > anemia, thrombocytopenia (<5%)

Pulmonary: Pneumonitis (idiosyncratic), fibrosis (<5%)

Other: Nodulosis, opportunistic infections (PCP, aspergillus, histoplasmosis cryptococcosis, Zoster, etc)

Usual Dosing Regimens: Therapy typically initiated at 7.5 mg/wk in a single dose; dose may be increased by 2.5 mg/wk at biweekly or monthly intervals. Typical dose range 7.5–15 mg/wk (maximum dose usually ≥25 mg/wk).

Monitoring:

Initial Evaluation: CBC, liver function tests (ALT, AST, GGT, alkaline phosphatase, albumin, bilirubin), urinalysis. Also, serum and RBC folate, serum B12, and serum ferritin if there is a clinical suspicion of deficiency. Chest radiograph ± pulmonary function testing if there is clinical suspicion of pulmonary disease. Consider screening for hepatitis B and C.

Follow-up: CBC, liver function tests, creatinine q2wk × 2, then q4wk (when patient is stable, this may eventually be increased to q6–8wk follow-up)

Hold Methotrexate and/or Evaluate if the Following Occur:

1) WBC < 3500/mm^3, or absolute PMN count <2000/mm^3
2) Platelet count < 150,000/mm^3
3) Liver function tests > 3× upper limit of normal or >2× on two visits
4) Mucosal ulcers
5) Severe GI upset or active GI bleed
6) Pulmonary symptoms (SOB, cough, chest pain, fever, abnormal chest radiograph)

Protocol for Azathioprine

Contraindications: Severe hepatic or hematologic disease, pregnancy, concomitant administration of allopurinol

Toxicity:

Heme: Dose-dependent leukopenia (approximately 2–8% with WBC < 2500/mm^3) and thrombocytopenia (0–1%)

GI: Nausea, vomiting, anorexia (approximately 10–15% of patients); lessened with divided dosages, and administration with or after meals. Increased liver function tests (approximately 1%)

Skin: Rash (approximately 2%)

Other: Increased risk of Infection (eg, zoster); risk of treatment-related malignancy (eg, lymphoproliferative) with large cumulative doses

Usual Dosing Regimens: Therapy typically initiated at ≤1.0 mg/kg/day (eg, ~50 mg/day). Dose may be increased at monthly intervals by ~0.5 mg/kg/day. Maintenance dose depends on efficacy and toxicity (particularly WBC count); usually <2.5 mg/kg/day.

Monitoring:

Initial Evaluation: CBC, liver function tests

Follow-up: CBC, liver function tests, q2–4wk

Hold Azathioprine and/or Evaluate if the Following Occur:

1) WBC < 3500/mm^3, or absolute PMN count < 2000/mm^3
2) Platelet count < 150,000/mm^3
3) Severe GI upset (nausea, vomiting, anorexia)
4) LFTs > 3× upper limit of normal or >2× on two visits
5) Skin rash

Protocol for Gold Therapy

Preparations:

Injectable: Aurothioglucose, gold sodium thiomalate

Oral: Auranofin

Toxicity: Translent nitritoid reaction (flushing, headache, etc.) may occur immediately post-dose
 Skin: Pruritic rash, oral ulcerations (~20%)
 Renal: Proteinuria (~20%)
 Heme: Thrombocytopenia > leukopenia (<5%)
 Oral Gold: Above reactions less common, diarrhea very common
Usual Dosing Regimens:
 IM Gold: Typically, therapy is initiated weekly (50 mg/wk, after test doses of 10 mg and/or 25 mg) until a total dose of 1000 mg has been received. The dosing interval is then increased to Q 3 or 4 wk.
 Oral Gold: 3 mg po, bid; maximum dose 9 mg/day
Monitoring:
 Initial Evaluation: CBC, urinalysis
 Follow-up: CBC, urinalysis before each injection
Hold Gold and/or Evaluate if the Following Occur:
 1) WBC < 3500/mm^3, or absolute PMN count < 2000/mm^3
 2) Platelet count < 150,000/mm^3, falling Hb or Hct
 3) Pruritic rash
 4) Mouth ulcers
 5) >trace proteinuria on dipstick (if consistent, check 24° urine)
 6) Oral gold: hold for persistent diarrhea

Protocol for D-Penicillamine Therapy

Factors Affecting Drug Levels: Renal function
Common Toxicities:
 Skin: Pruritic rash, oral ulcerations
 Heme: Leukopenia, thrombocytopenia
 Renal: Proteinuria
Uncommon Toxicities:
 Autoimmune: Pemphigus, myasthenia gravis, Goodpasture's syndrome, SLE-like syndrome
 Other: Severe bone marrow depression, bronchiolitis
Usual Dosing Regimens: Therapy is typically initiated at 125 mg or 250 mg/day, and then increased by 250 mg/day at monthly/bimonthly intervals; usual maximum dose ≤ 1000 mg/day.
Monitoring:
 Initial Evaluation: CBC, urinalysis
 Follow-up: CBC, urinalysis q2wk × 2, then CBC, urinalysis q4wk indefinitely (may increase in some patients to q6–8wk follow-up)
Hold D-Penicillamine and/or Evaluate if the Following Occur:
 1) WBC < 3500/mm^3, or absolute PMN count < 2000/mm^3
 2) Platelet count < 150,000/mm^3; falling Hb or Hct
 3) Pruritic rash
 4) Mouth ulcers
 5) >trace proteinuria on dipstick (if consistent, check 24° urine)

Protocol for Cyclosporine Therapy

Contraindications: Renal failure, uncontrolled hypertension, active infection, malignancy.
Increased Risk: Impaired renal function, hypertension
Factors Affecting   Threefold individual differences in bioavailability (affected by GI motility, etc).
 Drug Levels: ≠ absorption with food. CsA is metabolized by the hepatic P-450 system. Medications that ↑ CsA levels: Ca^{2+} channel blockers (diltiazem > verapamil, nicardipine; amlodipine, nifedipine have no effect), antibiotics (erythromycin, ketoconazole, fluconazole), metoclopramide, bromocriptine, androgens, oral contraceptives, methylprednisolone. Medications that ↓ CsA levels: rifampin, dilantin, phenobarbital, carbamazepine.
Toxicity:
 Renal: Acutely decreases glomerular filtration rate (reversible). Chronic high dose use may lead to irreversible decrease in renal function
 GI: Anorexia, nausea/vomiting, cramping/bloating
 Skin: Hypertrichosis (increased hair on face, arms, trunk), gingival hypertrophy
 Articular: Gout (CsA increases serum uric acid)

Immune: Potential for opportunistic infections (PCP, aspergillus, histoplasmosis, cryptococcosis, zoster, etc)

Neuro: Tremors, paresthesia, headache

Other: Hypertension (probably not involving renin-angiotensin system; therefore may want to use Ca^{2+} channel blockers, central sympathetic blockers, vasodilators, low-dose diuretics); hyperglycemia; ↑ alkaline phosphatase

Usual Dosing Regimens: Usually begun at 2–3 mg/kg/day, either as a single or split dose. May be increased; for autoimmune diseases, maximum dose is usually ≤5 mg/kg/day

Monitoring:

Initial Evaluation: Creatinine, blood pressure (BP)

Follow-up: Creatinine, BP; q2wk × 2, then q4wk

Hold Cyclosporine and/or Evaluate if the Following Occur:

1) Creatinine > 3.0, or an increase in creatinine of ≥30% over baseline (eg, if serum creatinine ↑ from 1.0 to 1.3 between visits)
2) Hypertension (BP > 160/90 mm Hg) or BP substantially increased from baseline
3) Infectious symptoms
4) Severe symptoms in other organ systems

Protocol for Cyclophosphamide Therapy

Contraindications: Pregnancy, history of malignancy, active infection

GI Nausea, vomiting, anorexia (highly emetogenic; prophylaxis useful)

Heme: Leukopenia (neutropenia, lymphocytopenia) > > ↓ Plt, anemia

GU: Hemorrhagic cystitis, risk of bladder cancer

Cancer: Increased risk, especially lymphoproliferative and bladder

Other: Alopecia (reversible), increased risk of infection (especially herpes zoster), infertility (premature ovarian failure)

Usual Dosing Regimens: Therapy typically initiated at ≤1.0 mg/kg/day (eg, ~50 mg/day). Dose may be increased at monthly intervals by ~0.5 mg/kg/day. Maintenance dose depends on efficacy and toxicity (particularly WBC count); usually <2.0 mg/kg/day.

Monitoring:

Initial Evaluation: CBC, creatinine, urinalysis

Follow-up: CBC, creatinine, urinalysis q4wk

Hold Cyclophosphamide and/or Evaluate if the Following Occur:

1) WBC < 3000/mm^3, or absolute PMN count < 1500/mm^3
2) Severe GI upset
3) Active Infection
4) Pregnancy
5) Hematuria

Chapter **10**

Physical Modalities in Management of Pain and Inflammation

Jeffrey K. Teraoka ■ Peter B. J. Wu

The successful treatment of musculoskeletal and rheumatologic conditions depends not only on specific administration of medications by the physician, but also on the judicious use of physical modalities given by a therapist or other health professional. The physician must be aware of the various treatment modalities available as well as their indications, contraindications, and techniques of administration. This chapter focuses on the different physical modalities available, with a brief summary of each, including the indications and contraindications for each as well as a general guideline that allows the primary physican to become more familiar in prescribing them appropriately for patients.

SUPERFICIAL HEAT

The use of heat in treating musculoskeletal diseases has existed in medical treatment since the beginning of modern day medicine. The basic premise for its effectiveness is that it provides analgesia through an increase in local blood circulation via vasodilation as well as reducing muscle tone and spasticity, increasing the elasticity of soft tissue, and perhaps enhancing healing through the increase in local circulation. Heat is transferred by one of three physical properties: convection, conduction, or radiation/conversion. *Superficial heat* refers to the transference of heat that does not extend deeper than the superficial layers of skin. Heat should be avoided in conditions of acute inflammation, trauma, or hemorrhage; areas of malignancy, edema, and ischemia; atrophic skin; and insensate tissues.[1]

Hot Packs

Hot packs exchange heat through conduction. Many forms are available, including gel-filled bags, hydrocollator packs containing silicon dioxide, *water-circulating heating pad,* and simple plastic or rubber bottles filled with warm water. Each form acquires a large heat capacity and releases the heat slowly to the tissues, thus minimizing burning and allowing a longer period of application without having to rewarm the material. Hydrocollator packs are kept in a hot water chamber until ready for use, wrapped in several layers of toweling, then applied to the area for 20 to 30 minutes. Electric heating pads and circulating water pads do not cool or heat spontaneously and therefore need to be monitored closely and limited to no more than 20 minutes at a time to prevent burning.[1, 2]

Heat Lamps

Heat lamps warm superficial tissues through transfer of radiant energy. A 250-watt bulb is usually used, with the lamp placed about 40 to 50 cm from the skin. Intensity can be adjusted by varying the distance between the patient and the lamp.

Hydrotherapy

Hydrotherapy (whirlpool) used circulating water at temperatures of 33° to 45°C to deliver massage, débridement, and heat through convection. Units can be large enough to accommodate the entire body (Hubbard tanks) or smaller, to treat only the affected extremity. More vigorous heating occurs with this type of therapy than with a stationary water bath because the warm water is in constant motion; this eliminates any insulation layer of cooler water against the skin. Hubbard tanks are often kept at 39°C or less; because the whole body is immersed, the core body temperature can be affected adversely if the temperature were higher. Smaller baths treating a single extremity can be elevated to 43° to 45°C. Hydrotherapy is an effective method for wound débridement. The gentle agitation, heat, and use of antiseptic solutions gently débride otherwise painful wounds and burns. Hydrotherapy is also used to help mobilize joints after cast removal and to mobilize soft tissues in muscle spasms and myofascial pain syndromes.[1]

Contrast Baths

Contrast baths provide effective relief of pain and muscle spasms through increased circulation by reflex hyperemia of the treated area. The extremity is soaked in alternating warm and cold baths for 1 to 5 minutes each for about four cycles. This treatment is also effective in reducing edema resulting from inflammation as well as in rheumatoid arthritis and reflex sympathetic dystrophy.[1]

Paraffin Baths

Paraffin baths use a container filled with melted wax and mineral oil heated to about 52° to 54°C. The mixture has a low thermal conductivity value, thus releasing the heat slowly and preventing burns despite the high temperature of the bath.[2] The wax also forms an insulating layer against the skin, which helps disperse the heat more evenly. There are two methods of treatment: continuous immersion and dipping. Continuous immersion elevates the temperature of the extremity more intensely and longer than the dipping method. Active synovitis and contractures are the best use of this modality.

DEEP HEAT: ULTRASOUND

Although several types of deep heating (diathermy) modalities exist, ultrasound is the one most commonly used. Ultrasound basically incorporates sound waves generated from piezoelectric crystals at a frequency of 0.8 to 1.0 mHz (too high for human perception). The sound is converted to heat that can penetrate the deeper tissues and heat deep muscle layers and tendons, fascia, synovium, and ligaments. The greatest heat production is at the bone–soft tissue interface; thus the muscle tissue, ligaments, and tendons nearest the bone are heated most intensely. The intensities used in clinical practice range between 0.5 and 2.0 watts/cm^2, and the applicator sizes are usually 5 to 10 cm. Ultrasound is usually given by direct contact with the skin (surface) with constant movement of the head transducer; this covers a larger area with less chance of burning. Indirect ultrasound can be used to treat an irregular surface (e.g., ankle, hand) by placing the ultrasound head in a container of degassed water, then submerging the affected part into the chamber and moving the head approximately 1 cm from the skin, around the body part without actual contact.[1]

Phonophoresis involves the use of medications or other agents mixed in with the coupling medium (gel) of the ultrasound application, theoretically allowing the ultrasound to *drive* the material or substance into the tissue past the skin barrier, avoiding the need for injections. Glucocorticoid creams and lidocaine are frequently used medications with this modality. It is most commonly used in rotator cuff tendinitis, lateral epicondylitis, and bursitis.

Ultrasound is indicated for use in degenerative joint disease (especially the hip), muscle spasms, tendinitis, and bursitis (subacute or chronic). Its use in acute states may cause increased inflammation. It can also be used to help stretch shortened muscles, tendons, and ligaments because the extensibility or elasticity of collagen increases with temperatures up to 45°C. It is best to use ultrasound in conjunction with a prolonged gradual stretch, maintaining the stretch until the temperature of the tissues has returned back to baseline.[1]

Ultrasound should not be used around any fluid-filled cavity or organ, such as the eyes, heart, and brain, or around abscesses or other infections, hematomas, gravid uteri, tumors, cervical ganglia, pacemakers, areas of stasis or ischemia, or the spine. It should also be avoided near artificial joint prostheses. Although not proven, metal implants can significantly reflect the heat to adjacent tissues, causing burns, or *melting* of the cement.[1]

COLD AGENTS

Cold is another superficial modality of therapy used to decrease swelling and pain, especially in the acute phase of an inflammatory disease or trauma. Cold decreases metabolic activity and inflammation as well as spasticity. Chilling initially causes a local reflex vasoconstriction with increased sympathetic tone. Below 15°C, subcutaneous vessels dilate. Subcutaneous temperatures can fall by 3° to 5°C within 10 minutes; deeper tissues decrease by at most 1°C after 10 minutes. Vasoconstriction decreases blood flow such that cooled tissues return to baseline temperatures more slowly than heated tissues.

Ice has a high heat capacity (ability to absorb heat). Treatments are usually maintained for 20 to 30 minutes, after which the skin may become irritated and uncomfortable. Iced massage consists of rubbing ice over the painful area to obtain analgesia (i.e., numbness after about 10 minutes).

Cooling with sprays (ethylene chloride, fluoromethanes), which cool by rapid evaporation against the skin, can be used to anesthetize a local area of pain, inflammation, or hemorrhage. It has also been used to decrease muscle spasms when used in conjunction with prolonged gentle stretching.

Ice is indicated with any acute condition, trauma being the most common indication because it decreases inflammation and edema and minimizes hypoxic and metabolic tissue damage. The well-known acronym *RICE* (*r*est, *i*ce, *c*ompression, and *e*levation) has earned its reputation in remedying most musculoskeletal injuries, including acute sprains, strains, and fractures. Ice is applied intermittently for the first 6 to 24 hours. After 24 hours, the use of ice versus heat is determined mainly by the bias of the practitioner as well as the effective symptomatic relief obtained by the patient rather than by any actual experimental rationale.

Prolonged and intensive cooling can cause tissue damage by vasoconstriction, especially in ischemic extremities as well as in Raynaud's phenomenon and Raynaud's disease. As with heat, use of cold in insensate areas should be carried out with caution.[1,2]

MASSAGE

Massage basically consists of rubbing, kneading, and pressing (i.e., manipulating) the soft tissues to help loosen them and decrease pain and stiffness. Massage can also help create a generalized relaxed state through its reflexive effects. It decreases edema, stretches scar tissue, and breaks up adhesions. Aside from the use of heat or cold, it is probably one of the oldest physical techniques. Its use had been traced back to ancient Egypt and Asia. Although medical technology has devised different types of equipment to facilitate massage, the best effects are still obtained through *hands-on* application because the practitioner's hands can monitor the patient's response and subsequently adjust the intensity and extent of delivery to the area of treatment. When massage is done with the motion applied toward the direction of the heart, venous return is facilitated to assist circulation as well as lymphatic drainage.

There are three classic types of massage. *Effleurage* consists of stroking or gliding motions, going along the muscle fibers or soft tissue planes. *Petrissage* uses a kneading and rolling motion over the soft tissue area. *Tapotement* uses a percussive motion across the generalized area of treatment. Other forms of massage have also become popular, such as *acupressure, reflexology*, and *shiatsu*, in which pressure is applied to the classic reflex points to restore energy flow, decrease pain, and promote a more relaxed state through reflex effects. *Cross-fiber massage* is another technique in which the motion is applied lightly across a ligament or tendon to help prevent adhesions from forming during the acute phase of recovery after injury, which helps the tissues (collagen fibers) heal in a unilateral direction, thus preserving motion and extensibility. *Deep friction massage* is done more vigorously to break up adhesions that have already formed from previous or chronic injury.

Massage should be avoided over malignancies, wounds, deep venous thromboses, and infections. It should be used with caution around calcified tissues or tendons, atrophic muscles, and skin grafts. Deep pressure massage done too vigorously over insensate or fragile areas can cause hematomas and rarely nerve damage. Despite these precautions, massage remains one of the most effective yet safe forms of therapeutic intervention.[3–5]

TRACTION

Traction is a modality in which stretching or pulling of the cervical or lumbar spine decreases pain and spasm by helping stretch the paraspinal musculature leading to realignment of the spine. It has been thought that this modality can distract the vertebral segments to impart a slight vacuum effect on the intervertebral discs, helping to *relocate* or reposition the disc into its proper confines. The minimal force (weight) for traction to impart any vertebral separation is 25 pounds, which causes a 2-mm distraction of the segment. Ten pounds is the minimal force needed to counterbalance the weight of the head. For the lumbar spine, the principles remain the same but require higher forces.[3]

Manual traction, as the name implies, is carried out by the therapist manually applying the traction force on the cervical spine. It is safer and more gentle, because the hands-on effect allows for close monitoring of the applied force. The exact amount of force used, however, cannot be determined. It is used initially to determine whether, in fact, the patient can tolerate the modality and also whether there has been any therapeutic effect to warrant further treatment.

Mechanical traction uses free weights or pulleys to create the force for traction (Figs. 10–1 and 10–2). Most home units use weights averaging about 20 pounds, which may not be adequate because only 10 pounds of actual traction is achieved; the other 10 pounds counterbalances the weight of the head. Home traction units, in fact, need close supervision by the therapist for proper pull and positioning. If not used correctly, home units inevitably fail because improper positioning causes more pain, misalignment, or both.[3]

Motorized traction provides consistent, measurable force on cervical or lumbar spine and can be applied continuously or intermittently. The patient can usually tolerate higher forces with intermittent traction. The effectiveness and safety depend mainly on close supervision by the therapist, but feedback from the patient regarding any pain or sensation of malignment is vital as well.

Neck position is crucial to the effectiveness of traction.[5, 6] Twenty degrees to 30 degrees of neck flexion has been shown to widen the intervertebral foramina (see Fig. 10–1). Twenty-four degrees has been shown to be the optimal angle of traction.[5] Neck extension should be avoided. Duration of treatment should be limited to 20 to 30 minutes, depending on the patient's tolerance. When using the intermittent mode, cycling should be 5 to 7 seconds *on* and 5 seconds *off* for 20 to 30 minutes. For most patients who are not obese and need traction of the lumbar spines, 50 pounds seems to cause posterior separation and 100 pounds causes both anterior and posterior widening.[7]

Traction can be used in subacute or chronic cervical or lumbar strains with or without radicular symp-

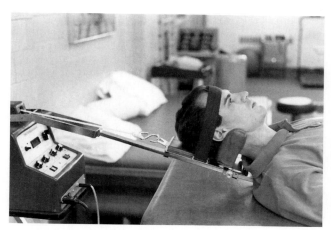

Figure 10–1. Mechanical cervical traction. Note angle of pull from machine approximately 20 degrees.

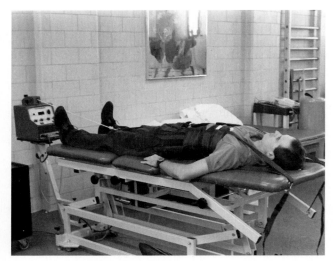

Figure 10–2. Mechanical lumbar traction.

toms. It may be used cautiously in true herniated disc disease; however, close monitoring and expertise in the use of the modality are mandatory. It should not be used with any suspicion of ligamentous instability, vertebrobasilar vascular disease, spinal infections or tumors, severe osteoporosis, inflammatory spondyloarthropathies including advanced rheumatoid arthritis, or any signs of myelopathy. Insufficient weight or tension and improper postioning are the most frequent reasons for traction to fail. Traction requires a therapist who is experienced in its use and keen in monitoring symptoms of discomfort. The prescription should include the neck position in 20 to 30 degrees of flexion; continuous versus intermittent; manual versus mechanical; duration (usually 20 to 30 minutes); and with the weight for cervical traction beginning at 10 pounds, advancing up to 35 pounds, and lumbar beginning at 50 pounds and advancing up to 100 pounds as tolerated.[3]

MANIPULATION

Manipulation is defined as passive manual treatment applied to specific joints and tissues to help facilitate movement, thus diminishing pain and re-establishing correct movement, balance, and alignment of the treated area. It involves the application of directed forces to the bones, joints, or both to overcome the restriction in motion. There are two main types of manipulation, defined by the amount of relative force and motion required to mobilize the segment. In *high-velocity, low-amplitude manipulation*, otherwise known as *thrusting* or *impulse manipulation*, the joint or abnormal segment is passively taken to the limit of movement (i.e., its *barrier*). A quick, controlled force or thrust is applied to the joint or segment in the direction of the restriction, which overcomes the barrier and frees the motion of the segment.

Low-velocity, high-amplitude manipulation also begins by bringing the joint segment to its barrier. Slowly applied force is directed at the barrier in a repeated *on-off* motion until the movement of the segment becomes freer. Repeated sessions are necessary to recover fully the unrestricted range of motion.

Muscle energy technique varies from the other thrusting techniques such that after the joint segment has been taken to its barrier, the force from the therapist is directed *away* from the restriction, against a voluntary isometric contraction exerted by the patient for 5 to 10 seconds. The patient then relaxes, and the therapist can then passively move the segment slightly beyond its previous barrier. With repetition, the barrier is displaced further until the restriction is overcome.

Myofascial release involves techniques similar to massage with gradual mobilization and stretching of the muscles and fascial connective tissue in the direction of the collagen fiber matrix, thereby lengthening the tissues, reducing spasm and restriction, and re-establishing muscle balance and alignment.

Manipulation can be used for all generalized musculoskeletal pain syndromes characterized by restricted joint motion, spasm, or localized tenderness. The gentler, more gradual techniques of low-velocity manipulation, myofascial release, and muscle energy do not carry significant risks if done correctly and therefore have lower contraindications. High-velocity manipulation, although remaining relatively safe if done by a skilled practitioner, does carry more risk of inducing pain. Contraindications include any possibility of malignancy, infection, acute inflammation, myelopathy, significant advanced bone disease including osteomalacia or osteoporosis, pregnancy, vertebral instability secondary to ligamentous injury, fractures, rheumatoid arthritis, and other active spondyloarthropathies. Hypermobility (i.e., excessive motion of the joint) is a contraindication for further manipulation. The isolated catastrophic cases of neurologic sequelae resulting from high-velocity manipulation have occurred in patients in whom the neck was extended during the manipulation or the maneuver was done too forcefully in a direction that injured the cervical vessels.[8–10]

Often after the first few treatment sessions, the patient actually feels worse with more pain, generalized discomfort, and restlessness. These symptoms usually resolve after several days to a week with anti-inflammatory drugs, ice, and gentle stretching exercises. If the treatments are effective, the patient achieves a more relaxed baseline before the next session. If not, the frequency of treatments can be extended out to allow more time to *recover*. If the patient continues to have pain that does not abate after a week, consideration must be given to stopping any further treatment or seeking another approach.

ELECTROTHERAPY

Electrotherapy has been used throughout history to help remedy various musculoskeletal conditions. Different modes of delivery, frequency, and equipment have been developed over the years to treat symptoms ranging from pain and spasm to atrophy.

Electrical Muscle Stimulation

Electrical muscle stimulation (EMS) has been used since ancient Greek times (using electric eels) through the present to help alleviate musculoskeletal pain and spasms as well as to facilitate muscle contraction and development of strength. There are a wide range of modalities of EMS, varying in the types of generators and currents used, type of waveform delivered, and the type and number of electrodes employed. Basically the principles and intended outcomes are the same. The success of treatment often depends on the individual's response after trying different forms of EMS as well as the therapist's expertise in technique. EMS theoretically helps relax muscles through the development of muscle fatigue after sustained or repeated contraction induced by the electrical stimulation. It has also been shown to increase the production of endorphins, to help circulatory stimulation and lymphatic drainage, and to promote muscle fiber recruitment. Aside from musculoskeletal conditions, it has been used in gynecologic problems, stress incontinence, ocular muscle spasms, and temporomandibular dysfunction. EMS should be avoided in patients with fractures, hemorrhagic states, phlebitis, and pacemakers.

Different types of currents delivered include galvanic or direct current (DC), pulsed galvanic or interrupted DC, faradic, and alternating current. Electrodes are usually applied as pads of various sizes to the affected muscle groups, especially the trapezius, rotator cuff, and paraspinal muscles. Muscles or tender points can also be stimulated by using a unipolar probe. Electrical stimulation should be considered as an adjunctive modality to help relieve pain and spasm in conjunction with an active exercise program.[11]

Transcutaneous Electrical Nerve Stimulation

Transcutaneous electrical nerve stimulation (TENS) uses electrical stimulation at a low intensity that theoretically blocks the transmission of pain from the spinal cord to the brain. The gate theory of pain generation underlies this modality. It states that afferent nociceptor transmission can be blocked before reaching the brain (where pain is consciously perceived). Pain sensation is transmitted more slowly than other sensory modalities because of the unmyelinated structure of the nociceptive C fibers. If two different sensory signals stimulate the internuncial cells of the substantia gelatinosa simultaneously, the non-nociceptive signal reaches the gate more quickly and is transmitted through to the brain, whereas the slower pain signal is blocked.[12] TENS provides the non-nociceptive afferent signal, thus blocking pain transmission. TENS has also been thought to stimulate the release of centrally acting endorphins, which also ameliorates pain perception.

The TENS unit consists of a signal generator with 2 to 4 leads. Intensity, frequency, and pulse wave characteristics can be modified on the unit. Current can be adjusted from 0 to 100 mA, pulse rates between 1 and 200 Hz, and pulse widths from 10 to 500 μs. Electrodes are placed adjacent to the painful area, often directing the current from an electrode pair across or crisscrossing the site (Fig. 10–3), or if used on an extremity, the leads are placed proximal to the site, (e.g., in an amputee with phantom pain). The placement of the electrodes is not specific; the therapist and patient must experiment and find the most effective configuration. The stimulus is usually initiated in a low-amplitude, high-frequency mode, with the intensity adjusted by the patient. High-amplitude, low-frequency modes can be tried on subsequent trials. The treatment is sustained for about 1 hour at a time; many patients, however, opt to wear the device for most of the day. Treatment is limited by battery life or skin irritation, not by any risk of significant bodily injury. With constant use, most patients seem to develop a tolerance to its effect, having to increase routinely either the intensity or the duration of application. Four to five initial trials are usually carried out under the direction of the therapist, and a personal unit is prescribed only after effective relief of pain is consistently achieved during trials.

TENS can be effective in nonspecific chronic back pain; pain from radiculopathies; neuropathic pain, as in reflex sympathetic dystrophy and diabetic neuropathy; myofascial pain syndromes and fibromyalgia; phantom pain; and post-surgical and obstetric pain. Studies vary widely with regard to its actual efficacy, with success rates ranging from 25% to 95%. Contraindications are few, mainly avoiding use in those with pacemakers, implantable defibrillators, significant arrhythmias, and pregnancy.[1]

Although the success rates are inconsistent, TENS can be an effective means of pain control when most other modalities or treatments have failed because it gives the patient a means of controlling his or her symptoms. A prescription for a TENS trial with the physical therapist usually determines whether the modality is further warranted.

BIOFEEDBACK

Biofeedback helps a patient gain an element of control over a physiologic process, whether it be muscular control (including spasms), pain, or other sensations. Even processes that are not classically considered under volitional control can be influenced by biofeedback (e.g., blood pressure, gastrointestinal motility, cardiac rhythm, seizures, and incontinence). The basic prin-

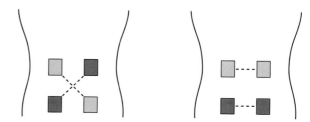

Figure 10–3. Configurations of transcutaneous nerve stimulation electrode awareness of afferent signals.

ciple involves a sensory signal or input, normally poorly perceived by the individual, which is augmented such that it can then be recognized and subsequently perceived consciously to effect a certain desired response. Visual and auditory feedback are the most common sensory modalities used; temperature, pressure, and other modalities have also been incorporated. Electromyography and imagery are probably the most common monitors used. Once a minimal response is achieved, further training can commence to effect more control. The patient can then gain control over more specific or isolated aspects of the process.[1] The self-induced change in the response itself can subsequently be used as the monitoring *device*. It is vital that the patient be attuned to and willing to go through the training process, and that the therapist is skilled in instituting the technique. The exact scientific mechanism for the effectiveness of biofeedback is yet to be determined. One common technique of biofeedback for muscle tension consists of having a patient contract various muscles to feel the sensation of *tension*, then voluntarily relax those muscles to feel the sensation of relaxation or easing of tension in those muscles. This exercise is repeated several times and then throughout different muscle groups ultimately to develop a conscious awareness of the sensation of tension or pain, such that the effect of control or regulation (i.e., conscious relaxation) (see Chapter 8) can be instituted. Biofeedback is somewhat similar to a servomechanism in which the action or output is monitored closely to regulate subsequent output, thus attaining a specific desired level of activity through feedback control (Fig. 10–4).

SUMMARY

Therapeutic modalities are an important component of therapy to help treat patients with various musculoskeletal disorders. The application of the various

modalities requires experience and proficiency in use as well as close monitoring of patient response. Whenever possible, an active exercise regimen should be the mainstay of therapy, with the use of modalities (i.e., passive therapy) as an adjunct to complete the treatment protocol. Careful regulation of the use of modalities is also essential; otherwise, a patient can become dependent on use of a modality and forego any active program that would otherwise help the patient take control of or adapt to the disorder.

ACKNOWLEDGMENT

Robert Anderson, RPT, Palo Alto VA Health Care Systems, for assisting with the photographs of traction (Fig. 10–1 and 10–2).

REFERENCES

1. Basford JR: Physical agents and biofeedback. In DeLisa JA, Gans BM, eds: Rehabilitation Medicine: Principles and Practice, 2nd ed. Philadelphia, JB Lippincott, 1993.
2. Lehman JF, deLateur BJ: Diathermy and superficial heat, laser and cold therapy. In Kottke FJ, Lehman JF, eds: Krusen's Handbook of Physical Medicine and Rehabilitation, 4th ed. Philadelphia, WB Saunders, 1990.
3. Geiringer SR, Kincaid CB, Rechtien JR: Traction, manipulation, and massage. In DeLisa JA, Gans BM, eds: Rehabilitation Medicine: Principles and Practice, 2nd ed. Philadelphia, JB Lippincott, 1993.
4. Cyriax JH: Textbook of Orthopaedic Medicine: Treatment by Manipulation, Massage and Injection, 10th ed. London, Bailliere-Tindall, 1982.
5. Basmajian JV, ed: Manipulation, Traction and Massage, 3rd ed. Baltimore, Williams & Wilkins, 1985.
6. Colachis SC, Strohm BR: A study of tractive forces and angle of pull on vertebral interspaces in the cervical spine. Arch Phys Med Rehabil 46:820–830, 1965.
7. Crue BL: Importance of flexion in cervical halter traction. Bull Los Angeles Neurol Soc 30:95–98, 1965.
8. Colachis SC, Strohm BR: Effects of intermittent traction on separation of lumbar vertebrae. Arch Phys Med Rehabil 50:251–258, 1969.
9. Bourdillon JF: Spinal Manipulation, 3rd ed. New York, Appleton-Century-Crofts, 1983.
10. Krueger BR, Okazaki H: Vertebral basilar distribution infarction following chiropractic cervical manipulation. Mayo Clin Proc 55:322–332, 1980.
11. Kahn J: Principles and Practice of Electrotherapy, 2nd ed. New York, Churchill Livingstone, 1991.
12. Melzack R, Wall PD: Pain mechanisms, a new theory. Science 150:971–979, 1965.

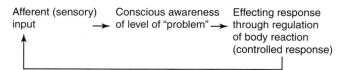

Figure 10–4. Biofeedback mechanism. Effecting a controlled bodily response through conscious awareness of afferent signals.

Chapter **11**

Record Keeping for Rheumatic Diseases

Ronald F. van Vollenhoven

Rheumatologic diseases are characterized and distinguished to a great extent by their chronic nature. As a result, accurate assessment of disease activity, severity, and functional status are paramount in determining whether (1) a response to treatment exists, (2) the response to treatment is sufficient in the clinical setting, and (3) other therapeutic approaches need to be considered. Medical records are also needed as the source documentation for issues pertaining to disability and employment status, which can have a significant impact on the patient's well-being. The role of the physician as patient advocate may require accurate records of disease characteristics and progression in these cases as well. Finally, the current emphasis on review of medical records as the basis for reimbursement compels an ever-increasing commitment of the physician to accuracy, completeness, and some degree of redundancy in medical record keeping.

SOAP—BENEFITS AND DEFICIENCIES

Although chart entries in the typical SOAP (subjective data, objective data, assessment, and plan) format are well suited for the documentation of acute events and diagnostic and therapeutic decisions at the time of the patient visit, they do not provide sufficient relevant documentation of the most important characteristics of chronic diseases. The main dimensions of chronic, rheumatic disease that need to be captured by the medical record in addition to the traditional SOAP note are outlined in Table 11–1 and include the following:

- At least one objective measure of disease activity
- An assessment of the severity of the disease
- An assessment of patient functional status (as relevant to the disease under consideration)
- An assessment of (usually irreversible) end-organ damage attributable to the disease (or its treatment)
- The cumulative treatment history for the disease in each patient

Depending on the specific disease, many different types of instruments have been developed that each capture one or more of these aspects. Although many such instruments are designed primarily as research tools and would be appropriate only in a specialty setting, some of them can be used by the primary care physician to improve greatly the quality of their medical records. These instruments are discussed subsequently, according to the disease in which they can be used.

RECORD KEEPING IN RHEUMATOID ARTHRITIS

The most important changes in understanding of and approach to rheumatoid arthritis (RA) are discussed elsewhere (see Chapter 25). Briefly, it has become increasingly clear that RA is associated with significant morbidity as well as decreased life expectancy,[1, 2] that cartilage and bone damage (which is irreversible) can develop early in the disease course,[3] and that treatment with disease-modifying antirheumatic drugs (DMARDs) can slow down the progression of such damage. The more traditional reliance on aspirin or nonsteroidal anti-inflammatory drugs (NSAIDs) is not likely to result in substantially better outcomes.[4–6] Moreover, the reliance on glucocorticoids in the treatment of RA—other than low-dose treatment (bridge therapy), the treatment of severe flares with or without extra-articular features, such as vasculitis or Felty's syndrome, or by intra-articular administration—has resulted in significant treatment-related morbidity and should generally be discouraged.[7] The medical record of a patient with RA needs to take into account five separate dimensions of the disease, each of which can be documented by various means.

Activity of Disease

Activity of disease typically refers to the degree of active synovial inflammation in the joints, the immunologically mediated process by which lymphocytes proliferate in the joint tissues, producing cytokines and effector pathways that lead to symptoms as well as joint distruction. Disease activity can be measured in several ways, and it is generally recommended not to rely on a single indicator but to use a combination of measurements.

Table 11–1. DIMENSIONS OF THE MEDICAL RECORD FOR CHRONIC RHEUMATIC DISEASES

Disease activity	How much inflammation is present? How much acute symptomatology can be attributed to this disease?
Disease severity	How severe or serious is this disease overall? What is the likely prognosis? How aggressive should treatment be?
Damage	How much, and what kind of, irreversible end-organ damage has occurred in this patient as the result of the illness or as the result of its treatment?
Quality of life	What is the quality of life for this patient? How much disability is present? What is the functional status?
Medication record	What medications have been used in the treatment of this patient's disease? What are the cumulative dosages?

JOINT COUNT

The record should reflect which joints are affected by the inflammatory process. Verbatim documentation is cumbersome and tends to be inaccurate. A printed stick-man with the joints marked, on which the affected joints are indicated, is commonly employed; a stamp with such a stickman can be obtained from the American College of Rheumatology. Either the joints that are swollen or the joints that are painful can be indicated; both approaches have advantages and disadvantages. A more quantitative approach is the tender joint count or swollen joint count; in this instance, the number of swollen or the number of painful joints is counted. Typically, 66 or 68 joints are evaluated, and forms for recording these are in widespread use, particularly in the setting of clinical research and clinical trials. For a primary care physician, however, this practice may still be impractical, and the 28-joint count is probably the best instrument to use (see Fig. 11–1 [all figures appear at the end of this chapter]).[8] This, instrument requires that the following joints are examined: all five metacarpophalangeal and proximal interphalangeal joints of the hands and the bilateral wrists, elbows, shoulders, and knees. Swelling, pain, or both could be recorded. Swelling is somewhat more objective. A disadvantage is that some swollen, painless joints may reflect chronic, noninflammatory pannus made up of abundant layers of synoviocytes, mononuclear leukocytes, and histiocytes and unlikely to change in medium-term follow-up.

JOINT SCORE

Scoring the degree to which joints are affected, for example, assigning 1, 2, or 3 points for each joint in terms of swelling (mild, moderate, severe), is also used extensively in research and trial settings, but it is likely that the added information in terms of severity is offset by the cumbersome and subjective nature of these assessments, the added time requirement, and the result-

ing statistical weakness. This scoring is therefore not recommended for primary care documentation purposes. Likewise, the use of gauges, rings, or even mercury baths to measure diameter, circumference, and volume of swollen joints is not recommended for day-to-day clinical use.

MORNING STIFFNESS

In addition to the joint count, it is generally helpful to record a measure of the patient's own assessment of RA activity. The duration of morning stiffness, best defined by patients as difficulty moving on awakening, is used most widely, is simple and intuitive, and is easy to record. In research settings, visual analogue scales of the patient's own assessment of disease activity are often employed.

BLOOD TESTS

A laboratory marker of disease activity should also be used, and either the erythrocyte sedimentation rate (ESR) or the C-reactive protein (CRP) can be chosen. A study[9] showed that these two acute-phase reactants can be used interchangeably, even though they might measure somewhat different aspects of the rheumatic inflammatory process. The ESR is more widely available and less expensive but requires immediate processing and may be influenced more by liver or renal disease and by concentrations of serum proteins (see Chapter 5). Other acute-phase reactants, such as serum amyloid A, are not widely used, and their cost is usually higher. These acute-phase reactants reflect disease activity only to a certain extent, and some patients with active synovial inflammation can have a normal ESR or CRP. A study of outcomes in RA has found a poor correlation of ESR with clinical measures of inflammation.[10]

Disease Severity and Prognosis

In RA, patients with positive rheumatoid factor, nodules, or erosions by x-rays have a worse prognosis.[11] These predictive markers of overall disease severity should be indicated clearly in the medical record. Preferably the entry on the record should reflect this important prognostic information. Thus, rather than simply writing *rheumatoid arthritis,* one should write *seropositive, nodular, erosive rheumatoid arthritis.* In this context, seropositivity or seronegativity reflects the positive or negative rheumatoid factor and not the antinuclear antibodies or other autoantibodies, which have limited prognostic significance.

Damage

The degree of damage attributable to the disease should be documented. In RA, this degree of damage is reflected by cartilage damage (apparent on x-ray films as joint space narrowing), bone damage (erosions), tendon laxity (leading to joint instability), tendon rupture (leading to loss of movement), and destruction of the periarticular structures (leading to deformities). All these end results of the inflammatory process must be described in the chart. They do not have to be repeated at every visit, but it may be helpful to have a separate entry reflecting damage that is updated annually.

Functional Status

The functional status of the patient needs to be documented periodically. The modified Stanford health assessment questionnaire (HAQ) disability index[12] can be completed by patients at semiannual intervals, but annual or biannual entries may suffice from a practical point of view. The HAQ disability index is simple, requires little time from the patient, and is available in many languages. It has been validated in a number of studies and is widely available. Other instruments intended to measure disability status, such as the SF-36, are more complex and, generally speaking, more suitable for research purposes than for a clinical practice setting.

Treatment History

Finally, the patient's cumulative treatment needs to be readily available in the medical record (see Fig. 11–2). This history is a requirement of hospital records under Joint Committee on Accredition of Hospitals (JCAHO) guidelines but is particularly relevant for RA because many treatments can be used over the course of time, and it may not be until years or decades later that it becomes important to be able to determine which treatments were used at what time and why they were discontinued. Thus, the record needs to reflect clearly each treatment with start and stop dates and a reasonably accurate assessment of total or cumulative dosage. Cumulative dosage has been used as a yardstick for treatment decisions in some situations. For instance, it has been recommended to discontinue parenteral gold treatment if no satisfactory response was obtained after a cumulative dosage of 1000 to 2000 mg, and after a cumulative dose of 5000 mg in a patient with an excellent clinical response, the drug could be discontinued.[13] The recommendation to perform liver biopsy after a cumulative dosage of methotrexate (of 1.5 or 2.0 g) is debated in the literature[14]; but in the most recent American College of Rheumatology guidelines, it is not endorsed.[15] Cyclophosphamide, albeit rarely used for RA, has long-term toxicities that are related to cumulative dosage, such as neoplasms of the bladder and bone marrow. For patients with RA, the medication record is ideally set up to reflect in separate categories analgesics, NSAIDs, glucocorticoids, DMARDs, and medications used to treat some of the common comorbidities of RA, such as gastroprotective agents, tricyclic antidepressants, and bone-protective or antiresorptive agents.

RECORD KEEPING IN OSTEOARTHRITIS

In osteoarthritis, the pain attributable to the disease tends to wax and wane, whereas the functional assessment may reveal a slow but inexorable increase. It is therefore important not only to document the main symptoms from visit to visit, but also the functional impact (see Figs. 11–3 and 11–4). The pain caused by osteoarthritis can be documented verbatim or reflected on a scale by the patient; both visual analogue scales (simply a line on which the patient indicates the degree of pain) and numerical scales serve the same end.

For fuctional impact, the appropriate test depends on the location of the arthritic process. Patients with hip or knee arthritis can be asked to walk 50 feet and the time be recorded. For osteoarthritis of the hands (distal interphalangeal, proximal interphalangeal, or carpometacarpal joints), the button time (seconds required to button and unbutton one shirt button) may be suitable.

To date, there are no effective serologic markers for osteoarthritis. It is likely, however, that in the future various such markers will become available, and if validated as markers of outcome, these should be included in the periodic assessment of these patients. The degree of osteoarthritis-related damage is most effectively documented by serial radiographs of the affected joints. For global functional assessment, the HAQ is ideally suited. The impact of osteoarthritis tends to have a slowly progressive course, and annual or biennial assessment is sufficient. The medication record for OA in the 1990s reflects analgesics and NSAIDs. This record could change with the introduction of new classes of agents with *chondroprotective* properties.

RECORD KEEPING IN SYSTEMIC LUPUS ERYTHEMATOSUS

Because of its multisystem nature, systemic lupus erythematosus (SLE) is a much more complicated disease to document than the diseases that primarily involve synovium. Generally speaking, the medical record needs to indicate the same dimensions referred to in previous paragraphs.

Lupus Activity

Lupus activity, in terms of the affected organ systems and their specific status should be recorded at each visit (see Fig. 11–5). Although the SOAP format may be appropriate for this, there is great divergence in the way various lupus manifestations present. Thus, lupus arthritis is primarily a patient-reported symptom, lupus rashes are easily noted on physicial examination, and nephritis or leukopenia may be evident only on laboratory examination. To avoid missing an important change in SLE symptoms, the record must include a list of lupus manifestations to date, with regular updates in terms of the status of each particular organ system affected.

A number of overall scoring systems for lupus activity have been proposed and are widely employed in research and clinical trial settings. These include the SLEDAI,[16] SLAM,[17] BILAG,[18] and others. It is not clear that recording these scores in the medical record is of major benefit in clinical practice, however, and the time needed to complete these instruments as well as the requirement of certain blood tests may be prohibitive in primary care. Computerized medical records may be able to compute lupus activity indices without additional time required for the physician, and this approach is currently being investigated. A global assessment by the physician on a scale of 1 to 100 is helpful.

Lupus Overall Severity

Overall severity of SLE (i.e., over the entire course of illness, rather than at a specific point in time) is a diffuse concept that has proved hard to define from a practical point of view. Katz and associates[19] developed a scoring system to reflect lupus severity. Whether this system will be beneficial to record is unclear as yet.

Damage

Damage attributable to SLE or to its treatment is one of the main reasons for morbidity, mortality, and declining quality of life in lupus patients. The importance of recording the cumulative damage is obvious, but a suitable format may be hard to find. It would be cumbersome to include a verbatim description in each chart note. It would be best to have a separate section in the medical record where damage is recorded cumulatively over time, similar to the diagnostic and medication information (see Fig. 11–6). This section requires some effort to set up, however. The SLICC damage index[20] may be helpful to arrive at a simple numerical score to indicate the total level of lupus-related cumulative damage.

Quality of Life

Quality of life in patients with SLE is often significantly diminished as a result of the impact of the illness itself as well as the treatment. To gauge quality of life, a disability score is important, but additional instruments to measure other aspects of life may need to be added, such as depression, fatigue, and overal function. The SF36, although lengthy, may provide helpful information even in the primary care setting.[21] This multiple-choice questionnaire takes the patient about 15 minutes to complete.

Medication History

Medication history is of crucial importance in the longitudinal documentation of SLE (see Fig. 11–6).

RECORD KEEPING IN SCLERODERMA

The cardinal manifestation of scleroderma is the abnormal skin, but the most serious consequences reflect disease in the heart, lungs, kidneys, or gastrointestinal tract. Therefore, the medical record needs to reflect all of these organ systems in an appropriate manner. In contrast to the illnesses discussed previously, scleroderma tends to have limited disease activity (although significant inflammatory activity can occur, particularly at the onset of the illness), but accurate recording of the more chronic changes is all the more important to identify patients in whom a previously stationary disease may be progressing to affect more seriously both the skin and the internal organs.

The degree of skin involvement can be ascertained by various skin scoring instruments, all of which rely on quantifying the disease in each of a number of regions. None of these systems are robust, however, and the main problem lies in distinguishing thickening of the skin resulting from edema (as seen in the early stages of scleroderma), thickening of the skin resulting of excessive collagen deposition (middle stage of the disease), and the less thick but taut, hidebound skin in the later stages of the disease. One useful semi-quantitative measure is the degrees of flexion to the palm lacking in the phalanges. A verbatim description of the skin involvement may still be the best option in this disease.

The involvement of internal organs needs to be documented in a longitudinal fashion. For example, the diffusing capacity of the lungs for carbon monoxide (generally believed to be most sensitive to sclerodermatous changes in the lungs) should be recorded in such a way as to allow comparisons from year to year.

RECORD KEEPING IN FIBROMYALGIA

Despite being one of the most common rheumatic conditions as well as being poorly understood, documentation of fibromyalgia is still in its infancy. Verbatim entries in the medical record usually reflect more of the frustration felt by both patient and physician than relevant medical facts. These data, however, can be analyzed in a fashion analogous to that outlined previously for other chronic diseases.

Activity of the Disease

The patient's main symptom, by definition, is widespread musculoskeletal pain. Therefore, it is not necessary to document this fact repeatedly. A quantitative measure of the pain should be obtained: This can be done most easily with a visual analogue scale, a horizontal line (marked with the numbers 0 and 100 on either side) on which the patient places a mark to indicate how severe his or her discomfort. The main purpose is to obtain this information consistently so as to obtain helpful information regarding changes in pain severity, disease course, and response to therapy. There is probably little use, if any, in a clinical practice setting to documenting numbers of tender points, dolorimetry results, or other more complex ways of recording disease activity. In patients with diagnoses of fibromyalgia, chronic fatigue syndrome (see Chapter 18), palindromic rheumatism, undifferentiated connective tissue disease, and other diagnoses with less defined criteria, it is crucial to be constantly ready to change the diagnoses to another entity if the clinical data or history warrant it.

Impact of Fibromyalgia on Daily Life

The impact of the disease on daily life must be documented, and for this, the HAQ disability index is suitable. However, because fibromyalgia is associated not only with functional impairment, but also frequently with abnormalities of sleep, mood, and other nonphysical factors, a more extensive instrument, such as the SF-36, might be considered. In clinical practice, however, these instruments are somewhat unwieldy.

Medication History

Medication history is as important in fibromyalgia as it is in other rheumatic diseases. Specific entries reflecting nonmedical interventions, such as physical therapy, acupuncture, TENS units, diathermy, massage, or chriopractic treatment as well as the use of nontraditional health food supplements and herbal remedies, should be added.

RECORD KEEPING IN ANKYLOSING SPONDYLITIS

Ankylosing spondylitis is another slowly progressive, chronic rheumatic disease, the documentation of which needs to be appropriate to the nature of the illness. The degree of inflammatory activity can best be gauged by an assessment of inflammatory symptoms, such as morning stiffness or global pain. The degree of impairment, which is likely to change slowly over time, is more important to quantify regularly. Flexion in the lumbosacral spine is usually measured by the Schober test (the increase in vertical distance between two points on the skin overlying the lumbosacral spine on maximal flexion) (see Chapter 3). Involvement of the thoracic spine can be gauged by measuring inspiratory chest wall excursion and involvement of the cervical-spine by measurement of the occiput-to-wall distance (with the patient standing straight, back against the wall). By the nature of the disease, these measurements do not have to be taken frequently, but they are helpful to follow the disease over 5, 10, or 20 years. The ultimate objective of management is to prevent so much neck and back fixed flexion that the patient can no longer see the horizon.

CONCLUSION

The general principles discussed in this chapter can be applied in a similar vein to other chronic rheumatic diseases. Although in some such diseases specialized instruments for measuring disease activity, severity, or damage have been used, these instruments are primarily intended for research. Most importantly, record keeping in rheumatic diseases requires assessments of *disease activity, severity, damage,* and *impact on function and quality of life.* Although the initial visits may be more time-intensive as a result, when following patients for extended periods of time, the well-kept records help in providing the patient with the best care possible, while allowing more time-efficient management in the long-term.

REFERENCES

1. Van der Grouche JP, Hazevoct HM, Cats A: Survival and cause of death in rheumatoid arthritis: Twenty-five year prospective follow-up. J Rheumatol 11:158, 1984.
2. Sherrer YS, Block DA, Mitchell DM, et al: The development of disability in rheumatoid arthritis. Arthritis Rheum 29:494; 1986.
3. Fuchs HA, Kaye JJ, Callahan LF, et al: Evidence of significant radiographic damage in rheumatoid arthritis within the first two years of disease. J Rheumatol 16:585, 1989.
4. Felson DT, Anderson JJ, Meenan RF: Use of short-term efficacy/toxicity trade-offs to select second-line drugs in rheumatoid arthritis. Arthritis Rheum 35:1117, 1992.
5. Wilske KR, Healey LA: Remodelling the pyramid: A concept whose time has come. J Rheumatol 16:565, 1989.
6. Felson DT, Anderson JJ, Meenan RF: The comparative efficacy and toxicity of second-line drugs in rheumatoid arthritis. Arthritis Rheum 33:1149, 1990.
7. Van Vollenhoven RF: Corticosteroids in rheumatic disease. Postgrad Med 103:137, 1998.
8. Smolen JS, Breedveld FC, Eberl G, et al: Validity and reliablility of the twenty-eight-joint count for the assessment of rheumatoid arthritis activity. Arthritis Rheum 38:38, 1995.
9. Wolfe F, Pew B, Harkness D: Which test is best: A comparative study of CRP and ESR in rheumatoid arthritis. Arthritis Rheum 39:S157; 1996.
10. Ward MM: Clinical measures in rheumatoid arthritis: Which are most useful in assessing patients? J Rheumatol 21:17, 1993.
11. Van der Heijde DM, Van Riel PL, Van Leeuwen MA, et al: Prognostic factors for radiographic damage and physical disability in early rheumatoid arthritis: A prospective study of 157 patients. Br J Rheumatol 31:519, 1992.
12. Pincus T, Callahan LF, Brooks RH, et al: Self-report questionnaire scores in rheumatoid arthritis compared with traditional physical, radiographic and laboratory measures. Ann Intern Med 110:259, 1989.
13. Furst DE: Rational use of disease-modifying antirheumatic drugs. Drugs 39:19–37, 1990.
14. Kremer JM, Alarcon GS, Lightfoot RW, et al: Methotrexate for rheumatoid arthritis: Suggested guidelines for monitoring liver toxicity. Arthritis Rheum 37:316, 1994.

15. Hassan W: Methotrexate and liver toxicity: Role of surveillance liver biopsy: Conflict between guidelines for rheumatologists and dermatologists. Ann Rheum Dis 55:273; 1996.
16. Bombardier C, Gladman DD, Urowitz MB, et al: Derivation of the SLEDAI: A Disease Activity Index for lupus patients. Arthritis Rheum 35:630, 1992.
17. Liang MH, Socher SA, Larson MG, Schur PH: Reliability and validity of six systems for the clinical assessment of disease activity in systemic lupus erythematosus. Arthritis Rheum 32:1107, 1989.
18. Symmons DPM, Coopock JS, Bacon PA, et al: Development and assessment of a computerized index of clinical disease activity in systemic lupus erythematosus. QJM 68:927, 1988.
19. Katz JD, Senecal JL, Rivest C, et al: A simple severity of disease index for systemic lupus erythematosus. Lupus 2:119, 1993.
20. Gladman DD, Ginzler E, Goldsmith C, et al: The development and initial validation of the SLICC/ACR damage index for SLE. Arthritis Rheum 39:363, 1996.
21. Ware JE, Sherbourne CD: The MOS SF-36 item short-form health survey (SF-36): Conceptual framework and item selection. Med Care 30:473, 1992.

Rheumatoid Arthritis: Form for Each Visit

Patient Identifiers:	Morning stiffness (minutes) _____
Today's date: _____	ESR or CRP _____

Dx: RA	Tender joints:*	Left	Right
S	MCP 1		
	MCP 2		
	MCP 3		
O	MCP 4		
	MCP 5		
	PIP 1		
A	PIP 2		
	PIP 3		
	PIP 4		
P	PIP 5		
	Wrist		
	Elbow		
Current Medications:	Shoulder		
	Knee		

* or swollen joints

Figure. 11–1. Example of a patient visit record for rheumatoid arthritis that includes an area for SOAP notes and a 28-joint checklist. SOAP, subjective data, objective data, assessment, and plan; MCP, metacarpophalangeal; PIP, proximal interphalangeal.

Rheumatoid Arthritis: Chart Form to be Updated Annually

DATES					
HAQ Disability Index					
Joint instability					
Tendon rupture					
Deformities					
Joint space narrowing					
Erosions					

Figure. 11–2. Example of an annual patient record for rheumatoid arthritis patients. Summary information on disease progression and medications can be entered by visit date and can quickly and easily be compared. HAQ, Health Assessment Questionnaire; DMARDs, disease-modifying antirheumatic drugs; IM, intramuscular; NSAIDs, nonsteroidal anti-inflammatory drugs.

Medication record		Dosage	Start date	Stop date	Why d/c'd?
DMARDs	Methotrexate				
	Sulfasalazine				
	Hydroxychloroquine				
	Gold (IM)				
	Azathioprine				
	Cyclosporin A				
	Other				
Corticosteroids	Prednisone				
	Other				
NSAIDs	_____				
	_____				
Other					
(e.g., analgesics,					
gastroprotective agents,					
antiresorptive agents, tricyclic					
antidepressants)					

Osteoarthritis: Form for Each Visit

Pt. Identifiers:

Today's date: _____

Dx: OA

S

O

Patient's pain assessment: _____

(0-100)

A

50-foot walk time: _____

(hip/knee)

P

Button & unbutton time: _____

(hand/wrist)

Figure. 11–3. Example of a patient visit record for osteoarthritis that includes an area for SOAP notes and disease progression measures.

Osteoarthritis: Chart Form to be Updated Annually

DATES					
HAQ Disability Index					
Recent X-ray finding					

Figure. 11–4. Example of an annual patient record for osteoarthritis patients. Summary information on disease progression and medications can be entered by visit date and can quickly and easily be compared. See Figure 11–2 for abbreviations.

Medication record	Dosage	Start date	Stop date	Why d/c'd?
NSAIDs _____ _____ _____				
Other (e.g., analgesics, gastroprotective agents, antiresorptive agents, tricyclic antidepressants)				

SLE: Form for Each Visit

Patient Identifiers:

Today's date: _____

Dx: SLE

S

O

A

P

Current Medications:

SLE symptoms present today (check if present, & comment)

General	Weight loss Fatigue Fever	GI	Abdominal pain Peritoneal signs
Skin & integument	Oral ulcers Periungual erythema Malar rash Photosensitive rash Discoid rash Rash, other Nail fold infarct Alopecia Vasculitis	Neurological	CVA TIA Neuritis Seizure Cognitive dysfunction Psychosis Dementia Organic brain syndrome Headache Meningitis
Eye	Cytoid bodies Retinal hemorrhage Episcleritis Papilledema	Musculo-skeletal	Myalgia Myositis Arthralgia Arthritis
RES	Lymphadeno- pathy Hepatomegaly Splenomegaly	Hematological	Leukopenia Lymphopenia Anemia Thrombocytopenia
Pulmonary	Dyspnea Pleuritic chest pain Abnormal exam	Renal	Proteinuria Hematuria Casts Pyuria
Cardiovascular	Raynaud's Hypertension Carditis		

Overall lupus activity, by physician (0-100): _____

Overall lupus activity, by patient (0-100): _____

Figure. 11–5. Example of a patient visit record for systemic lupus erythematosus that includes an area for SOAP notes, a symptoms checklist by organ system, and lupus activity indices. GI, gastrointestinal; CVA, cerebrovascular accident; TIA, transient ischemic attack; RES, reticuloendothelial system.

SLE: Chart Form to be Updated Annually

Check if present, or requiring treatment for at least 6 months:

DATES					
Cataract					
Retinal infarcts					
Cognitive impairment					
Major psychosis					
Seizures					
CVA					
Neuropathy (cranial or peripheral)					
Transverse myelitis					
GFR <50%					
Proteinuria >3.5 g/day					
End-stage renal disease					
Pulmonary hypertension					
Pulmonary fibrosis					
"Shrinking lung"					
Cardiomyopathy					
Valvular disease					
Chronic pericarditis (or pericardiectomy)					
Claudication					
Ischemic tissue loss					
Muscle atrophy					
Joint deformities					
Osteoporosis					
With fracture					
Avascular necrosis					
Permanent alopecia					
Premature gonadal failure					
Steroid-induced diabetes					

Medication record		Dosage	Start date	Stop date	Why d/c'd?
DMARDs	Methotrexate				
	Sulfasalazine				
	Hydroxychloroquine				
	Gold (IM)				
	Azathioprine				
	Cyclosporin A				
	Other				
Corticosteroids	Prednisone				
	Other				
NSAIDs	_____				
Other (e.g., analgesics, gastroprotective agents, antiresorptive agents, tricyclic antidepressants)					
Cytoxan					

Figure. 11–6. Example of an annual patient record for systemic lupus erythematosus patients. Sum-mary information on disease progression and medications can be entered by visit date and can quickly and easily be compared. CVA, cerebrovascular accident; GFR, glomer-ular filtration rate; see Figure 11–2 for other abbreviations.

Chapter **12**

Special Problems of Musculoskeletal Disease in the Elderly Patient

Michael M. Ward

The prevalence of many musculoskeletal diseases and of musculoskeletal complaints increases with age. Thus, the typical patient with a particular musculoskeletal condition or complaint is often elderly. Some musculoskeletal conditions may have atypical presentations in elderly patients. In addition, comorbid medical conditions and the many medications used to treat these conditions can complicate the management of elderly patients with musculoskeletal problems. Physical frailty, instability, falls, and immobility are also consequences of musculoskeletal aging. This chapter discusses these common problems in the care of elderly patients with musculoskeletal conditions.

ALTERED PRESENTATION OF MUSCULOSKELETAL DISEASES IN THE ELDERLY

In the evaluation of elderly patients, a broader range of possible diagnoses often must be considered than in younger patients. In the elderly, metastatic cancer, multiple myeloma, osteoporotic fractures, hyperparathyroidism and thyroid diseases must be considered in the differential diagnosis of musculoskeletal pain, whereas such conditions are less likely to be causes of musculoskeletal pain in young and middle-aged patients. The differential diagnosis of inflammatory polyarthritis in elderly patients should include thyroid disease, paraneoplastic conditions, and polymyalgia rheumatica as well as rheumatoid arthritis, connective tissue diseases, spondyloarthropathies, and crystal-induced arthritis.

Laboratory tests may be less helpful in identifying elderly patients with systemic inflammation. The erythrocyte sedimentation rate normally increases with age, and values of 30 to 40 mm/h are not unusual in healthy elderly persons. C-reactive protein concentrations can be a more specific measure of systemic inflammation in the elderly. Of healthy elderly persons, 5% to 15% have rheumatoid factor or antinuclear antibodies detectable in their serum. Although the concentrations of these autoantibodies in healthy patients tend to be low, titers of 1:160 or 1:320, are not uncommon.[1] Also, elderly patients more often have other medical conditions associated with rheumatoid factor seropositivity, such as chronic lung or liver disease, and are more often treated with medications that can induce antinuclear antibodies. These factors may complicate the evaluation process because positive test results for these autoantibodies are more likely to be false-positive in elderly patients than in younger patients. Testing for autoantibodies should therefore be selective in elderly patients and be performed only when other clinical findings are highly suggestive of a connective tissue disease.

The onset of rheumatoid arthritis in most elderly patients, as in most younger patients, involves the gradual development of polyarthritis in the small joints of the hands and feet. However, two alternative presentations may occur in a small number of elderly patients. One presentation involves the acute onset of polyarthritis, occasionally overnight, with severe pain and stiffness that involves proximal as well as distal joints. These patients may have diffuse swelling of the hands and feet. Patients with this type of explosive onset have been termed to have *benign rheumatoid arthritis of the elderly,* because such patients often experience remission within 1 year. Another way rheumatoid arthritis may present in the elderly is similar to polymyalgia rheumatica, with complaints of stiffness in the neck, shoulders, and hips, which evolves over months into a more typical peripheral polyarthritis. Patients who develop systemic lupus erythematosus later in life more commonly have pleuritis, pleural effusions, pericarditis, interstitial pulmonary fibrosis, and features of Sjögren's syndrome than do younger patients. They less commonly have alopecia, Raynaud's phenomenon, lymphadenopathy, neuropsychiatric manifestations, and hypocomplementemia.[2] Drug-induced lupus is also more common among elderly patients. Awareness of these altered clinical presentations can help facilitate diagnosis in elderly patients with musculoskeletal conditions.

DRUG-DISEASE INTERACTIONS IN ELDERLY PATIENTS

Although the treatment of musculoskeletal conditions in the elderly does not differ from the treatment of younger patients, the comorbid medical conditions commonly present in elderly patients can influence the choice of medications or limit treatment options. Elderly patients can also be more susceptible to the known toxicities of antirheumatic medications because of age-related alterations in drug metabolism or excretion or limitations in tissue resistance or repair mechanisms.[3] For example, age-associated decreases in hepatic or renal function may require reductions in the dosage of nonsteroidal anti-inflammatory drugs (NSAIDs), particularly those with long serum half-lives, such as naproxen, piroxicam, sulindac, salsalate, and long-acting preparations of indomethacin. Because most NSAIDs are highly protein bound, dose reductions are also indicated for patients with hypoalbuminemia. Dosages of acetaminophen should also be reduced in patients with decreased hepatic function. Elderly patients may also be more sensitive to the analgesic effects of narcotics, so that adequate analgesia may be obtained with the use of lower dosages of these medications than are needed in younger patients.

The most common antirheumatic drug–disease interactions in elderly patients are listed in Table 12–1. NSAID gastropathy is a serious concern and a major cause of morbidity and mortality among elderly patients.[4] The elderly may be more susceptible to NSAID gastropathy because age-associated decreases in prostaglandin-mediated gastric mucosal protection

mechanisms may be further compromised by NSAID treatment.[5] If NSAID therapy is required in a patient with a history of NSAID gastropathy, the risk of recurrence may be reduced by using nonacetylated salicylates or nabumetone rather than other NSAIDs or by adding misoprostil, an H_2-blocker, or a proton-pump inhibitor to the patient's medication regimen. NSAIDs that selectively or preferentially inhibit cyclooxygenase-2 hold promise for reducing the risks of gastrointestinal toxicity that accompany this class of medications.

Prostaglandins are also responsible for maintaining renal blood flow and glomerular filtration in settings of decreased effective circulatory volume and hyperreninemia. Therefore, NSAIDs may precipitate acute renal failure in elderly patients with congestive heart failure, nephrosis, decompensated cirrhosis, or hypovolemia.[6] NSAIDs may also cause sodium and water retention and lead to worsening of hypertension, peripheral edema, and congestive heart failure.

Some NSAIDs have particular drug–disease interactions. Moderate or high-dose salicylates may cause profound hearing loss in elderly patients who have mild presbycusis, often without the warning symptom of tinnitus. Manifestations of salicylism in the elderly include confusion, slurred speech, hyperactivity, hallucinations, seizures, and coma. Indomethacin can cause headache, confusion, cognitive dysfunction, depression, and paranoia, and its use is best avoided in the elderly. Phenylbutazone can cause similar central nervous system effects as well as aplastic anemia and should also probably be avoided in elderly patients.

Narcotic analgesics may cause excessive sedation and cognitive dysfunction in the elderly.[7] Elderly patients may also develop severe constipation or fecal impaction with these medications, and bowel regimens should begin along with any use of narcotics.

Tricyclic antidepressants are used to treat fibromyalgia and occasionally used for analgesia and insomnia. Elderly patients are particularly sensitive to the anticholinergic side effects of tricyclics and may commonly experience orthostatic hypotension, tachycardia, constipation, and urinary retention. Tricyclics with the least anticholinergic activity should be used. Tricyclic antidepressants may also cause cognitive dysfunction and excessive sedation in elderly patients, and patients should be carefully monitored for these side effects.

Systemic glucocorticoid treatment may worsen preexisting hypertension, diabetes mellitus, osteoporosis, muscle weakness, and glaucoma in elderly patients. Sodium retention may also worsen congestive heart failure. Glucocorticoids also increase the risk of infections, to which elderly patients may already be predisposed by diminished host defenses. Glucocorticoids may also cause a variety of central nervous system side effects, including agitation, psychosis, mania, and depression. These side effects may be more common in patients with dementia, and treatment with glucocorticoids may make mild psychiatric conditions more overt.

Although elderly patients may, in general, be more prone to side effects from antirheumatic medications, age is only a surrogate marker of the underlying physi-

Table 12–1. COMMON ANTIRHEUMATIC DRUG–DISEASE INTERACTIONS IN ELDERLY PATIENTS

Drug	Interactions
Nonsteroidal anti-inflammatory drugs	Gastritis, peptic ulcer disease, gastrointestinal bleeding
	Sodium and water retention
	Hypertension
	Acute renal insufficiency
	Cognitive dysfunction, confusion, depression
Narcotic analgesics	Cognitive dysfunction, confusion
	Constipation, impaction
Tricyclic antidepressants	Orthostatic hypotension
	Tachycardia
	Constipation
	Urinary retention
	Confusion, excessive sedation
	Blurred vision
Glucocorticoids	Skin atrophy
	Sodium and water retention
	Hypertension
	Hyperglycemia
	Myopathy
	Osteopenia
	Cataracts, glaucoma
	Increased risk of infections
	Insomnia, agitation, irritability
	Depression, mania, psychosis

ologic alterations that cause the predisposition to drug toxicity. Variation among elderly patients is great, and all are not equally susceptible to the side effects of antirheumatic medications.

Compliance with medication regimens may be decreased among elderly with comorbid conditions, such as dementia or depression, and by polypharmacy. Comorbid conditions may also make it difficult for elderly patients to comply with nonpharmacologic treatments. For example, stroke, severe obstructive pulmonary disease, angina, congestive heart failure, or depression may limit a patient's ability to participate in exercise programs and hamper efforts at rehabilitation.

DRUG-DRUG INTERACTIONS IN ELDERLY PATIENTS

Elderly patients may be particularly susceptible to drug-drug interactions because they are often taking several medications to treat varying medical conditions (see Chapter 9). The antirheumatic drugs most often involved in drug-drug interactions are NSAIDs (Table 12–2). Most NSAIDs bind tightly to protein, and their interactions with several other types of medications result from the displacement of these medications from protein-binding sites. Thus, the hypocoagulable effect of warfarin and the hypoglycemic effect of sulfonylureas may be enhanced, and the levels of free digoxin, penicillins, sulfonamides, phenytoin, and valproic acid may increase when NSAIDs are coadministered. NSAID treatment is usually contraindicated in patients receiving systemic anticoagulation because of the enhanced risk of bleeding when the hemostatic effects of platelet aggregation are inhibited. Concomitant use of NSAIDs and glucocorticoids or alcohol increases the risk of gastrointestinal bleeding. NSAIDs blunt the effects of several antihypertensive medications; this effect is greatest for β-blockers and diuretics but also occurs with vasodilators.[8] Use of NSAIDs together with loop diuretics may also increase the risk of acute renal failure by predisposing patients to intravascular volume depletion. Some NSAIDs increase serum levels of lithium by decreasing renal clearance of this medication.

Narcotic analgesics may interact with other medications affecting the central nervous system, including alcohol, tricyclic antidepressants, sedatives, hypnotics, and major tranquilizers, to cause excessive sedation, cognitive dysfunction, or coma. Elderly patients using these medications must be monitored closely when narcotic analgesics are introduced. Glucocorticoids have few interactions with other drugs but can cause profound hypokalemia when used with potassium-wasting diuretics.

INSTABILITY AND FALLS

One third of community-dwelling elderly persons sustain a fall each year.[9] Five percent of these falls result in a fracture, and an additional 5% result in soft tissue injury severe enough that the person seeks medical attention. Falls are the most common reason for restricted activity days in the elderly; are a marker of physical frailty; and are a predictor of hospitalization, nursing home placement, and death. Fear of future falls can have consequences as great or greater than those of the fall itself because it may lead to further restriction in activity, immobility, and depression.

Falls occur when the mechanisms responsible for postural stability cannot meet the physical requirements for movement through the environment (Table 12–3). Any environmental challenge that surpasses a person's ability to maintain an upright posture can result in a fall. Environmental factors, such as poor lighting, slippery or uneven surfaces, and obstacles, may be the primary cause in up to 40% of falls. Postural stability depends on proper functioning of an integrated system of sensory inputs from the visual, vestibular, and peripheral nervous systems; accurate processing of this sensory information in the central nervous system; and proper execution of compensatory movements by the musculoskeletal system. Defects or deficiencies in any of these three areas can lead to postural instability and falls.

Musculoskeletal problems contribute to postural instability by affecting either the afferent sensory input or the person's ability to move appropriately. Chronic

Table 12–2. NONSTEROIDAL ANTI-INFLAMMATORY DRUG INTERACTIONS

Mechanism	Drug	Effect
Displacement from protein-binding sites	Warfarin	Increased prothrombin time
	Sulfonylureas	Increased hypoglycemic effect
	Phenytoin	Increased blood level
	Valproic acid	Increased blood level
	Digoxin	Increased blood level
	Penicillins	Increased blood level
	Sulfonamides	Increased blood level
Decrease in renal excretion	Lithium	Increased blood level
Potentiation of adverse effects	Anticoagulants	Increased risk of bleeding
	Glucocorticoids	Increased risk of gastrointestinal bleeding
	Alcohol	Increased risk of gastrointestinal bleeding
	Loop diuretics	Increased risk of acute renal failure
Interference with drug action	Antihypertensives	Decreased antihypertensive effect
	Uricosurics (probenecid, sulfinpyrazone)	Decreased hypouricemic effect

Table 12–3. MECHANISMS RESPONSIBLE FOR POSTURAL INSTABILITY

Environmental factors
   Poor lighting
   Slippery/uneven surfaces
   Obstacles
Sensory system
   Visual impairment
   Vestibular disorders
   Auditory insufficiency
   Peripheral nervous system (e.g., peripheral neuropathy associated
     with diabetes mellitus)
Sensory processing—central nervous system
   Diminished cerebral perfusion
   Dementia
   Movement disorders (e.g., Parkinson's disease)
Musculoskeletal compensation
   Afferent sensory input/proprioception defects
   Inability to move appropriately
     Arthritis
     Muscle weakness
   Gait abnormalities
Orthostasis
Medications

arthritis in the hip, knee, or ankle or foot deformities may alter proprioception so that incorrect information about position sense is transmitted to the central nervous system. Hip extensor and knee extensor strength is required to maintain an upright posture. Weakness of these muscles, as a result of deconditioning, myopathy, or arthritis in surrounding joints, increases instability. Joint contractures at the hip or knee tend to displace the body's center of gravity anteriorly, requiring active muscle work to maintain balance. In this situation, muscle weakness or easy fatigability contributes to instability. Other factors that commonly contribute to postural instability include orthostasis and dehydration, dizziness of central or vestibular origin, conditions that decrease cerebral perfusion, dementia, Parkinson's disease, peripheral neuropathies, gait abnormalities, and defects in vision or hearing. Many medications, including antihypertensives, sedatives, tranquilizers, tricyclic antidepressants, and narcotics, are commonly implicated in falls.

Assessment of patients who fall should be directed at detecting reversible factors that may contribute to postural instability. A functional assessment that involves observation of the ways in which the patient rises and sits in a chair, turns, bends over, reaches up, and balances may be more insightful than a standard neuromuscular examination.[10] Interventions should be directed at correcting any reversible deficiencies. For patients with musculoskeletal impairments, physical and occupational therapy may be particularly helpful for gait training, strengthening of leg muscles, teaching of adaptive movements, and provision of properly fitted assistive devices such as canes or walkers. A home assessment by an occupational therapist can be cost-effective in identifying environmental obstacles and arranging for modifications such as handrails for support.

IMMOBILITY

Musculoskeletal problems are the most common reasons for elderly patients to be restricted to bed, chair, or wheelchair.[11] These problems include arthritis of lower extremity joints or the lumbar spine, hip fractures, vertebral compression fractures, and muscle weakness and deconditioning. Immobility owing to arthritis is most often the result of pain with activity. Joint effusions and soft tissue contractures can also contribute to arthritis-associated immobility by limiting the joint's range of motion, thereby placing the muscles that move the joint at a mechanical disadvantage and increasing the work of movement substantially. Other common causes of immobility include neurologic diseases, such as stroke, dementia, Parkinson's disease, myelopathy, and neuropathy; severe cardiovascular disease; and severe obstructive pulmonary disease. Immobility resulting from deconditioning may develop quickly in elderly patients hospitalized with an acute illness.

The complications of immobility are numerous, and many can be life-threatening. Immobility causes negative nitrogen and calcium balance, which can worsen muscle weakness and osteoporosis. Atelectasis, aspiration pneumonia, urinary tract infections, renal calculi, urinary incontinence, decubiti, venous thromboses, and pulmonary emboli can occur. Depression, sensory deprivation, and delirium are not uncommon. Because of the serious nature of many of these complications, attention should be directed at early identification of problems in ambulatory patients that may limit their rehabilitation potential if they become immobile. Efforts should be made to prevent functional decline in patients hospitalized with acute illnesses or to reverse rapidly any that develop. Because functional deficits that are less severe or of recent onset are more easily corrected than long-standing ones, rehabilitation should be started early in such patients.

The treatment of immobility resulting from musculoskeletal problems should begin with optimization of the treatment of any arthritis that may be present (Table 12–4). Consultation with a rheumatologist may be helpful in identifying an undiagnosed but treatable arthritis or in suggesting treatment alternatives. Pain should be controlled as best as possible. Treatments to improve sleep and depression can be useful adjuncts. Nutritional status, including vitamin sup-

Table 12–4. TREATMENT OF IMMOBILITY RESULTING FROM MUSCULOSKELETAL PROBLEMS IN THE ELDERLY

Identification of undiagnosed or diffuse arthritis or connective tissue
  diseases
Optimization of treatment for arthritis
Pain control
Treatment of depression
Improvement of sleep
Improvement of nutritional status
Exercise and physical therapy

Table 12–5. EXERCISE IN THE TREATMENT OF THE ELDERLY PATIENT WITH MUSCULOSKELETAL DISEASE
Range of motion
Stretch muscles
Maintain joint lubrication
Decrease fibrosis/adhesion
Strengthening
Improve joint stability
Increase function
Muscular and cardiovascular endurance

plements, should be optimized for patients to receive the most benefit from rehabilitative exercise programs.

Exercise is the key to reconditioning a deconditioned patient (Table 12–5) (see also Chapters 8 and 10).[12] Muscle strength may be lost at rates of up to 5% per day with immobility, but most of this can be recouped with exercise, even in elderly patients. Three types of exercises are used to treat deconditioning. Range-of-motion exercises are used to stretch muscles, allowing them to function at the lengths necessary to generate the most force during contraction. Range-of-motion exercises also maintain joint lubrication and decrease capsular fibrosis and adhesions. Soft tissue contractures resulting from fibrosis of tendons, ligaments, and joint capsules can occur quickly with immobility and often require prolonged rehabilitation to be reduced. Exercises to improve muscle strength are needed to provide additional joint stability and to protect joints by dissipating the forces generated across them with activity. Isometric exercises can be used to strengthen muscles surrounding painful joints. Lastly, exercises to improve muscular and cardiovascular endurance are needed to enable patients to perform the sustained work required by mobility. Rehabilitation in deconditioned patients is often a prolonged, strenuous, and at times frustrating process, and a patient's motivation is often the key to success.

REFERENCES

1. Slater CA, Davis RB, Shmerling RH: Antinuclear antibody testing: A study of clinical utility. Arch Intern Med 156:1421, 1996.
2. Ward MM, Polisson RP: A meta-analysis of the clinical manifestations of older-onset systemic lupus erythematosus. Arthritis Rheum 32:1226, 1989.
3. Gall EP, Higbee M: Pharmacologic therapy of rheumatic diseases. In Bressler R, Katz MD, eds: Geriatric Pharmacology. New York, McGraw-Hill, 1993, p 467.
4. Roth SH: NSAID gastropathy: A new understanding. Arch Intern Med 156:1623, 1996.
5. Solomon DH, Gurwitz JH: Toxicity of nonsteroidal anti-inflammatory drugs in the elderly: Is advanced age a risk factor? Am J Med 102:208, 1997.
6. Murray MD, Brater DC: Renal toxicity of the nonsteroidal anti-inflammatory drugs. Annu Rev Pharmacol Toxicol 32:435, 1993.
7. Ferrell BA: Pain management in elderly people. J Am Geriatr Soc 39:64, 1991.
8. Johnson AG, Nguyen TV, Day RO: Do nonsteroidal anti-inflammatory drugs affect blood pressure? A meta-analysis. Ann Intern Med 121:289, 1994.
9. Rubenstein LZ, Robbins AS, Schulman BL, et al: Falls and instability in the elderly. J Am Geriatr Soc 36:266, 1988.
10. Tinetti ME: Performance-oriented assessment of mobility problems in elderly patients. J Am Geriatr Soc 34:119, 1986.
11. Harper CM, Lyles YM: Physiology and complications of bed rest. J Am Geriatr Soc 36:1047, 1988.
12. Fiatarone MA, Evans WJ: The etiology and reversibility of muscle dysfunction in the aged. J Gerontol 48 (Spec):77, 1993.

Chapter **13**

The Child with
Joint, Limb, or Back Pain

Todd L. Lincoln

This textbook is directed primarily at problems confronted by primary care physicians in adult practice. However, for general practitioners who read this book, an understanding of the bone and joint problems of children is essential. Musculoskeletal complaints during childhood are common, yet evaluation is often challenging. Adolescents and older children are usually able to localize and characterize their pain, but younger children may present with unclear histories and nonspecific clinical findings. A familiarity with the wide assortment of congenital, developmental, infectious, neoplastic, and traumatic problems affecting pediatric patients is essential to identify the cause of pain and provide appropriate treatment.

JOINT AND LIMB PAIN

History

Parents and other caregivers provide the essential initial history when evaluating an infant or toddler with limb or joint pain. The description of irritability with limb movement (e.g., with diapering) or extreme guarding of the extremity (i.e., a *pseudoparalysis*) is indicative of an infant with limb pain. Features of septic arthritis or osteomyelitis should be specifically sought in infants and toddlers because the relative incidence of infection as a source of limb pain in this age group is high. A history of fever suggests a possible infectious cause; however, such a history can be absent, especially in neonates and young infants. Any recent illness should be noted because many common unassociated childhood illnesses can lead subsequently to osteomyelitis or septic arthritis. For example, varicella is known to predispose to streptococcal osteomyelitis. In the past, *Haemophilus influenzae* septic arthritis was a common complication of otitis media. Such infections are now increasingly rare since the introduction of the *H. influenzae* vaccination. Factors that are associated with an immunocompromised host response (e.g., long-term glucocorticoid use in a transplant patient or chemotherapy treatment in a leukemia patient) should also be clearly identified.

A history of recent trauma is nearly ubiquitous during the toddler and childhood years. Although such injuries may be the direct cause of the child's painful extremity, a high index for possible infection should nevertheless be maintained. In vivo studies in a rabbit model have demonstrated that the likelihood of establishing osteomyelitis with an equivalent inoculum of bacteria is greatly increased in the setting of preceding trauma.[1] In contrast, significant extremity trauma in pretoddlers is much less common, and should alert the nurse and physician to the possibility of child abuse. Thorough and accurate documentation of trauma in all children is essential to identify potential child abuse as well as to discourage overzealous investigation of innocent situations.

The acuity of the onset of symptoms is important to elicit. Although a rapid onset of pain in a child is more consistent with a traumatic, inflammatory, or infectious cause, whereas an indolent course increases the likelihood of a neoplasm, this generalization has limitations. For example, classic hematogenous osteomyelitis in children is described as an acute process with dramatic findings within the first week, but some children nevertheless present weeks or months after the onset of symptoms. The clinical course and radiographic changes of osteomyelitis in such long-standing infections mimic the findings of a tumor, and a biopsy often is necessary to differentiate infection from neoplasm. Traumatic injuries can also present within a variety of time frames. Children with minor injuries, such as a nondisplaced *toddler's fracture* of the tibia, may first present several days after a traumatic episode. Slipped capital femoral epiphysis of the hip can also be acute, subacute, or chronic and present from a few hours to a year from onset of symptoms.

A description of a characteristic variation of symptoms with time of day may add additional insight in the evaluation of children with limb or joint pain. Symptoms limited primarily to the early morning suggest a possible rheumatologic condition. Night pain and pain not associated with activity is classically described as an ominous finding, indicating a possible tumor. Although unilateral limb pain that wakes a child at night should heighten the suspicion for a tumor or infection, the description of bilateral leg pain in a 4- to 10-year-old child that is limited to the evening or nighttime is more reassuring. Such symmetric leg pain is characteristic of *growing pains*; however, this diagnosis should be made only after all other possibilities have been carefully considered. Severe lower back pain, worsened by spine flexion in an adolescent, can indicate the presence of spondylolisthesis.

Finally, common pain referral patterns should be well understood. Pain in the hip region may originate from the lumbar spine, intrapelvic region, sacroiliac joint, or knee. True hip joint pain is classically located in the medial groin area rather than laterally or posteriorly. Hip joint symptoms may also be referred to the medial aspect of the knee. To avoid disastrous consequences, careful evaluation of the child's hip should be routinely included in the evaluation of every child with complaints of knee pain. In the upper extremity, cervical spine pathology may lead to shoulder or arm pain, and shoulder pain is often referred to the medial aspect of the elbow. The history of pain in one musculoskeletal region must not dissuade careful investigation of adjacent anatomic areas.

Physical Examination

When examining infants and young children, a few clinical tips are useful to keep in mind. Simple observation looking for an abnormal posture or guarding of the extremity at rest should begin every physical examination. Rushing the evaluation and skipping this critical first step is likely to result in a fussy, crying patient and make accurate identification of the affected area far more difficult. Starting with areas distant to the suspected location of pain also eases the task of examining a crying child. Distraction techniques, such as bottle feeding an infant, allowing the parent to hold the child during the examination, or waiting for the infant to fall asleep before the physical examination, are additional useful clinical approaches.

Focal tenderness, deformity, and swelling characterize a fractured extremity. Pain from a displaced or angulated fracture is intense, and the child actively resists palpation, manipulation, or weight bearing on the injured limb. The examination may not be quite as evident when the fracture is nondisplaced. Bony injury can be easily distinguished from soft tissue or ligamentous injury in most cases by deliberate palpation of the bony anatomy. For example, firm palpation over the distal physis of the fibula elicits pain if a child has sustained a physeal fracture, whereas tenderness distal to the tip of the fibula indicates a ligamentous ankle sprain. Both of these injuries may have normal radiographs, and therefore accurate diagnosis and appropriate treatment rely entirely on the findings of a careful examination.

Warmth, swelling, and range of motion of each joint must be assessed. Positive clinical findings most likely indicate an infectious or inflammatory condition. The child with a septic hip classically presents firmly guarding the hip in a flexed, laterally rotated and abducted position in an attempt to decrease the intra-articular pressure and relieve pain. Likewise, the child with a septic knee tries to minimize intracapsular pressure by holding the joint in approximately 30 degrees of

flexion, vigorously resisting further flexion or extension. The intensity of pain relative to the degree of intra-articular effusion is important to note. A child with juvenile rheumatoid arthritis usually has more swelling and less pain than a child with septic arthritis.[2,3]

GAIT

Careful observation of a child's gait is also a key component in the physical examination of children with limb or joint pain. Children can be surprisingly adept at disguising their limp during an office physical examination, and some children may limp intermittently when fatigued. The first diagnostic decision is whether the gait pattern is antalgic or not. By definition, an *antalgic gait pattern* is *pain avoiding*. There are two primary methods that children with limb or joint pain use to achieve this goal. First, the velocity of the contralateral limb in swing phase is increased and the stride length is decreased to minimize the amount of time spent in single leg stance on the painful extremity. Second, children with hip pain often demonstrate a positive Trendelenburg gait pattern, leaning toward the affected side in single limb stance phase to diminish the joint reactive force.

A concerted attempt to define the anatomic source of an antalgic gait pattern should be made. Analyzing the motion of each joint independently (i.e., watching only the hip motion first, then the knee) helps simplify a complex gait pattern and clarifies which joint is leading to the gait abnormality. For example, by observing only the motion of the hip during the gait cycle, a decreased arc of hip motion and a corresponding increase in pelvic rotation become far more evident. Likewise, observing knee motion may highlight a circumduction gait pattern and help identify the knee region as the source of pain. Finally, the plantar aspect of the feet should not be overlooked when examining a child with a painful limp because unsuspected puncture wounds are not uncommon.

Children with a painless gait disturbance should not be confused with those who have an antalgic limp. Children with mild cerebral palsy commonly present for evaluation of a new limp. In such cases, a comprehensive birth and developmental milestone history should be obtained. Prematurity, low birth weight, neonatal distress, and developmental delay are common features in children with cerebral palsy. Increased reflexes, clonus, and upper extremity posturing with walking or running should be sought on physical examination. Children with early neuromuscular disease, such as muscular dystrophy, may also present because of a gait disturbance. A positive family history, coupled with hip extensor weakness and calf pseudohypertrophy, is indicative of this diagnosis. Assessment for Gowers' sign* should be

---

*Gowers' maneuver refers to a peculiar method of standing up from a seated position on the ground to compensate for hip extensor musculature weakness. It is characterized by the patient first assuming a quadripedal position, then *walking up* his or her lower extremities with his or her hands until standing. A positive *Gower's sign* denotes the dependence on this technique and is commonly seen in muscular dystrophy.

done if a myopathy is suspected. A painless limp may also be due to limb length inequality. Previously unsuspected developmental dislocation of the hip or congenital limb deficiencies, such as fibular hemimelia and congenital short femur, may be evident on closer inspection. Overall limb lengths can be estimated by measuring from the anterior-superior iliac spine to the ankle malleolus, although this method is notoriously inaccurate, and a scanogram radiograph should be obtained if any doubt remains.

Diagnostic Studies

LABORATORY TESTS

Blood tests are indicated if there is any suspicion of infection based on the history or physical examination. A white blood count (WBC) with differential cell count and a blood culture should be obtained in these cases; however, the limitations of these laboratory studies must be recognized. The poor sensitivity of a WBC is well known, and WBC is elevated in only about 25% of children with osteomyelitis or septic arthritis. An increase in polymorpholeukocytes and band cells is slightly more sensitive and is present with 65% of infected children.[4] Blood cultures are positive in only 40% to 50% of cases. The sensitivity of these blood tests in the neonate is even less. Microscopic examination of a blood smear of these blood specimens should be requested if a myelodysplastic disease, such as leukemia, is suspected.

An erythrocyte sedimentation rate (ESR) or a C-reactive protein (CRP) level is typically most helpful to evaluate for a possible infection. However, these studies are unreliable in the neonate. The ESR is elevated to greater than 20 mm/h in 92%, and the CRP is greater than 20 mg/L (2.0 mg/dL) in 98% of cases of infection.[5] As general indicators of active inflammation, neither ESR nor CRP is specific for osteomyelitis or septic arthritis; nevertheless, an elevated ESR or CRP in a child presenting with extremity pain should be considered secondary to osteomyelitis or septic arthritis until proven otherwise. CRP levels are purported by many centers to be more sensitive than ESR, with a more rapid peak reached in the setting of infection. CRP levels rise within 6 to 8 hours of the onset of tissue inflammation and reach a peak at 2 days. The ESR is less responsive and may be normal in the first 36 to 48 hours. Peak ESR values are attained by 4 days.[3, 5]

Lastly, a rheumatologic screening panel, such as a fluorescent antinuclear antibody, rheumatoid factor, and HLA-B27 level, should be obtained if a rheumatologic disease is suspected. Details regarding the interpretation of these screening tests are discussed elsewhere in this text (see Chapter 5).

MUSCULOSKELETAL IMAGING

Appropriate musculoskeletal imaging is also dictated by the specifics of the history and physical examination findings (see Chapter 4). Plain radiographs remain a standard component of the initial evaluation to identify fractures or tumors. The history and clinical findings are often nonspecific, and radiographs of the entire extremity are essential to eliminate the possibility of missing bone or joint pathology. Views of the contralateral extremity are sometimes helpful for comparison, especially for the practitioner who may not routinely evaluate skeletally immature patients. Fractures in children with open physes can be quite subtle; fracture patterns, such as a transphyseal fracture with no metaphyseal fragment, can be easily overlooked.

Early infection is difficult to identify with plain radiographs. The earliest radiographic finding of infection is obliteration of the normal soft tissue planes between muscle and fat and deep soft tissue swelling. Focal metaphyseal osteopenia or erosion is present in established osteomyelitis but is unlikely to be seen before a week from the onset of infection. An increased joint space or frank joint dislocation in the context of a painful range of motion is evidence for florid septic arthritis.

In many centers, ultrasound has become a mainstay in the evaluation of infants and children with extremity pain. Evaluation of the hip or shoulder is especially well suited for ultrasound study because intra-articular effusions are not readily apparent by physical examination alone. In contrast, an effusion in the knee, wrist, or ankle is often easily visible and less likely to require an ultrasound study for confirmation. With current ultrasound technology, 5 mL of fluid in the hip can be detected. Ultrasound is particularly suited for locating soft tissue abscesses or radiolucent foreign bodies. Relative to other modalities (e.g., computed tomography [CT] or magnetic resonance imaging [MRI]), ultrasonography is inexpensive and typically requires no sedation.

A triple-phase technetium bone scan is helpful to confirm the diagnosis of osteomyelitis, occult fracture, or bone tumor. Bone scans have been shown to have an 89% sensitivity and 94% specificity in the diagnosis of osteomyelitis[6]; however, results are not generally reliable within the first 24 to 48 hours from onset of infection. Pinhole collimation of particular regions of interest (e.g., the hip) increases the sensitivity of detecting and localizing asymmetric radionuclide uptake and should be specifically requested if the history or physical examination is suggestive. The accuracy of a bone scan is not affected by a prior needle aspiration of soft tissue or bone.[7, 8]

Bone scans are less helpful when evaluating neonates and infants with suspected osteomyelitis because a significant portion of these studies are falsely negative.[9] The usefulness of a bone scan is also limited for detecting septic arthritis. Isotope uptake on both sides of the joint is suggestive of septic arthritis; however, noninfectious causes of synovitis have similar findings.[6, 10] Other special nuclear medicine studies, such as a gallium or indium scan, are generally not warranted in most cases because these studies provide little additional yield, are time-consuming, and are expensive.

The use of MRI is another option in the evaluation of a child with a painful extremity. This modality is particularly suited for defining soft tissue and bone marrow abnormalities and is more sensitive than a bone scan for osteomyelitis within the first 24 hours of onset. Nevertheless, the availability, high cost (typically three times greater than a bone scan), and increased need for sedation of infants and young children limit the general use of MRI. Extensive, dramatic high signal changes on T2 images must be interpreted with caution because much of the signal change often represents surrounding reactive edema in bone rather than true extent of disease.

CT is an alternative to MRI when soft tissue abscess or a cortical bone abnormality is suspected. CT is the study of choice if fine detail of bony architecture is desired. Newer, high-speed spiral CT scanning units have significantly decreased the radiation exposure and time necessary to obtain images, simplifying its use in the pediatric population. Currently, imaging a single joint with CT can take as little as 10 minutes, compared with 1 hour with MRI. For fine soft tissue detail and identification of bone marrow abnormalities, however, MRI remains superior to CT.

Differential Diagnosis

Separating pediatric patients into four general age subgroups—infants (0 to 1 year old), toddlers (1 to 3 years old), children (4 to 11 years old), and adolescents (>11 years old)—provides a useful initial framework when evaluating the limping child. The list of likely causes of musculoskeletal pain changes somewhat as children mature; recognition of this change in disease incidence likewise sharpens one's clinical focus (Table 13–1). Although bone and joint infections occupy a central theme in the differential diagnosis of an infant or toddler with extremity pain, the incidence of such infections decreases with age. Instead, various developmental and traumatic causes increase in frequency as the cause of extremity pain during childhood and adolescence.

INFANTS (0 TO 1 YEAR OLD)

The initial concern when evaluating an infant with atraumatic limb or joint pain generally centers on the possibility of infection. Urgent evaluation for septic arthritis is indicated for any infant with a decreased, painful joint range of motion. Time is critical because loss of the normal glucosaminoglycan matrix of articular cartilage occurs within 8 hours after onset of a pyogenic joint infection.[11] A febrile infant whose hip is held in a characteristic position of flexion, lateral rotation, and abduction should prompt an immediate referral to an orthopaedic surgeon. Such ill-appearing infants typically warrant initial blood studies and screening radio-

Table 13–1. CAUSES OF EXTREMITY PAIN IN PEDIATRIC PATIENTS

	Infant	Toddler	Child	Adolescent
Infectious	Osteomyelitis Septic arthritis Psoas abscess	Osteomyelitis Septic arthritis Psoas abscess	Osteomyelitis Septic arthritis	Osteomyelitis Septic arthritis
Inflammatory	Caffey's disease		Juvenile rheumatoid arthritis Transient synovitis Acute rheumatic fever	
Traumatic	Birth fracture Battered infant	Fracture Sprains Nursemaid elbow Puncture wound	Fracture Sprains	Fracture Sprains Meniscal tear Slipped capital femoral epiphysis
Overuse			Stress fracture Calcaneal apophysitis Tibial tubercle apophysitis	Stress fracture Calcaneal apophysitis Tibial tubercle apophysitis Patellar tendinitis Iliotibial band friction Anterior knee pain
Osteochondrosis			Legg-Calvé-Perthes Capitellar osteochondritis Navicular osteochondritis	Osteochondritis (femoral condyle, talus)
Congenital/developmental			Discoid meniscus Tarsal coalition	Hip dysplasia Tarsal coalition
Neoplastic	Neuroblastoma	Rhabdomyosarcoma Leukemia Eosinophilic granuloma	Nonossifying fibroma Unicameral bone cyst Fibrous dysplasia Osteochondroma Eosinophilic granuloma Osteoid osteoma Osteogenic sarcoma Ewing's sarcoma Leukemia	Ewing's sarcoma Osteogenic sarcoma Eosinophilic granuloma Osteoid osteoma Osteoblastoma Aneurysmal bone cyst Chondroblastoma Osteochondroma
Miscellaneous			Growing pains Sickle cell crisis	Idiopathic juvenile osteoporosis Idiopathic chondrolysis of the hip

graphs followed by emergent hip joint aspiration and possible metaphyseal bone aspiration in an operating room setting. Aspiration should not be delayed by ultrasound or bone scan studies. Bone and joint aspiration is the most direct means to confirm the diagnosis, allows for early isolation of the infectious organism, and guides immediate definitive treatment (i.e., open surgical drainage of the hip). If the infant is not acutely ill and if the findings of the initial history and clinical examination do not warrant emergent aspiration, further diagnostic studies are indicated. A general algorithm for evaluating pediatric patients with suspected bone or joint infection is shown in Figure 13–1.

Concurrent osteomyelitis and septic arthritis should be suspected in infants. Metaphyseal blood vessels cross the physeal plate and penetrate the epiphysis in this age group, thereby providing organisms easy access into the joint from the adjacent metaphyseal bone. These crossing vessels disappear after the first year of life; however, concurrent osteomyelitis and septic arthritis of the shoulder, hip, ankle, and elbow can still easily develop in toddlers and older children because the metaphysis of these joints is located within the joint capsule. A high index of suspicion for a multifocal bone or joint infection at distant sites should also be maintained, particularly in the neonatal age group, in whom the incidence is highest.

A selective approach to surgical treatment of osteomyelitis and septic arthritis is advised. An 80% cure rate of isolated osteomyelitis treated with antibiotics and limb immobilization can be expected.[12] Surgical decompression and débridement for osteomyelitis is indicated if an abscess develops, if the child is severely ill, or if there has been a poor clinical response to 48 hours of antibiotics alone (e.g., persistent fevers, increased tenderness, and increased swelling). Chronic osteomyelitis with sequestrum formation also requires surgical débridement if a cure is to be expected. Although controversy remains, initial nonsurgical treatment is often appropriate for many cases of septic arthritis except with respect to the hip. Urgent surgical drainage of a septic hip is still mandatory, however, because detecting an effusion in these deep joints by clinical examination is unreliable, accurate needle aspiration is difficult to perform, and there is a risk of avascular necrosis of the femoral head with inadequate decompression. The most common organisms and current empirical antibiotic recommendations for osteomyelitis and septic arthritis are listed in Table 13–2.

Several alternative diagnoses can be confused with septic arthritis and osteomyelitis. Similar to hip sepsis, a psoas abscess leads to strenuous guarding against hip motion, especially extension. Significant delays in the diagnosis of a psoas abscess and exposure to unnecessary

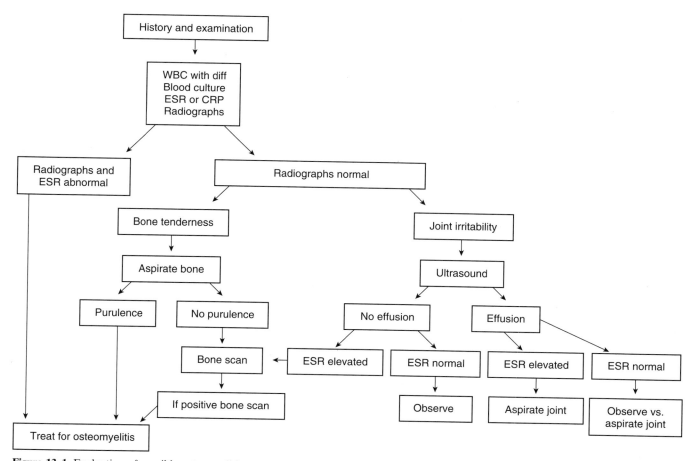

Figure 13–1. Evaluation of possible osteomyelitis or septic arthritis. WBC, with diff, white blood count with differential; ESR, erythrocyte sedimentation rate; CRP, C-reactive protein.

Table 13–2. LIKELY ORGANISMS AND ANTIBIOTIC CHOICE IN OSTEOMYELITIS AND SEPTIC ARTHRITIS

Age	Organism	Antibiotic
Osteomyelitis		
<4 wk	Group B streptococcus	Oxacillin plus gentamicin or cefotaxime
	Staphylococcus aureus	
	Gram-negative coliforms	
>4 wk	S. aureus	Oxacillin
		Cefazolin (if penicillin allergic)
		Clindamycin or vancomycin (if penicillin and cephalosporin allergic)
Septic Arthritis		
<4 wk	Group B streptococcus	Oxacillin plus gentamicin or cefotaxime
	S. aureus	
4 wk–4 y	S. aureus	Cefuroxime
	Group B streptococcus	
	Group A streptococcus	
>4 y	S. aureus	Oxacillin or cefazolin

procedures, such as hip aspiration or abdominal exploration, have been described.[13] An abdominal ultrasound or CT scan is helpful to avoid this error. Other rare noninfectious conditions, such as infantile cortical hyperostosis (Caffey's disease), can also mimic the fever, limb pain, and elevated ESR characteristic of infection.

Although less common than in older age groups, trauma may also explain the infant's extremity pain. Pseudoparalysis of the arm in newborns typifies a clavicle fracture, the most common bone fractured during vaginal delivery.[14] Fractures in the infant population heal rapidly and are generally painful for less than 1 week. As previously noted, potential child abuse should also be considered when evaluating any child with extremity trauma. The described mechanism of injury should be consistent with the fracture pattern seen (e.g., a direct blow to an extremity causes a transverse fracture, whereas a twisting injury causes a spiral fracture). Transphyseal fractures of the elbow or hip resulting in a dissociation of the epiphysis from the metaphysis, *corner fractures* of long bone metaphyses, posterior rib fractures, and multiple fractures present in various stages of healing all characterize the battered infant.[15, 16] Although recognition of these pathognomonic fractures is important, an isolated diaphyseal fracture of a long bone remains the most common injury pattern.[17]

As with all pediatric patients, the possibility of a bone or extremity soft tissue tumor should also be considered. Excluding metastatic neuroblastoma, however, neoplasms are distinctly unusual in the infant population.

TODDLERS (1 TO 3 YEARS OLD)

Osteomyelitis and septic arthritis remain a primary concern in toddlers with limb and joint pain. The con-

cerns and clinical findings of such infections are analogous to those described in the preceding section on infants, as is the suggested diagnostic algorithm.

In contrast to the infant patient population, fractures play an increasingly prominent role in the cause of extremity pain in the toddler age group. The most frequent mechanism of injury is from falling, often from a seemingly innocuous height. Because of the higher collagen content and lower mineral content of young children's bones, incomplete *greenstick* fractures are common. A torus (or *buckle*) fracture of the distal radius occurs frequently in the upper extremity and heals completely within 3 weeks with a simple wrist guard splint. A nondisplaced spiral fracture of the tibia (a *toddler's fracture*) can also occur after a minor fall and explain a toddler's reluctance to walk. Radiographs must often be scrutinized to recognize this minimal fracture and to distinguish it from the normal appearance of a nutrient vessel entering the cortical bone. In general, extremity fractures in this age group heal rapidly (within 3 to 4 weeks), and residual displacement or angulation at the fracture site is compatible with a full recovery because of the immense potential for bone remodeling with growth in children. Recurrent or multiple fractures should alert one to the possibility of child abuse or an underlying bone dysplasia, such as osteogenesis imperfecta.

Soft tissue sprains are less common than are fractures in this age group because of the relatively greater mechanical strength of tendons and ligaments compared with the physis. As noted previously, the physis should be carefully palpated to determine the site of maximal tenderness. Often, however, the toddler is uncooperative and fearful during the examination, and the clinical findings are equivocal. In such instances, it is prudent to treat the injury as a fracture and immobilize the extremity. The toddler should then routinely return at 10 days after the injury for repeat radiographs. At that time, periosteal new bone formation confirms whether a bony or physeal fracture has occurred.

One soft tissue injury that occurs with relative frequency is *nursemaid's elbow*. This subluxation of the annular ligament over the immature radial head is unique to this age group. The classic history includes a sudden jerk of the toddler's upper extremity by a parent, followed by an immediate reluctance of the toddler to move his or her elbow. The toddler holds the elbow flexed and in pronation and refuses to reach for toys or other objects during the examination. Unless there is an unmistakable history associated with the onset of symptoms, screening radiographs of the elbow are advised before manipulation of the extremity. Repeated attempts of *reducing* a presumed nursemaid's elbow when, in fact, a nondisplaced supracondylar humerus fracture is present both is cruel and risks conversion of the injury to a far more serious fracture pattern. Once alternative causes have been excluded, maximally flexing and forcibly supinating the elbow reduces a nursemaid's elbow. A palpable click and prompt relief of pain should be expected.

Unexplained musculoskeletal pain in a toddler should be conscientiously evaluated. Leukemia is the most common neoplasm in children younger than 16 years old and has a peak incidence between ages 2 and 5. Although the classic findings of leukemia include lethargy, fever, pallor, bruising, bleeding, and hepatosplenomegaly, the presenting complaint in approximately 20% of children is of musculoskeletal origin.[18] A delay in diagnosis is common and can be minimized by obtaining a complete blood count with differential and smear. Unexplained anemia and leukopenia necessitates prompt referral to an oncologist, and a bone marrow aspirate may be necessary. Other tumors that occur with relative frequency in toddlers include histiocytosis X and rhabdomyosarcoma, the most common soft tissue malignancy in young children.

CHILDREN (4 TO 11 YEARS OLD)

The diversity of possible causes of limb and joint pain continues to increase in children aged 4 to 11. Infection remains a prominent concern, as depicted previously. In addition, transient synovitis reaches a peak incidence in children between 3 and 8 years old and must often be distinguished from septic arthritis. Both entities result in a painful, diminished range of joint motion and a reluctance to bear weight on the extremity. A history of a recent viral infection, a lack of fever, and a normal ESR or CRP points toward transient synovitis rather than infection. However, the presence of fever, elevated WBC, or elevated ESR does not exclude the possibility of transient synovitis. In one series, 28% of patients with transient synovitis had an ESR greater than 20 mm/h, and 14% had a value greater than 30 mm/h.[19] A trial of anti-inflammatory medication and close follow-up is appropriate in such cases of presumed transient synovitis, with dramatic improvement in symptoms typical within 48 hours and complete resolution of symptoms expected within 10 days. Because the ESR can be normal in the first 36 to 48 hours of infection, an ultrasound study and referral to an orthopaedic specialist is warranted in cases in which joint examination causes marked pain.

Juvenile rheumatoid arthritis also occurs in this age group (commonly before age 5 years). As noted earlier, the joint pain in juvenile rheumatoid arthritis is typically less severe, and the amount of joint effusion is greater than found with septic arthritis.[2, 3] There is often a temporal pattern to the pain of juvenile rheumatoid arthritis, with characteristic morning stiffness resulting from edema collection in and around the inflamed joint. A child with pauciarticular rheumatoid arthritis should be routinely evaluated by an ophthalmologist for evidence of iridocyclitis, which initially causes no symptoms but can lead to blindness if untreated.

Acute rheumatic fever is an autoimmune response occurring 2 to 4 weeks after a streptococcal infection. In contrast to juvenile rheumatoid arthritis, the arthralgia is rapidly migratory and quickly responds to aspirin. Joint appearance mimics an acute septic arthritis with erythema, swelling, and tenderness.

Legg-Calvé-Perthes disease (i.e., idiopathic avascular necrosis of the proximal femoral epiphysis) should also be considered in children in this age group who present with hip or medial knee pain and a limp. The

typical child with Legg-Calvé-Perthes disease is a wiry, hyperactive boy between age 4 and 8 years old who is of Central European ethnicity. Clinical findings include an antalgic gait with a decreased hip range of motion, particularly internal rotation and abduction. Intermittent pain of variable severity can persist for up to 2 years, although complete healing of the femoral head from the avascular event can take up to 6 years. Plain radiographs usually suffice in making the diagnosis of Legg-Calvé-Perthes disease. MRI is infrequently necessary. Indications for nonsurgical versus surgical management of Legg-Calvé-Perthes disease remain in evolution, and this decision is best made by a pediatric orthopaedic surgeon.

Idiopathic avascular necrosis also occurs in the capitellum of the elbow (Panner's disease) and in the tarsal navicula (Kohler's disease) in this age group. These uncommon osteochondroses cause elbow and foot pain. Similar to Legg-Calvé-Perthes disease, plain radiographs are often diagnostic; however, MRI is occasionally necessary to establish the diagnosis in the early stages of disease.

Various fractures and sprains are common in this physically active age group, and overuse injuries are becoming increasingly prevalent along with the rise in participation in organized sports for children. Stress fractures of the tibia, fibula, and femur are most common. Triple-phase technetium bone scans are frequently helpful in diagnosing these injuries. Tibial tubercle apophysitis (Osgood-Schlatter disease) is a relatively common overuse injury and presents with focal tenderness and swelling directly over the anterior tibial tubercle. Repetitive jumping sports (e.g., basketball, jumping rope) commonly aggravate this condition, and activity modification is the mainstay of treatment. Activity-related heel pain from a calcaneal apophysitis (Sever's disease) is also common in children. Radiographs of the foot are normal, and treatment consists of activity modification, Achilles tendon stretching, and occasional short-term immobilization in a cast.

Finally, lower limb pain in children may be due to *growing pains*. This term is actually a misnomer because symptoms do not correlate with a period of peak growth. Children with growing pains complain of bilateral, deep aching pain in the calves, thighs, or popliteal fossa region. The pain is often worse in the evening or at night after a physically active day and can even be severe enough to wake the child from sleep. The pain responds to massage, heat, and analgesics and always resolves by morning. The physical examination is normal. Growing pains may be a psychogenic reaction pattern or indicative of a wider familial pattern of pain disorder.[20, 21] The diagnosis of growing pains should be one of exclusion, and one should always remain vigilant for signs of an occult neoplasm. Bone pain that lasts for more than 6 weeks without a clear explanation demands further diagnostic evaluation with a bone scan.

ADOLESCENTS (>11 YEARS OLD)

Although the preceding discussion of traumatic and overuse injury patterns is relevant for the adolescent age group as well, other diagnoses, such as Legg-

Calvé-Perthes disease and growing pains, are uncommon in adolescents. Instead a variety of additional diagnostic possibilities merit mention.

The most common painful hip disorder in adolescence is a slipped capital femoral epiphysis. Slipped capital femoral epiphysis reaches a peak incidence in adolescent boys at age 14 years and in girls at age 12 years. An endocrine evaluation is indicated in children who develop a slipped capital femoral epiphysis when younger than age 10 years or older than 16 years because an endocrinopathy frequently coexists.[22] Patients and families should be advised that the incidence of bilateral slipped capital femoral epiphysis is approximately 33%, and the clinician should be suspicious of an adolescent with a past history of a slipped capital femoral epiphysis who now presents with contralateral groin or knee pain. Besides pain, obligate external rotation of the hip when the hip is passively flexed during examination is suggestive of this diagnosis. Urgent surgery consisting of in situ screw fixation is recommended, preventing, it is hoped, the devastating consequences of avascular necrosis of the femoral head.

Hip pain and stiffness (especially internal and external rotation of the hip) can also be due to idiopathic chondrolysis. Idiopathic chondrolysis of the hip occurs five times more frequently in girls than boys and can be diagnosed radiographically by disuse osteopenia of the hip and a joint space narrowing of greater than 2 mm when compared with the contralateral hip. Treatment is directed toward maintaining hip motion and minimizing synovitis. In selected cases of recalcitrant severe cases, subtotal capsulectomy of the hip may be indicated. Referral to an orthopaedic surgeon is recommended.

Residual developmental dysplasia of the hip, a painless entity in infancy and younger childhood, may also be a source of hip pain during the teenage years. Abnormal mechanical load concentration within the dysplastic joint leads to early degenerative changes and symptoms of activity-related hip pain. A standing anterior-posterior pelvis radiograph demonstrates a variable decrease in acetabular coverage of the femoral head. Surgical reconstruction of the hip joint is determined based on symptomatic and radiographic criteria, with the goal of pain relief and maintaining the native hip joint for as many years as possible.

Knee pain is extremely common among adolescents, particularly in girls. The most common source of pain is referred from the patellofemoral joint and results in peripatellar and anterior knee pain with knee flexion activities, such as squatting, prolonged sitting, or descending stairs. Onset of pain is usually without a specific antecedent episode of trauma but may be temporally related to an increase in physical activity. Such knee pain should not be called *chondromalacia patellae* unless articular cartilage softening has been directly documented by surgical means. The term *anterior knee pain syndrome* should be adopted if a clear cause is not identified. Evidence for patellar maltracking should be sought on clinical examination, and overall mechanical alignment of the limb (such as the quadriceps angle and degree of femoral anteversion) should be recorded. Initial treatment is most often directed at strengthening

the vastus medialis oblique muscle as a means to normalize patellofemoral joint load. Referral of patients with anterior knee pain syndrome to a physical therapist is often fruitful. Approximately 75% of patients spontaneously improve, but the remainder may have symptoms throughout life. Surgical intervention remains highly controversial because no surgical procedure to date has been shown to alter this natural history definitively.[23]

A second common cause of seemingly atraumatic knee pain may be secondary to osteochondritis dessicans of the distal femoral epiphysis. Although the cause is unclear, most believe that this focal area of avascular necrosis is likely secondary to repetitive trauma. Symptoms include intermittent swelling of the knee and pain with activity. Physical examination often reveals tenderness on the femoral condyle and pain at 30 degrees knee flexion with the tibia internally rotated. A *notch* or *tunnel* view of the knee is frequently necessary to visualize the lesion, which is characteristically located on the lateral margin of the medial femoral condyle. Treatment can be either nonsurgical or surgical, depending on level of symptoms, size of fragment, and degree of fragment displacement. MRI evaluation of the knee often provides critical information regarding the prognosis for healing. Orthopaedic surgeons are most acquainted and capable of managing patients with osteochondritis dessicans.

Two of the gravest primary bone tumors most commonly occur during the adolescent years. The peak incidence of osteosarcoma is at age 14 years, and Ewing's sarcoma is most common at age 12 years. Malignant tumors occur most frequently at the level of the knee but naturally can be located at any other site as well. Suspicious bony or soft tissue lesions demand proper plain radiographs, a bone scan, and an MRI study. Evaluation and care of such patients is best left to tertiary referral centers where specialists in the medical and surgical management of musculoskeletal tumors are available.

BACK PAIN

Although the incidence of back pain during childhood is less than half that encountered in the adult population, the likelihood of identifying the cause of pain is far greater in the pediatric population. The list of possible causes is lengthy (Table 13–3), but the list of probable causes is narrowed by a complete history, physical examination, and appropriate diagnostic studies.

History

The precise location and nature of painful back complaints must be carefully probed and associated symptoms specifically queried. Back pain related to activity is less ominous than pain that is persistent and increasing in severity. Musculoskeletal back strain injuries present with complaints of acute paravertebral pain and tightness; this pattern of presentation becomes more

Table 13–3. CAUSES OF BACK PAIN IN PEDIATRIC PATIENTS

Congenital
    Syrinx
    Tether
    Diastematomyelia
Developmental
    Scoliosis
    Scheuermann's disease
Infectious
    Infectious spondylitis
    Discitis
    Vertebral osteomyelitis
    Tuberculous osteomyelitis
Inflammatory
    Ankylosing spondylitis
Traumatic
    Spondylolysis/spondylolisthesis
    Insufficiency fracture (e.g., steroids)
    Apophyseal fracture
    Disc herniation
    Muscle strain
Neoplastic
    Osteoid osteoma
    Hemangioma
    Osteoblastoma
    Giant cell tumor
    Eosinophilic granuloma
    Leukemia
    Neurofibroma
Visceral
    Urinary tract infection
    Hydronephrosis
    Ovarian cyst
    Inflammatory bowel disease

commonplace in older adolescence. Back pain that wakes a child from sleep at night is distinctly unusual and necessitates a complete evaluation and explanation. Additional features of the history that indicate a possible serious underlying cause include neurologic symptoms (dysesthesias, motor weakness, or a change in bowel or bladder function) and systemic symptoms, such as fevers, weight loss, atypical fatigability, and easy bruising. A painful scoliosis is also classically described as a worrisome presentation; however, studies have noted that up to one third of idiopathic scoliosis patients complain of back pain at some time during their medical care.[24] A final generally useful axiom is that the younger the patient with back pain, the more suspicious the clinician should be of a serious underlying cause.

A careful review of systems is a key component in the assessment of back pain in children. Recent respiratory infections or other bacterial infections may predispose to infectious spondylitis (discitis) in the preschool and young school-age child. The pain from a urinary tract infection may also masquerade as low back pain, as can the pain of adolescent female mittelschmerz. A directed family history may uncover potentially inheritable conditions, such as inflammatory bowel disease, ankylosing spondylitis, or spondylolisthesis. Finally, a social history seeking any psychosocial component to the patient's complaints is particularly appropriate when the history is unclear and the symptoms vague.

Physical Examination

Sagittal plane spinal contour is important to assess directly. Normal thoracic kyphosis is between 25 and 40 degrees and should be a gentle and flexible curvature. Loss of this normal kyphosis may be associated with pain and resultant palpable muscle spasm or a fixed structural abnormality from scoliosis. A rigidly increased kyphosis is typical of Scheuermann's disease as well as a variety of congenital spinal anomalies, such as a failure of normal anterior vertebral formation or segmentation. Assessing the patient while he or she bends forward and lies supine over a bolster highlights any fixed structural abnormalities of the spine. A scoliotic curve is highlighted by forward bending because of the asymmetric rib contour indicative of the three-dimensional rotation of scoliosis. A scoliosis that entirely disappears while lying on one's side is nonstructural and characteristic of a painful (*olisthetic*) scoliosis, similar to that seen with a herniated intervertebral disk.

Similarly, abnormal lumbar lordosis may be flexible or fixed. Abnormal thoracic kyphosis results in an increased lumbar lordosis, as the body attempts to normalize its center of gravity. For example, an adolescent with an increased thoracic kyphosis secondary to Scheuermann's disease has a compensatory hyperlordosis in the lumbar spine and presents with low back rather than upper back pain. A decrease, or flattening, of normal lumbar lordosis is noted with muscle spasm from a strain injury as well as congenital and developmental causes, such as congenital vertebral anomalies or spondylolisthesis.

Overall range of motion of the back provides an estimation of the degree of pain present. A young child who is reluctant to walk and refuses to bend forward to pick up a toy may have infectious spondylitis or, less commonly, spinal cord irritation from a tumor.

A thorough neurologic examination is mandatory. Radicular findings, such as focal motor group weakness and atrophy, sensory changes, reflex asymmetry, and a positive straight leg raise, should be searched for. Myelopathic signs, such as hyperreflexia, clonus, or ataxia, suggest spinal cord involvement rather than nerve root compression. Asymmetric foot size and a cavus foot deformity further support the possibility of a spinal cord abnormality (e.g., a tethered cord). A hairy skin patch or skin dimple along the back is often associated with congenital vertebral and intrathecal abnormalities and should prompt further investigation.

A general abdominal examination is also indicated whenever presented with a patient complaining of low back pain. Pelvic tenderness over the ovaries may reproduce the presenting complaints and warrant gynecologic referral. An abdominal mass should lead to further diagnostic imaging and referral to a specialist based on findings.

Diagnostic Studies

LABORATORY TESTS

Screening blood tests should be obtained whenever an infectious or inflammatory cause is suspected. Infectious spondylitis (discitis) causes an increased ESR in 80% of cases. CRP levels may be obtained as an alternative and, in contrast to the ESR, are a direct measure of an acute-phase reactant. An elevated WBC also suggests a possible infectious process. Inflammatory spondyloarthropathy, such as ankylosing spondylitis, is often associated with a positive HLA-B27 marker.

IMAGING

Radiographs are advised if any worrisome features of the history or clinical findings are present. Back pain in a child lasting for 4 weeks should be investigated radiographically. Minimal evaluation consists of an anteroposterior and a lateral view of the spine, although oblique views are also commonly helpful (e.g., the pars intra-articularis defect of spondylolysis is most easily seen on oblique projection). A coned-down radiograph should be obtained of any suspicious region identified on the initial screening radiograph.

A triple-phase bone scan is extremely helpful in situations in which initial radiographs are nondiagnostic, yet clinical concern remains high. Increased radionuclide uptake is seen with tumors, infection, and bony trauma. Although a *hot* bone scan is not specific, such a finding often confirms a previous clinical diagnostic suspicion or helps guide the physician in the choice of appropriate additional spinal imaging. Single-photon emission computed tomography (SPECT) is an additional nuclear medicine study that is often helpful in identifying occult spondylolysis in the lumbar spine.

Although not part of the evaluation of most children who present with back pain, CT and MRI are indicated whenever there is a need to elucidate spinal architecture further. CT provides optimal information about the bony elements of the spine, whereas MRI is better suited for soft tissue and marrow definition. CT best visualizes fractures of the spine as well as certain tumors (e.g., osteoid osteoma). Three-dimensional reconstruction of CT images is often quite helpful in clarifying complex congenital spine anomalies. CT scans also can show a variety of intervertebral disc or spinal cord abnormalities; however, MRI typically provides more detailed images. In addition, MRI is generally more sensitive for identifying most types of neoplastic processes.

Differential Diagnosis

The assortment of possible causes of back pain in children is outlined in Table 13–3. Several of these causes merit specific discussion. Infectious spondylitis has been referred to as *discitis*, based on the classic involvement of the intervertebral disc space as seen by disc space narrowing and vertebral end-plate irregularity on plain radiographs as well as increased radionuclide uptake in the intervertebral region on bone scan. More advanced imaging techniques, such as MRI, have suggested that *discitis* more likely is an infectious process that begins in the relatively avascular vertebral end-plate and secondarily affects the intervertebral disc.[25] Therefore, infectious spondylitis is a more appropriate term, indicating both the components of vertebral osteomyelitis and the intradiscal infection. Infectious spondylitis occurs most commonly in the toddler and young child age groups and classically presents with a refusal to walk or bend forward. Initial radiographs may be unrevealing, whereas a bone scan is most often diagnostic. Although still controversial, most clinicians believe that use of antistaphylococcal antibiotics and bed rest leads to the most rapid resolution of symptoms. Biopsy is not indicated, unless the child does not rapidly respond to treatment or unless a possibility of tumor lingers. The prognosis for full recovery is excellent, even in cases of untreated infectious spondylitis.

As mentioned earlier, intermittent minor musculoskeletal pain is a relatively common occurrence with *scoliosis*. However, unremitting pain and neurologic signs are not common occurrences. Such findings demand a thorough evaluation. MRI usually is the study of choice. MRI is also indicated in many cases in which the curve pattern is atypical, such as a high magnitude curve in a child younger than 10 years old or a left-sided thoracic curve (most idiopathic thoracic curves are right-sided).

Scheuermann's disease is characterized by a rigid increase in thoracic kyphosis. Although the cause remains unsettled, the kyphosis of Scheuermann's disease is secondary to a decrease in anterior vertebral body growth and results in a series of wedge-shaped vertebra. It is not seen before age 10 years. Adolescents present because of pain over the gibbus or for cosmetic concerns. Clinical findings include an increased kyphosis that does not correct over a bolster, a compensatory hyperlordosis of the lumbar spine, and a forward shot appearance of the head. Radiographs are diagnostic. In mild cases, an exercise program emphasizing back, hamstring, and pectoralis stretching is appropriate. If 2 or more years of spinal growth is expected and the kyphosis measures 50 degrees or greater, full-time use of a brace until skeletal maturity is recommended. Surgical indications include kyphosis greater than 75 degrees or unacceptable cosmesis. An orthopaedic surgeon should have a principal role in managing Scheuermann's disease.

Spondylolysis is defined by a defect in the pars intra-articularis and is caused by repetitive flexion and extension of the lumbar spine. An increased incidence is found in gymnasts, divers, football linemen, baseball pitchers, rowers, and weight lifters. The presenting complaint is pain that is aggravated by activity, particularly with back extension movements. Patients present with decreased lumbar spinal mobility secondary to pain and tight hamstring muscles. Oblique radiographs and occasionally a bone scan or SPECT study are often necessary to establish the diagnosis.

Any forward slippage of the vertebra because of instability is called *spondylolisthesis*. Spondylolisthesis in children can be dysplastic (developmental elongation of the pars intra-articularis) or isthmic (stress fracture of the pars intra-articularis from repetitive trauma). Spondylolysis and spondylolisthesis in children occur at the fifth lumbar vertebra, as opposed to the fourth lumbar vertebra as seen in adult degenerative spine conditions. Progressive spondylolisthesis is associated with an early age of onset, greater than 50% forward slippage, female gender, and a dysplastic cause.

Treatment of painful spondylolysis or spondylolisthesis in children initially consists of activity modification and nonsteroidal anti-inflammatory medication. Recalcitrant pain is treated with a custom-molded lumbar orthosis. Surgical fusion is indicated for spondylolisthesis of greater than 50% or for unremitting pain. Surgical attempts to repair acute spondylolysis remain controversial. Referral to an orthopaedic surgeon is prudent during the management of spondylolysis and spondylolisthesis.

Finally, a variety of neoplastic processes exhibit a predilection for the spine. *Hemangioma, eosinophilic granuloma,* and *giant cell tumor* characteristically occur in the vertebral body. In contrast, *osteoid osteoma, osteoblastoma,* and *aneurysmal bone cysts* are more commonly found in the pedicle, lamina, and spinous processes of the spine.

REFERENCES

1. Morrissy RT, Haynes DW: Acute hematogenous osteomyelitis: A model with trauma as an etiology. J Pediatr Orthop 9:447–456, 1989.
2. Scott P, Ansell B, Huskisson E: Measurement of pain in juvenile chronic polyarthritis. Ann Rheum Dis 36:186–187, 1977.
3. Morrissy RT: Bone and joint sepsis. In Morrissy RT, Weinstein SL, eds: Lovell and Winter's Pediatric Orthopaedics, Vol I. Philadelphia, Lippincott-Raven, 1996, pp 579–624.
4. Morey B, Peterson H: Hematogenous pyogenic osteomyelitis in children. Orthop Clin North Am 6:935, 1975.
5. Unkila-Kallio L, Kallio MJT, Eskola J, Peltola H: Serum C-reactive protein, erythrocyte sedimentation rate, and white blood cell count in acute hematogenous osteomyelitis of children. Pediatrics 91:59–62, 1994.
6. Howie D, Savage J, Wilson T, et al: The technetium phosphate bone scan in the diagnosis of osteomyelitis in childhood. J Bone Joint Surg Am 65:431, 1983.
7. Canale ST, Harkness RM, Thomas PA, Massie JD: Does aspiration of bones and joints affect results of later bone scanning? J Pediatr Orthop 5:23–26, 1985.
8. McCoy J, Morrissy R, Seibert J: Clinical experience with the technetium-99 scan in children. Clin Orthop 154:175, 1981.
9. Herndon W, Alexieva B, Schwindt M, et al: Nuclear imaging for musculoskeletal infections in children. J Pediatr Orthop 5:343–347, 1985.
10. Sundberg S, Savage J, Foster B: Technetium phosphate bone scan in the diagnosis of septic arthritis in childhood. J Pediatr Orthop 9:579, 1989.
11. Smith L, Schurman DJ, Kajiyama G, et al: The effect of antibiotics on the destruction of cartilage in experimental infectious arthritis. J Bone Joint Surg Am 69:1063, 1987.
12. Gillespie WJ, Mayo K: The management of acute hematogenous osteomyelitis in the antibiotic era: A study of the outcome. J Bone Joint Surg Br 63:126–131, 1981.
13. Smith S, Lenarz L, Mollitt DL, Golladay ES: The sore psoas: A difficult diagnosis in childhood. J Pediatr Surg 17: 975–978, 1982.
14. Levine M, Holroyde J, Woods JR Jr, et al: Birth trauma: Incidence and predisposing factors. Obstet Gynecol 63:792–795, 1984.
15. Kempe C, Silverman F, Steele B, et al: The battered-child syndrome. JAMA 181:17–24, 1962.
16. Kleinman P, Marks S, Blackburn B: The metaphyseal lesion in abused infants: A radiographic-histopathologic study. AJR Am J Roentgenol 146:895–905, 1986.
17. King J, Diefendorf D, Apthorp J, et al: Analysis of 429 fractures in 189 battered children. J Pediatr Orthop 8:585–589, 1988.
18. Rogalsky RJ, Black GB, Reed MH: Orthopaedic manifestations of leukemia in children. J Bone Joint Surg Am 68:494–501, 1986.
19. Del B, Champoux A, Bockers T, et al: Septic arthritis versus transient synovitis of the hip: The value of screening laboratory tests. Ann Emerg Med 21:1418, 1992.
20. Nash J, Apley J: "Growing pains": A clinical study of non-arthritic limb pains in children. Arch Dis Child 26:134, 1951.
21. Oster J: Recurrent abdominal pain, headache and limb pains in children and adolescents. Pediatrics 50:429–436, 1972.
22. Loder RT, Wittenberg B, DeSilva G: Slipped capital femoral epiphysis associated with endocrine disorders. J Pediatr Orthop 15: 349–356, 1995.
23. Nimon G, Murray D, Sandow M, Goodfellow J: Natural history of anterior knee pain: A 14- to 20-year follow-up of nonoperative management. J Pediatr Orthop 18:118–122, 1998.
24. Ramirez N, Johnston CE, Browne RH: The prevalence of back pain in children who have idiopathic scoliosis. J Bone Joint Surg Am 79:364–368, 1997.
25. Ring D, Wenger DR: Magnetic resonance-imaging scans in discitis. J Bone Joint Surg Am 76:596–601, 1994.

Chapter **14**

Rheumatic Diseases and the Pregnant Woman

Mark C. Genovese ■ Maurice L. Druzin

This chapter provides guidance to the primary care physician regarding the management of the patient with rheumatic disease during pregnancy. Although not designed to supplant the referral to an obstetrician and rheumatologist, it should help the primary care physician to better understand the management strategies being employed by the consultants and to better predict potential dangers. Each rheumatic disease conveys different risks to both the fetus and the mother. Although most who suffer from rheumatoid arthritis (RA) tend to have disease improvement during pregnancy, patients with systemic lupus erythematosus (SLE) may experience worsening. Not only do the underlying diseases typically fluctuate during pregnancy, but also most patients need to have their medications adjusted or discontinued at confirmation of pregnancy, if not before conception. The adjustment of the medical regimen may lead to an increase in disease activity. The safety of many of the medications used in the treatment of rheumatic diseases has not been established in pregnancy and requires the guidance of experts.

A significant portion of this chapter is devoted to outlining the changes that one might expect in individual disorders, including SLE, antiphospholipid syndromes, RA, seronegative spondyloarthropathies (ankylosing spondylitis, psoriatic arthritis, Reiter's syndrome), and systemic sclerosis.

SYSTEMIC LUPUS ERYTHEMATOSUS

Of the rheumatic diseases, SLE is the disease most often exacerbated by pregnancy. SLE is an autoimmune disease characterized by involvement of multiple organ systems (see Chapter 27). Disease may be limited to skin involvement, such as photosensitivity, malar rash, discoid lupus, and aphthous ulceration, or may result in internal organ involvement, such as pleuropericarditis, nephritis, or cerebritis. The disease itself commonly affects approximately 40 out of every 100,000 people worldwide with an annual incidence of approximately 5 per 100,000. It commonly affects people in their 20s and 30s, and women are affected more frequently than men with a 9 : 1 ratio.

It is generally believed that pregnancy results in increased disease activity in women with SLE. The degree to which pregnancy increases disease activity has been a matter of debate. Typically, one can expect a patient with SLE to flare approximately once every 2 years, particularly with manifestations including constitutional symptoms, musculoskeletal involvement, and cutaneous involvement.[1] Data suggest that the number of flares is often increased in SLE patients during pregnancy, occurring in up to 60% of SLE patients during pregnancy for a rate of approximately 1.6 per patient-year.[2, 3] Flares in disease activity in SLE patients during pregnancy are represented by constitutional symptoms, renal abnormalities, cutaneous manifestations, and musculoskeletal involvement. Patients with SLE need to be followed quite closely by their primary care physician, rheumatologist, and obstetrician.

Risks of Pregnancy in Systemic Lupus Erythematosus

Many risks have been identified for both the mother and the fetus, including worsening of SLE activity, loss of pregnancy, preterm birth, and neonatal lupus. The degree of disease activity at time of conception is a significant predictor of disease activity and flare during pregnancy. Women with little or no activity at the start of pregnancy are less likely to have a flare of disease than those with active disease at time of conception.[4, 5] The sudden discontinuation of medications at the time pregnancy is diagnosed may lead to increased activity or disease flare. For this reason and for the safety of the fetus, it is often safer to plan pregnancies during periods of disease remission and to make judicious adjustments to medications before conception. A more extensive discussion of the safety of many of the rheumatic drugs used to treat SLE is found later.

RENAL DISEASE

Of particular importance for the SLE patient who is pregnant or considering pregnancy is the status of her renal function. Patients with no evidence of renal disease or those whose renal disease is in remission generally do well during pregnancy and do not experience a worsening of renal function. However, it has been reported that 8% to 30% of patients with SLE will develop transient but reversible decrease in renal function.[6] Some patients go on to develop severe and permanent renal dysfunction. A creatinine clearance level in the mother of less than 50 mL/h or a serum creatinine level of greater than 1.4 increases the risk of renal deterioration and obstetric complications.[7]

The differential diagnosis of proteinuria during pregnancy presents a challenge. The presence of protein in the urine may represent SLE flare in renal disease, or it may represent preeclampsia (pregnancy-induced hypertension). In some instances, it can be exceedingly difficult to differentiate between the two. Baseline measures for blood pressure, urine protein, and complement (C3, C4, CH50) are useful even though the diagnosis must be made on clinical grounds.

RISK TO THE FETUS

The fetus is also at increased risk during pregnancy in the SLE patient. Variables in the mother that play a role in the health of the fetus include the following:

- Lupus activity at the time of conception
- Lupus organ involvement (renal disease, pulmonary disease, central nervous system involvement)
- Presence of antiphospholipid antibodies
- Presence of maternal autoantibodies, such as anti-SSA (Ro) and anti-SSB (La).

SLE activity at the time of conception may lead to an increased risk of fetal loss; overall, it is believed that the outcome of pregnancy is improved if SLE is quiescent at time of conception. In individuals with renal disease, there is an increased risk of preeclampsia, intrauterine growth retardation, preterm delivery, and fetal loss. Women who suffer from central nervous system or pulmonary involvement may themselves be at risk for serious complications and are more likely to have preterm deliveries. In addition, the presence of antiphospholipid antibodies increases the risk of fetal loss and intrauterine growth retardation (a deeper discussion of antiphospholipid antibody syndromes follows).

NEONATAL LUPUS

Neonatal lupus describes neonatal abnormalities involving the skin, liver, cardiac conduction system, and blood. It may develop in the setting of many illnesses, including RA and Sjögren's syndrome. The syndrome of neonatal lupus is associated with the presence of the maternal autoantibodies anti-SSA and anti-SSB. If the mother is anti-SSA or anti-SSB positive, she should be alerted to the risk of the fetus developing neonatal lupus. It is believed that these maternal autoantibodies cross the placenta and injure the developing fetus. The most serious complication of neonatal lupus is congenital heart block (third-degree heart block), a rare phenomenon affecting the developing cardiac conduction system. Although the noncardiac manifestations of neonatal lupus, such as transient rash and thrombocy-

topenia, are reversible and tend to resolve by the sixth month of life, congenital heart block is irreversible and often requires the placement of a pacemaker. The resolution of the noncardiac symptoms occurs concurrently with the loss of maternal autoantibodies in the fetus.

ANTIPHOSPHOLIPID ANTIBODY SYNDROME

The antiphospholipid antibody syndrome is characterized by venous and arterial thrombosis, autoimmune thrombocytopenia, and recurrent fetal loss. The syndrome is often subdivided into *primary antiphospholipid syndrome,* which occurs in patients with no other autoimmune disease, and *secondary forms,* which occur in patients with an underlying connective tissue disease. Approximately 25% of SLE patients have antiphospholipid antibodies present, either the lupus anticoagulant or the anticardiolipin antibody. The lupus anticoagulant is usually identified by an elevation in the activated partial thromboplastin time (aPTT). A mixing study is then done to exclude factor deficiencies and to identify the presence of an in vitro inhibitor of coagulation. Subsequently, a dilute Russell viper venom time (dRVVT) or a kaolin clotting time (KCT) assay is run to confirm the presence of the lupus anticoagulant. Alternatively, anticardiolipin antibodies are identified by the use of an enzyme-linked immunosorbent assay (ELISA). The presence of either the lupus anticoagulant or anticardiolipin antibodies confirms the antiphospholipid antibody syndrome and may confer risks for both the mother and the fetus. High levels of antiphospholipid antibodies are associated with both thrombosis and fetal loss. In the future, additional assays, such as those for β_2-glycoprotein, may be available and might help further differentiate patients who are at highest risk for complications related to antiphospholipid antibodies.

Clinically, the history of either venous or arterial thrombosis in the mother or the history of fetal loss may indicate the presence of antiphospholipid antibodies. Although first-trimester spontaneous abortion is common among women in the general population, antiphospholipid antibodies increase the risk of fetal loss in the second and the third trimesters of pregnancy. This loss may occur secondary to placental insufficiency mediated by placental-vascular pathology, chronic inflammation, or thrombosis.[8] In addition, preeclampsia, intrauterine growth restriction (retardation), preterm delivery, and maternal venous and arterial thrombosis may occur secondary to the antiphospholipid antibody syndrome.

The following scenarios of patients with antiphospholipid antibody syndrome should be helpful in sorting out therapy for these cases:

- A woman with antiphospholipid antibodies without prior history of thromboembolic disease or fetal loss is usually treated with low-dose aspirin (81 mg/d). This therapy is both inexpensive and relatively safe.
- If the woman has high antibody titers based on laboratory evaluation, she can be started on low-dose subcutaneous heparin, with or without low-dose aspirin.

- Women who are antiphospholipid antibody positive with a history of recurrent second-trimester or third-trimester fetal loss should be treated with low-dose subcutaneous heparin and low-dose aspirin.
- If antibody titers are high, the woman is often fully anticoagulated with unfractionated or low-molecular-weight heparin.
- In women who are found to be antiphospholipid antibody positive and have had prior evidence of a thromboembolic event, full anticoagulation is used and should probably be continued as lifelong therapy. Warfarin (Coumadin) is teratogenic and so is not used during pregnancy.

In addition to pharmacologic interventions, patients with antiphospholipid antibodies require close obstetric monitoring. Patients with antiphospholipid antibody syndrome are at increased risk of serious complications, both maternal and fetal, including death. Events are not limited only to the term of pregnancy; the patient is at increased risk during the postpartum period (6 weeks) as well. Patients need to be actively counseled regarding risks, and women with prior history of arterial thromboembolism should probably be discouraged from becoming pregnant.

RHEUMATOID ARTHRITIS

RA is an autoimmune disease characterized by polyarticular arthritis usually in a symmetric fashion. In addition, the disease may be marked with extra-articular manifestations, including vasculitis, nodule formation, lung involvement, and neuropathy (all more thoroughly reviewed in Chapter 25). In contrast to SLE, 75% of patients with RA have a remission during pregnancy. Improvement in disease activity during pregnancy portends few if any risks for the mother. Given the lack of risk to the mother, it is important for the primary care provider to focus attention on avoidance of potential risks to the fetus.

Experience has suggested that women who improved during a previous pregnancy are likely to improve during subsequent pregnancies.[9] Most patients experience improvement early in the pregnancy, and additional improvements in disease activity have been seen in the second and third trimesters. Improvement tends to be sustained throughout the pregnancy.[9, 10]

The improvement in disease activity during pregnancy in women with RA is often followed by an equally large increase in disease activity in the postpartum period. Most women develop active arthritis or disease recurrence in the postpartum period.[9] In one study, it was found that recurrence of symptoms of RA occurred in 81% (82 of 101) of patients within the first 4 months of the postpartum period.[11]

The most interesting hypothesis to explain the change in RA activity during pregnancy is related to disparity in maternal/fetal histocompatibility (HLA) antigens in the major histocompatibility complex (MHC). A maternal immune response against fetal HLA antigens might be responsible for the decrease of arthritis during pregnancy. Investigators examined the disparity between a child's paternal HLA antigens and the mother's HLA antigens and found that when there was a maternal-fetal disparity in HLA class II MHC antigens HLA-DR and HLA-DQ, significant reductions in disease activity occurred.[10] Possible mechanisms for this reduction include (1) a maternal antibody response to paternal HLA antigens, (2) induction of suppressor T cells after exposure to fetal HLA antigens leading to suppression of the maternal immune response, or (3) fetal HLA peptides affecting the maternal T-cell repertoire and maternal immune response.[9]

There is no evidence of an increased rate of premature births, spontaneous abortions, or low birth weight among pregnant women with RA.[9] Given that the disease itself conveys little risk to the mother or fetus during pregnancy, it is important to avoid potential exogenous risks to the fetus. Use and avoidance of potentially dangerous medications are outlined later.

SERONEGATIVE SPONDYLOARTHROPATHY

Pregnancy occurring in patients with a seronegative spondyloarthropathy has been poorly studied in the past. The seronegative spondyloarthropathies are made up of a group of similar illnesses: *ankylosing spondylitis, psoriatic arthritis, Reiter's syndrome,* and *inflammatory bowel disease.* These disorders have in common an absence of rheumatoid factor (thus seronegative), inflammatory arthritis (often in an asymmetric distribution), a predilection for the development of sacroiliac involvement (spondyloarthropathy), and inflammation of tendinous insertions (enthesopathy) that may lead to calcification and fusion. Detailed descriptions of the seronegative spondyloarthropathies are presented in Chapter 26. There have been some case reports and series of patients reported with pregnancy and seronegative spondyloarthropathy. However, whether a pregnant patient with one of these disease improves or gets worse during pregnancy, or has a flare after pregnancy, is difficult to predict.

Most studies indicate that ankylosing spondylitis can worsen during pregnancy, especially in the later trimesters. Also, it appears that a postpartum flare, similar to that seen in RA, is common. Patients with a spondyloarthropathy with accompanying features such as psoriasis, ulcerative colitis, and peripheral arthritis, appear to have a different course during pregnancy.[12] In this group, disease activity subsides, only to recur in the postpartum period. These studies were undertaken with small numbers of patients, and drawing broad conclusions is difficult.

SCLERODERMA

The illness of systemic sclerosis (scleroderma) is not as common as RA or SLE. Systemic sclerosis is classified as either diffuse (skin involvement extending beyond the hands and face) or limited (see Chapter 28).

The disease itself affects approximately 75,000 to 100,000 people in the United States with an annual incidence of approximately 4 to 12 people per million.[13] This disorder affects women more than men in a 4 : 1 ratio. The mean age of onset is in the early 40s. Given the infrequent nature of the disease and the age of onset, not many women with systemic sclerosis become pregnant. Nevertheless, it is quite possible that a primary care provider will care for one or more patients with systemic sclerosis and will need to counsel them on the risks of pregnancy.

Overall, scleroderma is relatively stable throughout pregnancy. Raynaud's phenomenon tends to improve, whereas arthralgia and gastroesophageal reflux tend to worsen during pregnancy. Some symptoms may be difficult to distinguish as being related to scleroderma or pregnancy because gastroesophageal reflux, arthralgias, and edema could be ascribed to pregnancy alone.

Renal Crisis in Scleroderma

One of the most serious complications of systemic sclerosis is renal crisis. This condition tends to be an early complication in a small number of patients with diffuse scleroderma. It can be a possible complication of pregnancy in systemic sclerosis. It is not a frequent complication. Should scleroderma renal crisis develop in patients who are not pregnant, angiotensin-converting enzyme (ACE) inhibitors are considered the treatment of choice. However, during pregnancy the use of ACE inhibitors has been shown to lead to fetal renal impairment and oligohydramnios and thus is contraindicated. At least one investigator has used ACE inhibitors for the treatment of scleroderma renal crisis in pregnancy,[14] but the use of ACE inhibitors is warranted only when the potential benefits clearly outweigh the risks to the fetus.

Fetal Risk in Scleroderma

Although maternal disease activity in systemic sclerosis does not appear to change in most cases of pregnancy, the outcome of the fetus appears to be significantly affected by systemic sclerosis. Pregnancy in scleroderma was more likely to result in small-for-gestational-age infants (10%) than RA (4%) or normal controls (2%).[15] In a prospective study of 50 women with 67 pregnancies, patients with late diffuse scleroderma had a high frequency of miscarriage. There was a high frequency of premature births: 26% of the whole group and 40% of the pregnancies in women with early diffuse disease.[16] These abnormalities may be related to the occurrence of fibrosis of the placenta.

Women with scleroderma should be counseled about their increased risk for miscarriage and premature birth. Should the patient become pregnant, she should be followed closely because of the high frequency of premature births. The patient should also be followed closely for the development of high blood pressure or proteinuria, possible signals of the onset of renal crisis.

MEDICATION USE DURING PREGNANCY

The adjustment of medications in the rheumatic patient during pregnancy is exceedingly difficult. Termination of medications that have kept a disease process in remission or under control can result in immediate or delayed flare of disease. This situation may prove dangerous for the mother, the fetus, or both. Adjustments must be made such that medications with any potential teratogenicity are avoided but without endangering the health or life of the mother. Once conception is being considered or pregnancy confirmed, it is important to initiate the use of prenatal vitamins. Their use, particularly the use of folic acid, has been associated with decreased incidence of neural tube defects. All women who could potentially become pregnant should be taking at least 0.4 mg of folic acid supplementation daily.

Many changes take place in women during pregnancy regardless of the presence or absence of a connective tissue disease. These changes may significantly affect the way medications are processed in the body. Total body fluid increases and is accompanied by increased plasma volume and decreased albumin. These changes affect drug distribution and drug binding, leading to a greater percentage of drug being available in the free (unbound), pharmacologically active form. All of these changes may result in an altered physiologic response to medications. For this reason, attention needs to be paid to the use of medications in the pregnant patient.

In addition to the maternal metabolism of medication, the placenta plays a significant role in influencing fetal exposure. The placenta forms both a barrier and a conduit between the mother and the fetus. Medications can cross the placenta through a variety of processes: diffusion, facilitated diffusion, active transport, and special transport processes.[17] Molecules most likely to cross the placenta are small, non-ionic, and lipid soluble.[17] Placental transfer may be affected by the maternal placental vasculature, which has been shown to be abnormal in some rheumatic diseases, such as SLE. Once medications are transferred across the placenta, their effects are determined by fetal metabolism, which differs depending on the stage of development.

Categories of Drugs Used in Pregnancy

NONSTEROIDAL ANTI-INFLAMMATORY DRUGS

Nonsteroidal anti-inflammatory drugs (NSAIDs) are the most frequently prescribed medication in rheumatic diseases (see Chapter 9), but they are generally avoided in pregnancy. The use of NSAIDs can result in problems for both the mother and the fetus. Potential risks include maternal and fetal bleeding related to platelet inhibition. This risk increases significantly in the last weeks of pregnancy secondary to blood loss or hemorrhage during delivery. The inhibition of prostaglandin synthesis in the infant may result in premature closure or constriction of the ductus arteriosus, causing pulmonary hypertension. In addition, NSAIDs may result in prolongation of pregnancy, prolongation of labor, reduction of amniotic fluid, and transient reduction of fetal renal function.[17]

Aspirin and indomethacin are the best-studied NSAIDs. Aspirin has been found to cross the placental membrane. Data from more than 14,000 women who took aspirin during the first 4 months of pregnancy suggest that there is no increased risk of congenital malformation.[18] Although aspirin is typically avoided in higher dosages during pregnancy, it has been used in low dosage (<150 mg but usually 81 mg/d) for the prevention of preeclampsia. Given conflicting data in the published literature, the decision to start low-dose aspirin for the prevention of preeclampsia is controversial and is best left up to the discretion of the patient's obstetrician. As mentioned previously, low-dose aspirin has also been studied in the treatment of antiphospholipid antibody syndrome and is an accepted treatment.

Knowledge of the safety and dangers of using indomethacin during pregnancy comes from studies looking at the use of indomethacin as a tocolytic (agent to delay labor). Indomethacin does cross the placental barrier but does not appear to be associated with congenital malformation.[17] Oligohydramnios, fetal renal impairment, and premature closure of the ductus arteriosus are associated with its use. The impairments in fetal renal function and in the decrease in amniotic fluid appear to be reversible when the indomethacin is stopped.

The overwhelming evidence from previous studies suggests that, as a group, NSAIDs potentially have significant risks to both the mother and the fetus. If NSAIDs (other than low-dose aspirin for preeclampsia or for antiphospholipid antibody syndrome) are given during pregnancy, they should be given in the lowest possible dosages and for the shortest length of time possible. Intensive fetal surveillance for evidence of premature closure of the patent ductus arteriosus and decreased amniotic fluid should be instituted. NSAIDs should be avoided during the last trimester given the potential risks outlined.

GLUCOCORTICOIDS

The most commonly used glucocorticoids are prednisone and prednisolone, and the lowest possible dosage is used to avoid side effects. The same is true regarding the use of glucocorticoids during pregnancy. Evidence suggests that, although not resulting in congenital deformity, long-term use of glucocorticoids during pregnancy (>20 mg/d of prednisone) can result in increased frequency of preterm births.[19]

The effects of glucocorticoids on the fetus depend on the agent in question. Although prednisone crosses the placenta, it is not converted to its active form prednisolone by the fetal liver. Prednisolone, an active agent, is converted to prednisone in the placenta. Approximately only one tenth of the maternal level of prednisolone is passed on to the fetus. Therefore, prednisone and prednisolone are possibly the two safest glucocorticoids for use in pregnancy.

The other glucocorticoids are less commonly used. Dexamethasone and betamethasone are rarely used in the treatment of connective tissue diseases because they are known to cross the placenta and have effects on the fetus. They are used, however, to enhance fetal lung development in preterm delivery.

Adverse complications are associated with prednisone use. The use of greater than 10 mg/d of prednisone during lupus pregnancy may lead to increased risk of hypertension, hyperglycemia, and possibly preterm birth.[19] The use of prednisone in pregnant women with antiphospholipid antibody syndrome has resulted in higher morbidity, including preeclampsia and prematurity.[20]

DISEASE-MODIFYING ANTIRHEUMATIC DRUGS

Disease-modifying antirheumatic drugs (DMARDs) are a wide-ranging group of medications, and as a whole they are generally avoided if possible during pregnancy. Similarly, patients of childbearing age with rheumatic diseases should be urged to use an effective means of birth control to avoid potential risks to the fetus while they are taking these types of medications. If a patient taking a DMARD is contemplating or planning pregnancy, these agents are usually stopped. The risks of the medication to the fetus vary based on the class of the medication being used and the timing of the exposure.

SULFASALAZINE

Sulfasalazine is an agent used most often in inflammatory arthritis and inflammatory bowel disease. The agent itself is 5-aminosalicylic acid bound to sulfapyridine. For the most part, it goes undigested and unabsorbed until reaching the large bowel, where it is split by bacteria. The majority of the 5-aminosalicylic acid is excreted in the feces, while the sulfapyridine is absorbed, metabolized in the liver, and later excreted in the urine. Sulfasalazine and its components cross the placenta, but no evidence of teratogenicity has been found, and this agent may be used in pregnancy.

ANTIMALARIAL AGENTS

Antimalarial agents, such as hydroxychloroquine (Plaquenil) and chloroquine, have modest efficacy and are used in a variety of disorders, including SLE and RA. Both agents have long half-lives and are stored within the body. Studies in both animals and humans have suggested that chloroquine passes through the placenta. Although not classified as a teratogen, inner ear and retinal toxicity has been seen in animals, and there are a few case reports in humans.[17]

Hydroxychloroquine has been less well studied, but potential retinal toxicity may limit the use of this agent during pregnancy as well. Some data suggest that in patients with severe SLE, it is safer for both mother and fetus to continue hydroxychloroquine during pregnancy than to stop it.[21–23] Theoretical risks do exist, however, and the decision to continue hydroxychloroquine during pregnancy must be left to the guidance of the treating obstetrician, rheumatologist, and ultimately the mother.

GOLD SALTS

Gold salts are used almost exclusively for the treatment of inflammatory arthritis. Gold salts are usually administered intramuscularly as the oral versions are infrequently used. Overall, the use of gold salts during pregnancy has been poorly studied. In animals, it appears that congenital malformations and growth retardation can be seen. In humans, most studies suggest that no abnormalities have thus far been reported. Because of the limited data, gold salts are usually discontinued during pregnancy.

METHOTREXATE

Over the last decade, methotrexate has become one of the most frequently used agents in RA. In pregnancy, however, the medication can have devastating consequences. In animals, the use of methotrexate has resulted in fetal death and congenital malformations. In humans, methotrexate has been used as an abortifacient, and its use in pregnant women can result in spontaneous abortion and congenital malformations. For these reasons, the use of methotrexate is contraindicated in pregnancy and in women of childbearing age who are not using a suitable method of birth control.

AZATHIOPRINE

Azathioprine (Imuran) is used extensively as an immunosuppressive agent. It is used frequently in conjunction with glucocorticoids as an adjunct and as a steroid-sparing agent. It is occasionally used in inflammatory arthritis but more commonly prescribed in SLE and vasculitis. Experience with azathioprine in animals has suggested that in high dosages it is teratogenic.[17] In humans, azathioprine has been shown to cross the placenta in small amounts. Azathioprine requires conversion in the liver to its active metabolite, 6-mercaptopurine. Because the fetal liver is unable to convert azathioprine to its active form, the fetus should have some degree of protection. The best studies regarding the use of azathioprine in pregnancy are based on data from renal transplant recipients. The cumulative data suggest that there is only a small risk of congenital anomalies or growth retardation in patients on higher dosages. If azathioprine is used during pregnancy, monitoring for toxicity should take place every 4 weeks, based on reports of leukopenia and thrombocytopenia

in some infants at birth.[24] Tests for monitoring should include complete blood count, platelets, and liver function tests. Consensus opinion suggests that azathioprine can be used in pregnancy, but treatment should be reserved for situations in which the benefits clearly outweigh the potential risks.

CYCLOPHOSPHAMIDE

Cyclophosphamide (Cytoxan) is an alkylating agent and has been used extensively as an antitumor agent. In the care of the patient with rheumatic disease, it has been found effective in the treatment of vasculitis and lupus nephritis. In animal studies, cyclophosphamide is a teratogen and is known to produce birth defects. There are reports of pregnant women with SLE exposed to cyclophosphamide; the majority of reports suggest that there is a high risk for fetal malformation, with those risks being the greatest during the first trimester.[17, 24] Given the high risk to the fetus, cyclophosphamide is contraindicated during pregnancy and should be avoided unless the mother has life-threatening disease activity.

CYCLOSPORIN A

Cyclosporin A has traditionally been used as an immunosuppressive agent in organ transplantation. It is, however, being used more frequently in the treatment of rheumatic diseases, including RA and SLE. In animal models, dose-related nephrotoxicity and teratogenicity have been reported. In humans, cyclosporin A is known to cross the placenta and may lead to growth retardation and premature birth.[17, 24] Overall, there is limited experience with pregnancy and cyclosporin A use in patients with rheumatic diseases, and there are no studies to assess the long-term effects of this medication on the fetus. As with many of the other immunosuppressive medications outlined previously, this medication is best avoided except in situations in which the benefits can clearly be shown to outweigh the potential risks.

Decisions About Medication Use

The decision to use any of the aforementioned medications during pregnancy can be difficult because there is potential risk to the fetus with almost any agent. As has already been suggested, it is best to avoid all unnecessary medication during pregnancy. The problem in the case of patients suffering from rheumatic diseases is that often the medications are necessary to keep the disease under some degree of control. The U.S. Food and Drug Administration (FDA) rates medications and their suitability for use in pregnancy. The rating of an *A* indicates that controlled studies in women show no evidence of risk. A *B* indicates that there is no evidence of risk in humans. Either human studies show no risk, whereas animal studies do, or human studies have not been done, and animal studies suggest no danger. A *C* suggests that risk cannot be ruled out. Animal studies either show evidence of risk for the fetus or have not been done, and human studies have not been done. Medications in this group should be given only if the potential benefit justifies the risk. A *D* indicates evidence of risk for the human fetus. Drugs in this group may still be used in life-threatening situations. The rating of an *X* indicates that the medication is contraindicated in pregnancy, and the risks outweigh any potential benefit. Table 14–1 lists the FDA ratings for the medications discussed here.

SCREENING STUDIES IN PREGNANCY

In addition to the adjustments in the medical regimen that must be made at or before pregnancy, other screening studies should be considered. When the patient with a rheumatic disease is considering pregnancy or becomes pregnant, a number of laboratory studies should be performed (Table 14–2). At the least, these tests provide a baseline for comparison should problems develop later in the pregnancy, but more importantly, they may help provide guidance as to the risks to the mother or fetus. Pregnancy in patients with rheumatic diseases is a prototype for demonstrating that close communication between all providers—the obstetrician, the rheumatologist, and the primary care physician—avoids confusion, duplication, and unnecessary expense in laboratory testing.

In Chapter 5 the use of laboratory tests is outlined more extensively. Electrolytes, renal function, liver function, complete blood count, and urinalysis provide insight into the presence or absence and degree of disease activity. Should the urinalysis show an active sediment or protein loss, a 24-hour collection should be obtained. The 24-hour collection better quantifies the degree of renal function (creatinine clearance) and the degree of protein loss (useful for comparison should preeclampsia develop).

Fluorescent antinuclear antibody, although a test sensitive for lupus, is also present in a variety of other autoimmune diseases. If it has not been previously checked, it should be obtained at this point. The anti–double-stranded DNA is a more specific marker of lupus. It should be checked in SLE patients because it may indicate the possibility of renal involvement and, in some cases, the degree of renal activity.

Anti-SSA and anti-SSB are autoantibodies fre-

TABLE 14–2. SCREENING TESTS TO CONSIDER FOR THE PREGNANT PATIENT WITH A CONNECTIVE TISSUE DISEASE

Fluorescent antinuclear antibody
Anti-ds DNA
Anti-SSA (Ro)
Anti-SSB (La)
C3, C4, CH50
Electrolytes
Renal function
Liver function tests
Complete blood count with platelets
Urinalysis
Anticardiolipin enzyme-linked immunosorbent assay
Activated partial thromboplastin time
Dilute Russell viper venom time

quently seen with Sjögren's syndrome, although they may accompany RA or SLE. In this situation, they are checked because of their association with neonatal lupus. The aPTT, anticardiolipin, and DRVVT are tests used to check for antiphospholipid antibody syndromes. Elevations in these tests are associated with fetal loss and thrombotic complications. Measurements of complement utilization (C3, C4, CH50) indicate disease activity in SLE. In this situation, it may help to differentiate preeclampsia from a flare in lupus.[25]

CONCLUSION

Each of the rheumatic diseases conveys different risks to both the fetus and the mother. This chapter provides guidance to the primary care physician regarding the management of the rheumatic patient during pregnancy. It provides a framework for the primary care physician to better understand the management strategies being employed by the obstetrician and rheumatologist. It also points out the dangers to watch for and the potential risks of some of the medications frequently used in the care of the rheumatic patient.

Table 14–1. FOOD AND DRUG ADMINISTRATION PREGNANCY RATING

Medication	Rating
Glucocorticoids (prednisone and prednisolone)	B
Sulfasalazine	B
Hydroxychloroquine	C
Gold sodium thiomalate	C
Cyclosporin A	C
Azathioprine	D
Cyclophosphamide	D
Methotrexate	X

REFERENCES

1. Petri M, Genovese M, Engle E, Hochberg M: Definition, incidence, and clinical description of flare in systemic lupus erythematosus. Arthritis Rheum 34:937–944, 1991.
2. Petri M, Howard D, Repke J: Frequency of lupus flare in pregnancy: The Hopkins Lupus Pregnancy Center experience. Arthritis Rheum 34:1538–1545, 1991.
3. Ruiz-Irastorza G, Lima F, Alves J, et al: Increased rate of lupus flare during pregnancy and the puerperium: A prospective study of 78 pregnancies. Br J Rheumatol 35:133–138, 1996.
4. Estes D, Larson DL: Systemic lupus erythematosus and pregnancy. Clin Obstet Gynecol 8:307–321, 1965.
5. Tozman ECS, Urowitz MB, Gladman DD: Systemic lupus erythematosus and pregnancy. J Rheumatol 7:624–632, 1980.
6. Druzin ML, van Vollenhoven RF: Systemic lupus erythematosus and pregnancy. Ann Med Intern 147:265–273, 1996.
7. Jones DC, Hayslett JP: Outcome of pregnancy in women with moderate or severe renal insufficiency. N Engl J Med 335:226–232, 1996.

8. Salafia CM, Parke AL: Placental pathology in systemic lupus erythematosus and phospholipid antibody syndrome. Rheum Dis Clin North Am 23:85–97, 1997.
9. Nelson JL, Ostensen M: Pregnancy and rheumatoid arthritis. Rheum Dis Clin North Am 23:195–212, 1997.
10. Nelson JL, Hughes KA, Smith AG, et al: Maternal-fetal disparity in HLA class II alloantigens and the pregnancy-induced amelioration of rheumatoid arthritis. N Engl J Med 329:466–471, 1993.
11. Oka M: Effect of pregnancy on the course of rheumatoid arthritis. Ann Rheum Dis 12:227–229, 1953.
12. Ostensen M, Husby G: A prospective clinical study of the effect of pregnancy on rheumatoid arthritis and ankylosing spondylitis. Arthritis Rheum 26:1155–1159, 1983.
13. Seibold JR: Connective tissue diseases characterized by fibrosis. In Kelley WN, Harris ED Jr, Ruddy D, Sledge CB, eds: Textbook of Rheumatology, 5th ed. Philadelphia, WB Saunders, 1996, pp 1133–1162.
14. Steen VD: Scleroderma and pregnancy. Rheum Dis Clin North Am 23:133–147, 1997.
15. Steen VD, Conte C, Day N, et al: Pregnancy in women with systemic sclerosis. Arthritis Rheum 32:151–157, 1989.
16. Steen VD, Brodeur M, Conte C: Prospective pregnancy (PG) study in women with systemic sclerosis (SSc). Arthritis Rheum 39:S151, 1996.
17. Ostensen M: Optimisation of antirheumatic drug treatment in pregnancy. Clin Pharmacokinet 27:486–503, 1994.
18. Slone D, Heinonen OP, Kaufman DW, et al: Aspirin and congenital malformations. Lancet 1:1373–1375, 1976.
19. Petri M: Hopkins Lupus Pregnancy Center: 1987 to 1996. Rheum Dis Clin North Am 23:1–13, 1997.
20. Cowchock FS, Reece EA, Balaban D, et al: Repeated fetal losses associated with antiphospholipid antibodies: A collaborative randomized trial comparing prednisone with low-dose heparin treatment. Am J Obstet Gynecol 166:1318–1323, 1992.
21. Parke AL, Rothfield NF: Antimalarial drugs in pregnancy—the North American experience. Lupus 5(suppl 1):S67–69, 1996.
22. Parke A, West B: Hydroxychloroquine in pregnant patients with systemic lupus erythematosus. J Rheumatol 23:1715–1718, 1996.
23. Buchanan NMM, Toubi E, Khamashta MA, et al: Hydroxychloroquine and lupus pregnancy: Review of a series of 36 cases. Ann Rheum Dis 55:486–488, 1996.
24. Ramsey-Goldman R, Schilling E: Immunosuppressive drug use during pregnancy. Rheum Dis Clin North Am 23:149–167, 1997.
25. Mascola MA, Repke JT: Obstetric management of the high-risk lupus pregnancy. 23:119–132, 1997.

Chapter **15**

Overuse Injuries

Peter Brukner ■ Gordon O. Matheson

O veruse injuries have become more common in the past two decades, resulting from an increased participation in exercise as well as an increased volume of training in all sports. Any repetitive activity can lead to an overuse injury. Injury occurs when repetitive microtrauma overloads the capacity of a tissue to repair itself. The body's response includes acute, and often chronic, inflammation with structural changes to the tissue. The first challenge to the practitioner is accurate diagnosis. The second is accurate treatment. The third and most difficult challenge is to determine why the overuse injury has occurred and what steps are now necessary to ensure that the injury does not recur.

Diagnosis depends on a comprehensive history that includes the onset, nature, and site of the pain; factors related to training; and technique. On examination, careful palpation should be performed to determine which anatomic structures are affected. It is often helpful to ask patients to perform the maneuver that reproduces their pain. Inflammation is usually associated with swelling, redness, increased temperature, and tenderness. If superficial structures are inflamed, these signs can be present. However, inflammation of deeper structures may not necessarily demonstrate these signs. The basic treatment of overuse injuries involves relative rest, that is, avoidance of aggravating activities while maintaining fitness; the use of ice and various electrotherapeutic modalities; soft tissue techniques; nonsteroidal anti-inflammatory drugs (NSAIDs); and, most importantly, well-designed rehabilitation protocols.

CAUSES OF OVERUSE INJURIES

A cause must be found for every overuse injury. The cause may be quite evident, such as a sudden doubling of training quantity, poor footwear, or an obvious biomechanical abnormality. Alternatively the cause may be more subtle, such as running on an uneven surface, muscle imbalances, or a leg length discrepancy. The causes of overuse injuries are usually divided into *extrinsic factors,* such as training, surfaces, shoes, equipment, and environmental conditions, and *intrinsic factors,* such as malalignment, leg length discrepancy, muscle imbalance, muscle weakness, lack of flexibility, and body composition. The many possible predisposing factors are show in Table 15–1.

FIVE MOST COMMON CLINICAL PRESENTATIONS OF OVERUSE INJURIES

Rotator Cuff Tendinitis

Rotator cuff tendinitis is a common cause of shoulder pain in athletes. It may be *primary,* as a result of simple overuse, or *secondary,* (i.e., altered shoulder mechanics, such as impaired scapulohumeral rhythm or impingement). The predisposing factors to rotator cuff tendinitis are shown in Figure 15–1. Tendinitis, with resultant inflammation and swelling of the rotator cuff tendons, causes impingement of the cuff beneath the coracoacromial arch and further aggravation of the tendinitis. This cycle explains why this condition may become chronic, particularly in the competitive athlete who does not reduce the aggravating activity. Rotator cuff tendinitis can be associated with subacromial bursitis, decreasing further the subacromial space.

The athlete with rotator cuff tendinitis complains of pain with overhead activity, such as throwing, swimming, and overhead shots in racquet sports. Activities undertaken at less than 90 degrees abduction of the arm are usually pain-free. There may also be a history of associated symptoms of instability such as recurrent subluxation.

Examination shows tenderness over the supraspinatus tendon proximal to or at its insertion into the greater tuberosity of the humerus. Active movement reveals a painful arc on abduction between approximately 70 and 120 degrees. For the athlete with rotator cuff tendinitis, symptoms can be reproduced with the impingement test (Fig. 15–2) as well as at the extremes of passive flexion. Pain also occurs with resisted contraction of the supraspinatus, which is best performed with resisted upward movement with the shoulder joint in 90 degrees abduction, 30 degrees horizontal flexion, and internal rotation.

The treatment of rotator cuff tendinitis should be considered in two parts. The first part is the treatment of the tendinitis itself. This involves avoidance of the aggravating activity, local application of ice, NSAIDs, and electrotherapeutic modalities (e.g., ultrasound, interferential stimulation, laser and magnetic field therapy). The purpose of this phase of treatment is to reduce pain and inflammation. If this regimen has limited success, a

Table 15–1. OVERUSE INJURIES: PREDISPOSING FACTORS	
Extrinsic Factors	**Intrinsic Factors**
Training errors	Malalignment
Excessive volume	Pes planus (flatfoot)
Excessive intensity	Pes cavus (high arch)
Rapid increase	Rearfoot varus
Sudden change	Genu valgum (knock-knee)
Excessive fatigue	Genu varum (bowleg)
Inadequate recovery	Patella alta (high patella)
Faulty technique	Femoral neck anteversion
Surfaces	Tibial torsion
Hard	Leg length discrepancy
Soft	Muscle imbalance
Uneven	Muscle weakness
Shoes	Lack of flexibility
Inappropriate	Generalized muscle tightness
Worn out	Focal areas of muscle thickening
Equipment	Restricted joint range of motion
Inappropriate	Sex, size, body composition
Environmental conditions	Psychological factors
Hot	
Cold	
Inadequate nutrition	

training errors. Muscular action stabilizes the glenohumeral joint during movement, and impaired scapulohumeral rhythm may predispose to rotator cuff tendinitis. Decreased rotator cuff strength or an imbalance between the internal and external rotators of the shoulder must be assessed. Treatment involves strengthening of the external rotators (teres minor, infraspinatus, posterior deltoid) because they are usually relatively weak compared with the internal rotators (subscapularis, anterior deltoid, pectoralis). Posterior capsular tightness may be associated with reduced rotator cuff strength. Stretching of the posterior capsule may be helpful.

Freestyle and butterfly swimmers are particularly liable to rotator cuff tendinitis because they develop excessive strength of the internal rotators of the shoulder, resulting in excessive internal rotation of the head of the humerus. This excessive internal rotation reduces the subacromial space. The closer approximation of the greater tuberosity to the acromions is thought by many to cause impingement of the rotator cuff tendons and to reduce blood supply (the *wringing-out* effect) to this tissue.

SHOULDER INSTABILITY

Rotator cuff tendinitis often occurs secondary to shoulder instability, which should always be considered in any patient who presents with symptoms typical of rotator cuff tendon problems. If the presence of instability is not recognized, rotator cuff tendinitis is likely to

glucocorticoid injection into the subacromial space often is helpful and may reduce the athlete's symptoms sufficiently to begin a rehabilitation program.

The second part is the correction of associated abnormalities, including glenohumeral instability, muscle weakness or incoordination, soft tissue tightness, and

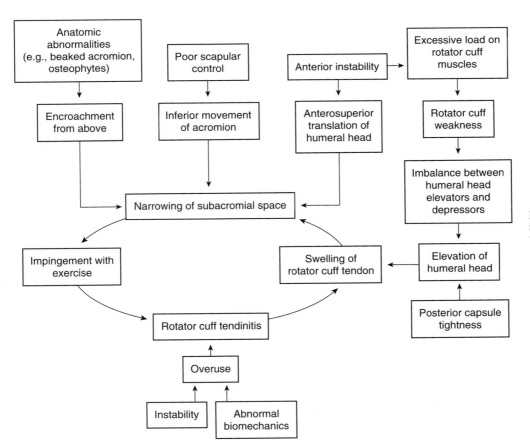

Figure 15–1. Predisposing factors in the development of rotator cuff tendinitis.

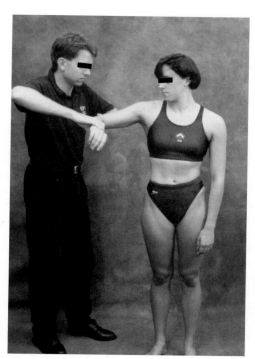

Figure 15–2. Physical examination for shoulder impingement.

recur on return to the sport. Anterior glenohumeral instability may be post-traumatic, as a result of an acute episode of trauma causing anterior dislocation or subluxation, or atraumatic, as a result of gradual development of instability in response to repeated microtrauma.

In post-traumatic instability, the patient usually reports a specific incident, commonly a moderately forceful abduction and external rotation injury. After this episode, the patient reports that the shoulder has not returned to normal. The atraumatic type of shoulder instability is common in athletes, especially those involved in repeated overhead activities, such as baseball pitchers, javelin throwers, swimmers, and tennis players. As a result of repetitive stress, the anterior capsule of the shoulder joint becomes *stretched*, leading to anterior instability. The athlete with atraumatic anterior instability may present with shoulder pain, or the first clinical evidence of the presence of instability may be an episode of subluxation.

The symptoms of anterior instability may include recurrent dislocation or subluxation and shoulder pain. The shoulder pain is usually the result of impingement of the rotator cuff tendons because of anterior translation of the humeral head, *silent subluxation*. This problem is aggravated by the weakened rotator cuff muscles, which, in turn, may lead to failure of humeral head depression during abduction. Recurrent episodes of impingement result in a rotator cuff tendinitis.

EXAMINATION FOR SHOULDER INSTABILITY. When examining the shoulder, it is important to note the presence of generalized ligamentous laxity, such as the amount of passive external rotation. Full assessment of the power of all the primary and secondary muscles controlling the shoulder should also be per-

formed as well as palpating for tenderness. With anterior instability, the patient usually notes that the shoulder dislocates or subluxes in abduction and external rotation. The degree of anterior shoulder laxity can then be assessed with the anterior drawer test (Fig. 15–3). The apprehension test (Fig. 15–4) is also an indicator of anterior instability. If the examiner's thumb is placed behind the humeral head to push it forward, this may aggravate the athlete's apprehension and confirm the diagnosis of anterior instability. Conversely, posterior pressure on the humeral head may reduce apprehension. Magnetic resonance imaging (MRI) reliably demonstrates the presence of associated bony lesions as well as soft tissue abnormalities of the labrum, the capsule, and the associated tendons.

TREATMENT. With the post-traumatic type of anterior shoulder instability, conservative measures consisting of an intensive strengthening program may be unsuccessful in relieving symptoms of instability, and surgical treatment may be required (see Chapter 16). A number of different procedures are available, but in athletes, particularly those in whom the dominant throwing arm is involved, the underlying mechanical lesion should be corrected.

In treating the atraumatic type of instability, an intensive rehabilitation program is often successful. The most important component of this is strengthening of the dynamic stabilizers (rotator cuff muscles) and scapular stabilizing muscles with particular emphasis on the muscles opposing the direction of the instability. Rehabilitation of the unstable shoulder joint should always begin by reducing inflammation. Until pain-free range of motion is achieved, rehabilitation is limited to

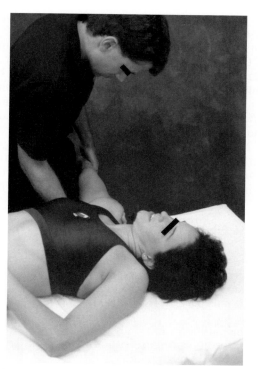

Figure 15–3. Anterior drawer test for anterior glenohumeral instability.

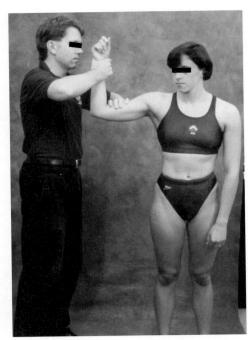

Figure 15–4. Apprehension test associated with glenohumeral instability.

isometric contractions of the adductor, rotator cuff, and scapular stabilizing muscles. As range of motion is achieved, exercises are advanced, with the emphasis on scapular stabilizing exercises through range of motion. Given full range of pain-free movement, specific rotator cuff strengthening exercises are added. Eventually, more functional, sport-specific exercises are prescribed before permitting gradual return to full sporting activity. All exercises must be pain-free. If pain develops, the exercise program should be reduced.

In the rehabilitation of the athlete with impingement, the primary consideration is to improve rotator cuff strength to aid humeral head stabilization. In the rehabilitation of impingement secondary to instability (either traumatic or atraumatic), adequate dynamic stabilization of the scapula must be obtained. In addition, the muscles opposing the instability must be strengthened. Multidirectional instability is best managed by strengthening the entire rotator cuff and surrounding glenohumeral musculature as well as avoiding activities involving movements at the limits of range of motion.

Lateral Elbow Pain

Lateral elbow pain is a common overuse syndrome related to excessive wrist extension. Although this condition has been called *tennis elbow,* it is more common in non–tennis players. It has also been referred to as *lateral epicondylitis,* an inappropriate term because the site of the pathology is usually just below the lateral epicondyle, and the primary pathology is often degenerative rather than inflammatory.

The primary pathologic process involved in this condition is degeneration of the extensor carpi radialis bevis (ECRB) tendon, usually within 1 cm of its attachment to the common extensor origin at the lateral epicondyle. Histologically, there is an invasion of fibroblasts and vascular granulation tissue termed *angiofibroblastic hyperplasia.* This granulation tissue has a large number of nociceptive nerve endings, which may explain why the lesion is so painful. With continued use, these degenerative changes may result in the development of microscopic tears and scarring within the tendon. Conversely, a tear may be the primary pathology, with degenerative change being secondary. Because this is primarily a mechanical process, it might be termed *tendinosis* rather than tendinitis. An inflammatory component may be present as a result of exacerbation of the underlying lesion, probably secondary to microscopic tearing.

Other conditions that cause lateral elbow pain include synovitis of the radiohumeral joint, radiohumeral bursitis, and entrapment of the posterior interosseous nerve as it passes through the supinator muscle. These conditions may exist by themselves or in conjunction with extensor tendinitis. Extensor tendinitis occurs in association with any activity involving repeated wrist extension against resistance, including sporting activities, such as tennis, squash, and badminton, as well as occupational and leisure activities, such as carpentry, bricklaying, sewing, knitting, and carrying suitcases.

There are two distinct clinical presentations of this condition. The most common is an insidious onset of pain, which occurs after unaccustomed activity involving repeated wrist extension. This pain occurs typically after a person spends the weekend laying bricks or using a screwdriver. It is also seen after prolonged sewing or knitting. It may occur after the use of a new tennis racquet, or after a heavy training session.

The other clinical presentation is sudden onset of lateral elbow pain associated with a single instance of exertion involving the wrist extensors, for example, lifting a heavy object or attempting a hard backhand in a tennis match with too much reliance on the forearm and not enough on the trunk and legs. The insidious onset is thought to correspond to microscopic tears within the tendon, whereas the less common acute onset may correspond to a macroscopic tear of the tendon.

On examination, the maximal area of tenderness is approximately 1 cm distal to the lateral epicondyle in the ECRB tendon. Typically the pain is reproduced by resisted wrist extension, especially with the wrist pronated and radially deviated (Mills' test). Resisted extension of the wrist producing pain is the most reliable diagnostic test.

TREATMENT

The basic principles of treatment of soft tissue injuries apply: control of pain and inflammation, restoration of flexibility and strength, treatment of associated causative factors, and a program of gradual return to activity with added support and correction of the predisposing factors. Soft tissue therapy is performed at the site of the lesion and to adjacent tight or thickened tissues. Direct massage at the site of the lesion can be performed. Stretching of the ECRB muscle and associated wrist extensors should be performed regularly.

A muscle strengthening program should be commenced as soon as pain permits, beginning with isometric contraction of the wrist extensors. When this can be performed without pain, gradual progression to concentric and then eccentric exercises should occur. The most important factor to be avoided is excessive or unaccustomed activity.

Regardless of the cause, counterforce bracing appears to reduce the forces on the extensor tendons. The brace, usually a nondistensible band fastened with Velcro, should be applied during the rehabilitation process and on return to the aggravating activity. Many patients mistakenly assume that the brace should be applied over the painful area itself, but the correct site is in the upper forearm, approximately 10 cm below the elbow joint. The brace should be applied firmly.

Glucocorticoid injection is frequently used in the treatment of tennis elbow. However, with appropriate management as indicated these agents can be avoided. The indications for glucocorticoid injection in this condition include failure of an appropriate rehabilitation program after 3 months or localization of pain to the lateral epicondyle, possibly resulting from periostitis. Glucocorticoid and local anesthetic agents should be injected around the ECRB tendon, directly over the point of maximal tenderness. For a guide to injection, see Chapter 6. Glucocorticoid injections should be regarded as one component of the treatment program and followed by appropriate rehabilitation.

Occasionally, particularly in cases with a long history of lateral elbow pain, the treatment program mentioned fails to resolve the patient's symptoms. Failure of conservative treatment after 12 months is a reasonable indication for surgery. Surgery involves excision of the degenerative tissue within the ECRB tendon.

Anterior Knee Pain

Anterior knee pain is the most common presenting symptom in clinical sports medicine practice. Common causes of pain include patellofemoral syndrome; patellar tendinitis; quadriceps tendinitis; fat pad impingement; and, in the adolescent, Osgood-Schlatter disease. *Patellofemoral syndrome* is the term used to describe a constellation of symptoms that include pain in the peripatellar region with or without cartilage changes to the undersurface of the patella. This condition was formerly known as *chondromalacia patellae*. Although macroscopic chondral pathology is seen reasonably frequently at arthroscopy, a causal relationship between the pain and arthroscopic findings has not been established, and the vast majority of patients do well with conservative treatment.

During knee flexion, the patella moves in the groove formed by the femoral condyles and comes to lie in the intercondylar notch. Its excursion is controlled by the quadriceps muscles and, in particular, the vastus medialis obliquus. During flexion, different areas of the articular surface of the patella come into contact with the femur in a sequential manner. The mechanism of pain production in patellofemoral syndrome has not been fully established, but possible sites include inflammation of peripatellar soft tissues and synovium, articular cartilage, or subchondral bone. Activities that increase the load on the patellofemoral joint, such as squatting, downhill running, or walking downstairs, aggravate this condition. A number of factors may predispose to patellofemoral syndrome and are listed in Table 15–2.

Training factors (e.g., increased repetition and intensity, hills, stairs, or squats) increase the load on the patellofemoral joint and are usually found in combination with other predisposing factors. Squats and loads placed on the quadriceps muscle at the extremes of flexion often precipitate patella and femoral pain. The patient with patellofemoral syndrome complains of pain with distance running, pain going up and (particularly) down stairs or hills, and pain with prolonged sitting (*theatre sign*). Other symptoms, such as crepitus, swelling, pseudolocking, and *giving way,* are common.

During clinical assessment, it is important for diagnostic purposes to reproduce the patient's anterior knee pain. This is usually done with either a double or single leg squat. It is essential to asses the relationships between the patella and the femur and the patella and its surrounding soft tissues. The clinician should assess the position of the patella in relation to the femur, assessing the tilt, rotation, and glide and passive movement of the patella in all directions (medial, lateral, superior, inferior).

The patella should sit approximately midway between the two condyles. The most common abnormality is a laterally placed patella with restricted medial glide. The medial and lateral patellar borders should be of equal height. Another common abnormality is a depressed lateral border; this is called a *lateral tilt.* The

---

TABLE 15–2. PREDISPOSING FACTORS TO THE DEVELOPMENT OF PATELLOFEMORAL SYNDROME

Abnormal biomechanics
  Excessive pronation
  Femoral anteversion (internal femoral torsion)
  High small patella (patella alta)
  Increased Q angle*
Soft tissue tightness
  Muscles
    Gastrocnemius
    Hamstrings
    Rectus femoris
    Iliotibial band
  Lateral structures
    Lateral retinaculum
    Iliotibial band
    Vastus lateralis
Muscle dysfunction
  Vastus medialis obliquus
  Hip abductors/external rotators (gluteus medius)
Training
  Distance running
  Hills, stairs

*Angle between line of pull of quadriceps muscle and line of patellar tendon.

long axis of the patella should be parallel with the long axis of the femur, and deviation is described as rotational abnormality. The superior and inferior pole of the patella should lie in the same plane. The abnormality seen most commonly in this axis is called *inferior tilt* and clinically results in the inferior pole being difficult to palpate as it is embedded in the infrapatellar fat pad.

Assessment of the status of the vastus medialis obliquus is essential. Evidence of wasting may be present. This wasting may be bilateral if the condition is congenital or unilateral if it is acquired as a result of surgery, disuse, or injury. It is important also to assess the timing of the vastus medialis obliquus contractions to ensure that it is synchronous with the rest of the quadriceps mechanism.

Examination of the hip is also an important component of the clinical assessment of patellofemoral pain. In particular, the strength and control of the gluteus medius should be assessed. Hip pain is often referred to the knee. Any weakness or incoordination has to be rectified as part of the treatment program.

TREATMENT

The first priority of treatment is to reduce any acute inflammation that may be present. This reduction is achieved with a combination of rest from aggravating activities, ice, NSAIDs, and electrotherapeutic modalities (e.g., ultrasound, laser, electrical stimulation). Taping can have an immediate pain-relieving effect. The aim of taping in the management of patellofemoral syndrome is to correct the abnormal position of the patella in relation to the femur. The main effect of this taping is mechanical, although neural or proprioceptive effects may also contribute. Taping is an effective interim measure to relieve patellofemoral pain while other biomechanical abnormalities (e.g., vastus medialis obliquus weakness, excessive pronation) are being corrected. The most commonly used technique involves taping the patella with a medial glide (Fig. 15–5).

The effect of taping should always be assessed im-

mediately after the tape is applied. A pain-provoking activity, such as a single or double leg squat, should be performed immediately before the taping and performed again after taping. If the tape has been applied correctly, the post-taping squat is painless. If pain is still present, the tape should be altered, possibly including a component for tilt or rotation or both.

If patients are able to perform strengthening exercises pain-free without tape, exercises alone are sufficient to correct the abnormality. Most people, however, require tape to perform the exercises and, initially, to continue their sporting activities. Acute cases of patellofemoral syndrome may initially need tape applied 24 hours per day until the condition settles.

Exercises are progressed from non–weight bearing through partial weight bearing to full weight bearing. Functional exercises are then commenced with steadily increasing load and difficulty. The aim is to achieve a carryover from functional exercises to functional activities. Because fatigue is probably a major consideration in a patient with a wasted vastus medialis obliquus, small numbers of exercises should be performed frequently throughout the day. Graded vastus medialis obliquus exercises, performed under the supervision of a physical therapist, are the mainstay of treatment.

Stretching of tight lateral structures, such as the lateral retinaculum, is beneficial. This stretching is best done in a side-lying position with the knee flexed. The patella is glided medially using the heel of the hand for a sustained stretch. Attention must also be paid to stretching other tight muscles, such as the quadriceps, hamstrings, calf, and iliotibial band.

The need for surgery in patellofemoral syndrome has been almost eliminated as a result of the improved understanding of its cause and the introduction of the vastus medialis obliquus strengthening and taping program. The only indication for surgery in this condition is failure of an appropriate conservative management program. In the presence of clinically and arthroscopically demonstrable chondromalacia patellae, chondroplasty may be performed. The previously popular procedure known as *lateral retinacular release* is now rarely necessary but, if performed, requires appropriate postoperative rehabilitation with an emphasis on vastus medialis obliquus control.

Shin Pain

Shin pain is an extremely common complaint among athletes. The term *shin splints* has been used in the past to describe the pain along the medial border of the shin commonly experienced by runners. It is, however, necessary to make a more precise pathologic diagnosis, and therefore the term *shin splints* should be avoided. Shin pain generally arises from injury to one of three structures: bone, tenoperiosteum, or muscle compartment. These three types of injuries can usually be distinguished on the basis of history, examination, and investigations. Two or all three of these conditions may exist together.

One of the major causes of all three injuries is ab-

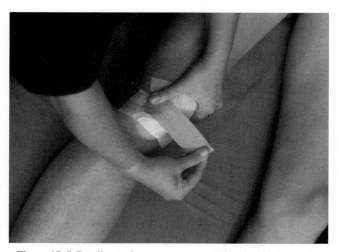

Figure 15–5. Patellar taping to correct medial glide of the patella.

normal biomechanics. Shin pain occurs in athletes with both extremes of foot type. A rigid, cavus (high arch) foot has limited shock attenuation, thus increasing the impact pressure on the bone. In athletes with excessively pronated feet, the muscles of the superficial and deep compartments are required to contract harder and longer eccentrically to resist pronation after heel strike. On toe-off, they then work hard concentrically to accelerate supination. With fatigue, these muscles fail to provide the normal degree of shock absorption. This mechanism may lead to the development of a stress fracture or tenoperiostitis and exacerbates a tendency to develop compartment syndromes.

The athlete with excessive pronation has a tendency to develop lateral shin pain, especially when pronation occurs during toe-off. During this phase, the peroneal muscles contract strongly to stabilize the foot for propulsion. The repetitive force of contraction of the fibula may lead to stress fracture. Tight calf muscles, which commonly occur as a result of hard training, restrict ankle dorsiflexion and increase the tendency for excessive pronation, leading to increased internal rotation of the tibia.

STRESS FRACTURE OF THE TIBIA

The athlete with stress fracture of the tibia presents with gradual onset of shin pain, aggravated by exercise. If the offending activity is not discontinued, pain may occur with walking, at rest, or even at night. Examination reveals localized tenderness over the tibia, usually in the distal third. Biomechanical examination may show a rigid, cavus foot incapable of absorbing load or an excessively pronating foot causing excessive muscle fatigue. Reduced impact absorption results.

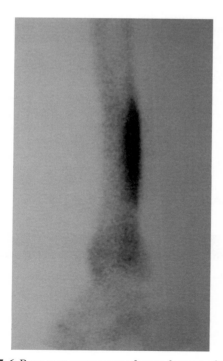

Figure 15–6. Bone scan appearance of stress fracture of the tibia.

Most stress fractures of the tibia are located on the medial border of the tibia and are accompanied by obvious tenderness. The typical bone scan appearance of a stress fracture of the tibia is shown in Figure 15–6. As with other overuse injuries of bone, the full continuum of excessive bone stress is observed, from bone strain to stress reaction and stress fracture.

The treatment of stress fracture of the tibia involves a period of modified rest (sometimes requiring a period of non–weight bearing on crutches for pain relief) before the pain settles. During this time, the patient should avoid the offending activity but may maintain fitness by cycling, rowing, or swimming. This period lasts 4 to 8 weeks. There should be a gradual progression in the quantity of the exercise performed over the following month.

It is important to determine which factors have precipitated the stress fracture. The most common causes are excessive training and biomechanical abnormalities. In women, reduced bone density as a result of hypoestrogenemia secondary to athletic amenorrhea can contribute.

TENOPERIOSTITIS

The patient with tenoperiostitis complains of pain along the medial border of the tibia that usually decreases after warming up. The athlete can often complete the training session, but pain gradually recurs after exercise and is worse the following morning. On examination, there is commonly an area of tenderness along the medial border of the tibia that may extend along the entire tibia or may be as little as 2 cm in length. This tenderness usually occurs at the junction of the lower third and upper two thirds of the tibia. There may also be tenderness and induration within the fascia just posterior to the medial border. Excessive pronation is often present.

Initial treatment is to reduce inflammation by the use of rest, NSAIDs, ice, and electrotherapeutic modalities. The most effective treatment involves deep soft massage; correction of biomechanical abnormalities, such as with orthoses; and strength and endurance training of the lower leg musculature. The athlete should recommence training on alternate days only, wearing appropriate footwear and running on shock-absorbent surfaces.

COMPARTMENT SYNDROME

The lower leg has a number of muscle compartments each enveloped by a thick inelastic fascia. As a result of overuse, these muscle compartments may become swollen and painful, particularly if there is excessive scarring of the fascia. There are two common compartment syndromes seen in runners. The deep posterior compartment, containing flexor hallucis longus, flexor digitorum longus, and tibialis posterior, is usually associated with posteromedial tibial pain. Occasionally a separate fascial sheath surrounds the tibialis posterior muscle forming an extra compartment that is particularly liable to provoke symptoms. The other compartment syndrome commonly seen in runners is the anterior compartment syndrome.

Deep posterior compartment syndrome typically presents as an ache in the region of the medial border of the tibia or as chronic calf pain. The patient describes a feeling of tightness or a bursting sensation, and pain increases with exercise. There may be associated weakness and paresthesia, which may be indicative of nerve compression. Small muscle hernias occasionally occur along the medial or anterior borders of the tibia after exercise.

The bone scan appearance may be normal, or it may show a linear uptake similar to that of tenoperiostitis. The definitive test for this condition is a compartment pressure test. To measure deep posterior compartment pressures, a catheter is inserted from the medial aspect through two layers of fascia. If deep compartment syndrome is being considered as a diagnosis, referral to a specialist should be considered before attempting to measure compartment pressures.

Treatment consists initially of a conservative regimen of reduced exercise and deep soft tissue therapy. Assessment and correction of any biomechanical abnormalities, especially excessive pronation, must be included. If this conservative treatment fails, surgery is indicated. Fasciotomy (release of the fascial sheath around the compartment) alone is insufficient because the sheath reforms. It is necessary to perform a fasciectomy (removal of the fascial sheath) in addition to the fasciotomy.

The anterior compartment contains the tibialis anterior, extensor digitorum longus, extensor hallucis longus, and peroneus tertius muscles. Pain during exertion is felt lateral to the anterior border of the shin. There may be reduced sensation in the first web space. Examination is normal, or there may be palpable generalized tightness of the anterior compartment with focal regions of excessive muscle thickening. It is also important to assess the plantar flexors, especially soleus and gastrocnemius. If these antagonists are tight, they may predispose to anterior compartment syndrome. Isotopic bone scan is usually negative in this condition. Diagnosis is confirmed with compartment pressure testing. Treatment is based on the same principles as for the deep posterior compartment. Surgery may be required after failure of conservative treatment, especially if sensory symptoms persist.

Pain in the Region of the Achilles Tendon

Pain in the region of the Achilles tendon is a frequent presenting symptom, especially among distance runners. Injury to the Achilles tendon itself is the most common cause of injury in this region, but other structures in the area can also be the source of pain. The retrocalcaneal bursa, which lies between the posterior aspect of the calcaneus and the insertion of the Achilles tendon, and the Achilles bursa, which lies between the insertion of the Achilles tendon and the skin, are two bursae that, when inflamed, may produce symptoms either in isolation or in conjunction with Achilles tendon injuries.

The Achilles tendon is the combined tendon of the gastrocnemius and soleus muscles. The tiny plantar muscle also inserts into the Achilles tendon. The tendon is surrounded by a paratendon (peritendon, not a synovial sheath), a thin layer of collagen that is continuous with the fascia of the muscle and the periosteum of the calcaneus. The tendon has a relatively poor blood supply, but its low metabolic rate enables it to carry heavy loads under tension for long periods of time without ischemic damage. The relative avascularity and low metabolic rate may explain why the tendon is slow to heal when injured.

Injury to the Achilles tendon occurs when a load applied to the tendon, either in a single episode or, more often, over a period of time, exceeds the ability of the tendon to withstand it. Factors that may predispose to Achilles tendon injury are increase in activity (mileage, speed, gradient), decrease in recovery time between training sessions, change of surface, change of footwear (e.g., lower heeled spike, shoe with heel tab), poor footwear (e.g., inadequate heel counter, increased lateral flaring, decreased forefoot flexibility), excessive pronation (increased load on gastrocnemius/soleus complex to resupinate the foot for toe-off), poor muscle flexibility (e.g., tight gastrocnemius), and decreased joint range of motion (restricted dorsiflexion).

Achilles tendinitis is associated with the development of local edema and a disruption of the ground substance with minimal disruption to the tendon fibers. This may eventually progress to separation of the tendon fibers and later to focal degeneration and granulation. Achilles tendinitis is classified into grades I, II, III, or IV. The classification is shown in Table 15–3 with appropriate guidelines for activity.

Achilles tendinitis is a condition that responds well if appropriate treatment is instituted at an early stage. If the athlete disregards symptoms and continues training, severe tendon pathology may develop. In that case, treatment and rehabilitation can take up to 6 months or even require surgery. The first aim of treatment is to reduce the local pain and inflammation. This is achieved with NSAIDs, ice, and electrotherapeutic modalities

TABLE 15–3. CLINICAL GRADING OF ACHILLES TENDINITIS AND GUIDELINES FOR ACTIVITY	
Relationship of Symptoms to Activity	**Guidelines for Activity**
I Pain after running only	Continue activity during treatment; ice after activity
II Pain before and after running; pain gradually lessens during a run	Receive treatment; modify activity (e.g. decreased mileage, no hills, decreased speed)
III Pain with activity causing decrease in volume	Receive treatment; rest from aggravating activity; cross-training
IV Pain during everyday activities (pain worsening or progressing)	Rest for longer period; longer rehabilitation program (minimum 3 months); surgery may be required if no improvement with rehabilitation.

(e.g., high voltage galvanic stimulation [HVGS], magnetic field therapy). A heel raise should be used (in both shoes) to reduce the load on the tendon. The next step is to restore full extensibility of the tendon. This step is especially important in chronic Achilles tendinitis, in which postinflammatory adhesions have formed between the tendon and the paratendon. It is important to apply ice to the site of the lesion in a position of pain-free stretch for 10 minutes after treatment. Self-stretching programs are also important.

Initially, it is important to rest from aggravating activities until pain and inflammation settle. A strengthening program may be commenced when the following criteria are met: full pain-free stretch, no morning pain or stiffness, no pain on walking, and no pain with calf raise. The treatment program then aims to increase the strength of the tendon to enable it to tolerate the required load without injury. Eccentric exercises form the basis of the strengthening program for the Achilles tendona and should be used with the supervision of experienced physical therapists. Eccentric loading of the musculotendinous unit promotes collagen formation throughout the tendon, thereby increasing the elastic and tensile properties of the tendon. Eccentric exercises have the potential to cause damage if performed inappropriately or excessively. The exercises should be preceded by an adequate warm-up and stretch, commenced at a low level and progressed gradually. The patient should progress to the next exercise only when the previous activity is pain-free during and after the activity. Initially, eccentric exercises probably should not be performed on consecutive days. During the rehabilitation program, it may be appropriate to alternate days of activity (e.g., bike, jog) with days of eccentric strengthening.

With intense treatment and rest from aggravating activity, Achilles tendinitis may respond relatively quickly (e.g., 4 to 8 weeks), especially if the symptoms have not been present for more than 1 or 2 months. Long-standing Achilles tendinitis may require an intense rehabilitation program of up to 6 months.

As with any overuse injury, secondary prevention is an important component of the treatment. The factors predisposing to the Achilles tendon injury must be identified and corrected. Generalized tightness of the calf muscles predisposes athletes to the development of Achilles tendon injuries and needs to be corrected with a structured stretching program. Reduced range of motion in the ankle or subtalar joints also places increased load on the Achilles tendon. Mobilization of these joints may be necessary.

Abnormal foot biomechanics, such as excessive pronation, is a common predisposing factor to Achilles tendon injuries. A biomechanical assessment is an essential part of the examination, and treatment with orthotics may be indicated. Attention should also be paid to the athlete's shoes. Inadequate rear-foot support and control may be a predisposing factor. This factor may be due to the design of the shoe or its age. The shoe should be assessed and recommendations regarding appropriate footwear given.

Activity may be resumed gradually when local tenderness has settled. On return to activity, a heel raise should be used to reduce the load on the Achilles tendon (both shoes). Jogging should be commenced and gradually increased, provided that there is no pain during or after exercise. When the patient is able to jog comfortably for 45 minutes, speed can be gradually increased. Later, sprint work and hill running may be slowly introduced. The athlete should be particularly wary of doing track work in spikes with low heels.

Occasionally, conservative management of Achilles injury, such as Achilles tendinitis or partial tears of the Achilles tendon, may fail. This failure is more common in patients with long-standing symptoms, those who persist in full training despite their injury, and those with predisposing factors that have not been corrected. In these cases, surgery may be indicated. The rehabilitation program, particularly for severe Achilles tendon injuries, is a slow, lengthy program. Surgery is indicated only when there is failure to progress in the rehabilitation program. Surgery should not be considered unless appropriate conservative management of at least 3 months has failed to improve the condition.

Surgery of the patient with chronic Achilles tendon injury involves incision of the paratendon and release of adhesions, removal of any areas of degenerative tissue, and repair of any partial tears. Surgery needs to be followed by an intense rehabilitation program, involving eccentric strengthening, for at least 3 months before return to sport.

CONCLUSION

Overuse injuries occur in "weekend warriors" and poorly conditioned individuals trying to do too much, too soon. The same principles apply as those used in the highly tuned competitive athlete. Algorithm D gives a general overview of the acute noninflammatory problems that affect these individuals.

BIBLIOGRAPHY

Brukner P, Khan K: Clinical Sports Medicine. New York, McGraw-Hill, 1993.

Harries M, Williams C, Stanish WD, Micheli LJ, eds: Oxford Textbook of Sports Medicine. Oxford, Oxford University Press, 1995.

Hawkins RJ, Misamore GW, eds: Shoulder Injuries in the Athlete. New York, Churchill Livingstone, 1996.

Reid DC: Sports Injury Assessment and Rehabilitation. New York, Churchill Livingstone, 1992.

Renstrom PAFH, ed: Sports Injuries: Basic Principles of Prevention and Care. Oxford, Blackwell Scientific Publications, 1993.

Renstrom PAFH, ed: Clinical Practice of Sports Injury Prevention and Care. Oxford, Blackwell Scientific Publications, 1994.

Appendix

Algorithm D: Acute Noninflammatory Articular Conditions

If the articular condition is acute and noninflammatory, the provider should determine whether fracture is present or further investigation is needed.

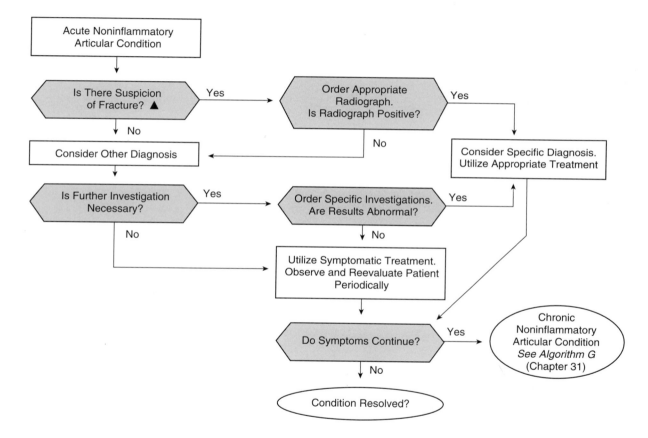

Acute Noninflammatory
Articular Condition

Is There Suspicion
of Fracture? ▲ → Yes → Order Appropriate
Radiograph.
Is Radiograph Positive? → Yes

No

Consider Other Diagnosis ← No

Consider Specific Diagnosis.
Utilize Appropriate Treatment

Is Further Investigation
Necessary? → Yes → Order Specific Investigations.
Are Results Abnormal? → Yes

No

No

Utilize Symptomatic Treatment.
Observe and Reevaluate Patient
Periodically

Do Symptoms Continue? → Yes → Chronic
Noninflammatory
Articular Condition
See Algorithm G
(Chapter 31)

No

Condition Resolved?

From Lipsky PE: Algorithms for the diagnosis and management of musculoskeletal complaints. Am J Med 103(6A):55S, 1997.

Chapter **16**

Trauma—Management by the Primary Care Physician and the Orthopaedic Surgeon

Marc A. Samson ▪ Michael F. Dillingham ▪ Gary S. Fanton

It is estimated that one third of all visits to primary care physicians and up to 50% of emergency department visits are a result of acute or chronic musculoskeletal injuries. As the role of primary care physicians continues to grow in the current health care system, so does the amount of musculoskeletal pathology in their practices. This chapter guides the primary care physician as to how to diagnose and manage acutely these conditions and when an appropriate referral is indicated.

MUSCULOSKELETAL INJURIES

Evaluation of musculoskeletal injuries should include examination of joint stability, deformity, and function. The most accurate examination is usually obtained as soon as possible after the acute injury. Over time, muscle spasm, joint effusion, and discomfort increase, which makes ligamentous laxity more difficult to detect and dislocations more difficult to reduce. Therefore, it becomes imperative that the physician treating these injuries provides an expedient and accurate assessment followed by quick and appropriate treatment.

An injury to a ligament is commonly called a *sprain,* whereas an injury to the musculotendinous unit is termed a *strain.* Sprains are generally classified as mild, moderate, or severe depending on the degree of the disruption of the ligament's fibers. The greater the degree of disruption of the fibers, the greater the likelihood of joint instability and the greater the severity of injury. A simple grading system from I to III is used to signify the degree of instability and ligament injury (Table 16–1, Fig. 16–1). Strains are generally classified as acute or chronic, again with a grading system from I to III to describe the severity of the injury (see Table 16–1).

The primary care physician must consider all medical possibilities when diagnosing a musculoskeletal injury. In addition, medical illnesses, such as rheumatologic conditions, may masquerade as athletic injuries. For example, the first manifestation of rheumatoid arthritis

may follow a knee or ankle injury. Furthermore, some patients may attribute the early stages of pseudogout or gout to a strained knee or ankle.

Before examining the patient with an acute musculoskeletal injury, the physician should elicit a detailed history. The patient should be questioned specifically whether there is a prior history of injury, about the mechanism of injury, whether a pop or snap was heard or felt, and whether there was an immediate or delayed onset of pain and swelling. If the injury is to the lower extremity, the relationship to weight bearing should be determined. If the injury is to the upper extremity, it is helpful to know if the injured limb is the dominant one. The responses to these questions help the examiner form a working differential diagnosis and direct the physical examination. Table 16–2 outlines many common musculoskeletal injuries.

Radiographs can be useful when evaluating musculoskeletal injuries. A few general principles should be considered. At least two views (anteroposterior and lateral) should always be obtained because injuries are not always apparent on a single view. In some instances, it is helpful to obtain comparison views of the contralateral extremity. This is especially true for children who have areas of radiolucency in the epiphysis, which are frequently difficult to differentiate from acute injuries.

Shoulder Injuries

As this chapter discusses traumatic injuries, a more expansive review of the shoulder is in Chapter 15. Examination of the acute shoulder injury should include evaluation of the bony structures, musculotendinous units, and neurovascular structures. The purpose of the examination is to evaluate for deformity, limitation of function, and instability.

One of the most common injuries to the shoulder is the acromioclavicular joint sprain. It usually follows a blow to or fall on to the shoulder, which forcibly separates the acromion from the clavicle. The patient usually complains of well-localized and severe pain over the

Table 16–1. CLASSIFICATION AND TREATMENT OF SPRAINS AND STRAINS

Grade	Classification	Description	Treatment
Sprain (Injury to Ligament)			
I	Mild	Minimal disruption of fibers, minimal or no instability	Symptomatic
II	Moderate	Mild-to-moderate instability	Symptomatic, consider protection with brace
III	Severe	Complete disruption of fibers, gross instability	Symptomatic, consider surgery
Strain (Injury to Musculotendinous Unit)			
I	Mild	No gross disruption of fibers	Symptomatic
II	Moderate	Partial disruption of fibers	Symptomatic, consider protection with brace/splint or surgery for tendon tear
III	Severe	Complete disruption of fibers	Symptomatic, consider surgery for tendon tear

From Callahan LR, Dillingham MF: Common sports injuries. In Noble J, Green H, eds: Textbook of Primary Care Medicine, 2nd ed. St Louis, Mosby-Year Book, 1996.

acromioclavicular joint and has difficulty with abduction or cross-body motion. The findings on examination and treatment differ with the degree of sprain. In general, grade I (nondisplaced, incomplete) and II (minimally displaced) sprains reveal little deformity and are managed easily with nonsteroidal anti-inflammatory drugs (NSAIDs) and a compression sling for comfort. Patients with grade III, IV, V, or VI sprains (complete displacement) should be referred to an orthopaedist for possible surgical management.

A fracture of the clavicle results from a direct blow to the bone or a fall on the ipsilateral shoulder. Standard radiographs usually confirm this diagnosis. Unless complicated, this fracture can usually be managed with a sling or figure-of-eight bandage and pain management. If the injury involves the acromioclavicular joint, if the clavicle tents the overlying skin, or if any neurovascular injury is suspected, a prompt referral is advised.

A rotator cuff tendon tear may result from a fall, or it may occur from minimal trauma. The patient frequently complains of pain and weakness of the shoulder and occasional inability to raise the arm. Examination usually reveals weakness of the rotator cuff muscles and pain with abduction or forward flexion beyond the scapular plane. This injury usually requires a referral to the orthopaedist.

Dislocation of the glenohumeral joint is another commonly encountered injury. This injury is usually traumatic in nature and can occur anteriorly, inferiorly, or posteriorly. The anterior dislocation is the most common. The patient presents with severe pain, inability to move the arm, and deformity of the shoulder girdle. Before attempting a closed reduction, evaluation of the axillary nerve, which innervates the deltoid muscle as well as the skin lateral to the shoulder, should be performed. A popular method for reduction is the traction and countertraction maneuver. In this technique, the physician applies steady constant traction to the affected arm in approximately 30 degrees of abduction, while pressuring the humeral head into the joint by gentle rotation. The assistant anchors the patient's trunk with a sheet around the chest providing countertraction. Once relocated, postreduction anteroposterior, lateral, and axillary x-ray views should be obtained to confirm reduction and rule out associated fractures. Initial treatment should consist of a sling or shoulder immobilizer, ice, and adequate pain management.

Wrist and Hand Injuries

A fracture of the scaphoid bone is frequently seen after a fall on an outstretched hand. The examiner should suspect this type of fracture in any patient with tenderness in the anatomic snuffbox. Initial radiographs may be negative. It is wise for the treating physician to have a high index of suspicion, place the patient in a thumb spica splint, and refer the case to an orthopaedist.

Gamekeeper or skier's thumb is an acute sprain of the ulnocollateral ligament of the thumb. This injury typically occurs when the thumb is forcibly abducted. On initial examination, the ulnar aspect of the metacarpophalangeal joint may appear swollen, and there may be localized tenderness over the ulnocollateral ligament. In cases in which there is no radiographic evidence of fracture, the examiner may assess stability by stressing the ulnocollateral ligament and comparing laxity to the contralateral thumb. If the sprain is stable, treatment is a special thumb cast or splint and NSAIDs. If a complete tear is suspected, referral to an orthopaedist is advised.

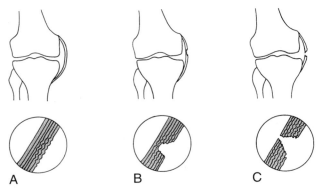

Figure 16–1. Ligamentous sprains vary in severity. A, First degree. B, Second degree. C, Third-degree sprain, which indicates complete rupture. (From Callahan LR, Dillingham MF: Common sports injuries. In Noble J, Green H, eds: Textbook of Primary Care Medicine, 2nd ed. St Louis, Mosby-Year Book, 1996, p 1206.)

Table 16–2. MUSCULOSKELETAL INJURIES

Region and Injury	History/Symptoms	Physical Examination	Tests/Treatment
Shoulder			
Acromioclavicular separation	Acute injury: pain and possible deformity over top of shoulder at acromioclavicular joint	Localized tenderness, possible deformity, distal clavicle displacement	X-ray: Grade II: symptomatic treatment; grade III or greater: orthopaedic consultation
Rotator cuff tear	Fall on outstretched arm or acute overload of cuff; pain over lateral shoulder, occasional difficulty in arm abduction	Pain or weakness on external rotation and abduction	X-ray to rule out fracture; MRI if complete surgical repair required
Instability, anterior or posterior/subluxation	Pain with overhand maneuver, possible *dead arm* when throwing, occasional sense of instability	Possibly consistent with cuff irritation or weakness; positive apprehension sign, either anterior or posterior; findings of joint laxity	Orthopaedic consultation to determine further treatment, including possible rehabilitation and surgical treatment
Elbow and wrist			
Medial ligament sprain	Pain during play	Tenderness over the ligament and with valgus stress; possible clinical instability	Stress X-rays, MRI. Grade I or II: rehabilitation and rest; grade III (complete or near-complete tear): orthopaedic consultation and surgery
Navicular fracture	Fall on outstretched hand	Tenderness in anatomic snuffbox	X-ray: Consider immobilization; if fracture present or symptoms present, orthopaedic referral
Lumbar spine			
Spondylolysis	Low back pain and stiffness; occasional buttock, leg, or thigh pain; occasionally associated with radiculopathy	Tenderness to palpation; occasional muscle spasm; pain with rotation and extension; increased lordosis	X-rays; if results equivocal, bone scan and/or MRI. If positive, orthopaedic consultation
Discogenic pain (annular tear, disc protrusion)	Any of the following: low back pain, buttock pain, thigh, or leg pain, possible radicular pain	Midline tenderness to palpation; possible increased pain with forward flexion; possible positive straight leg raise	X-rays. Rest, ice, NSAIDs; if symptoms are severe or persistent, orthopaedic or physiatry referral
Knee			
Injury to ligament			
Anterior cruciate ligament	A sense of giving way, often associated with pop, subsequent swelling, and pain	Effusion, positive Lachman's test, positive anterior drawer test; frequent joint line pain	Possible MRI. Non–weight bearing and immobilization briefly for symptoms; acute arthroscopic surgery
Posterior cruciate ligament	Generally a fall on the proximal tibia; acute or subacute onset; posterior (popliteal space) knee pain	Positive posterior drawer test (may evolve over hours or days); possible effusion, possible popliteal area pain	Initial treatment is symptomatic; orthopaedic consultation, generally nonsurgical
Medial and lateral collateral ligaments	Occasional sense of tearing with a sense of acute tibial displacement and subsequent pain	Local tenderness, instability on stress testing, frequent hamstring guarding	Possible MRI. Immobilization or crutches for comfort; grade I: symptomatic treatment; grade II or III: orthopaedic consult
Injury to cartilage			
Meniscal tear (medial or lateral)	Usually joint line pain, occasionally clicking, popping, or locking	Joint line tenderness, possible effusion, possible positive McMurray test	MRI. Symptomatic treatment; possible orthopaedic consultation for arthroscopy
Foot/ankle			
Ankle sprain (medial-syndesmotic)	Ankle inverted, everted or forcibly plantar flexed	Swelling and pain to palpation over involved ligaments	X-ray to rule out fracture. Ice, crutches, compression, possible acute immobilization; if severe, orthopaedic consultation

MRI, magnetic resonance imaging; NSAIDs, nonsteroidal anti-inflammatory drugs.

Knee Injuries

The knee is the most frequently injured joint with which the primary care physician may be confronted. As with the shoulder, the knee should be evaluated for deformity, limitation of function, loss of motion, stability, and localization of tenderness. Assessment should also be made for joint effusion.

The anterior cruciate ligament (ACL) is one of the most commonly injured structures of the knee. Injury to this ligament frequently occurs in sports requiring jumping, quick directional change (cutting), or rapid deceleration. The patient usually complains of a pop and may feel as if the knee is going to give way. If the examiner evaluates the knee before swelling has occurred, the examination is usually more diagnostic. Findings indicative of an ACL injury include a positive Lachman's test, anterior drawer test, and pivot shift test (Box 16–1). Once swelling has occurred, the examination is less reliable. It is important to have the patient as com-

Box 16–1. USEFUL TESTS FOR INJURIES TO THE KNEE

Drawer Sign

The patient lies supine on the examination table with the knee flexed at 90 degrees, with the foot resting flat on the table with muscles relaxed. The examiner then grasps the proximal portion of the tibia and pulls forward. The examiner may choose to sit on the patient's foot to anchor it. Forward motion exceeding 1 cm is thought to reflect a positive test, indicating anterior instability of the knee and a torn cruciate ligament.

Lachman Test

The patient lies supine on the examination table with legs outstretched. The examiner places one hand on the anterior distal femur and the other on the posterior proximal tibia. The examiner lifts up on the tibia while applying counterforce to the femur. Forward motion on the tibia exceeding 1 cm is a positive test indicating anterior knee instability and a torn cruciate ligament.

Pivot Shift Test

The patient lies supine with the knee held in flexion. One of the examiner's hands is placed at the knee with the thumb over the lateral joint line. The other hand is placed under the heel. The knee is then extended by the examiner while applying mild valgus and internal rotation stress to the knee. If the lateral joint line demonstrates excessive motion, the test is positive for cruciate instability.

---

fortable as possible while examining the injury; a pillow placed under the knee to encourage muscular relaxation is often helpful. Joint aspiration of a tense effusion is sometimes helpful, and evidence of a hemarthrosis is highly suggestive of an ACL tear. Radiographs are necessary to rule out associated fractures. If an ACL injury is suspected, NSAIDs, ice, immobilization, compressive dressing, and an acute referral to an orthopaedist for diagnostic testing (magnetic resonance imaging) and possible ligament reconstruction are recommended.

Meniscal injury may accompany a tear of the ACL or may occur as an isolated injury. This frequently results from a twisting injury. The finding of joint line tenderness in the patient complaining of knee pain, especially if associated with a pop or click, supports this diagnosis. Radiographs are generally not helpful. Arthroscopic surgery and possible repair are indicated for many patients with meniscal tears. Meniscal repair may reduce the future possibility of clinical osteoarthritis.

Injuries to the medial and lateral collateral ligaments are also frequent knee injuries. The medial collateral ligament is injured by lateral (valgus) force to the knee, especially with the affected foot planted. The athlete complains of pain and swelling medially, and the ligament is tender to the palpation at the site of injury. Applying valgus stress to the knee in 30 degrees of flexion confirms laxity. Radiographs may demonstrate an associated avulsion fracture. If the tear is grade I or grade II (see Table 16–1 and Fig. 16–1), immobilization in flexion with early protected mobilization, ice, and NSAIDs is indicated. A grade III sprain may or may not require surgical repair; therefore referral to an orthopaedist is advisable.

Foot and Ankle Injuries

One of the most common athletic injuries is the ankle sprain; however, several other injuries might mimic this condition. A true sprain is a stretching or tearing of the ligaments. The most common type of ankle sprain is an inversion sprain, in which the plantar surface of the foot rolls in. This results in damage to the lateral ligament complex, especially the anterior talofibular ligament. The patient complains of pain over the lateral ankle, and swelling usually develops quickly in the area anterior to the lateral malleolus. If there is difficulty with weight bearing or bony tenderness, a radiograph should be obtained to rule out a fracture. On examination, the most important finding is point tenderness over the injured ligament. Testing for stability usually is not critical to acute diagnosis. Initial treatment should consist of elevation, ice, and compression. If the sprain is determined to be mild, this treatment followed by appropriate rehabilitation should suffice.

Less commonly, sprains to the deltoid ligament (medial) and tibiofibular ligament (syndesmosis) occur. The mechanism is an eversion injury as opposed to the more common inversion injury. Both are significant injuries and often require immobilization, prolonged treatment, and occasionally surgery. Any complex sprain, which does not respond quickly to treatment, should be referred to an orthopaedist.

Some ankle injuries initially diagnosed as simple sprains represent other pathology. Two injuries the physician needs to be aware of are those affecting the Achilles tendon and the peroneal tendons; (see also Chapter 15). The patient with an acute Achilles tendon tear frequently hears a pop and has pain but is able to continue walking. Attempts to stand on the toes are unsuccessful. A Thompson test confirms the diagnosis. To perform this maneuver, the patient either kneels on a chair with the calf pointing up or lies prone on the examination table. The examiner then gently squeezes the calf muscle. If the tendon is intact, the foot passively plantar flexes. Lack of this passive flexion signals a positive Thompson test and thus a rupture of the Achilles tendon.

A second injury that masquerades as an ankle sprain is the subluxation of the peroneal tendons. This injury occurs when the foot is fixed and the leg is forcibly rotated. The peroneal tendon tears free of its anchoring retinaculum and subluxates anteriorly, over the lateral malleolus. If the examiner holds the foot in neutral position and asks the patient to resist eversion, the tendon may subluxate anteriorly. If the diagnosis is made promptly, successful treatment with several weeks of casting may suffice. If the diagnosis is delayed or the disorder recurs, surgery may be required.

In general, acute injuries to the foot are much less common than overuse injuries. Two injuries that deserve mention are the hyperextension injury of the metatarsophalangeal joint of the great toe (turf toe) and the Lysfranc sprain. In the former, the patient complains of pain in the first metatarsophalangeal joint, with tenderness and swelling of the joint. Treatment is symptomatic with NSAIDs and rest. The Lysfranc sprain represents a midfoot sprain of the tarsal metatarsal joint. This sprain may require prolonged metatarsal immobilization, rest, and possibly surgery. Comparison standing anteroposterior radiographs may be diagnostic. Foot and ankle fractures are relatively uncommon in primary care practice, but when they do occur, they frequently need surgery. Acute management of foot and ankle fractures should include immobilization, elevation, ice, and prompt orthopaedic evaluation.

Spine Injuries

Athletic injuries of the spine fall into two major groups: the neck and lower back. Neck or cervical spine injuries are potentially the most serious and life-threatening of the musculoskeletal injuries. Any severe neck injury should be treated as a medical emergency, with the suspension of the athletic event if necessary until the neck can be protected and the patient transported safely.

Most injuries to the cervical spine result in transient neuropraxia. The athlete may complain of altered sensation and motor function in the upper extremity and occasionally the lower extremity. The paresthesia resolves spontaneously usually within minutes. Also common is the burner or stinger syndrome. This represents a stretching injury of the brachial plexus of compression of the nerve root at the foramen. The athlete complains of burning pain radiating down the shoulder, upper arm, and hand associated with weakness of muscles, such as the deltoid and the biceps. Symptoms generally resolve spontaneously over minutes or hours. Return to athletic action is not allowed until normal strength and sensation have returned.

The lumbar spine is frequently a site of pain and injury for athletes and nonathletes alike. Although muscle strains do occur, it is important to look for other common causes of lumbar pain. Disc herniation and annular tears are frequent causes of pain. They are frequently associated with radiculopathy. There may be pain on flexion or tenderness with midline palpation of the spine at the involved level.

Patients with spondylolysis, or a stress fracture of the pars interarticularis, may have acute low back pain. This injury is most common in teenage athletes involved in gymnastics, football (especially linemen), or weight lifting. It is also commonly associated with diminished range of motion of the lumbar spine and tight hamstrings. Physical findings may include pain on spinal extension while standing on the single leg on the side of the defect (positive one-legged hyperextension test), on rotation, and during palpation over the irritated area. Radiographs confirm a defect of the pars interarticu-laris seen on the oblique lumbar view (fracture of neck of the Scotty dog). Rest (i.e., cessation of the aggravating sport) is the treatment of choice, and occasionally immobilization is required. If the defect has progressed to become a spondylolisthesis, or translation of the vertebral body, consultation with a spine specialist is advised.

REHABILITATION

Once an injury has occurred and the initial treatment plan has been instituted, the physician should think ahead to the need for rehabilitation. The primary goal of rehabilitation should be to return the patient to activity as soon and as safely as possible.

In the initial 24 to 48 hours after a musculoskeletal injury, acute treatment may be carried out according to the mnemonic PRICE: Protection from further injury is accomplished by cessation of activity and using a splint for immobilization. Rest prevents further injury and allows the injury to begin healing. Ice is a potent anti-inflammatory by decreasing swelling, pain, and muscle spasm. Ice should be applied for periods of less than 15 minutes with an equal period without ice. Compression, usually in the form of an elastic bandage, limits swelling and may provide some support to the injured tissue. Elevation helps to decrease swelling.

After definitive diagnosis and acute therapy, the actual rehabilitation process begins. Rehabilitation should be sport, athlete, and injury specific; a program should be individually designed for each patient depending on the sport in which he or she participates. Therefore, attention needs to be paid to general conditioning as well as local rehabilitation of the injured limb. Flexibility, strength, proprioception, and endurance must be addressed. Modalities that may be employed include ice and heat, ultrasound, electrical stimulation, and iontophoresis.

CHILDREN

The child's skeletal immaturity predisposes to injuries not encountered in the older athlete (see Chapter 13). The epiphyseal plate, the cartilaginous growth center of the bone, is the weakest portion of a growing bone and is commonly injured. Such injuries are common and can affect growth and alignment of the limb, so careful evaluation is required. Physical examination should always include palpation of the epiphysis. Tenderness of the physis is diagnostic for physeal injury. Depending on the type and extent of epiphyseal injury, treatment ranges from closed reduction to open reduction and internal fixation.

OLDER PATIENTS

Patients older than 65 years old have the same injury profile as younger patients except in three areas. First, active weight-bearing exercise such as jogging is associated with better bone density in the general skeleton in younger patients. This, in turn, offers some protection against compression fractures of the vertebral spine and hip, especially when compared to the risk of fracture encountered by sedentary age-matched groups.

Second, a warm-up period is mandatory for older patients to minimize tendon injuries. The combination of tendinopathies and degenerative processes predisposes older patients to muscle and tendon injuries when compared to younger ones. A complete warm-up is essential to facilitate injury prevention.

Third, exercise can aggravate existing osteoarthritis of the knee, hip, and lower spine. However, exercise, weight control, and increased muscle strength, which ultimately serve to protect the joints, usually offset such aggravation.

CONCLUSION

As primary care musculoskeletal medicine continues to expand, the primary care physician is confronted with increasing numbers of musculoskeletal injuries. Early diagnosis and prompt treatment minimize patient discomfort and morbidity.

BIBLIOGRAPHY

Apple DF, Hayes WC: Prevention of Falls and Hip Fractures in the Elderly. Rosemont, IL, AAOS, 1993.
Callahan LR, Dillingham MF: Common sports injuries. In Noble J, Green H, eds: Textbook of Primary Care Medicine, 2nd ed. St. Louis, Mosby-Year Book, 1996.
Grana WA, Kalenak A, eds: Clinical Sports Medicine. Philadelphia, WB Saunders, 1991.
Greenspan A: Orthopedic Radiology: A Practical Approach, 2nd ed. New York, Raven Press, 1992.
Hoppenfeld S: Physical Examination of the Spine and Extremities. East Norwalk, CT, Appleton-Century-Crofts, 1976.
Snider R: Essentials of Musculoskeletal Care. Rosemont, IL, AAOS, 1997.
Strauss RH, ed: Sports Medicine, 2nd ed. Philadelphia, WB Saunders, 1991.
Thabit G III, Micheli L: Orthopedic disorders of the extremities. In Burg FD, Ingelfinger JR, Wald ER, eds: Current Pediatric Therapy. Philadelphia, WB Saunders, 1993.

Chapter **17**

The Skin and Musculoskeletal Diseases

Elizabeth C. W. Hughes ■ Susan M. Swetter

CUTANEOUS CLUES TO RHEUMATOLOGIC DISEASE

In evaluating a patient with rheumatologic disease, there are many subtle, nonspecific skin findings that may help to determine the cause of musculoskeletal disease. Cutaneous findings may also help to predict the course of preexisting disease. A fundamental understanding of the approach to evaluating the skin is essential for recognition of rheumatologic disorders.

Nails and Periungual Skin

The nails and periungual skin may provide useful clues to underlying musculoskeletal disease. The feet should also be examined because skin findings are not restricted to the hands. In fact, manicuring frequently alters the appearance of the hands and fingernails, obscuring or confounding cutaneous manifestations of systemic disease.

The classic finding of the nail unit in scleroderma, dermatomyositis, or systemic lupus erythematosus (SLE) is prominent periungual capillary loops or telangiectasias on the proximal nail fold (Fig. 17–1). Careful examination reveals that there is actually dropout of some capillaries with concomitant dilation of the remaining small vessels.[1] These can be seen most easily with the +40 lens of an ophthalmoscope if a dissecting microscope is not available. Dilated capillary loops can be found in patients with all forms of autoimmune rheumatic disease. Dilated periungual capillary loops in a patient with discoid lupus erythematosus (LE) may signal progression to systemic disease.[2] Hemorrhages of the nail bed may also be seen, but the differential diagnosis in this situation also includes endocarditis and trauma.

More common but less specific are periungual edema and erythema as well as hypertrophy of the cuticles. Periungual erythema, often with scaling, may accompany the rash of acute LE or dermatomyositis (Fig. 17–2).[3] These periungual changes, however, are most commonly caused by irritant hand dermatitis and chronic paronychia. Patients with autoimmune disease are at risk of other dermatoses secondary to skin break-

down; if the nail changes do not resolve with treatment of the systemic disease, a secondary dermatosis should be considered.

Nails can be sensitive barometers of systemic illness, but their slow growth (average of 1 mm of growth per month) means that abnormalities of the nail plate may not be apparent for some time after an acute inflammatory insult. Beau's lines are white horizontal grooves in the nail plate that represent temporary disruptions in nail growth during acute illness or metabolic stress (Fig. 17–3).[4] These lines usually curve in the same direction as the lunula and are usually present on all fingernails and toenails. If the illness is prolonged or severe enough, there may be a complete horizontal break in the nail plate. New nail growth occurs if the underlying illness is controlled. The nail changes in psoriasis are different and are discussed later.

Patients with recurrent Raynaud's phenomenon or vascular compromise may have pits in the tips of the fingers or toes and may even have partial loss of the tip of the digit as a result of underlying ischemia.[5] The nails often show an exaggerated longitudinal curvature and may overhang the tip of the finger. Frank ulceration of the fingertip is not necessary to produce this change. In the setting of severe ischemia, there may be complete loss of the distal digit, including the nail. Patients with systemic sclerosis and CREST syndrome (calcinosis cutis, Raynaud's phenomenon, esophageal dysfunction, sclerodactyly, and telangiectasia) are especially prone to this condition.

Photosensitivity

Photosensitivity is the hallmark of several autoimmune rheumatologic diseases. It is important to note the distribution of the lesions when evaluating a patient with a photoexacerbated skin eruption. Common sun-exposed areas are the dorsal hands, extensor forearms and distal upper arms, lateral neck, cheeks, chin, nose, and forehead. The scalp may also be involved, particularly if the patient has any degree of hair loss. Relatively photoprotected areas are the upper lip, submental chin and upper neck, interdigital spaces of the hands, and upper eyelids. If the findings of photosensitivity are asym-

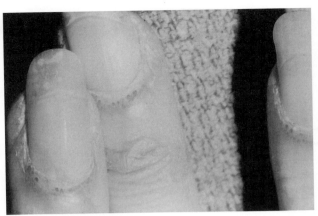

Figure 17–1. Periungual capillary loops. (Courtesy of Stanford University Department of Dermatology.)

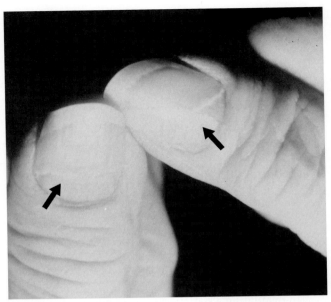

Figure 17–3. Beau's lines (*arrows*). (Courtesy of Stanford University Department of Dermatology.)

metric, the amount of time spent in a car or in a sunny room in a stationary position may be relevant. Window glass does not block all types of ultraviolet radiation, so the patient's main sun exposure may occur while riding in a car or sitting at a desk in front of a window.

Poikiloderma

Poikiloderma describes the combination of atrophy, telangiectasia, and pigmentary alteration, and it most commonly occurs in sites of chronic sun damage, particularly the neck and chest (Civatte's poikiloderma). Dermatomyositis commonly causes exaggerated poikilodermatous changes of sun-exposed areas and can also induce these changes in nonexposed, sun-protected skin.[6]

Malar Rash

The malar rash of acute LE may be simulated by dermatomyositis, in addition to several common conditions, such as rosacea, seborrheic dermatitis, contact dermatitis, polymorphous light eruption, and phototoxic

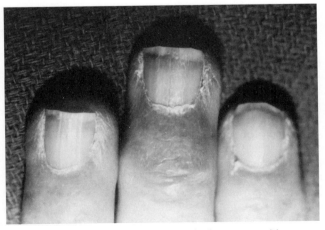

Figure 17–2. Periungual changes in dermatomyositis.

drug eruption. Patients with these other dermatoses often have erythema of the nose and are not limited to the *butterfly* distribution of the classic malar rash. Presence of autoimmune rheumatologic disease does not eliminate the possibility of other causes of malar rash or photosensitivity. A patient with rosacea typically has frequent flushing, in association with extreme temperatures or ingestion of spicy foods or alcohol. The degree of erythema is variable and transient, often resolving in a matter of minutes. The flushing and telangiectasias of rosacea are usually accompanied by erythematous papules or pustules, which are absent in LE. Seborrheic dermatitis typically shows waxy, yellowish scale in addition to erythema, and it involves the eyebrows and alar creases, areas generally spared in LE. Polymorphous light eruption typically begins in the spring or early summer and gradually improves with repeated exposure to sunlight. Patients with polymorphous light eruption may have pronounced local discomfort in sun-exposed skin, but they are rarely systemically ill. Phototoxic drug eruptions and contact dermatitis may appear similar to LE, but careful history of oral and topical medications should differentiate the two conditions.

Alopecia

Nonscarring hair loss may occur in patients with rheumatologic disease, particularly when the disease is flaring or poorly controlled. *Telogen effluvium* is the typical pattern of nonscarring hair loss.[7] The patient generally reports diffuse hair shedding but may appear to have a full head of hair to the examiner. A pull test yields several easily extracted hairs with club-shaped, depigmented bulbs. The shedding begins approximately 2 to 3 months after the acute illness and persists for 1 to 6 months. However, telogen effluvium may become chronic if the rheumatologic disease is not easily controlled. In either case, the patient should be reassured that this hair loss is not permanent and will not result in baldness. Cytotoxic medications used to treat rheumatologic disease may also cause transient, diffuse hair shedding (*anagen effluvium*).

Scarring alopecia occurs in discoid LE and localized morphea. In these cases, areas of partial or complete baldness are observed on the scalp. The follicular markings are lost and replaced by atrophic scar. Scarring alopecia causes permanent hair loss; any treatment is directed toward halting the destructive inflammatory process and not toward restoring lost hair.

Subcutaneous Nodules

Several musculoskeletal diseases are accompanied by subcutaneous nodules. The clinical findings are nearly identical in each case—firm, subcutaneous nodules that are typically the same color as surrounding uninvolved skin but may have a slightly yellow or white hue. The consistency helps differentiate the cause of the nodule. Firm nodules are usually the result of deposition of calcium or crystalline material in the skin. Rheumatoid nodules are soft and compressible; cysts or lipomas are somewhat rubbery. Nodules resulting from deposition of solid material (e.g., monosodium urate crystals or calcium salts) can ulcerate and discharge chalky material (Fig. 17–4). Although these nodules are not painful when the overlying skin is intact, ulceration is usually accompanied by pain.

Vasculitis

Cutaneous vasculitis can be associated with many autoimmune rheumatologic conditions, including lupus erythematosus, rheumatoid arthritis, and dermatomyositis, although primary vasculitides may also have skin and joint manifestations. Vasculitis is classified by the size of vessel involved: small vessel vasculitis refers

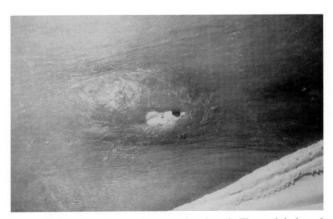

Figure 17–4. Calcinosis cutis in systemic sclerosis. The nodule has ulcerated and is discharging calcium salts. Tophi of gout can also exude white, chalky material. (Courtesy of Stanford University Department of Dermatology.)

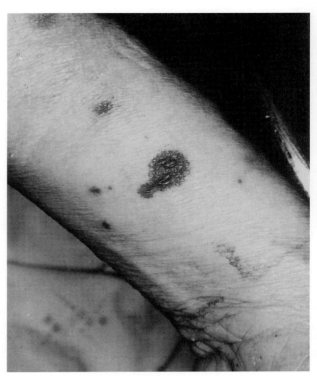

Figure 17–5. Palpable purpura.

to inflammation mainly of dermal vessels (capillaries), medium vessel vasculitis affects vessels in the subcutis (arterioles, venules, and small arteries), and large vessel vasculitis refers to vasculitis of large arteries.[8] Small and medium vessel vasculitis may show cutaneous manifestations; large vessel vasculitis generally spares the skin (see Chapter 27).

The hallmark of cutaneous vasculitis is palpable purpura—nonblanching, deeply erythematous, violaceous, or ecchymotic papules or plaques (Fig. 17–5). Palpable purpura most commonly occurs in the setting of small vessel leukocytoclastic vasculitis. It may be accompanied by nodules, bullae, pustules, or extensive skin necrosis, although these findings are more typical of medium vessel vasculitis.[9, 10] Another manifestation of cutaneous small vessel vasculitis is urticarial vasculitis (Fig. 17–6). This form of vasculitis consists of edematous, erythematous or dusky red-purple, partially blanchable plaques, which simulate urticaria but persist for longer than 24 hours.[11]

The classic example of a small vessel vasculitis is Henoch-Schönlein purpura; other causes include SLE, rheumatoid arthritis, hepatitis B or C infection, medications, human immunodeficiency virus (HIV) infection, and malignancy.[12] Other organs with rich supplies of capillaries, including the kidney, gastrointestinal tract, and joints, may be involved with small vessel vasculitis, but between 40% and 50% of patients have no systemic symptoms. Approximately 50% of patients with small vessel vasculitis have no discernible cause for the condition (*idiopathic leukocytoclastic vasculitis*).

In medium vessel vasculitis, cutaneous findings include a reticulate, nonblanching, dusky red vascular pat-

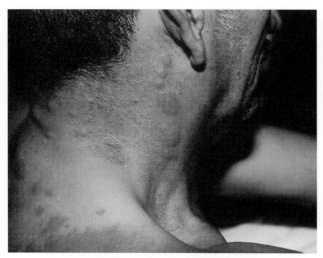

Figure 17–6. Urticarial vasculitis.

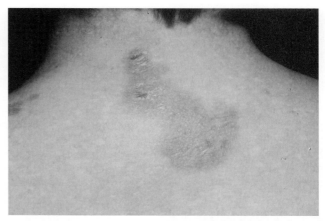

Figure 17–7. Papulosquamous lesion in lupus erythematosus. (Courtesy of Stanford University Department of Dermatology.)

tern of the skin, termed *livedo reticularis*. There may also be palpable or nonpalpable purpura, bullae, necrosis, nodules, and ulceration. Numerous other organ systems may be involved. Polyarteritis nodosa, Wegener's granulomatosis, and allergic granulomatous angiitis (Churg-Strauss) are examples of this condition. Livedo vasculitis is the most common cutaneous manifestation of the antiphospholipid syndrome (see Chapter 14).[13] Several noninflammatory conditions typified by vascular occlusion, such as thrombotic thrombocytopenic purpura, calciphylaxis, and cholesterol emboli, may show cutaneous findings indistinguishable from those of medium vessel vasculitis.

RHEUMATOLOGIC DISEASES WITH PROMINENT CUTANEOUS FINDINGS

Lupus Erythematosus

There are three commonly recognized cutaneous forms of LE: acute, subacute, and chronic. Although the American College of Rheumatology criteria for SLE define only four specific cutaneous and mucosal findings, in practice the cutaneous manifestations of LE are myriad.[7] In addition to the malar, discoid, and photosensitive rashes, patients with lupus may also have papulosquamous, hypertrophic, or bullous lesions or panniculitis. Any of these lesions may occur in a patient with LE, despite the type or degree of disease. Likewise, an individual with lupus may have cutaneous manifestations only and never develop systemic disease, or may develop cutaneous lesions after years of systemic involvement.

The classic malar rash of acute LE consists of edema and erythema of the upper cheeks and bridge of the nose, sometimes accompanied by fine scale. The rash may extend to other parts of the face, such as forehead and chin, although the alar creases and nasal tip are usually spared. The photosensitive rash has a similar appearance of erythema and edema and occurs in photo-

exposed sites, such as the anterior, upper chest (also referred to as the *V of the neck*), the extensor forearms, and the dorsal hands. Ultraviolet B radiation (290 to 320 nm) is primarily responsible for the photosensitivity in systemic lupus.[14]

Subacute cutaneous LE often manifests with papulosquamous lesions, typified by thin erythematous plaques with adherent scale and follicular plugging. They may be mistaken for psoriasis or eczema (Fig. 17–7). The plaques often have curved borders with central clearing, giving an annular or arcuate appearance (Fig. 17–8). The lesions occur on both photoexposed and photoprotected skin but are most common on the trunk. Although the appearance is similar to the early form of discoid lupus,

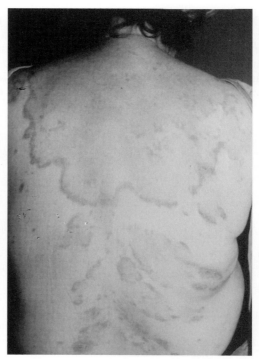

Figure 17–8. Subacute cutaneous lupus. (Courtesy of Stanford University Department of Dermatology.)

these lesions do not lead to scarring, hyperpigmentation, or alopecia. Half of all patients with subacute cutaneous LE eventually meet the criteria for SLE. In this subgroup, arthritis is the most common extracutaneous finding; renal and central nervous system disease occur less often than in patients who present initially with systemic disease. Patients with subacute lupus are often antinuclear antibody (ANA) negative, but most do produce anti-Ro (SS-A) antibodies, with or without producing anti-La (SS-B), although repeated testing may be necessary to detect these antibodies.[16, 17]

Lesions of discoid LE begin as erythematous plaques with adherent scale and follicular plugging, termed *carpet tack* scale. Late lesions are sharply demarcated and have an atrophic, hypopigmented, scarred center with a hypopigmented and hyperpigmented border. Discoid lesions can involve any cutaneous or mucosal surface and have a predilection for the external ear in patients with SLE.[18] If present on the scalp, discoid lupus leads to permanent scarring alopecia.

Chronic discoid lesions typically occur without systemic involvement, although 5% to 10% of patients with SLE present with discoid lesions.[2] Approximately 50% of patients with chronic discoid LE have lesions limited to the head, neck, or both. Spontaneous remission occurs in about half of these patients, although the scarring and alopecia are irreversible.[19] Individuals may also have widespread cutaneous discoid lupus involving the skin above and below the neck; in these cases, spontaneous remission occurs in fewer than 10% of patients. In addition, individuals with disseminated discoid lupus lesions are more likely eventually to develop systemic lupus than are patients who have discoid lesions limited to the head and neck. Squamous cell carcinoma may develop in active discoid lesions that are present for many years. Nonhealing ulcers or changing discoid lesions should be evaluated carefully to exclude carcinoma.

Hypertrophic lupus, which occurs in approximately 2% of patients with cutaneous lupus, has several manifestations.[20] It may appear as thick hyperkeratotic scale overlying erythematous plaques, as individual scaling papules or nodules, or as diffuse hyperkeratosis. The most common sites of hypertrophic lupus are the face, palms, soles, and extensor surface of the upper and lower limbs. If the hyperkeratosis occurs on the hands or feet, it causes keratoderma, which may limit the mobility of digits.

Lupus panniculitis, also called *lupus profundus,* has an incidence similar to that of hypertrophic lupus. It appears as firm, partially mobile, subcutaneous nodules. Typical lesions of discoid lupus may overlie lesions of lupus profundus or may occur elsewhere on the same patient. The nodules heal with atrophy and may ulcerate. Typical locations are the buttocks, thighs, cheeks, and upper arms. The prognosis of patients with lupus profundus is similar to those with chronic discoid lupus.[21]

Tumid lupus, also called *lupus erythematosus tumidus,* is characterized by sharply demarcated, markedly edematous, erythematous to violaceous papules and plaques without follicular plugging or significant scaling.[20] The lesions may present in an annular or polycyclic pattern and occur mainly on the face.

Bullous lesions occur in fewer than 5% of patients with lupus and usually occur in patients with acute SLE or subacute cutaneous lupus.[20] There are two different causes for blistering in lupus lesions. In one form, there is extensive destruction of the basal layer of the epidermis, causing separation of the epidermis from the dermis. Patients with this form of blistering have tense or flaccid bullae on an erythematous base, with occasional central necrosis, giving a clinical appearance similar to erythema multiforme or toxic epidermal necrolysis. Bullae may also be due to the production of specific autoantibodies directed against the basement membrane zone of the skin. Patients with this form of blistering most commonly have tense vesicles or bullae, similar to patients with bullous pemphigoid.

Changes of the oral mucosa may be nonspecific. Erosions and shallow ulcerations usually appear as red patches and often have no necrosis, although deeper ulceration is possible. Typical discoid lesions may also occur on mucous membranes, leaving central atrophy, scarring, and hypopigmentation and hyperpigmentation of the border of the ulcer. Similar lesions can affect the vermilion of the lips.

Vasculitis can occur in patients with lupus erythematosus. The clinical appearance is identical to the other forms of vasculitis previously discussed.

Dermatomyositis

The pathognomonic clinical findings of dermatomyositis are Gottron's papules and the heliotrope rash. Gottron's papules occur in up to 80% of patients with dermatomyositis at some point in the course of their disease.[6] The lesions are erythematous-to-violaceous papules that occur over bony prominences, particularly small joints of the hands (metacarpal, proximal interphalangeal, and distal phalangeal joints) (Fig. 17–9). If these papules become atrophic and telangiectatic, they are referred to as *Gottron's sign.* Gottron's papules can generally be distinguished from the papulosquamous or photoexacerbated rash of SLE, which also occurs on the dorsal hands but predominantly affects the skin between the joints. The heliotrope rash is a lilac-to-violaceous, edematous plaque of the periorbital skin, particularly the upper eyelid.

There are numerous less specific cutaneous manifestations of dermatomyositis, many of which show overlap with LE. Poikiloderma and ill-defined erythematous, nonscaling patches in a photodistributed pattern are frequently seen.[22] There may be similar findings in photoprotected areas. Erythema may also be present in the malar region, in which case there may be strong similarity to acute lupus erythematosus. Proximal nail fold erythema, telangiectasias, or infarcts and cuticular hypertrophy, often in conjunction with Gottron's papules, are common.[5] Diffuse nonscarring alopecia, either with or without poikiloderma or scale of the scalp, may also be present.

Several uncommon cutaneous findings may also be seen in dermatomyositis. Mucin deposition in the dermis is usually detected only histologically; occasion-

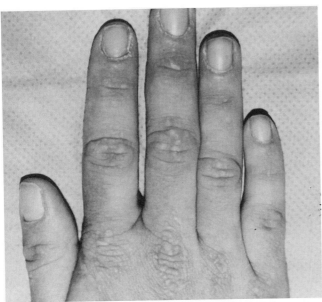

Figure 17–9. Gottron's papules. (Courtesy of Stanford University Department of Dermatology.)

ally, there is clinically apparent infiltration of the skin.[22] Subcutaneous and periarticular calcium deposition occurs particularly in children with dermatomyositis.[23] These deposits occur most commonly around the muscles most affected by the myopathy (the proximal muscle girdles of the shoulder and pelvis) and over bony prominences. Patients with overlap syndromes may have prominent sclerosis, particularly of the digits and distal extremities. Discoid lupus lesions and rheumatoid nodules have also been reported in patients with dermatomyositis.

Disorders Characterized by Cutaneous Sclerosis

The terminology of sclerosing disorders of the skin is somewhat confusing. There are three primary sclerosing disorders which affect the skin: *systemic sclerosis, CREST syndrome,* and *morphea/scleroderma.* Overlap syndromes encompassing features of LE and dermatomyositis also exist. The pathognomonic feature is tight, immobile skin that cannot be lifted away from the underlying subcutaneous fat by gently pinching the skin. The skin is referred to as *bound-down* and lacks normal creases and dermatoglyphics (fingerprints). This change is often most remarkable on the hands and feet, which may have the appearance of being encased in wax.

Systemic sclerosis involves both the skin and the internal organs. The sclerosis of the skin typically begins insidiously as a perceived firmness and eventually progresses to the features described previously. In systemic sclerosis, the induration involves the trunk, particularly the upper thorax, more prominently than in other forms of sclerosis, but distal extremities are usually affected as well.[5] This central sclerosis can limit movement of the neck and rib cage, and perioral involvement gives a pinched appearance to the face. The oral aperture may be decreased, sometimes substantially, even though the patient is frequently unaware of this change. Involvement of the hands leads to sclerodactyly with contractures. Raynaud's phenomenon, digital infarcts, and pitted scars of the fingertips may be present as well as the nail fold and cuticle changes discussed previously.[7]

Patients with systemic sclerosis also may have a variety of nonsclerotic skin changes.[24] Depigmentation is common on the trunk and is characteristically patchy, with normally pigmented or hyperpigmented macules found within patches of depigmentation. Patients may also have diffuse hyperpigmentation alone. Ulceration may occur at sites of minor trauma or overlying joint contractures. These ulcerations are slow to heal, probably because there is relative vascular compromise in areas of sclerosis. As in CREST syndrome, there may be telangiectasias and calcinosis cutis.

The majority of clinical characteristics of CREST syndrome involve the skin. There is a broad overlap with systemic sclerosis because calcinosis cutis, Raynaud's phenomenon, sclerodactyly, and telangiectasias occur in both disease states. The sclerosis in CREST syndrome is much more likely to be limited to the hands and feet than in other forms of systemic sclerosis. Ulceration may occur at sites of trauma or calcinosis, as in systemic sclerosis.

Localized scleroderma defines a heterogeneous group of disorders.[25] The key finding in all types is an indurated plaque of bound-down skin, occasionally with a shiny surface and a violaceous or faintly erythematous border. If the plaque occurs on hair-bearing skin, there is overlying scarring alopecia. There are several patterns of localized scleroderma. The term *morphea* refers to a limited number of round or oval sclerotic plaques that may be distributed on any area of the skin (Fig. 17–10). Patients with numerous, widespread plaques and papules are said to have generalized morphea. The plaque may be linear, which is termed *linear scleroderma.*

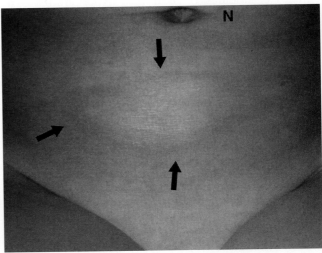

Figure 17–10. Morphea. Small oval patch on the lower abdomen (*arrows*). N, navel. (Courtesy of Stanford University Department of Dermatology.)

When a plaque of linear scleroderma crosses a joint, it may cause reduced range of motion or even immobility. Linear scleroderma may be accompanied by atrophy of subcutaneous structures, including fascia, muscle, and bone; in extreme cases, there may be hemiatrophy of a limb or of the face. In these cases, the atrophy of the subcutaneous structures is permanent, despite possible remission of subcutaneous sclerosis.

Mixed Connective Tissue Disease

All of the cutaneous findings in mixed connective tissue disease can be seen in other autoimmune rheumatologic disorders, including LE, systemic sclerosis, and dermatomyositis. Common cutaneous manifestations include edema of the fingers and hands, Raynaud's phenomenon, sclerodactyly, and the periungual changes. Lesions mimicking all forms of cutaneous lupus, malar rash, and Gottron's papules also occur.[26]

Rheumatoid Arthritis

Although many dermatologic conditions may coexist with rheumatoid arthritis (RA), the classic lesion is the rheumatoid nodule[27] (see Chapter 25). These nodules are soft, compressible subcutaneous nodules that lack any change in surface texture or color. They range in size from less than 1 cm in diameter to several centimeters, and they usually occur near a joint. Rheumatoid nodules are present in 20% to 25% of patients with RA but are not pathognomonic for rheumatoid arthritis. Similar-appearing nodules may also occur in LE, dermatomyositis, or granuloma annulare.

A distinctive type of vasculitis can also occur in patients with RA, usually in patients with high titers of rheumatoid factor.[27] This vasculitis is classified based on the severity, rather than on the size of vessel involved (small, medium, or large). Mild vasculitis shows digital infarcts, petechiae, and livedo reticularis. Moderate vasculitis is characterized by palpable purpura of the legs and buttocks. Severe rheumatoid vasculitis has palpable purpura with cutaneous necrosis and ulcerations. Patients with severe vasculitis are systemically ill and have a mortality rate of approximately 30%.[28]

Pyoderma Gangrenosum

Pyoderma gangrenosum is associated with many systemic diseases, most commonly RA, inflammatory bowel disease, and myeloproliferative disorders. In fact, it is not unusual to see the triad of inflammatory bowel disease, arthritis, and pyoderma gangrenosum. Up to 50% of cases of pyoderma gangrenosum are idiopathic, however, with no identifiable, underlying disorder.[29]

Pyoderma grangrenosum begins as extremely tender, erythematous plaques, usually with overlying pustules. These plaques break down rapidly, usually over a matter of days. The resultant ulcers have necrotic, purulent material at the base with characteristic undermined, overhanging edges and a violaceous or erythematous border (Fig. 17–11). The ulcers are often bizarrely shaped. Other variants of pyoderma gangrenosum include bullous, pustular, and vegetative forms. Pyoderma gangrenosum can occur on any cutaneous or mucosal surface. Pyoderma gangrenosum demonstrates the phenomenon of pathergy, whereby the ulcers are exacerbated or initiated by trauma. Attempts at débridement or grafting may actually worsen pyoderma gangrenosum. Treatment with sulfones or cytotoxic drugs can be useful in some patients.

Psoriasis

Psoriasis affects at least 1% of adults in the United States. The usual age of onset is in early to mid adulthood, although people of all ages, including children, may be affected. Six percent to 15% of all patients with psoriasis have associated arthritis.[30] Psoriatic arthritis is seronegative, but patients may have rheumatoid arthritis and psoriasis simultaneously, in which case there may be cutaneous stigmata of both conditions. The activity of the skin disease does not parallel the activity of arthritis in psoriasis. In fact, patients with severe psoriatic arthritis may have no demonstrable skin disease. However, patients with extremely severe cutaneous psoriasis are somewhat more likely to have arthritis than patients with a limited amount of skin involvement.

As with cutaneous manifestations of LE, there are a myriad of skin findings in psoriasis.[31] The classic lesion is a well-demarcated erythematous plaque surmounted by silvery, adherent scale (Fig. 17–12). The thickness of both the plaque and the scale may vary greatly; in partially treated or well-emolliated psoriasis, there may be no scale. The classic areas of involvement are the extensor surfaces of the extremities (particularly the elbows and knees), the scalp, the umbilicus, the sacrum, the penis, and the gluteal cleft. Psoriasis may affect any cutaneous or mucosal surface, including the palms and

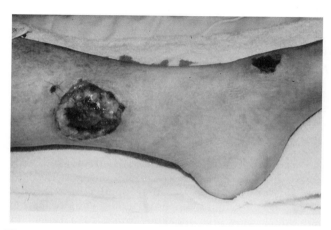

Figure 17–11. Pyoderma gangrenosum. (Courtesy of Stanford University Department of Dermatology.)

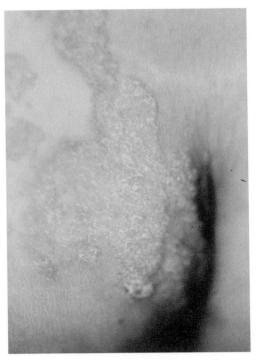

Figure 17–12. Psoriasis. Classic scaling patches near the anus.

soles.[32] In the mouth, geographic tongue is believed to be a manifestation of pustular psoriasis.

The most common type of psoriasis is the plaque form described previously, but there are several other patterns. Guttate psoriasis describes diffusely distributed, small, thin psoriatic papules, which usually appear suddenly, often after a streptococcal upper respiratory tract infection. Many patients who present initially with guttate psoriasis eventually develop the more typical plaque form of psoriasis, although some patients maintain a guttate pattern. Psoriasis may also be pustular, in which case the erythematous plaques are covered by small sterile pustules. This variant often affects the palms and soles but may occur anywhere. Psoriasis may be erythrodermic, that is, diffusely erythematous with little or no scaling, discrete papules, or plaques. However, thicker plaques are often observed in typically involved areas, such as the elbows, knees, and scalp. Psoriasis may also be distributed in the groin and intertriginous areas, in which case it is called *inverse psoriasis*. On the genitalia, scaling may be minimal or absent. Psoriasis can be very inflammatory and cosmetically disfiguring in one area while sparing other body sites. It is not uncommon to see patients with diffuse and severe scalp or nail involvement but little or no psoriasis elsewhere.

The classic nail changes in psoriasis are distal onycholysis (lifting of the nail plate from the nail bed), coarse pits, and spotty yellow discoloration of the nails that simulates a drop of oil trapped under the nail (Fig. 17–13).[33] Other changes include scaling of the nail bed, which may give the appearance of a fungal infection, and diffuse erythema and scaling of the periun-

gual skin. Psoriasis may also progress to destroy the entire nail plate. In up to 75% of patients with psoriatic arthritis, nail disease precedes the onset of arthritis, and 85% of patients with psoriatic arthritis have nail involvement at some point. Nail involvement in psoriasis is quite common, whereas arthritis is relatively rare, so generalizations about a patient's likelihood to develop arthritis should not be made on the basis of nail involvement.

Medications used to treat psoriatic arthritis may or may not affect skin lesions. Methotrexate, sulfasalazine, and cyclosporine can be beneficial for both skin and joint disease, whereas systemic retinoids, ultraviolet B light, and psoralens plus ultraviolet A light (PUVA) have no effect on arthritis. Arthritis treatment with gold or antimalarials has no effect on the cutaneous involvement. The use of systemic glucocorticoids in skin psoriasis is problematic because patients treated with systemic glucocorticoids often have dramatic rebound flares, which may be difficult to control when the steroids are discontinued.[31] In addition, rebound flares often require additional systemic steroids, leading to an escalating cycle of steroid use.

Reiter's Disease

Although Reiter's disease consists of a triad of clinical findings that do not involve the skin, there are distinctive cutaneous findings.[34] The lesions have a similar appearance to psoriasis—erythematous plaques with adherent scale or, occasionally, pustules. Keratoderma blennorrhagica describes thick scaling plaques on the palms and soles, often with pustules. The scale has a distinctive yellow or yellow-red color. In circumcised men, balanitis circinata presents as a thin, erythematous plaque with fine scale on the glans penis; in uncircumcised men, there may be more prominent vesicles, pustules, or erosions. Patients may have scaling plaques on the extensor extremities that mimic psoriasis. Painless erosions and shallow ulcerations of the mouth may be observed in patients with Reiter's disease.

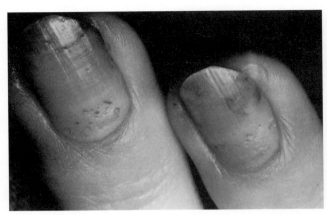

Figure 17–13. Psoriasis of the nail. (Courtesy of Stanford University Department of Dermatology.)

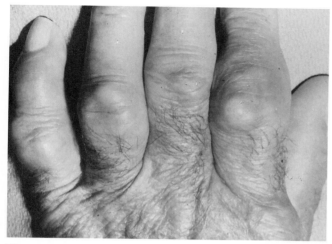

Figure 17–14. Gouty tophi. (Courtesy of Stanford University Department of Dermatology.)

Gout

Cutaneous signs of gout are easily recognized. In cases of acute gout, there may be erythema, warmth, and tenderness of the affected joint, simulating cellulitis.[35] Tophi, signs of long-standing disease, are subcutaneous nodules that usually are painless and have no overlying epidermal change except for a slight yellow or white color (Fig. 17–14). Occassionally the tophi can rupture, with a chalky-white discharge and potential ulceration, similar to that shown in Figure 17–4. This situation can be extremely painful.

SUMMARY

Clinical recognition of various cutaneous findings can aid in the diagnosis of several rheumatologic disorders. Skin biopsy and additional immunofluorescence or serologic studies are diagnostic for many of the conditions described herein.

REFERENCES

1. Tosti A: The nail apparatus in collagen disorders. Semin Dermatol 10:71–76, 1991.
2. Sontheimer RD, Provost TT: Lupus erythematosus. In Sontheimer RD, Provost TT, eds: Cutaneous Manifestations of Rheumatic Diseases. Baltimore, Williams & Wilkins, 1996, pp 1–71.
3. Samitz MH: Cuticular changes in dermatomyositis. Arch Dermatol 110:866–867, 1974.
4. Daniel CR, Sams WM, Scher RK: Nails in systemic disease. Dermatol Clin 3:465–483, 1985.
5. Goodfield MJD: The skin in systemic sclerosis. Clin Dermatol 12:229–234, 1994.
6. Callen JP: Dermatomyositis. Dis Mon 33:237–305, 1987.
7. Laman SD, Provost TT: Cutaneous manifestations of lupus erythematosus. Rheum Dis Clin North Am 20:195–212, 1994.
8. Piette WW: Primary systemic vasculitis. In Sontheimer RD, Provost TT, eds: Cutaneous Manifestations of Rheumatic Diseases. Baltimore, Williams & Wilkins, 1996, pp 177–232.
9. Jennette CJ, Milling DM, Falk RJ: Vasculitis affecting the skin. Arch Dermatol 130:899–906, 1994.
10. Callen JP: Vasculitis. In Callen JP, Jorizzo JL, et al, eds: Dermatological Signs of Internal Disease, 2nd ed. Philadelphia, WB Saunders, 1995, pp 31–39.
11. Gammon WR: Urticarial vasculitis. Dermatol Clin 3:97–105, 1985.
12. Gibson LE: Cutaneous vasculitis: Approach to diagnosis and systemic associations. Mayo Clin Proc 65:221–229, 1990.
13. Nahass GT: Antiphospholipid antibodies and the antiphospholipid antibody syndrome. J Am Acad Dermatol 36:149–168, 1997.
14. Cohen MR, Isenberg DA: Ultraviolet irradiation in systemic lupus erythematosus: Friend or foe? Br J Rheumatol 35:1002–1007, 1996.
15. Gilliam JN, Sontheimer RD: Subacute cutaneous lupus erythematosus. Clin Rheum Dis 8:343–352, 1982.
16. Sontheimer RD, Maddison PJ, et al: Serologic and HLA associations in subacute cutaneous lupus, a clinical subset of lupus erythematosus. Ann Intern Med 97:664–671, 1982.
17. Provost TT, Watson R, Simmons-O'Brien E: Significance of the anti-Ro (SS-A) antibody in evaluation of patients with cutaneous manifestations of a connective tissue disease. J Am Acad Dermatol 35:147–169, 1996.
18. Tuffanelli DL: Discoid lupus erythematosus. Clin Rheum Dis 8:327–341, 1982.
19. Callen JP: Lupus erythematosus. In Callen JP, Jorizzo JL, et al, eds: Dermatological Signs of Internal Disease, 2nd ed. Philadelphia, WB Saunders, 1995, pp 3–12.
20. Mascaro JM, Herrero C, Hausmann G: Uncommon cutaneous manifestations of lupus erythematosus. Lupus 6:122–131, 1997.
21. Watanabe T, Tsuchida T: Lupus erythematosus profundus: A cutaneous marker for a distinct clinical subset? Br J Dermatol 134:123–125, 1996.
22. Adams-Gandhi LB, Boyd AD, King LE: Diagnosis and management of dermatomyositis. Compr Ther 22:156–164, 1996.
23. Roberts LJ, Fink CW: Childhood polymyositis/dermatomyositis. Clin Dermatol 6:36–46, 1988.
24. Perez MI, Kohn SR: Systemic sclerosis. J Am Acad Dermatol 28:525–547, 1993.
25. Ghersetich I, Teofoli P, et al: Localized scleroderma. Clin Dermatol 12:237–242, 1994.
26. Gilliam JN, Prystowsky SD: Mixed connective tissue disease syndrome. Arch Dermatol 113:583–587, 1977.
27. Jorizzo JL, Daniels JC: Dermatologic conditions reported in patients with rheumatoid arthritis. J Am Acad Dermatol 8:439–457, 1983.
28. Jorizzo JL, Greer KE, Callen JP: Miscellaneous disorders with prominent features involving the skin and the joints. In Callen JP, Jorizzo JL, et al, eds: Dermatological Signs of Internal Disease, 2nd ed. Philadelphia, WB Saunders, 1995, pp 40–54.
29. Powell FC, Su WPD, Perry HO: Pyoderma gangrenosum: Classification and management. J Am Acad Dermatol 34:395–409, 1996.
30. Stern RS: Psoriasis. Lancet 350:349–350, 1997.
31. Goodfield M: Skin lesions in psoriasis. Baillieres Clin Rheumatol 8:295–316, 1994.
32. Larko O: Problem sites: Scalp, palm and sole, and nail. Dermatol Clin 13:771–777, 1995.
33. Scher RK: Psoriasis of the nail. Dermatol Clin 3:387–394, 1985.
34. Calin A: Keratodermia blennorrhagica and mucocutaneous manifestations of Reiter's syndrome. Ann Rheum Dis 38(suppl): 68–72, 1979.
35. Schumacher HR: Crystal-induced arthritis: an overview. Am J Med 100(suppl 2A):46S–52S, 1996.

Part II

APPROACH TO THE PATIENT WITH MUSCULOSKELETAL PAIN

Chapter 18

Differential Diagnosis of Soft Tissue and Joint Pain

Edward D. Harris, Jr. ■ David J. Schurman
Mark C. Genovese ■ Peter B.J. Wu

The processes of examining joints and periarticular structures were introduced in Chapters 2 and 3. Once a diagnosis has been made of a specific entity, the approach to management can be defined according to guidelines described in the chapters of Part III. This chapter provides the physician with help in diagnosis of specific musculoskeletal disorders.

DIFFUSE SOFT TISSUE AND MUSCLE PAIN

Diffuse soft tissue and muscle pain is associated with both inflammatory and noninflammatory diseases of soft tissues. Soft tissue rheumatic processes represent a diverse group of disorders involving muscle, tendon, ligament, and bursae. A careful history and a detailed examination often lead to the correct diagnosis of a local, regional, or generalized musculoskeletal problem. Improvement after conservative and symptomatic management is often seen. The majority of these problems can be dealt with in the primary care physician's office. In some situations, referral to a specialist can be useful when the diagnosis remains unclear, or when initial conservative management has failed.

Polymyalgia Rheumatica

Before 1970, polymyalgia rheumatica (PMR) (referred to as *Horton's syndrome* in the medical literature) was rarely diagnosed. It then became appreciated that the syndrome of pain (more than weakness) in the shoulder and hip girdles, mild fevers, fatigue, anemia of chronic disease, and elevated acute phase reactants in serum represented an entity that was exquisitely responsive to relatively low doses of glucocorticoid therapy and, in a minority of patients, was associated with biopsy-proven giant cell arthritis found in branches of the temporal artery.[1, 2] After 10 years or more of physician education about PMR and temporal arthritis, the pendulum has swung toward premature diagnoses of PMR and excessive use of glucocorticoids without exclusion of other diseases. As of 1999, PMR is still over-

diagnosed. Only as a last resort should prednisone therapy be given as a therapeutic trial in vague syndromes of diffuse pain associated with a high erythrocyte sedimentation rate (ESR) or C-reactive protein. In the absence of renal disease, a patient with an ESR greater than 100 mm/h might have a severe active infection, a malignancy, or vasculitis; in such cases, infection or malignancy should be ruled out first.

To complicate diagnosis, it has become evident in the last 25 years that PMR-like syndromes can develop in some patients with an already established connective tissue disease, such as rheumatoid arthritis. Treatment of this syndrome and its companion, giant cell arthritis, are discussed in detail in Chapter 27.

Erythema Nodosum

Erythema nodosum means "painful red nodules." They appear exactly as this in many cases, most often on the extensor surfaces of the lower legs. The pathology is acute, and chronic inflammation of the subcutaneous tissue along with vascular proliferation in the dermis occurs. More often appearing in women than men, it is a manifestation of sarcoidosis in about half of the cases.[3] Other causes include indolent infection with tuberculosis, coccidioidomycosis, and histoplasmosis and reactions to drugs, including sulfa-containing drugs and oral contraceptives. When one of these lesions appears over a joint, it may be falsely thought of as indicating synovial inflammation.

Myofascial Pain Syndrome

Myofascial pain syndrome is a common problem marked by myofascial trigger points. The *myofascial trigger point* is defined as a small area within a tight band of skeletal muscle fibers that can give rise to characteristic referred pain. In contrast to tender points in fibromyalgia, myofascial trigger points have a tendency to reproduce consistent referred pain in a distinctive distribution in individual muscles. The pathophysiology of myofascial trigger points remains unknown, and biopsy specimens of the involved site have never revealed pathologic features. One theory, the *energy crisis hypothesis,* suggests that there is an increased energy consumption with a decreased energy supply in the muscle fibers of a myofascial trigger point region that results in the contracture of a bundle of muscle fibers (i.e., tight band formation).[4] Alternatively, it has been suggested that excessive acetylcholine release in the dysfunctional end-plate with the interaction of the spinal cord mechanism might be responsible for myofascial trigger point and taut band formation.[5]

Treatment of myofascial pain syndrome should be directed at identifying the trigger points and tight bands in involved muscles, then inactivating them. Spraying the trigger point with a vapocoolant, such as ethyl chloride, followed by active or passive stretching for the involved muscles can be beneficial. The insertion of a small-gauge needle into the trigger point and injection of a local anesthetic, such as lidocaine, is also an effective means of relieving pain.

Fibromyalgia

In the absence of firm diagnostic criteria, fibromyalgia cannot yet be labeled as a discrete entity. Although described as a syndrome, many patients given the diagnosis have incomplete or somewhat different manifestations than are put forth as classic criteria. It is characterized by fatigue, stiffness, and widespread musculoskeletal pain and tenderness. The syndrome itself can occur independently or as a secondary process in patients with other connective tissue diseases, such as rheumatoid arthritis or systemic lupus erythematosus (SLE). Although the basal symptoms can be precipitated through lack of sleep, strenuous exercise, or emotional stress, there can be a multitude of somatic complaints that can be manifest in individuals with the diagnosis of fibromyalgia. It is best thought of as a central pain state without a well-defined source, in which the aches and pains that others may brush aside are amplified to a bothersome level, and the quality of life becomes substantially diminished. This problem is not rare. It may affect 3% of the population, it is more common in women, and its prevalence increases steadily from late teens to the 80s, especially in women.[6]

Patients with fibromyalgia, both men and women, are usually functional citizens, working despite their pain but desperate to be relieved of their agony. They get out of bed in the morning stiff and miserable, convinced that they have not slept more than a few hours. Their muscles hurt; their skin is tender. Often, cramping abdominal pain and the urge to defecate on awakening lead to a small loose bowel movement, a process that can be repeated often during the day. They can have a day that is productive but painful, punctuated sometimes by migraine headaches or tension headaches. Once, earlier in their lives, they were able to exercise but no more. Even a fast walk produces the feeling that they are "hitting the wall" as would a marathon runner, and after exercise they feel "wiped out." They rarely are

overweight, often have cold intolerance, find it progressively more difficult to concentrate, and easily become irritable. Premenstrual symptoms are markedly amplified. A tolerant spouse is stressed by their problems; a less forgiving and less flexible one may leave home. Antidepressants of various types, including low-dose amytriptyline at bedtime, may have been prescribed; a small cohort responds, but most do not.

On examination, these patients have a normal blood pressure, although it is reported that some have an exaggerated increase in systolic blood pressure in response to a sustained isometric hand grip. The remainder of the examination is marked by normal findings with the exception of tender points at various tendinous insertions: the back of the neck, near the sternoclavicular and sternomanubrial joints, medial border of the scapula, gluteal muscles and near the greater trochanter, and epicondyles of the elbow and knees (Fig. 18–1). Less tender are large muscle bundles, such as the quadriceps, gastrocnemius, and deltoids. Laboratory tests are similarly normal. In particular, acute-phase reactants, thyroid and liver function tests, and glucose tolerance are normal unless the patients

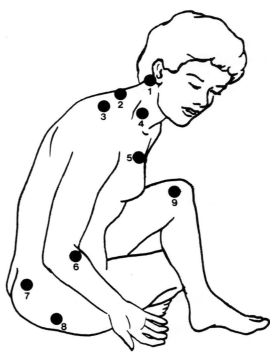

Figure 18–1. Tender point locations. The nine paired tender points recommended by the 1990 American College of Rheumatology Criteria Committee for establishing a diagnosis of fibromyalgia are (*1*) insertion of nuchal muscles into occiput; (*2*) upper border of trapezius—midportion; (*3*) muscle attachments to upper medial border of scapula; (*4*) anterior aspects of the C5, C7 intertransverse spaces; (*5*) second rib space about 3 cm lateral to the sternal border; (*6*) muscle attachments to lateral epicondyle—about 2 cm below bony prominence; (*7*) upper outer quadrant of gluteal muscles; (*8*) muscle attachments just posterior to greater trochanter; and (*9*) medial fat pad of knee proximal to joint line. A total of 11 or more tender points in conjunction with a history of widespread pain is characteristic of the fibromyalgia syndrome. (From Bennett RM: The fibromyalgia syndrome. In Kelly WN, Harris ED, Ruddy S, Sledge CB, eds: Textbook of Rheumatology, 5th ed. Philadelphia, WB Saunders, 1997, p 513.)

had preexisting abnormalities of these systems. Cardiovascular fitness tests are often abruptly halted without electrocardiographic abnormalities by the patients because of diffuse pain and exhaustion. Fibromyalgia can last for years and cannot be perceived as self-limiting.

Fibromyalgia must be suspected in patients who present with the symptoms and examination just described. In an effort to define the process more rigidly, the American College of Rheumatology produced guidelines in 1990 that specify

Widespread pain of 3 months or more.

Pain in axial distribution, on both left and right sides of the body and both above and below the waist.

Pain present in at least 11 of 18 specified tender point sites (see Fig. 18–1) on digital palpation (with force required to blanch a fingernail).

Although the diagnostic criteria are imperfect, they have provided researchers with a basic starting point in the study of this disorder and provide guidelines for the practitioner. Physicians need to be precise in evaluation and diagnosis because patients referred to rheumatologists with a diagnosis of fibromyalgia can be found to have one of the following instead:

• Diffuse connective tissue disease
• Early spondyloarthropathy or sciatica
• Multiple sclerosis
• Depression
• Hypothyroidism
• Inflammatory bowel disease
• Inflammatory or metabolic myopathy
• PMR
• Chronic fatigue syndrome (CFS)
• Myofascial pain syndromes

The underlying cause of fibromyalgia has been elusive. More studies of the possible cause of fibromyalgia have been performed than, perhaps, any other illnesses. Almost every metabolic system has been implicated. The pathophysiology of the disorder is unknown. Early studies focused on the hypothesis that the principal abnormality was in the areas of increased tenderness. However, biopsies of tender points have generally demonstrated histologically normal muscle.[7]

It has been suggested that an up-regulation of *N-methyl-D-aspartate* (NMDA) receptors is related to a dysregulation of substance P release at peripheral nerve sites. Another study has noted parallels with low insulin growth factor in these patients and has documented symptomatic improvement during administration of growth hormone. One month of growth hormone therapy costs about $1500. Another hypothesis that has been tested and reported in abstract form is that fibromyalgia is caused by muscle ischemia resulting from increased vascular resistance, low blood volume, and normotension; beneficial results were reported with treatment with clonidine and diltiazem (confirmation of these data is essential). It certainly seems probable that chronic stimulation of the nervous system by an as yet unknown substance sensitizes the central neural structures involved in pain perception.[8]

Fibromyalgia is a complex syndrome with a considerable variation of symptoms among patients. Effective treatment is, needless to say, difficult.[9] Education emphasizing that this is not a crippling or potentially fatal disorder is important. Education should be done concurrently with the use of acetaminophen and nonsteroidal anti-inflammatory drugs (NSAIDs) to reduce pain. More importantly, however, is the implementation of a long-term strategy to improve the patient's sleep pattern, increase energy, and decrease achiness. The plan should feature the use of exercise and good sleep hygiene. Exercise should start with stretching and gentle strengthening, then progress slowly to aerobic conditioning. Antidepressants may provide a useful adjunct because many patients with fibromyalgia also suffer some degree of mood disturbance. Selective serotonin reuptake inhibitors (SSRIs) may help improve mood, whereas tricyclic antidepressants, such as amytriptyline and nortriptyline, may also help modulate the sleep cycle. Muscle relaxants, such as cyclobenzaprine (Flexeril), orphenadrine (Norflex), and carisoprodol (Soma), also may be useful in helping patients initiate and escalate the exercise and stretching regimen. Narcotic-based analgesics should not be used in the treatment of fibromyalgia.

Chronic Fatigue Syndrome

Chronic fatigue syndrome (CFS) is worth special emphasis in the differential diagnosis of generalized pain. CFS currently is defined by a working case definition developed under the leadership of the Centers for Disease Control and Prevention.[10] Patients diagnosed with CFS should have (1) severe, debilitating fatigue that usually comes on suddenly after an infectious illness, persists or relapses for 6 months or more, or is new or of a definite onset; (2) symptoms that are not truly relieved by rest, leading to greatly diminished function at work and in social situations; (3) four or more specific, associated symptoms (impaired memory or concentration, sore throat, tender cervical or axillary lymph nodes, muscle pain, multi-joint paint, new headaches, unrefreshing sleep, and postexertional malaise); and (4) symptoms that cannot be attributed to a group of specific organic and psychiatric conditions often associated with fatigue. The last-mentioned criterion is particularly difficult because CFS patients are often depressed, and it is debated whether depression or CFS comes first in these patients.

CFS is estimated to be present in fewer than 0.3% of patients in primary care clinics, making it a diagnosis less common than that of fibromyalgia.[11] CFS patients are more often women with good education but, in contrast to fibromyalgia, tend to be young. Objectively, they are not depressed or hypochondriacs. There is not the central up-regulation of the hypothalamic-pituitary-adrenal axis in CFS that is found in depression. In addition, antidepressant medication rarely provides relief of symptoms. Over time, with physician and family support and treatment with modalities used in fibromyalgia, there is gradual improvement in most patients.

Glucocorticoid Withdrawal

The human body is extraordinarily sensitive to small changes in circulating glucocorticoids. The consequence is not so much severe life-threatening Addison's disease, but rather the more common, less spectacular syndrome of glucocorticoid withdrawal when a relatively small dose of prednisone, for example, is tapered too quickly. Symptoms of glucocorticoid withdrawal may resemble the symptoms of the primary disease. For example, the patient with PMR who is relieved of musculoskeletal pain associated with increased acute-phase reactants by 20 mg of prednisone each day may develop musculoskeletal pain when the drug is withdrawn. This reflects not the underlying disease, but rather the body's reaction to glucocorticoid withdrawal. Successful prednisone tapering may, for example, require lowering of the *weekly* total dose of prednisone by no more than 1.0 mg.

Bone Diseases

Any excessive new bone formation is often symptomatic. Thus, patients with *Paget's disease* have diffuse bony pain in affected bones, most often the skull, pelvis, and tibia. They may have noted an increased hat size and bowing of the legs or *saber shins.* A diagnosis can usually be made by plain radiographs. This process can mimic metastatic cancer in bone (particularly from the prostate). Although serum calcium and phosphorus are usually normal, serum alkaline phosphatase can be up to 20 times normal.

Osteomalacia, the metabolic bone disease caused by an inadequate [calcium × phosphorus] product in blood (see Chapter 35), often causes diffuse pain in bones of the extremities, chest wall, and back. In contrast, *osteoporosis* is symptomatic only when compression fractures of the spine or stress fractures in the fibula or tibia occur. Fluoride toxicity can present as diffuse bone pain; sodium fluoride is used occasionally as therapy for osteoporosis.

Patients with lung tumors or hypoxemic states who have periosteal new bone proliferation *hypertrophic osteoarthropathy* (HOA) have pain at proliferative sites that are almost always at the distal ends of long bones. Careful examination reveals that tenderness is present on compression of distal bones, not the joint. These patients gain relief from elevation of the affected extremity (one man with painful tibiofibular disease from HOA only obtained relief by standing on his head on a pillow placed on the floor in a corner of a room).

The possibility that vague bone pain can represent *cancer* must always be kept in mind by the inquiring physician. Metastatic disease is more common than a primary malignancy of bone. Paget's disease of bone degenerates into osteogenic sarcoma from time to time, particularly in those with active disease. A relatively abrupt increase in localized bone pain in pagetic patients should be a red flag suggesting either a fracture or malignant degeneration of the bone disease.

Growth Pains and Ligamentous Laxity

Growing pains are principally symptomatic in adolescents and young adults and are not an uncommon cause of diffuse joint pains. Discomfort is primarily related to exercise. The patient usually awakens feeling fine and tolerates exercise well but then has postexertional pain in weight-bearing joints.[12] Often the patient is a young man in a phase of rapid growth in height. On examination, no synovitis or thickening of the joint capsule is noted. Muscle bulk is often less than normal in the extremities, and hyperextension and an excessive medial-lateral motion of the knees can be found. Laboratory test results are normal. Therapy is physical. Isotonic exercises to build up both small and large muscle groups are appropriate.

ACUTELY ILL PATIENTS WITH POLYARTHRITIS AND POLYARTHRALGIA

Different algorithms apply to differential diagnosis when symptoms involve more than one joint. The explanation for this is simple and based on the fact that polyarticular disease is usually caused by either inflammatory or infiltrative processes. One useful classification of polyarthritis is separating entities by whether or not there is associated *fever.* Fever is caused either by endotoxin and related compounds released by infectious agents or by the host's own cytokines (e.g., interleukin-1) being produced in response to an infectious agent, tumor, or idiopathic inflammation.

Polyarthritis and Fever

Every patient with fever and polyarthritis should have a prompt, complete evaluation by a physician to find an infection that can be specifically treated. Essentials of such an evaluation include a complete review of systems and thorough questioning about recent travel, hiking, eating, and exposure to other sick people. While blood, urine, sputum, cultures, and serologic tests are being taken, appropriate imaging studies should be obtained. Even in the absence of anemia, a bone marrow for histology and culture must be considered. In addition to standard metabolic panels, ESR or C-reactive protein, and a complete hemogram, it is important to assay for rheumatoid factor, antinuclear antibodies, and the electrophoretic pattern of serum proteins. This full work-up should be completed within several days.

INFECTIOUS CAUSES

BACTERIA. The hematogenous spread of bacteria can produce septic arthritis in more than one joint at the same time. Polyarticular sepsis is an important diagnosis to make because specific antibiotic treatment must be instituted immediately (see Chapter 33). History and physical examination should focus on possible entry sites for bacteria, including puncture wounds, abrasions, evidence of intravenous drug use, or concurrent infection in other organs (e.g., the lungs or kidney). There is almost always excess synovial fluid in a septic joint, and the most accessible joint (usually the knee, if it is involved) must be aspirated and the fluid sent for culture, Gram stain, crystals, and cell count. Blood cultures are essential as well. Infection by pyogenic organisms (e.g., *Staphylococcus aureus*) that involves more than one joint carries a high mortality rate, a fact that justifies parenteral antibiotic treatment, even if there is only a small likelihood that a bacterial infection is present. As noted in Chapter 33, infection by *Neisseria gonorrhoeae* can present as a migratory tenosynovitis, a monarthritis, or a polyarticular and systemic infection. Bacterial endocarditis rarely produces septic joints; occasional patients with subacute bacterial endocarditis have a reactive, sterile synovitis with only mild inflammation. The same can be said for arthritis associated with *Neisseria meningitidis*. Bacteria are not found in these synovial fluid samples, and the number of white blood cells can vary substantially. Lyme disease is an infectious process. If a patient with fever and arthritis in more than one joint has a history of a round, pink skin lesion that expanded and may have been related to a tick bite or has Bell's palsy or a cardiac conduction defect (heart block), Lyme disease must be high on the differential diagnosis (see Chapter 33).

MYCOBACTERIA AND FUNGI. Joint infection by mycobacteria or fungi is often indolent and not accompanied by fever. The joint can be cool but with boggy soft tissue palpable and relatively little effusion. Synovial needle biopsy (or open biopsy) may be needed to make the diagnosis.

HUMAN IMMUNODEFICIENCY VIRUS. Infection with human immunodeficiency virus (HIV) may be associated with a transient, mild synovitis during the first several weeks of infection when a patient may have a flu-like syndrome. Later, in more established disease, HIV infection can be associated with an aggressive Reiter's syndrome or reactive arthritis involving large joints of the lower extremity.

OTHER VIRAL INFECTIONS. Parvovirus B19 outbreaks usually occur in the late winter and spring. A number of symptomatic patients have a polyarthritis, which is symmetric (classically involving the small joints of the hands, knees, wrists, and ankles), generalized, and of short duration. It can be associated with a chronic anemia and rarely with short-lived aplastic anemia. Rarely a B19 infection can evolve into a chronic arthritis (usually oligoarthritis) that resembles rheumatoid arthritis and even more rarely is linked to vasculitis.[13] The finding of parvovirus in synovium of patients with rheumatoid arthritis has led to the hypothesis that parvovirus is a cause of rheumatoid arthritis. An immunoglobulin M (IgM) antibody can be detected in serum for 2 or 3 months after the initial infection. In addition to arthritis, children have erythema infectiosum during early parvovirus B19 infection. This mild skin eruption occurs on the malar prominences of the face, giving a *slapped cheek* appearance. In otherwise normal persons, no treatment is necessary. In immunocompromised individuals, intravenous IgG is sometimes indicated.

Hepatitis C infection is being recognized more frequently as a causative agent in vasculitis, particularly purpura or organ dysfunction generated by cryoglobulins. This virus has much lymphotrophic activity, and this is probably responsible for its associations with rheumatic disorders. Polymerase chain reaction assays can give a semiquantitative report of viral load in infected patients. Before treatment of any connective tissue disease with immunosuppressive agents or methotrexate, hepatitis C assays should be obtained because, when the drug is discontinued for any reason, there is often a vigorous return of inflammation.[14]

Another virus that has been linked to rheumatoid arthritis as a potential causative agent is the Epstein-Barr virus (EBV). Antibody titers against this agent are higher in patients with rheumatoid arthritis than in normal subjects, but there is no sound evidence that EBV is part of the cause. Occasional patients with fever, adenopathy, and pharyngitis that are the manifestations of infectious mononucleosis caused by EBV have mild-to-moderate arthralgias without significant synovitis. Similar syndromes with pain exceeding swelling or inflammation are noted in other viral diseases, including rubella, adenovirus, and coxsackie.

The arthritis associated with hepatitis B infection is a sterile one that reflects immune complex deposition causing inflammation in synovial tissue. It is noted before the jaundice appears, and the pain subsides as the bilirubin rises above 2 to 3 mg/dL.

Systemic Noninfectious Diseases

The following is a useful aphorism: *A patient with an ESR that is greater than 100 mm/h has a severe infection, vasculitis or systemic connective tissue disease, or malignancy.*

MALIGNANCY

Malignancies that present with fever and synovitis are usually well advanced at presentation. Exceptions are lymphomas, particularly angiocentric lymphomas, and certain organ tumors, such as adenocarcinoma of the lung or renal cell carcinoma. Angiocentric lymphomas frequently mimic vasculitis at presentation because the malignant cells, usually B-cell derivatives, in blood vessels cause widespread microthromboses and infarctions. Tissue biopsy is required to make a definitive diagnosis. There is some evidence that EBV infection is related to this kind of vasculitis.[15] Other malignancies that mimic vasculitis because of purpura and tissue infarction include heavy chain disease, Waldenstrom's macroglobulinemia, and multiple myeloma.

SYSTEMIC CONNECTIVE TISSUE DISEASE

The worrisome *rheumatic* diseases that have febrile and severe presentations are listed subsequently, with the more difficult to diagnose shown first.

The classification and description of vasculitis are outlined in Chapter 27. *Polyarteritis* is the most difficult of these conditions to diagnose and, as well, is the most difficult to treat effectively. The presence of hypertension, hematuria, or asymmetric neurologic symptoms may indicate that this necrotizing process is present. Early biopsy of involved organs is indicated; those most often generating positive histopathology include muscle, peripheral nerve, kidney, and testis. Invasive or noninvasive angiograms should be ordered to explore possible vascular involvement of organs, such as the bowel, heart, or brain. Vasculitic involvement of arteries in muscle usually presents as muscle pain rather than weakness.

The remarkable specificity of antineutrophil cytoplasmic antibody (c-ANCA) for *Wegener's granulomatosis* has made the diagnosis of this entity significantly easier,[16] especially considering that the biopsy specimens of sinuses or lung often are reported to show acute and chronic inflammation without discrete evidence for vasculitis. The *Churg-Strauss syndrome* is marked by eosinophia and eosinophil-laden granulomatous disease of the lungs.

Giant cell arthritis, including *Takayasu's arthritis,* must be suspected if it is to be diagnosed. When it appears as classic temporal arthritis, with scalp tenderness, jaw claudication, and dilated, tender temporal arteries in a person older than 50 years, it is relatively easy to diagnose. However, giant cell arthritis can present differently, including as a myocardial infarction, an acute dementia, and an acute abdomen. Biopsy or angiograms may show the telltale smooth narrowing of arteries that helps in diagnosis.

In *hypersensitivity angiitis* (leukocytoclastic angiitis), palpable purpura is often present (Fig. 18–2), providing accessible biopsy opportunities. Unless a clear-cut cause is obvious, tests for cryoglobulins and hepatitis C must be ordered; hepatitis C can generate the cryoglobulins, which, in turn, can induce palpable purpura. *Henoch-Schönlein purpura,* presenting as palpable purpura, abdominal pain, and gastrointestinal bleeding, is seen more often in children than in adults. As mentioned previously, in palpable purpura, assays for cryoglobulinemia, hepatitis C, and HIV-1 should be obtained.

ANTIPHOSPHOLIPID ANTIBODY SYNDROME

The complications in pregnancy induced by antiphospholipid antibodies are discussed in Chapter 14. Antiphospholipid antibodies are not an uncommon finding in SLE and can by inducing thromboses of small blood vessels, increase the morbidity of this disease. This is one of the few syndromes in which the autoantibodies actually cause the pathology, rather than being secondary to it. Synovitis is rare in primary antiphospholipid antibody syndromes, but in patients with fever,

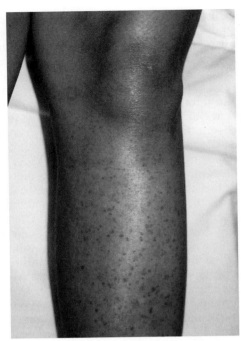

Figure 18–2. Palpable purpura associated with hepatitis C–induced cryoglobulinemia.

thrombocytopenia, and clinical evidence for thrombosis in one or more vessels or minor features such as livedo reticularis, leg ulcers, or migraine headaches, the titer of antiphospholipid antibody should be ordered. An approach to the ordering of these studies is outlined in Chapter 5.

ADULT-ONSET STILL'S DISEASE

Adult-onset Still's disease (AOSD) is a systemic inflammatory illness accompanied by the hallmark signs of spiking fever, rash, and polyarthritis. In fact, it is the presentation of systemic juvenile rheumatoid arthritis (Still's disease) in the adult. AOSD is a diagnosis of exclusion. The clinical features include a high spiking fever to 39°C in the evenings, usually accompanied by a sore throat and rash. The rash has been classically described as an evanescent, salmon-colored eruption. More generally, it is noted to be a subtle, nonconfluent, erythematous, maculopapular eruption occurring most often on the torso and the upper extremities. The musculoskeletal manifestations are prominent with arthralgia, myalgia, and an oligoarticular or polyarticular arthritis commonly affecting the knees, wrists, ankles, and small joints of the hands. Lymphadenopathy and hepatosplenomegaly are among other common manifestations. Laboratory tests usually reveal an elevated white blood count to greater than 15,000/mm³, high ESR, mild anemia, and hepatocellular dysfunction. An elevation in the serum ferritin level may be helpful in the diagnosis.[17]

Many of these patients do well. The disease has a waxing and waning course. Twenty percent of patients do well with NSAIDs alone. The remainder require at least a short course of glucocorticoids. Of patients 5 or more years from the initial diagnosis, 50% no longer are receiving therapy, have less disability than patients with rheumatoid arthritis or SLE, and have similar socioeconomic status to same-sex siblings.[17]

SYSTEMIC LUPUS ERYTHEMATOSUS, DERMATOMYOSITIS, POLYMYOSITIS, RHEUMATOID ARTHRITIS, AND MIXED CONNECTIVE TISSUE DISEASE

SLE is the most difficult condition to diagnose because it can present so often in unusual syndromes. Although most commonly the disease presents with fatigue, mild fever, photosensitivity, arthralgia, and a malar rash, it is known that severe headache, psychosis, cardiomyopathy, glomerulonephritis, seizures, and hemolytic anemia can be isolated presentations of this autoimmune disease (see Chapter 27).[18] Deposition of immune complexes within vascular walls generates inflammation. Antinuclear antibodies should be positive in 98% of cases. Leukopenia in a clinical setting where leukocytosis should be expected can be an indication of SLE.

RA rarely presents initially as an acute febrile illness. Once established, however, especially in patients with high titers of rheumatoid factor and acute-phase reactants, RA can have febrile crises (see Chapter 25). Signs of muscle inflammation (i.e., an elevated creatine kinase) in the presence of proximal muscle weakness is sound evidence for myositis, although all of the connective tissue diseases (i.e., SLE, scleroderma, RA) can have myositis as a major manifestation (see Chapter 29). An overlap syndrome, mixed connective tissue disease (MCTD), can present as a mixture of RA, SLE, scleroderma, or myositis; alternatively, it can appear predominantly as only one of these syndromes. The diagnosis should be considered when there is an overlap of symptoms and signs. MCTD is defined by a laboratory parameter: high titers of serum antibodies against ribonuclear proteins.[19]

ACUTE RHEUMATIC FEVER

Acute rheumatic disease is rarely seen de novo in adults. However, the diagnosis should be suspected in any person with an acute febrile illness, migratory polyarthritis, and pain in joints out of proportion to inflammation.

SUBACUTE OR CHRONIC DISEASE ASSOCIATED WITH ARTHROPATHY

Patients with subacute or chronic disease associated with arthropathy do not present acutely to hospitals or emergency departments; they are seen more often in outpatient facilities. They can have complaints referable to many organ systems not clearly related to joints. Many patients have known diagnoses that have no immediate association in the physician's or patient's mind with the arthritis. In addition, any of the processes

described previously in the differential diagnosis of acute febrile illnesses may present in indolent fashion, including sepsis, vasculitis, and malignancy as well as less severe processes.

Amyloidosis

Although there are at least 15 different amyloid proteins that are expressed clinically as multiple clinical syndromes ranging from Alzheimer's disease to familial polyneuropathy, joint involvement is associated primarily with AL, the amyloid generated by abnormal lymphocytes and dysproteinemias, and with the amyloid derived from β_2-microglobulin in patients with chronic renal failure.[20] In AL disease, renal failure, cardiomyopathy, and, less often, neuropathy and a boggy synovitis are the usual presentations. Carpal tunnel syndrome can be caused by amyloid. In patients with renal disease, usually on dialysis, a syndrome of joint pain, carpal tunnel syndrome, and osteonecrosis is seen with β_2-microglobulin in the tissues, including synovium. The amyloid that usually develops in patients with long-standing rheumatoid arthritis is derived from the acute-phase reactant protein, serum amyloid A (SAA) protein.

The diagnosis of amyloid can be made conclusively only by examination of tissues using Congo Red and other stains. Treatment is difficult at best. Therapy with anticancer drugs is often initiated, with little evidence for significant beneficial effects. Colchicine has been advocated as an adjunctive therapy, based on its capacity to prevent proteins from being released from cells after biosynthesis.[21]

Behçet's Disease

About half of patients with Behçet's disease, a painful and chronic syndrome, have arthritis, especially when the disease is active.[22] Of those, around half have more than one joint involved. Synovial analysis shows moderate inflammation. The major clinical features are recurrent, painful, aphthous mouth and genital ulcerations, posterior uveitis or retinal vasculitis, pathergic responses to skin pricks, deep vein phlebitis, and aseptic meningitis. The pathology is an immune-mediated vasculitis. Treatment is by glucocorticoid palliation and, in severe cases, by using cytotoxic agents, such as chlorambucil, methotrexate, and cyclosporine.

Crystal Synovitis

Calcium pyrophosphate deposition disease (CPPD) can mimic RA when it appears as a subacute polyarticular disease. Pathologically the offending crystals activate synovial lining cells to produce cytokines similar to those found in rheumatoid arthritis (see Chapter 30). Therefore, when the synovial lining is chronically exposed to calcium pyrophosphate deposition disease crystals, the end result is a synovitis similar to rheumatoid arthritis. Chronic tophaceous gout can have the same effect but is more unusual in developed countries since the beginning of widespread use of allopurinol to control serum urate levels.[23]

Endocrine Syndromes

Almost every endocrine disease has manifestations within connective tissue, a fact that emphasizes the impact of hormones as well as cytokines on bones and joints. Rarely are these effects acute, but in all of them there can be substantial morbidity.[24]

DIABETES MELLITUS

Slow, progressive contractures of flexor tendons in the palm are associated with dermal fibrosis that is similar to scleroderma. This limitation of finger extension is linked with duration of diabetes mellitus and retinal and vascular complications. Calcific peritendinitis of the shoulder that can lead to adhesive capsulitis is more common in diabetics than in the general population. Microvascular disease can lead to resorption of toes in these patients (diabetic osteolysis), and neurovascular disease can produce rapid destruction of joints with much associated new bone proliferation (Charcot joint). Diffuse idiopathic skeletal hyperostosis (DISH) is manifest more in diabetics than in most others. This process of new bone proliferation in the axial skeleton and pelvis can produce a clinical picture that resembles seronegative spondyloarthropathy and causes much limitation of activities and discomfort in these patients.

HYPERPARATHYROIDISM

Marked osteoporosis, a syndrome of painless muscle weakness, and a predisposition to developing CPPD are associated with hyperparathyroidism. In secondary hyperparathyroidism generated by chronic renal disease, an erosive process involving the hands, clavicle, and axial skeleton can be found.

HYPERTHYROIDISM

Soft tissue swelling, clubbing, and periostitis of metacarpal joints are seen in Graves' disease in rare instances. Painless myopathy in hyperthyroidism is promptly reversed by corrective therapy. Because anti-DNA antibodies are found in many Graves' disease patients, this diagnosis should be ruled out in patients with an autoantibody profile suggestive of SLE but with no clinical findings to support the diagnosis of SLE.

HYPOTHYROIDISM

An interesting association with hypothyroidism is with the excess accumulation of thick, almost gelatinous, synovial fluid, sometimes linked with CPPD. Patients with relatively acute Hashimoto's thyroiditis can have a synovitis that resembles mild rheumatoid disease. Hypothyroidism has a predilection to develop

carpal tunnel syndrome. In untreated hypothyroidism, there can be elevated creatine kinase levels in plasma not associated with clinical muscle disease.

ACROMEGALY

The reason that hands grow bigger in acromegaly is not that bones are growing longer; growth plates are closed in adults and are not reactivated by growth hormone or other stimuli. Rather, articular cartilage in all joints begins to proliferate, as does a propensity to develop osteophytes at joint margins. The abnormal hyaline cartilage develops fissures, and osteoarthritis develops. CPPD is more common in acromegaly than in the normal population, and the carpal tunnel syndrome develops in as many as 50% of acromegalics because there is no room for proliferating soft tissue in the wrist into which to expand.

Erosive Inflammatory Osteoarthritis

Erosive inflammatory osteoarthritis has features of both osteoarthritis and an inflammatory synovitis, such as rheumatoid arthritis.[25] It has the following characteristics:

- Peak appearance in middle-aged women, whose mothers have had similar problems
- Restriction largely to proximal interphalangeal joints, distal interphalangeal joints, first carpometacarpal joint, and knees
- On physical examination, Heberden's nodes with decreased range of motion of the distal interphalangeal joints, bony ankylosis, and proliferation at the proximal interphalangeal joints with little evidence for synovitis

Despite the absence of palpable synovitis and the presence of accentuated distal interphalangeal joint disease, normal ESR, and negative tests for rheumatoid factor, these patients frequently are given an erroneous diagnosis of rheumatoid arthritis.

Familial Mediterranean Fever

Familial Mediterranean fever is a rare episodic syndrome that rarely involves more than three joints. The majority of cases are in Sephardic Jews. The arthritis occurs when the patient develops attacks of fever, peritonitis, or pleuritis. The synovitis is not erosive, but there can be periarticular demineralization. Data support the use of colchicine (0.5 to 2.0 mg/d) to decrease the frequency of attacks and to postpone the complication of amyloidosis, which affects numerous patients.

Hemochromatosis

Hemochromatosis is an iron overload syndrome in which the excess deposits of ferrous/ferric ions in articular cartilage interfere with the normal anionic charge distribution in this sensitive tissue, creating a milieu for CPPD and osteoarthritis to develop. Hemochromatosis always should be ruled out when a patient presents with osteoarthritis in an unusual joint (e.g., metacarpophalangeal joints, shoulders, ankles, elbows). In some individuals, the appearance of CPPD and osteoarthritis can be the presenting symptoms, before liver, pancreas, or cardiac involvement becomes symptomatic.[26]

Hemoglobinopathies

In homozygous SS disease, the microvascular occlusions caused by the rigid cell membranes can occasionally induce a destructive arthropathy similar to that seen in rheumatoid arthritis. In most patients, however, the joint symptoms reflect osteonecrosis and periosteal new bone formation near or in condyles of long bones.

Hemophilic Arthropathy

Hemophilic arthropathy refers to the heritable deficiency of factor VIII (or, less frequently, factor IX) that frequently results in bleeding into joints as synovium is mildly traumatized during normal functions. The iron in the red blood cells, in addition to becoming deposited in cartilage and creating conditions for osteoarthritis to develop, is sufficient to stimulate synovial cell proliferation resembling rheumatoid arthritis. The resulting joint destruction can be rapid and complete, with striking loss of function. Large joints are involved much more frequently than small ones.

Intermittent Hydrarthrosis

Intermittent hydrarthrosis, similar to palindromic rheumatism, is an episodic syndrome. Seen in young women, frequently adolescents, it is characterized by weakly inflammatory synovitis with significant effusions in the knees primarily (Fig. 18–3). There is discomfort and stiffness, but no proliferative synovitis develops, and there are no residual abnormalities between attacks (weeks to months). Biopsy specimens of synovium show a mild inflammation, dilated capillaries and venules, and minimal synovial proliferation.

Multicentric Reticulohistiocytosis

Although multicentric reticulohistiocytosis is an extremely rare syndrome, it is interesting because of its relevance to the pathogenesis of joint destruction in rheumatoid arthritis. It is marked by infiltration into the synovium of multinucleate lipid-laden histiocytes that produce large amounts of metalloproteases. There are small nodular skin lesions on the hands containing the same cells. The destructive *lesions* in the hands produce an *opera glass hand (main en lorgnette),* another name for *arthritis mutilans.*

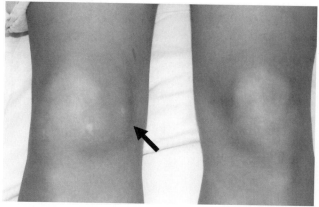

Figure 18–3. Intermittent hydrarthrosis. This 17-year-old woman had periodic flares of swelling in the right knee, with return to normal after several days of observation, rest, and application of cold. Joint fluid consistently revealed 2500 to 4000 white blood count; no organisms were cultured, crystals were not seen. The loss of concavity (*arrow*) below the medial border of the patella is a sign of intra-articular fluid, 10 to 20 mL.

Parkinson's Disease

Few physicians generally think of joint deformities in association with Parkinson's disease, but along with tremor or rigidity or both in this process, there is a predilection for developing swan-neck deformities of the fingers. The difference between this abnormality and that related to inflammatory synovitis is the lack of any soft tissue swelling at any of the joints.

Polychondritis

Polychondritis is a rare syndrome but fascinating because of evidence that it involves an autoimmune attack on articular cartilage and fibrocartilage. This process, often referred to as *relapsing polychondritis,* begins most often in middle age and has an equal sex distribution, in contrast to most diffuse autoimmune syndromes that are more common in women. Symptoms usually begin with symptomatic inflammation of the cartilage of the ear (Fig. 18–4). The entire ear except for the earlobe can be red and tender. Polyarthritis, nasal or tracheal chondritis, episcleritis, and pulmonary inflammation secondary to bronchial cartilage collapse and secretion accumulation are additional common manifestations.

Reactive Arthritis

Reactive arthritis syndromes are the *B27-associated syndromes.* Although often presenting as back pain and stiffness with evidence for sacroiliitis, reactive arthritis can present as peripheral joint disease primarily involving large joints. A Schober test is often positive (Fig. 18–5). In all patients with arthritis, a careful history should be taken to identify back pain, a recent gastroenteritis (Reiter's syndrome), any crusting or proliferative

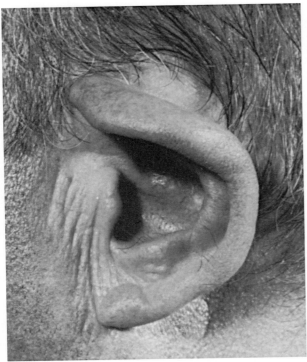

Figure 18–4. Distortion and collapse of the external ear in a patient with relapsing polychondritis. (From Hochberg MC: Relapsing polychondritis. In Kelly WN, Harris ED, Ruddy S, Sledge CB, eds: Textbook of Rheumatology, 5th ed. Philadelphia, WB Saunders, 1997, p. 1405.)

lesion suggestive of psoriasis, or chronic diarrhea or abdominal cramping (reactive arthritis associated with ulcerative colitis or Crohn's disease). Rarely (<1 in 50,000), a patient may have both rheumatoid arthritis and a reactive arthritis. Enteric infections are complicated occasionally by inflammatory joint disease. Arthritis (in large joints) can follow infections with *Yersinia enterocolitica, Campylobacter jejuni, Salmonella, Shigella,* and *Chlamydia* species.

PAIN IN OR AROUND ONE JOINT

When a patient complains of the acute onset of pain in or around one joint, the first questions must be: "Did you hurt yourself?" "Have you done anything in the past few days to put a strain on that joint?" "What have you been doing in the past several days?" The reason for these questions is to rule in or out the possibility that this pain represents a tissue response to overuse or direct trauma (see Chapters 15 and 16). Tendinitis and bursitis are the most frequent diagnoses made. It is crucial to rule out an intra-articular process because an acute painful joint may represent one of the few rheumatologic emergencies—infection in the joint space. Acute gout is in second place in the list of concerns, principally because there are effective treatments for gout that can minimize morbidity.

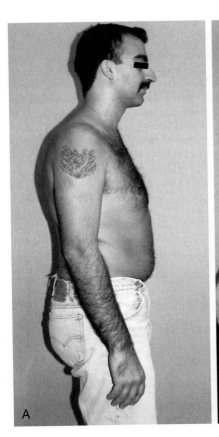
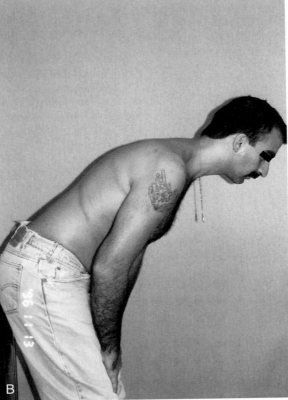

Figure 18–5. *A,* This 42-year-old Iranian man developed Reiter's syndrome after a severe *Salmonella* infection. Back pain, conjunctivitis, and scaling lesions of keratodermia blenorrhagica were the manifestations. He appears normal in the upright position. *B,* When attempting forward flexion with knees straight, he lacks flexibility of the lumbar spine. His Schober test measurements (see Chapter 2 and 26) moved from 10 to 12 cm. The normal flexion moves skin markings from 10 to at least 14 cm.

INTRA-ARTICULAR CAUSES OF MONARTICULAR ARTHRITIS

Sepsis

The septic joint is a medical emergency. For many reasons, few of which are known, the knee is most often the site. This may be related to the greater surface area of synovium in this joint. Most septic joints are seeded from hematogenous spread. Predisposing factors, with simple examples of the condition, are as follows (see also Chapter 33):

- Joint with a proliferative synovitis
  - Rheumatoid arthritis
  - Psoriatic arthritis
- Immunocompromised state
  - Acquired immunodeficiency syndrome (AIDS)
  - Chemotherapy for malignancy
  - Immunoglobulin deficiency
- Diabetes mellitus
- Sexual promiscuity
- Intravenous drug use
- Septicemia from another source
  - Pneumonia
  - Cellulitis
- Direct penetration
  - Rose thorn from kneeling in a garden
- Advanced age
- Alcoholism
- Joint prosthesis

A great many septic joints are not recognized until weeks after the process begins. One factor is the anatomy. Joint sepsis begins in the synovium. The synovium is surrounded by a thick, collagenous joint capsule and overlying subcutaneous tissue and skin. Although the infection generates synovial fluid and inflammation, there can be virtually no warmth or redness observed in the overlying skin until days after the infection begins. Warm, red skin over part of a painful joint implies that the pathology may be cellulitis or a process such as erythema nodosum rather than synovial inflammation. A useful finding on physical examination is that when synovium is involved in the area of a painful joint, passive as well as active motion of the joint is painful, whereas in subcutaneous inflammation, passive motion may not generate an increase in pain, but active motion is exquisitely painful. The varieties of infection and treatment are outlined in Chapter 33.

Gout

Gout can mimic infection and vice versa (see Chapter 30). Gout usually occurs in middle-aged and older persons because serum urate rises with age and with medications (e.g., thiazide diuretics) taken more by older patients. As well, it takes years for tissue deposits to form once serum urate has risen above normal levels. Gout as a cause of monarthritis should be suspected in the following contexts:

- Previous attacks of acute arthritis in the same joint
- Coexisting diabetes and hypertension in a man
- Recent heavy alcoholic intake
- Recent vigorous exercise or dehydration
- Family history of gout
- Salicylate ingestion (>100 mg to <1.2 g/d)

Although there are other more rare causes, many of which are hereditary and others of which are related to less commonly used drugs (e.g., cyclosporine), the above-listed situations are the most commonly found predisposing factors.

Pseudogout, caused by an inflammatory response to CPPD crystals that are shed from sites in cartilage, is generally not as acute as gout. Exceptions to this, for obscure reasons, include the acute painful inflammation of wrist joints in elderly women who often have CPPD crystals seen on examination of joint fluid and degenerative changes in wrist bones seen on radiographs, with or without visible chondrocalcinosis (see Chapter 31).

It is difficult to overemphasize the importance of aspiration and analysis of joint fluid when a patient presents with acute monarthritis. The details of joint, fluid analysis are outlined in Chapter 6. The minimum essential analyses are as follows:

OBSERVATION. Is the fluid clear, pale yellow, and transparent (normal), or does it have various degrees of cloudiness representing cellular elements (abnormal)? Blood (not related to a traumatic tap) means hemorrhage from synovial vessels. In effusions secondary to acute trauma that have fat globules visible, fracture of the subchondral bone into marrow is a concern.

GRAM STAIN. Although sensitivity is not 100% even for bacterial pathogens, Gram stain provides rapid indication of infection.

CULTURE. A few cubic centimeters of fluid should be immediately injected into a sterile tube for culture for bacteria, including *N. gonorrhoeae.*

WHITE BLOOD CELL COUNT AND DIFFERENTIAL. The following rough guides are useful:

- 200 to 1500 cells/mm^3: Trauma or osteoarthritis.
- 1500 to 15,000 cells/mm^3: Moderate inflammation, seen occasionally in gout and more commonly in pseudogout. Of the septic processes, gonococcal infection is more likely to have only moderate numbers of cells, in contrast to infection by organisms such as *S. aureus* or *Streptococcus pyogenes,* which generate high numbers (usually >40,000/mm^3) of white blood cells in synovial fluid.
- >15,000 cells/mm^3: Moderate to severe inflammation. When the cell count in synovial fluid exceeds 50,000/mm^3, the possibilities for diagnosis other than sepsis or gout become diminishingly small. The exception to this is severe and preexisting rheumatoid arthritis. Even in the most intense infections of the joint, white blood cell counts rarely exceed 100,000 cells/mm^3 because plasma leaking from inflamed synovial vessels dilutes the cells.

The percentage of polymorphonuclear leukocytes in synovial fluid almost always is proportional to the total white blood cell count. In fluid containing fewer than 500 cells/mm^3, the percentage of monocytes may equal that of granulocytes, but the great majority of cells are granulocytes once the counts exceed 5000 to 10,000/mm^3.

CRYSTAL EXAMINATION. Although crystals may be visible on a wet mount without using a polarized microscope, the polarization of light through a wet preparation viewed through an oil immersion lens offers the best chance of seeing the needle-shaped sodium urate crystals or the rhomboid, less birefringent crystals of CPPD.

Other Causes of Monarticular Arthritis

None of the following present often as acute synovitis, but each can be a monarticular phenomenon. Rarely, RA or psoriatic arthritis presents as monarthritis. More commonly, Lyme disease or one of the varieties of reactive arthritis (e.g., Reiter's syndrome, ankylosing spondylitis, and the arthritis of inflammatory bowel disease) presents as monarticular arthritis. In children, a form of juvenile arthritis associated with vision-threatening iridocyclitis may present as monarticular disease. An inflammatory but sterile synovitis is seen occasionally in bacterial endocarditis or associated with *N. meningitidis* infections. In adolescents, a usually benign syndrome of knee swelling called *intermittent hydrarthrosis* (see Fig. 18–3) can present as monarticular arthritis; white blood cell count in synovial fluid is non-inflammatory. Although it rarely presents acutely, pigmented villonodular synovitis is usually a monarticular disease dominated by substantial swelling of the joint (usually the knee) often out of proportion to pain. The joint fluid is often bloody or even dark, resembling crankcase oil, a reflection of chronic hemorrhage into the joint. Sarcoidosis can involve one joint, usually in the lower extremity, and is associated with cystic areas of destruction in surrounding bone.

Osteoarthritis, particularly of the hip, begins usually as monarticular disease, and this applies also to degenerative disease of the thumb and knee.

It is estimated that about 10–15% of hip replacement arthroplasties performed each year in the United States are initiated because of osteonecrosis of this joint. Osteonecrosis develops as death of bone marrow and trabecular elements caused by direct microvascular injury, subclinical microthromboses, fat embolism, or gas embolism. Osteonecrosis is clinically associated with glucocorticoid administration, ethanol abuse, hip fracture or dislocation, Gaucher's disease, liver disease, hemoglobinopathy, gout, and radiculopathy.

SOFT TISSUE RHEUMATISM

Soft tissue rheumatism represents a group of diverse entities involving muscle, tendon, ligament, and bursa. As a group, it accounts for some of the most frequent complaints encountered by primary care clinicians. Soft tissue rheumatism can also account for as much as 25% of all hospital consultations for the rheumatic disorders and be responsible for a significant loss of working days annually. There are no universally accepted diagnostic criteria for soft tissue rheumatic conditions; thus the prevalence of soft tissue rheumatism is difficult to obtain. PMR, erythema nodosum, myofascial pain syndrome, fibromyalgia, CFS, and metabolic bone disease have been outlined earlier in this chapter.

Minor injury and inflammation of soft tissue can cause significant pain and dysfunction. The soft tissue structures mentioned are common sites of nociceptive pain stimuli and functional impairment in patients with soft tissue injuries (see Chapters 7 and 15). As a group, these conditions are often misunderstood and neglected because patients and physicians often attribute the symptoms to arthritis. A careful history and detailed physical examination are the keys to the diagnosis of soft tissue rheumatism, whereas extensive laboratory testing and radiographs are not particularly helpful.

Local soft tissue conditions can also be categorized into tendinitis, bursitis, entrapment neuropathy, and enthesopathy. Local conditions in the shoulder include rotator cuff tendinitis, subacromial bursitis, adhesive capsulitis, impingement syndrome, and bicipital tendinitis. In the elbow, they include olecranon bursitis and lateral and medial epicondylitis. In the wrist and hand, they include deQuervain's tenosynovitis and carpal tunnel syndrome. In the hip, they include trochanteric bursitis and ischial bursitis. In the knee, they include prepatellar bursitis, patellar tendinitis, and anserine bursitis. Regional conditions may include myofascial pain syndrome. Well-known generalized conditions include fibromyalgia and CFS. In the following descriptions of specific syndromes, no mention of hand and wrist problems is made; these are covered in Chapter 23.

Tissue Response to Injury

Acute injury to soft tissues results in an inflammatory response and subsequent repair processes. Three stages of soft tissue response are observed after acute injury in the soft tissues: inflammatory stage, proliferative stage, and maturation stage.[27] The inflammatory stage begins immediately after acute injury. Its course can run from 2 days to 2 weeks. Inflammatory mediators are released from injured cells and evoke a cascading response, which subsequently results in swelling and edema.

Rest is the mainstay of treatment of any injury in the inflammatory stage. This can be achieved by taping, splinting, or casting as well as, most importantly, by avoidance of the provocative activities. Ice, elevation, and compression are used as adjuncts to limit inflammation (see Chapter 15). NSAIDs can be used to reduce the inflammation and the associated pain. Analgesics can also be provided for pain.

The second stage of repair after injury is the proliferative stage.[27] It lasts 1 to 2 weeks, during which time collagen is produced by fibroblasts, and blood vessels are stimulated to grow into the injured area. These products are immature and disorganized and thus are susceptible to further injury. Recurrent injury can occur if the provocative activities are resumed too early.

Passive range of motion and active but pain-free mobilization aid remodeling of newly produced collagen tissue, help prevent adhesions, and reduce edema. It also prevents disuse atrophy and contracture and promotes tissue healing. Modalities such as a heat pad, electrical stimulation, and ultrasound can be used in physical therapy once the acute phase has subsided. NSAIDs may also be helpful in alleviating symptoms, acting as analgesics at this stage rather than as anti-inflammatories.

The third stage of repair after injury is the maturation stage and continues for 6 to 12 weeks. Fibroblasts help remodel the injured site by producing organized collagen.

Flexibility exercises and strengthening exercises, starting with isometric contractions followed by a gradually escalating exercise program, should be started. Muscle tissue responds to exercise with an increase in mass and strength. Although the response to injury is similar in muscle, tendon, and ligament, muscle fibers have the ability to regenerate. New muscle fibers can be seen within days after injury to replace the injured fibers that are being removed by macrophages. Scar tissue results if the rate of collagen exceeds new myofibril formation.

Shoulder Pain

The shoulder itself is a complicated structure and actually consists of many joints, including the acromioclavicular joint, sternoclavicular joint, scapulothoracic joint, and glenohumeral joint. Paramount in its design is the need for stability in multiple planes of motion (see Chapter 3). The rotator cuff, a soft tissue structure composed of tendons from various muscle groups (supraspinatus, subscapularis, teres minor, and infraspinatus), is chiefly responsible for providing that stability. Subsequently a large number of soft tissue disorders involving the shoulder are related to abnormalities or inflammation within the rotator cuff or surrounding bursae. Different areas of localized pain in the shoulder and their anatomic correlations are shown in Figure 18–6.

Inflammation of the tendons that compose the rotator cuff can occur for many reasons. Inflammation may occur after repetitive use or overuse, secondary to trauma including impingement, and related to crystalline deposition and calcification. It is the most common cause of shoulder discomfort and may, in turn, lead to secondary inflammation of the subacromial bursa and the bicipital tendon. Some patients may present with complaints of persistent pain with motion, whereas others complain of pain or tenderness to palpation or just while lying on the shoulder in bed. Rotator cuff injury associated with overuse syndromes is reviewed in Chapter 15.

Although the diagnosis of the type of shoulder problem can usually be made from the patient's history,

the physical examination is essential to confirm initial suspicions. The examination should start with simple observation: How is the arm held? Does the patient appear to be able to move it? With the shoulder disrobed, is there evidence of a winged scapula (no longer tethered to the back by muscle, suggesting muscular dystrophy, myositis, or muscle tear); a bulge along the humerus (suggesting a torn biceps tendon); or atrophy of the deltoid or the rotator cuff, particularly in comparison to the other shoulder?

Palpation is the next maneuver. Does palpation elicit tenderness and pain over the tendons, bursae (subacromial and deltoid), or joints? Tenderness and pain usually imply tendinitis, bursitis, or arthritis. The goal is to assess the limits of motion with abduction/adduction, flexion/extension, and internal/external rotation of the shoulder. Pain on passive range of motion often suggests arthritis or soft tissue impingement. When range of motion lessens with active motion, soft tissue injury or inflammation should be suspected. Particularly useful to assess rotator cuff inflammation or injury is active motion against resistance. Resistance to abduction isolates the supraspinatus, whereas resistance to internal rotation isolates the subscapularis and bicipital tendon. Resistance to external rotation stresses the infraspinatus and teres minor. A thorough examination including these maneuvers should help the physician differentiate between arthritis, tendinitis, and bursitis. Rotator cuff tendinitis itself is covered extensively in Chapter 15. Variations on rotator cuff tendinitis, including impingement syndrome, adhesive capsulitis, and bicipital tendinitis, are covered subsequently.

REFLEX SYMPATHETIC DYSTROPHY

Reflex sympathetic dystrophy (RSD) is often confused with joint disease, particularly in its early stages and when it involves the shoulder. Its cause is unknown but is clearly related in some fashion to the sympathetic nervous system. Relatively minor trauma often triggers reflex sympathetic dystrophy. It begins with diffuse swelling, pain, erythema of skin, and radiographic evidence of demineralization of all or part of an extremity. If left untreated, atrophy can develop, and the involved arm or lower leg becomes cold and shiny with atrophy of muscles and skin. Recovery during the early stages is possible with proper pain control, nerve blocks, and high doses of anti-inflammatory drugs. In the atrophic stage, therapy is often futile. Evaluation and management of injured joints and those associated with overuse are covered in Chapters 15 and 16.

ROTATOR CUFF IMPINGEMENT SYNDROME

A particular variant of rotator cuff tendinitis has come to be known as *impingement syndrome*. Rotator cuff impingement syndrome represents a syndrome in which the rotator cuff and the subacromial bursa become impinged or caught beneath the anterior edge of the acromion. This disorder has been stratified into three stages: inflammation, degeneration, and attrition.[28] Stage I involves edema and hemorrhage in the

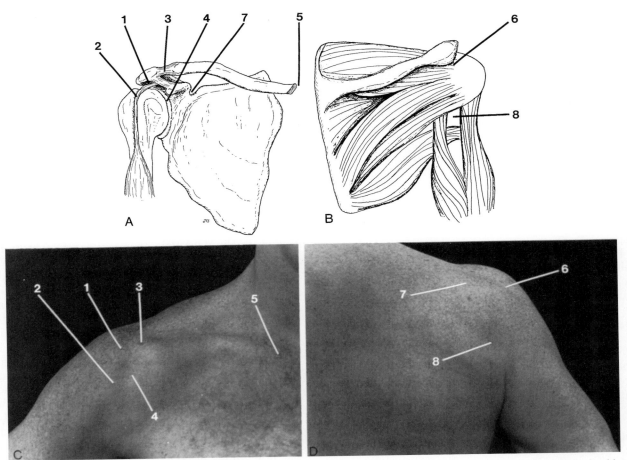

Figure 18–6. Musculoskeletal (*A* and *B*) and topographic (*C* and *D*) areas localizing pain and tenderness associated with specific shoulder problems. *1,* Subacromial space (rotator cuff tendinitis/impingement syndrome, calcific tendinitis, rotator cuff tear). *2,* Bicipital groove (bicipital tendinitis, biceps tendon subluxation and tear). *3,* Acromioclavicular joint. *4,* Anterior glenohumeral joint (glenohumeral arthritis, osteonecrosis, glenoid labrum tears, adhesive capsulitis). *5,* Sternoclavicular joint. *6,* Posterior edge of acromion (rotator cuff tendinitis, calcific tendinitis, rotator cuff tear). *7,* Suprascapular notch (suprascapular nerve entrapment). *8,* Quadrilateral space (axillary nerve entrapment). These areas of pain and tenderness frequently overlap. (From Evaluation of the patient. In Kelly WN, Harris ED, Ruddy Sledge CB, eds: Textbook of Rheumatology, 5th ed. Philadelphia, WB Saunders, 1997, p 414.)

rotator cuff. It usually occurs in younger individuals (<25 years old) who are active, particularly those with excessive overhead arm use. Stage II represents progression from inflammation to fibrosis and tendinitis. This progression tends to occur in the 25- to 40-year-old group after repeated episodes of mechanical impingement. Stage III, the final stage of impingement syndrome, involves rotator cuff tears, biceps rupture, and bony change. This stage tends to occur in individuals older than age 40 after repeated impingement. In addition, patients with significant inflammatory disease of the shoulder joint (e.g., rheumatoid arthritis) may accelerate quickly to stage III.

Patients suffering from impingement syndrome usually complain of either isolated pain and tenderness along the anterior edge of the acromion or of diffuse pain along the lateral aspect of the acromion. One helpful maneuver in assessing for rotator cuff tendinitis and impingement syndrome is the impingement sign illustrated in Figure 18–6.

Plain radiographs can be obtained to look for crystalline deposition or for bony pathology, such as sub-

acromial sclerosis or cystic changes involving the greater tuberosity. Early on, there are few changes; however, late in disease, change can become more apparent. Magnetic resonance imaging has also been widely used to investigate the underlying pathology of tendinitis and partial or complete tears of the rotator cuff.

Treatment in early stages usually involves rest and the use of NSAIDs. Stretching of the posterior capsule of the shoulder and strengthening of the rotator cuff can be useful. An injection of glucocorticoid into the subacromial bursa is usually effective and can be performed if the patient does not respond to an exercise program. Surgical consultation should be obtained for patients with rotator cuff tears or for patients with tendinitis who fail to respond to conservative treatments.

ADHESIVE CAPSULITIS

Adhesive capsulitis, also known as *frozen shoulder,* is characterized by a significant loss of range of motion in the glenohumeral joint. It can occur after repetitive or even single trauma, or it can be related to other periarticular inflammatory conditions, such as rotator cuff tendinitis, subacromial bursitis, and bicipital tendinitis. It rarely occurs before age 40 and is found more often in women than in men. Most patients are in the later decades of life. It is associated with restricted motion of the glenohumeral joint with both active and passive motion, with pain occurring at the extremes of motion.

Clinically the patient presents with loss of range of motion and with discomfort in the shoulder. Activities of daily living, such as dressing, grooming, and personal hygiene, become difficult because of the pain and the limitation in the range of motion of the shoulder. Physical examination shows gross limitations of the shoulder movement in virtually all planes of motion, with external rotation and abduction being the most affected.

The treatment initially involves pain control with the use of NSAIDs or analgesics. A progressive mobilization program to restore function should be started that includes pendulum swing and circular swing exercises. Strengthening exercises are also important and can be performed as short arc movement using an elastic band within the pain-free range. If it can be identified, the underlying problem should be corrected.

BICIPITAL TENDINITIS

Bicipital tendinitis commonly occurs in conjunction with primary impingement or inflammation of the rotator cuff.[28] Given the intimate relationship of the biceps tendon with the rotator cuff, trauma or inflammation to one often elicits difficulties in the other. The patient usually presents with a history of repetitive overhead arm use and anterior shoulder pain, which is worse with motion.

Physical examination reveals local tenderness at the bicipital groove. The area of tenderness moves as the arm is abducted and externally rotated. Pain can often be reproduced as the tendon moves under the examiner's fingers. Yergason's maneuver (e.g., supination of the forearm against resistance, with the elbow at 90 degrees) usually elicits pain over the bicipital tendon. Alternatively, pain may be reproduced at the bicipital groove when a patient places his or her hands on the head and abducts the arms (Ludington's sign) or by flexing the shoulder against resistance with the elbow extended (Speed's test).

Patients usually respond to rest, moist heat, ultrasound, and NSAIDs. Gentle passive and active range-of-motion exercise can be helpful and should be introduced slowly. Glucocorticoid injection into the bicipital tendon sheath may be considered; however, surrounding neurovascular bundles and the potential risk of tendon rupture if glucocorticoids are injected into tendons make this somewhat risky (see Chapter 6). Alternatively, a glucocorticoid injection can be given in the subacromial bursa and may provide some benefit with less risk. Although bicipital tendinitis can occur independently, it may occur in relation to a coexisting rotator

cuff tendinitis, and therapy should be designed to have an impact on both.

Elbow Pain

OLECRANON BURSITIS

Olecranon bursitis is the inflammation of the bursa that overlies the olecranon process of the ulna. It commonly occurs related to trauma and underlying rheumatic processes. Some cases are either directly or indirectly related to strenuous activities, whereas others are related to repetitive direct pressure on the bursa. Occasionally a septic bursitis develops. The patient complains of pain at the posterior aspect of the elbow, which is aggravated by flexion of the elbow past 90 degrees. Local swelling and redness are usually present.

Physical examination discloses a boggy, swollen, and tender olecranon bursa; the range of motion of the elbow is normal. This finding may help when trying to distinguish bursal inflammation from an effusion within the joint itself. Aspiration of the bursa is necessary to rule out infection, and fluid should be sent for a cell count, crystal examination, Gram stain, and culture. If an infection is present, the most common cause would be *S. aureus*, requiring antibiotic treatment. Otherwise, a compression bandage is recommended to help prevent recurrence of swelling. An injection of a glucocorticoid, such as 20 mg triamcinolone hexacetonide, should also be considered if the Gram stain is negative because this can lead to dramatic improvement. The periodic application of ice and the use of an elbow pad can help prevent recurrence and offer protection. If infection persists or bursitis becomes recurrent, surgical excision of the bursa may be required.

LATERAL EPICONDYLITIS

Lateral epicondylitis is commonly known as *tennis elbow*. As reviewed in Chapter 15, it is not related to tennis in the majority of patients. Most cases are caused by occupational stress rather than racket sports. The patient may present with pain on the extensor aspect of the forearm that becomes localized to the area of lateral epicondyle. Resisted wrist extension typically reproduces the symptoms. Local tenderness at the lateral epicondyle, or slightly distal to it, helps establish the diagnosis.

The initial treatment is rest to reduce inflammation; however, total immobilization is discouraged so as to prevent muscle atrophy and loss of strength. A cock-up splint can be provided to maintain the wrist in 20 degrees of extension and should be worn for up to 2 weeks. Ice and NSAIDs can be useful to control pain and inflammation. After the initial phase, passive wrist extensor stretches should be implemented. Active wrist exercises are then gradually introduced. Modalities, such as ultrasound, phonophoresis, high-voltage galvanic stimulation, and transcutaneous electrical nerve stimulation, can be incorporated to improve pain control and soft tissue mobility. A counterforce brace or

Approach to the Patient with Musculoskeletal Pain

tennis elbow band can be prescribed to be worn during activities. It has been demonstrated that use of the brace results in an increase in the wrist extension and the grip strength as well as a decrease of symptoms.[29] Local glucocorticoid injection can be added if the treatment progress is slow or the patient is unable to participate in active therapy secondary to pain and inflammation.

MEDIAL EPICONDYLITIS

Medial epicondylitis is popularly known as *golfer's elbow*. The patient presents with complaints of pain at the medial aspect of the elbow. Resistance to wrist flexion and pronation reproduces pain. Local tenderness at the medial epicondyle, or slightly distal to it, confirms the diagnosis. The treatment principles for lateral epicondylitis can be similarly applied in treating medial epicondylitis. A splint can be fabricated to maintain the wrist in 10 degrees of flexion to provide relative rest in the acute phase. Passive stretching of the wrist flexors can be started as the pain abates. Active wrist exercises should be introduced slowly with an attention to the wrist flexors and pronators.

Hip and Buttock Pain

TROCHANTERIC BURSITIS

Trochanteric bursitis is a common problem. Patients present with pain over the greater trochanter. Discomfort can be aggravated by climbing stairs or by lying on the affected side. Physical examination discloses tenderness over the greater trochanter, which can sometimes be exacerbated with hip flexion, abduction, and external rotation. Treatment includes rest, NSAIDs, and glucocorticoid injection.

ISCHIAL BURSITIS

Patients typically complain of buttock pain, which is persistent throughout the day, and patients may find it extremely difficult to sit on one side of the buttock. Physical examination discloses a tender ischial tuberosity. Treatment consists of NSAIDs, stretching of the hamstrings, aspiration of the bursa, and glucocorticoid injection.

Knee Pain

PREPATELLAR BURSITIS

Prepatellar bursitis is also known as *housemaid's knee*. It frequently occurs after direct trauma, such as a fall, or after persistent kneeling at work or prayer. The patient usually presents with swelling and mild pain at the lower aspect of the patella that extends just proximal to the tibial tuberosity. It can often be misdiagnosed as a joint effusion (see Chapter 2).

Physical examination reveals local swelling and tenderness. Erythema and warmth are found less often. Aspiration of the bursa should be performed to rule out infection because this site can frequently become infected after trauma. Conservative treatment measures should be used, including ice, NSAIDs, a knee pad, and avoidance of kneeling. If conservative measures fail, and infection has been excluded, glucocorticoid injection is usually effective.

PATELLAR TENDINITIS

Patellar tendinitis is also known as *jumper's knee*. It usually results from repetitive overloading of the patellar tendon. The patient presents with pain at the inferior aspect of the knee, aggravated by stair climbing, running, or activities such as basketball and tennis. Physical examination frequently discloses a tender patellar tendon at the inferior pole of the patella. Treatment consists of rest, NSAIDs, therapeutic modalities, stretching exercises for the quadriceps, and general lower extremity strengthening.

ANSERINE BURSITIS

The anserine bursa lies near the insertion of the tendons of the gracilis, sartorius, and semitendinosus muscles on the anterior-medial side of the proximal tibia. Patients complain of pain on the anterior-medial aspect of the knee. On examination, an area of tenderness is found 2 inches below the knee, medial to the tibial tuberosity. Treatment of anserine bursitis consists of rest, ice, NSAIDs, and strengthening exercises for the hamstrings. Local injection of glucocorticoids can be effective in reducing pain and inflammation.

Pain in the Foot and Ankle

Because disorders of the foot and ankle are both common and complex, two sections of Chapter 21, one written by an orthopaedic surgeon and one by a podiatrist, are devoted to these topics.

The Appendix to this chapter presents a review of several soft tissue problems.

REFERENCES

1. Vecchio P: Is it arthritis? Beware the mimics. Aust Fam Physician 27:17–20, 1998.
2. Lawrence RC, Helmick CG, Arnett FC, et al: Estimates of the prevalence of arthritis and selected musculoskeletal disorders in the United States. Arthritis Rheum 41:778–799, 1998.
3. Cancrini C, Angelini F, Colavita M, et al: Erythema nodosum: A presenting sign of early onset sarcoidosis. Clin Exp Rheumatol 16:337–339, 1998.
4. Simons DG: Clinical and etiological update of myofascial pain from trigger points. J Musculoskeletal Pain 4:93–121, 1996.
5. Hong CZ, Torigoe Y, Yu J: The localized twitch responses in responsive bands of rabbit skeletal muscle fibers are related to the reflexes at spinal cord level. J Musculoskeletal Pain 3:15–33, 1995.
6. Bennett RM: The fibromyalgia syndrome. In Kelley WN, Harris ED Jr, Ruddy S, Sledge CB, eds: Textbook of Rheumatology, 5th ed. Philadelphia, WB Saunders, 1997, pp 511–520.
7. Bengtson A, Henrickson KG, Larsson J: Muscle biopsy in fibromyalgia. Scand J Rheumatol 15:1–6, 1986.

8. Weigent DA, Bradley LA, Blalock JE, et al: Current concepts in the pathophysiology of abnormal pain perception in fibromyalgia. Am J Med Sci 315:405–412, 1998.

9. Alarcon GS, Bradley LA: Advances in the treatment of fibromyalgia: Current status and future directions. Am J Med Sci 315:397–404, 1998.

10. Goshorn RK: Chronic fatigue syndrome: A review for clinicians. Semin Neurol 18:237–242, 1998.

11. Jain SS, DeLisa JA: Chronic fatigue syndrome: A literature review from a physiatric perspective. Am J Phys Med Rehabil 77:160–167, 1998.

12. Oberklaid F, Amos D, Liu C, et al: "Growing pains": Clinical and behavioral correlates in a community sample. J Dev Behav Pediatr 18:102–106, 1997.

13. Balkhy HH, Sabella C, Goldfarb J: Parvovirus: A review. Bull Rheum Dis 47:4–9, 1998.

14. Phillips PE: Viral arthritis. Curr Opin Rheumatol 9:337–344, 1997.

15. Isoda K, Mizutani H, Nishiguchi T, et al: EB virus-related angiocentric T-cell lymphoma. Int J Dermatol 37:39–41, 1998.

16. Schleiffer T, Burkhard B, Klooker P, et al: Clinical course and symptomatic prediagnostic period of patients with Wegener's granulomatosis and microscopic polyangiitis. Ren Fail 20:519–532, 1998.

17. Sampalis JS, Esdaile JM, Medsger TA, et al: A controlled study of the long-term prognosis of adult Still's disease. Am J Med 98:384–388, 1995.

18. Lahita RG: Clinical presentation of systemic lupus erythematosus. In Kelley WN, Harris ED Jr, Ruddy S, Sledge CB, eds: Textbook of Rheumatology, 5th ed. Philadelphia, WB Saunders, 1997, pp 1028–1039.

19. Bennett RM: Mixed connective tissue disease and other overlap syndromes. In Kelley WN, Harris ED Jr, Ruddy S, Sledge CB, eds: Textbook of Rheumatology, 5th ed. Philadelphia, WB Saunders, 1997, pp 1065–1078.

20. Husby G: Treatment of amyloidosis and the rheumatologist: State of the art and perspectives for the future. Scand J Rheumatol 27:161–165, 1998.

21. Hawkins PN: The diagnosis, natural history and treatment of amyloidosis. The Goulstonian Lecture 1995. J R Coll Physicians Lond 31:552–560, 1997.

22. Benamour S, Zeroual B, Alaoui FZ: Joint manifestations in Behcet's disease: A review of 340 cases. Rev Rheum Engl Ed 65:299–307, 1998.

23. Wise CM, Agudelo CA: Diagnosis and management of complicated gout. Bull Rheum Dis 47:2–5, 1998.

24. McGuire JL, Lambert RE: Arthropathies associated with endocrine disorders. In Kelley WN, Harris ED Jr, Ruddy S, Sledge CB, eds: Textbook of Rheumatology, 5th ed. Philadelphia, WB Saunders, 1997, pp 1499–1513.

25. Solomon L: Clinical features of osteoarthritis. In Kelley WN, Harris ED Jr, Ruddy S, Sledge CB, eds: Textbook of Rheumatology, 5th ed. Philadelphia, WB Saunders, 1997, pp 1383–1393.

26. Lambert RE, McGuire JL: Iron storage disease. In Kelley WN, Harris ED Jr, Ruddy S, Sledge CB, eds: Textbook of Rheumatology, 5th ed. Philadelphia, WB Saunders 1997, pp 1423–1429.

27. Pitner MA: Pathophysiology of overuse injuries in the hand and wrist. Hand Clin 6:355–364, 1990.

28. Thornhill TS: Shoulder pain. In Kelley WN, Harris ED Jr, Ruddy S, Sledge CB, eds: Textbook of Rheumatology, 5th ed. Philadelphia, WB Saunders, 1997, pp 413–438.

29. Stonecipher DR, Catlin PA: The effect of a forearm strap on wrist extensor strength. J Orthop Sports Phys Ther 6:184–189, 1984.

Approach to the Patient with Musculoskeletal Pain

Algorithm D: Acute Noninflammatory Articular Conditions

If the articular condition is acute and noninflammatory, the provider should determine whether fracture is present or further investigation is needed.

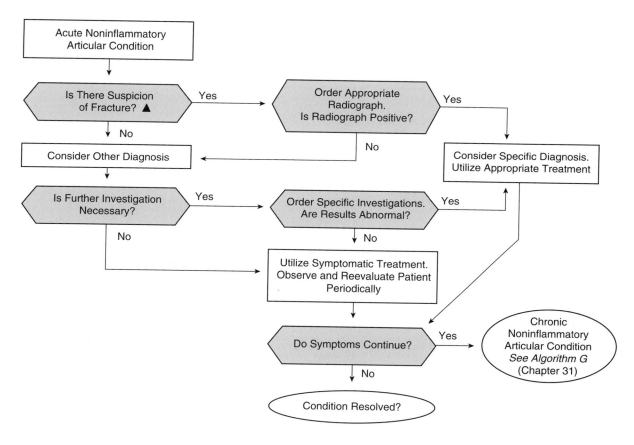

Reprinted with permission from Lipsky PE: Algorithms for the diagnosis and management of musculoskeletal complaints. Am J Med 103(6A): 55S, 63S, 1997.

Table 18A–1. CHARACTERISTICS OF COMMON LOCALIZED NONARTICULAR DISORDERS

Shoulder	Rotator cuff tendinitis (subacromial bursitis)	• Aching and discomfort in subdeltoid region
		  -associated with night pain
		  -aggravated by abduction of arm
		• History of repetitive and strenuous upper limb activity (may be absent in elderly)
		• Onset may be acute or chronic in any age group
		• Consider rotator cuff tear when weakness or wasting is present

	Bicipital tendinitis	• Pain over anterior aspect of shoulder exacerbated by resisted elbow flexion or suppination • Occurs at any age • Night pain is rare • Associated with overuse
	Capsulitis (frozen shoulder)	• Deep pain in shoulder with decreased active and passive movement • Insidious onset in persons >40 yr • Associated with night pain
Elbow	Tennis elbow (lateral epicondylitis)	• Pain and tenderness over lateral epicondyle of the humerus, impairing grip • Aggravated by resisted dorsiflexion of the wrist • Often brought on by overuse in persons >30 yr
	Golfer's elbow (medial epicondylitis)	• Pain and tenderness poorly localized to the medial epicondyle of the humerus • Aggravated by resisted wrist flexion • Associated with overuse
	Olecranon bursitis	• Localized swelling and pain over the olecranon • Pain is usually not aggravated by movement ▲ • 25% of cases may be infected (usually with *Streptococcus aureus*)
Wrist and Hand	deQuervain's tenosynovitis	• Insidious onset of pain over radial aspect of the wrist during pinch grip • Most common in women 30–50 yr old • Related to repetitive strain and chronic overuse
	Trigger finger	• Pain over the flexor tendon of the finger with intermittent locking of the digit in flexion • Related to stenosing tenosynovitis of the flexor tendons of the finger or thumb • Related to overuse trauma from repetitive gripping
	Dupuytren's contracture	• Nodular thickening of the palmar fascia, drawing fingers into flexion of the MCP joints • Usually minimal associated pain

Hip	Trochanteric bursitis	• Deep aching pain on lateral aspect of hip and thigh • Pain is aggravated by activity, often present at night, related to position • More frequent in women • Movement of hip usually normal
Knee	Prepatellar bursitis	• Circumscribed, painful swelling anterior to the patella • Related to recurrent trauma ▲ • May be infected
	Anserine bursitis	• Pain over the medial aspect of the upper tibia
Ankle and Foot	Achilles tendinitis	• Pain, swelling, tenderness near the insertion of the Achilles tendon • Aggravated by dorsiflexion of the ankle • Related to repetitive trauma
	Plantar fasciitis	• Pain on the under surface of the heel on weight bearing • Aggravated by dorsiflexion of the toes • Radiographs may show a plantar spur • Related to repetitive trauma • Related to repetitive trauma

▲ = Requires immediate diagnosis and treatment.

Approach to the Patient with Musculoskeletal Pain

Low Back Pain

Elaine S. Date

Approach to the Patient with Musculoskeletal Pain

Low back pain is a common diagnosis, but causes and efficacy of treatment of low back pain, particularly conservative management techniques, are not clearly understood. The low back should be approached as a complex structure that contains pain generators, but it has been well documented that structural abnormalities can be found in patients without low back pain.[1, 2] This fact makes low back pain a challenging condition to treat. Guidelines have been established for treatment of acute nonspecific low back pain by the Agency for Health Care Policy and Research (AHCPR)[3] and for nonspecific low back in the workplace.[4] This chapter is a practical guide to aid the primary care physician in evaluating the patient with acute or chronic low back pain with an exacerbation and making a clinical diagnosis. It also briefly covers the ordering of certain diagnostic tests and treatment alternatives as well as when to refer a patient. More detailed explanations of back pain related to degenerative disease of intervertebral discs and osteoarthritis of the spine are found in Chapter 32.

ANATOMY

The lumbar spine is made up of five lumbar vertebrae and the sacrum. The typical lumbar vertebra is illustrated in Figure 19–1. Each lumbar vertebra has three functional components: the vertebral bodies, the neural arches, and the bony process (spinous and transverse).[5] The lumbar vertebrae bear weight, the neural arches (the lamina and pedicles) surround and protect the neural elements, and the spinous and transverse processes serve as anchors for muscles in the back. The facet joints or zygapophyseal joints are synovial joints, and they are made up of the inferior articular process from the vertebrae above and the superior articular process from the vertebrae below. One can also approach the intervertebral complex of the spine as a three-joint complex as defined by Kirkaldy-Willis and Burton,[6] with the intervertebral disc and two facet joints making up the three parts.

The lumbar disc is illustrated in Figure 19–2. The surrounding fibers or annulus fibrosus, which consists of fibrocartilaginous tissue and fibrous protein, contains the nucleus pulposus, which is a gelatinous material. The outermost fibers of the annulus fibrosus attach to the vertebral bodies and the epiphysial ring and the inner portion of the fibers, which pass from one cartilage endplate to the other.

CAUSES OF LOW BACK PAIN

There are numerous proposed causes of low back pain, some of which are poorly understood. It is logical to break down the possible causes into the following categories:[5] (1) spondylogenic, (2) neurogenic, (3) viscerogenic, (4) vascular, (5) psychogenic, (6) referred, and (7) mechanical.

Spondylogenic Causes

Disc related: Annular tear, disc protrusion/disc disruption, painful degenerative disc disease, herniated nucleus pulposus.
Structural: Spondylolisthesis with or without instability.
Facet joint inflammation/arthropathy.
Traumatic fracture: From a fall or motor vehicle accident. It is also common to see compression fractures in postmenopausal women with minimal trauma (e.g., coughing or sneezing).
Tumors: Primary bone tumors or metastatic, commonly from breast or prostatic cancer.
Sprain/strain: Ligamentous or muscular, or a combination of both.
Seronegative spondyloarthropathies: Ankylosing spondylitis, Reiter's syndrome, psoriatic arthritis.
Nonspecific acute low back pain: The vast majority of patients with low back pain recover spontaneously within 2 weeks. It is not clear whether this is due to ligamentous or muscular strain, or possibly even disc trauma, but often medical care is neither sought nor needed in these cases.

Neurogenic Causes

Lumbar radiculopathy from nerve root inflammation/ denervation: This can be in itself due to a herniated nucleus pulposus, lateral stenosis, or endocrine causes, such as a diabetic radiculopathy. Infectious causes, such as herpes radiculopathy, have also been reported.
Spinal stenosis: Stenosis is caused by degenerative joint disease with facet hypertrophy and alterations in

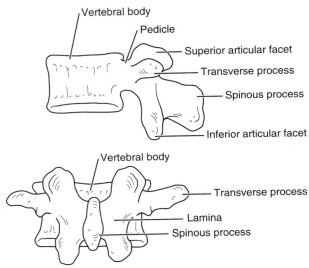

Figure 19–1. Lumbar vertebrae (lateral and anteroposterior views).

disc and soft tissues, such as the ligamentum flavum, and cause a decrease in the diameter of the spinal canal. This, in turn, causes a mechanical pressure on the neural structures, which can be manifested as localized low back pain often radiating to one or both lower extremities.

Peripheral nerve entrapment: Although unusual, peripheral nerve entrapments, such as tibial or peroneal neuropathies, can present as a radicular pain and referred low back pain. Electromyography and nerve conduction studies are useful in these cases in confirming the diagnosis.

Viscerogenic Causes

Gastrointestinal: Referred pain from pancreas or less commonly the colon. If clinically suspected, for example, an amylase test should be ordered.

Genitourinary: Referred pain from the kidneys, bladder, prostate, or uterus. It is appropriate to order a prostate-specific antigen in men older than 40 years old and ascertain that all women have had a recent gynecologic examination if the cause of back pain is not otherwise obvious.

Vascular Causes

Aneurysm: Abdominal aortic aneursyms can present as low back pain. In patients older than 50 years old,

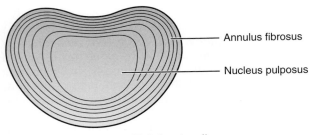

Figure 19–2. Lumbar disc.

the physician should listen for abdominal bruits on the first visit.

Peripheral vascular disease: Vascular claudication can present with symptoms similar to neurogenic claudication.

Psychogenic Causes

Particularly in patients with chronic low back pain or if there are other significant stress factors, psychological factors may either impede recovery or play a significant role in the disease process.

Referred Pain

A number of structures surrounding the spine can act as pain generators and be described as *low back pain.* Sacroiliitis from inflammation or arthropathy of the sacroiliac joints can present as low back pain, as can hip pain from causes such as osteoarthritis and a vascular necrosis.

Mechanical Causes

Although some clinicians use the term *mechanical low back pain* to describe *nonspecific low back pain,* it may be better to define mechanical low back pain as originating from a true mechanical source that places abnormal stresses on the spine. Examples include significant leg length discrepancy, which places abnormal forces on the spine because of an altered gait, and an antalgic gait secondary to a injured knee or plantar fasciitis.

HISTORY

Evaluation of the low back pain patient requires a thorough history that has many components. Important factors to note in the history and possible associated diagnoses include the following:

1. *Onset of pain:* Was the onset sudden (e.g., during or immediately after lifting a heavy object), after a motor vehicle accident, or of gradual onset (e.g., after repeated stooping or turning)? Was there an associated *pop?* Although there are exceptions to the rule, sudden-onset low back pain after lifting, bending, or Valsalva maneuver is discogenic.

2. *Specifics of symptoms:* Where is the pain? Is it sharp, dull, continuous, or intermittent. Does it radiate? It is especially important to note whether or not there is associated leg pain (sciatica), which is discussed in greater detail later. Weakness, especially if in a specific myotomal pattern, warrants an immediate referral to a spine specialist. Numbness or tingling, if in a dermatomal pattern, is suspicious for a neurogenic cause.

What makes the pain better or worse? Pain increased with sitting or forward bending is often associated with disc disease, and pain with extension is associated with posterior element loading. Pain with walking is commonly seen with spinal stenosis, particularly if the pain is relieved with forward bending or sitting. Pain with any type of activity (flexion/extension, coming up to neutral position after flexing forward) may indicate spinal instability. Exacerbation of pain with coughing, sneezing, or Valsalva maneuver typically is associated with disc pain. Morning pain or stiffness can be seen with a rheumatologic process (degenerative joint disease, spondyloarthropathy), whereas night pain is a flag to rule out metastatic disease. These are general guidelines only because there is no specific symptom linked with any particular syndrome or disease process. If bladder, bowel, or sexual dysfunction is present, especially bladder or bowel incontinence of sudden onset, a cauda equina syndrome (compression of the cauda equina), a surgical emergency, must be ruled out. Does the pain cause waking from sleep? Night pain is of concern. Malignancy must be ruled out. Poor sleep patterns are also associated with fibromyalgia.

3. *Previous diagnostic work-up:* Previous plain films of the lumbar spine, magnetic resonance imaging (MRI), computed tomography (CT), myelogram, electromyography and nerve conduction studies, bone scan, and somatosensory evoked potentials can all be helpful in the making the diagnosis.

4. *Previous and current treatment:* Included here are medications, physical therapy, chiropractic manipulation, injections, and surgery.

5. *Previous history of injury to the low back or the cervical spine.*

6. *Work and employment history:* Return to work rates depend on whether or not the back pain occurred on the job. If this is a workman's compensation case, the case can be quite complex, and referral to a spine specialist or occupational medicine physician should be considered.

7. *Other constitutional symptoms:* Fever, weight loss or gain, severe fatigue, joint pain, abdominal pain, and pelvic pain can all indicate a systemic process or primary process underlying spine pain. Depression or other psychological symptoms may either compound the underlying cause or be a reactive depression owing to chronic pain.

PHYSICAL EXAMINATION

The spine examination is quite specific. It may not be practical for the primary care physician to perform an entire spine examination, but essential components of a full spine examination are outlined.

1. Vital signs, including patient's height and weight.
2. General appearance: Are there abnormal pain behaviors, such as excessive grimacing or an exaggerated limp?
3. Lumbar spine examination:
   a. *Inspection:* The physician should look for scoliosis, listing, and obvious deformities.
   b. *Palpation:* The physician palpates various areas of the spine and on either side of the spine for tenderness. Spinous processes, interspinous spaces, associated lumbar paraspinals, over the iliac crest, greater trochanters, sacroiliac joints, and sciatic notches are palpated. At times, a step-off is palpable in spondylolisthesis; decreased intervertebral spaces can be obvious in severe compression fractures.
   c. *Range of motion of the lumbar spine:* The physician observes the range of the lumbar spine (not the hips) in forward flexion, extension, and right and left lateral bending. Disc disease usually is exacerbated with forward flexion, as are other anterior compartment abnormalities, such as compression fractures. Extension often exacerbates posterior element disease. Patients with lateral disc herniations have difficulty bending to the side away from the herniation because this puts more pressure on the opposite side of the disc. Range of motion can be rated as a percentage of expected normal range for the individual's age, sex, and general flexibility.
   d. *Straight leg raise:* Although there are a number of tests for nerve root tension, the straight leg raise is probably the most commonly used. The patient must be lying supine with both legs fully extended. The examiner then lifts the leg (with knee kept extended) off the examining table. Generally, if the patient experiences pain in the back radiating down the leg when it is between 30 and 70 degrees, this is considered a positive test for nerve root inflammation or radiculopathy. By dorsiflexing the ankle, the examiner puts increased tension on the nerve, and this should increase the patient's pain if positive. A positive crossed straight leg test (pain in the involved extremity when the opposite leg is lifted while extended) usually indicates a central disc herniation.
   e. *Femoral stretch test:* With the patient in prone position, the leg is flexed at the knee and extended passively at the hip. With a high lumbar (L2–L4) or femoral neuropathy, pain can be reproduced down the anterior thigh toward the knee.
4. Examination of extremities:
   a. *Hip examination:* Hip range of motion (passive flexion, external and internal rotation) and FABER's test (flexion/abduction/external rotation of the hip to see if pain is elicited) should be performed to rule out hip pathology. Hip x-rays are indicated if the hip appears to be associated with the low back pain.
   b. *Leg lengths:* Leg lengths can be measured from the anterior-superior iliac spine to medial malleolus or, in the heavier patient when it is difficult to palpate the anterior-superior iliac spine reliably, from the umbilicus to the medial malleolus. A discrepancy of greater than 1.5 cm is generally thought to create enough abnormal mechanical forces to create back pain. Shoe lifts can be helpful in compensating for leg length discrepancies.
   c. *Leg circumferences:* Side-to-side differences between the thigh or calf indicates atrophy from a neurogenic source. There is no rule as to what makes a difference significant, but in general a greater than 1.0-cm difference in the nondomi-

nant leg should alert the examiner to a possible radiculopathy or other neurogenic cause.

5. Neurologic

a. *Manual muscle testing by major muscle groups:* Usually the smaller (more distal) muscle groups are more sensitive to testing because they are easier for the examiner to overcome on strength testing, whereas large muscle groups, such as the hamstrings, take a significant amount of denervation or atrophy for the examiner to detect weakness. The physician should test each muscle group with the muscles in the position of maximal contraction. Weakness in specific myotomal patterns indicates a radiculopathy: for example, for L4, knee extensors, hip adductors: L5, knee flexors, ankle dorsiflexors, ankle everters, great toe dorsiflexion (extensor hallicus longus); and S1, hip extensors, toe plantar flexors. Because ankle plantar flexors (gastrocsoleus) are strong in most people, it is not useful to examine by manual muscle testing. Instead the physician should have the patient balance on the physician's hands or the clinic counter and attempt to do toe raises on each leg separately. Normally a patient should be able to do toe raises easily; fatigue or inability to do 10 toe raises on one side may indicate a S1 radiculopathy.

b. *Sensation:* The physician can test for sensation with pinprick and soft touch in the lumbar and S1 dermatomes.

c. *Muscle stretch reflexes:* The physician should test the knee jerk (L4), medial hamstrings (L5), and ankle jerk (S1). Side-to-side discrepancy may indicate a radiculopathy. Bilaterally depressed reflexes may be consistent with a patient's age, peripheral neuropathy, or spinal stenosis.

d. *Upper motor neuron tests:* Positive Babinski's sign or ankle clonus (especially in the patient older than 50 years) indicates a higher lesion and the need for appropriate clinical testing and investigation.

e. *Gait:* Gait observation can demonstrate subtle weakness in particular muscle groups or even indicate pathology outside of the low back, such as a spastic gait or ataxic gait. Having the patient heel and toe walk is a quick test for strength of ankle dorsiflexors and plantar flexors.

6. *Vascular:* The peripheral pulses should be checked to rule out vascular insufficiency; the physician should listen for abdominal or femoral bruits.

7. *Genitourinary:* A rectal examination and pelvic examination (in women) should be done if pelvic or anorectal sources of pain are suspected.

8. *Functional tests:* By checking certain functional skills the examiner can obtain quick assessment of muscle strength and coordination. The physician should have the patient go from squatting to standing. Also the physician should assess the ability to do an abdominal crunch or trunk extension to assess spine support musculature.

9. *Nonorganic physical tests:* These are tests described by Waddell et al.[9] Three out of five positive nonorganic signs can be used as a screen to identify patients who need a psychological assessment. The tests are easy to conduct.

a. Tenderness, superficial or nonanatomic: If the patient's skin is tender to light pinching over the low back or is tender to deep palpation over a widespread nonanatomic distribution, this is considered a positive test.

b. Simulation: If a patient has low back pain with axial loading (with compression over the head) or with pelvic rotation (with the shoulders and pelvis passively rotated with the feet together), this is considered a positive test.

c. Distraction: If a patient has pain with supine straight leg raise, but has no pain while the physician is performing a sitting straight leg raise (e.g., while doing manual muscle strength testing), this is considered a positive sign.

d. Regional disturbances: Weakness or sensory loss in a nonanatomic, widespread distribution (e.g., an entire leg) is considered a positive test.

e. Overreaction: Overreactive pain behaviors, such as moaning, excessive sweating, and collapsing, during the examination is considered as a positive test.

DIAGNOSTIC WORK-UP

There is much controversy over the extent of diagnostic work-up that should be performed in a patient with acute versus chronic low back pain. In the patient with nonspecific acute low back pain, the AHCPR[3] recommends patient education and avoidance of debilitation in the early stages. If there are neurologic findings from an obvious disc herniation, it is reasonable to refer to a spine specialist for further diagnostic work-up and possible treatment. It is not unreasonable in a patient without neurologic findings but with pain for 4 weeks to proceed with plain radiographs of the lumbar spine to rule out unusual pathology (e.g., metastatic disease, spondylolisthesis). Typically, anteroposterior and lateral views are a sufficient screen; obliques and coned down views can always be ordered later if there is any suspicion of pathology. This approach, at least in the majority of patients, avoids the added exposure to radiation and expense from unnecessary views. Laboratory work-up is indicated if there is suspicion of systemic disease. Usually, an erythrocyte sedimentation rate with complete blood count is sufficient as a screen for possible inflammatory diseases or infectious processes (see Chapter 26).

If a disc herniation is strongly suspected and sciatica and neurologic symptoms persist for 4 weeks, it is reasonable to order an MRI scan. At this point, surgical management is a consideration, as well as more aggressive conservative management, such as an epidural injection. MRI is needed before a referral to a spine specialist. When there is no neurologic involvement and unusual pathology, such as a malignancy, is not suspected, the spine specialist can make the decision whether or not MRI or another radiologic test, such as a computed tomography scan or myelogram, would be clinically useful or necessary.

Electromyography and nerve conduction studies can be useful for diagnostic work-up of lumbosacral radiculopathy[10]; it is a sensitive electrophysiologic test as opposed to a structural test, such as MRI. Within days of an injury, nerve conduction studies can detect a peripheral nerve entrapment. An abnormal long latency response called the H-reflex usually indicates an S1 radiculopathy. It takes 3 weeks to obtain the abnormal findings associated with denervation in limb muscles with the needle examination. Somatosensory evoked potentials, although useful for certain disease processes, such as myelopathy and demyelinating diseases, is not proven to be sensitive for detection of nerve root involvement in lumbar radiculopathy.

TREATMENT

Conservative Management

Initial care in the patient with nonspecific acute low back pain by the AHCPR guidelines should consist of patient education and comfort. Nonsteroidal anti-inflammatory agents can be useful in the initial management; opioids should be avoided because they have not been shown to be more effective. Undue back irritation should be eliminated, and aerobic conditioning (e.g., swimming or stationary biking) can help avoid deconditioning. As per the AHCPR guidelines, modalities such as manipulation, traction, physical modalities such as massage and diathermy, acupuncture, and injections have no proven efficacy in acute nonspecific low back pain. A review of the literature[11] for acute nonradicular low back pain suggests that a brief period of bed rest is appropriate, and physical therapy for acute low back pain seems to be useful. Long-term exercise, particularly when it is reinforced at work, appears to be beneficial for prevention of low back pain. Any patient with low back pain for longer than a few weeks benefits from referral to a physical therapist for back education, techniques for prevention of back injury, and exercises to help strengthen the musculature that supports the spine. Literature review[12] for chronic low back pain (nonradicular) indicates that functional restoration appears to be appropriate for selected patients, but the ability to predict which patients will respond does not yet exist. Intervention with therapeutic exercise and physical therapy is indicated in any patient who is motivated to participate.

The efficacy of injections, such as epidural injections, in the management of low back pain has also been reviewed.[13] Although few controlled studies exist, it appears that epidural injections are efficacious for patients with certain lower extremity radicular pain syndromes. In general, patients with more acute (<6 months' duration) and more lumbar pathology appear to respond better to epidural injections. Epidural injections need to be used carefully but can assist in the management of a select group of patients with acute or subacute low back pain or even chronic low back pain with exacerbation.

Conservative treatment of spinal stenosis has also been shown to include intensive exercise effectively.[14]

In certain cases, surgical management for decompression and sometimes fusion can assist in alleviating symptoms and signs associated with spinal stenosis, although the surgical risks may be too high in certain groups of elderly patients. A full discussion of surgical options in degenerative disease of the spinal is presented in Chapter 32.

REFERRALS

The management of the low back pain patient is often challenging, and the literature is still quite sparse in terms of effective conservative management. Many spine centers are well equipped to evaluate and service patients with acute-to-chronic low back pain. Often a physiatrist who is specifically trained in the spine evaluates the patient and handles the conservative rehabilitation program. Referrals are made to the spine surgeon in appropriate cases. Immediate referrals should be made to a surgeon in cases of possible cauda equina syndrome. If there is any question as to the management of the patient, a spine specialist can monitor the patient's pain and neurologic status and refer to a surgeon when necessary.

REFERENCES

1. Jensen MC, Brant-Zawadzki MN, Obuchowski N, et al: Magnetic resonance imaging of the lumbar spine in people with low back pain. N Engl J Med 331:69–73, 1994.
2. Wiesel SW, Tsourmas N, Feffer HL, et al: A study of computer-assisted tomography: 1. The incidence of positive CAT scans in an asymptomatic group of patients. Spine 9:549–551, 1984.
3. Bigos S, Bowyer O, Braen G, et al: Acute Low Back Problems in Adults. Clinical Practice Guideline No. 14; AHCPR Publication No. 95-0642. Rockville, MD, Agency for Health Care Policy and Research, Public Health Service, U.S. Department of Health and Human Services, 1994.
4. Task Force on Pain in the Workplace, Fordyce WE, ed: Back Pain in the Workplace. Management of Disability in Nonspecific Conditions. Seattle, International Association for the Study of Pain Press, 1995.
5. McCulloch J, Transfeldt E: McNab's Backache, 3rd ed. Baltimore, Williams & Wilkins, 1997.
6. Kirkaldy-Willis WH, Burton CV, ed: Managing Low Back Pain, 3rd ed. New York, Churchill Livingstone, 1992.
7. Borenstein DG, Wiesel SW: Low Back Pain: Medical Diagnosis and Comprehensive Management. Philadelphia, WB Saunders, 1989.
8. Schofferman JA: Diagnostic decision making. In White AH, Schofferman JA, eds: Spine Care: Diagnosis and Conservative Management. St. Louis, Mosby, 1995, pp 41–51.
9. Waddell G, McCulloch JA, Kummel E, Venner RM: Nonorganic physical signs in low-back pain. Spine 5:117–125, 1980.
10. Wilbourn AJ, Aminoff MJ: AAEE minimograph #32: The electrophysiologic examination in patients with radiculopathies. Muscle Nerve: 11:1099–1114, 1988.
11. Scheer SJ, Radack KL, O'Brien DR: Randomized controlled trials in industrial low back pain relating to return to work: Part 1. Acute interventions. Arch Phys Med Rehabil 76:966–973, 1995.
12. Wheeler AH, Hanley ENJ: Nonoperative treatment for the low back pain: Rest to restoration. Spine 20: 375–378, 1995.
13. Spaccarelli KC: Lumbar and caudal epidural injections. Mayo Clin Proc 71:169–178, 1996.
14. Nelson BW, O'Reilly E, Hogan M, et al: The clinical effects of intensive, specific exercise on chronic low back pain: A controlled study of 895 consecutive patients with one-year followup. Orthopedics 18:971–981, 1995.

Neck Pain

Eugene J. Carragee

eck, shoulder, and interscapular pain associated with cervical spine problems is common. It is found to have a lifetime incidence of 60% to 80% in adults on retrospective questioning. In some studies, 15% to 20% had suffered from neck and shoulder problems in the last 12 months. In a large study of industrial workers, 12% reported neck and upper spine symptoms daily. The prevalence appears to increase with age and physically demanding labor. In the overwhelming majority of cases, these symptoms cause no specific impairment or disability. In a small percentage of people, neck pain may be associated with significant functional loss. Even in these situations, however, most patients do not have clear pathologic findings in the spine or surrounding tissues, and in most cases, the cause of the neck pain is never definitively determined. In a small minority of patients, clear pathology associated with the patients' symptoms is found. More occasionally, neurologic injury or true instability can be demonstrated.

This field is complicated by the subjective nature of most cervical complaints and the presence of worker's compensation or personal injury claims. In a study of Swiss accident insurance records, most neck complaints had claims resulting from motor vehicle accidents, and more than 80% of these were classified as *soft tissue injuries*.[1] The evaluation of these cases cannot be made in a vacuum, and the emotional, social, and legal implications of the patient's situation often loom large in the clinician's understanding of the illness. The literature is divided, with many researchers pointing to the clear epidemiologic evidence connecting litigation and secondary gain with complaints of neck pain. Other workers, in smaller cohort studies, fail to find the psychological and social factors playing a significant role in case-by-case analyses. The possible causes of neck pain are legion. This chapter considers three commonly encountered cervical spine–related clinical presentations: degenerative cervical spine disease, rheumatoid disease of the cervical spine, and the whiplash syndromes.

DEGENERATIVE CERVICAL SPINE DISEASE

Natural History

Most patients with degenerative changes of the cervical spine never seek medical care for this problem. Of those who do, three primary clinical situations are encountered. The first of these is the *axial pain syndromes*, in which the patient has mainly neck, interscapular, or shoulder pain or all three. The others are *cervical radiculopathy* and *myelopathy syndromes*. In these cases, the patient may have varying degrees of neck pain but also has either root (radiculopathy) or spinal cord (myelopathy) irritation or compression. Neck pain in most patients without specific cause has a relatively benign course. Although the symptom is common, it is most likely associated with degenerative changes of the intervertebral discs or facet joints. Most of those patients do quite well without specific intervention.

Cervical radiculopathy resolves completely after one episode without recurrence in about approximately half of the cases. In one study, despite a nearly 20-year follow-up, no patients went on to develop a myelopathy in the long term, although 25% did have persistent or worsening root symptoms.[2]

The natural history of myelopathic patients is much less benign. Patients with only mild disability have the best prognosis with long-term care. Of patients with significant spinal cord dysfunction, there is little chance that these signs or symptoms will regress spontaneously without operative intervention.[3]

History

Patients with simple neck pain often describe a *crick* in their neck or some onset of pain after repetitive motions, sitting, or working. Workers at computer terminals, including typists or transcriptionists, and people doing assembly line work with small components may notice problems associated with the requirements of prolonged static posture. These symptoms are common and may occur with or without associated radiographic changes. Patients presenting with pain after significant motor vehicle accidents are discussed later under the whiplash syndrome.

Usually, degenerative conditions are worsened by activities that stress the neck and cervical spine. Persistent unremitting pain even at rest should alert the physician to possibly more serious underlying problems, such as infection or tumor. In the absence of these serious space-occupying lesions, a significant emotional or psychological disturbance should be considered when pain is disproportional to the findings.

Approach to the Patient with Musculoskeletal Pain

The location of the discomfort may be helpful. Cervical facet pain at the higher regions of C2 and C3 often occurs along the upper neck, head, forehead, and temple region. Research mapping out the sclerotome pain associated with different cervical facets has produced the distributions given in Figure 20–1.[4] Each progressively caudal segment appears to refer pain further down the neck to the interscapular region.

Occasionally, eye, ear, nose, and throat symptoms may be associated with cervical disease. These symptoms may be related to irritation of the sympathetic nerve plexuses anterior to the vertebrae in the cervical spine. Occasionally, difficulty swallowing may occur with large anterior cervical osteophytes compressing the esophagus. This difficulty can also result from compression of the cranial nerves that coordinate swallowing. Rarely, patients may lose consciousness because of compression of the vertebral arteries. Conversely, pain from distant structures may radiate to the neck. These include the pain of cardiac ischemia, Pancoast tumors, and esophageal problems.

Nerve root compression is most common at the C6–C7 roots. Pain from irritation of these roots characteristically radiates down the arm to the forearm and hand. C5 root irritation usually radiates to the area of the deltoid in a cape distribution, and C8 irritation radiates to the forearm along the ulnar border to the small and great fingers. It is important to understand the anatomy of the cervical spine, wherein the nerve root compressed by a disc lesion usually affects the lower root. Therefore, at a C5–C6 disc, the C6 nerve root is compressed. The nerve root exiting between C7 and T1 is the C8 nerve root. The T1 nerve root exiting below the T1 pedicle is rarely involved. Occasionally, patients may complain of difficulty walking, *dizziness*, or dead feeling in their legs. These may all be indications of cervical cord compression.

In evaluating patients with neurologic symptoms that may be referable to the neck, it is important to remember conditions that may mimic cervical radiculopathy or myelopathy, including peripheral nerve problems at the brachial plexus, carpal tunnel, or cubital tunnel. In patients with long track signs, multiple sclerosis, amyotrophic lateral sclerosis, and normal pressure hydrocephalus must be considered. In addition, small strokes, particularly infarcts of the internal capsule, may produce bilateral upper motor neuron signs and symptoms. These usually have no sensory loss and are often associated with poorly controlled hypertension.

Physical Findings

The physical examination in patients with simple mechanical neck pain is often unhelpful. Occasionally, there is a decrease in volitional neck motion or tenderness to palpation posteriorly. In these patients, the neurologic examination is usually normal. The lower extremity reflexes should be checked for spasticity in all patients evaluated with neck troubles. A new finding of hyperreflexia, adductor reflexes, or clonus at the ankles should prompt a thorough investigation for cord compression.

Cervical radiculopathies are usually not subtle. Pain radiating down to the hand usually directs the examiner to the appropriate levels. A quick screening examination for each of the nerve roots may be summarized as follows: C5–C6 innervates the deltoid, C6 innervates the wrist extensors, C7 innervates the triceps, C8 innervates the finger flexors, and T1 innervates the intrinsic muscles in the hands. The Spurling sign is a test for exacerbation of radicular symptoms. In this test, the patient rotates and bends the head laterally toward the involved side. If this increases pain, a test is considered positive and thought to reflect cervical root compression. Similarly, neck extension and, occasionally, rotation toward the involved side may increase the symptoms. Abducting the arm and flexing the elbow may relieve symptoms of root compression because tension is taken off the middle cervical roots. This maneuver is also helpful in differentiating between shoulder and cervical processes. Shoulder pain is usually made worse with abduction and external rotation of the shoulder, but the pain in cervical radiculopathy is usually lessened with this motion.

Lower extremity weakness may be subtle in patients with myelopathy. The combination of loss of proprioception and weakness may give the patient an apparently severe ataxia. The gait is characteristically wide based, and sometimes foot slapping is seen. The upper extremities may have upper motor neuron or lower motor neuron findings or some combination of these depending on the level of cord compression. Occasionally a *L'hermitte* sign may be elicited with head flexion or extension in patients with cervical myelopathy wherein the patient may complain of an electrical sensation into the arms and legs.

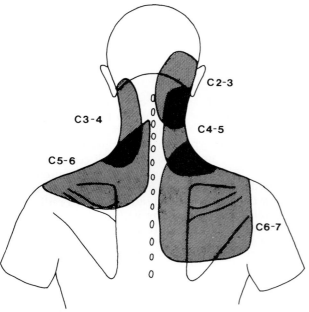

Figure 20–1. A map of the characteristic areas of pain referred from cervical zygapophyseal joints of C2–C3 to C6–C7. (From Dwyer A, Aprill C, Bogduk N: Cervical zygapophyseal joint pain patterns: I. Study of normal volunteers. Spine 15:453–454, 1990.)

Further evaluation of myelopathic changes in the upper extremity include the Hoffmann sign, which involves flicking the distal middle finger and looking for contraction of the thumb across the palm. This sign is indicative of upper motor neuron disease in the midcervical level. The upper cervical levels can be assessed with a scapulohumeral reflex wherein the reflex hammer is brought down on the scapular spine and acromium causing a jerk upward of the shoulder. This reflex is thought to be due to compression at the upper cervical levels (C1–C3). Cranial nerve function and the jaw jerk reflex should be checked. If this reflex is also hyperactive, the pathology probably is to be found intracranially or is due to a metabolic disease causing global spasticity.

Radiographic Examination

Plain radiographs are rarely helpful in the evaluation of neck pain because progressive degenerative changes are found with age in most people. Signs of segmental instability with an S-shaped spine may be found, however, and may be evidence of infection or metastatic disease. Because plain radiographs do not reliably depict the space available for neural elements, computed tomography (CT), myelography, and magnetic resonance imaging (MRI) scanning are usually recommended for those investigations. Most cases of cervical radiculopathy respond in relatively short order to the passage of time and supportive measures. In the absence of indications of myelopathy or severe motor loss, MRI scanning in all patients with cervical radicular complaints is not recommended. In most instances, these conditions improve. Myelography and CT myelography have the advantage of being more dynamic studies. During myelography, the patient can flex and extend the neck. The movement of the individual segments and discs can be seen at times to compress the spinal cord or roots. Conversely MRI and CT scan are usually static tests that do not reflect changes with motion. Some new MRI scanning techniques can show flexion and extension of the cervical spine in real time and may be an important diagnostic tool in the future.

The findings on CT and MRI scanning of the cervical spine must be interpreted with caution. Some degenerative changes appear with age in virtually all individuals. In asymptomatic control patients, MRI scanning revealed a 25% prevalence of major abnormalities found on MRI in patients older than 40 years of age. Therefore, a clear correlation of the patient's complaints, physical findings, and radiographic testing is of paramount importance. The MRI scan is a useful tool in eliminating the possibility of more serious or occult processes, such as infections, tumor, multiple sclerosis, Chiari malformations, syrinx, and hydrocephalus.

Electrophysiologic Examination

In some cases, the diagnosis of radicular or myelopathic complaints remains uncertain even after sophisticated imaging studies have been performed. Electromyelogram, nerve conduction velocity study, or somatosensory evoked potential may be helpful in these instances. These examinations are most helpful in evaluating patients who have multiple structural abnormalities on the imaging studies and the clinician suspects only one level may be presently asymptomatic. It takes as long as 4 weeks for electromyelogram abnormalities to be manifest, and ordering this test before the passage of that much time may not be useful. The electromyelogram and nerve conduction velocity studies may disclose peripheral neuropathy.

Treatment

NONOPERATIVE TREATMENT

Nonoperative treatment is the rule for most patients with cervical spine problems. In most cases, neck pain and cervical radiculopathy syndromes are self-limited, and the patients recover in a matter of weeks. Treatment with nonsteroidal anti-inflammatory drugs is often advocated, but there is no clear advantage over acetaminophen in most patients. Some patients may benefit from the use of a soft collar or sometimes a more rigid orthosis if there is evidence of chronic segmental instability. Physical therapy is often advocated, and this treatment has included passive modalities for pain control as well as active modalities, such as strengthening and stretching exercises. Simple neck pain is often treated with chiropractic manipulation, and in the absence of neurologic signs, this is often reported to be helpful. As with the other nonoperative modalities, there does not appear to be compelling evidence that chiropractic manipulation is specifically effective in these cases, however.

OPERATIVE TREATMENT

The indications for surgery in patients with degenerative cervical spine disease appear to vary by practice, geographic location, and patient expectations. Primary care physicians need to be aware of alternative approaches used by their surgical colleagues. Cervical myelopathy with significant impairment is probably the clearest indication for aggressive operative treatment. Neck pain with only degenerative changes found on imaging studies and no neurologic loss probably has the weakest indication.

For cervical radiculopathies, the usual indications for surgery include (1) continuing radicular pain after 6 to 12 weeks of nonoperative care, (2) progressive neurologic loss, and (3) association with any degree of myelopathy. The imaging and electrophysiologic studies should correlate exactly with the physical findings and patient complaints. Experience has shown that the chances of successful outcome are less if these guidelines are not followed. The choice of anterior or posterior procedures for cervical spine pathology is controversial.

ANTERIOR APPROACHES. Controversy exists regarding the best management of degenerative cervical disc disease. There are proponents of anterior surgery, including a discectomy and fusion with or without instrumentation. Others recommend anterior discectomy alone, particularly in patients without myelopathy and with only single-level disease. It is not clear which treatment is the best. Most patients with a true cervical radiculopathy treated with either of these methods apparently do quite well. Between 60% and 90% of patients are significantly improved. Better results are seen in patients with radiculopathy of shorter duration, younger patients, patients without worker's compensation issues being involved, and nonsmoking male patients.

The diagnosis of cervical myelopathy requires a surgeon with significantly more experience. In cases of significant myelopathy, the entire vertebral body at one or several levels may need to be removed and the anterior spine reconstructed. Some patients may require both an anterior and a posterior decompression to address the problem adequately. In general, patients who have any degree of kyphosis in the involved segments should have at least an anterior approach as part of their operative treatment.

POSTERIOR APPROACHES. Posterior approaches in primary neck pain syndromes without neurologic involvement are unlikely to be helpful. There is probably no appropriate role for cervical laminectomy or laminoplasty in these patients. In patients with lateral disc herniation and a well-maintained cervical lordosis, a small cervical laminotomy may be an effective treatment. Central disc herniations are technically difficult to correct from the posterior approach, and laminectomy is probably not indicated. Patients with diffuse spinal canal stenosis with myelopathy and an accompanying radiculopathy may be helped by a posterior approach if the patient has a well-maintained cervical lordosis.

Complications

The most frequent complication of anterior cervical discectomy and fusion is persistent pain at the bone-graft site. This pain can be minimized by careful technique, by avoiding large grafts, or by using bone-graft substitutes. Patients often have difficulty swallowing for some period of time after surgery, particularly if previous surgery had been performed. Because these surgeries are frequently performed, most surgeons have sufficient experience with the anatomy to avoid damage to the vital structures in the neck, such as the carotid artery and jugular vein, esophagus, trachea, larynx, and spinal cord. These still occur, albeit with a low frequency.[5] In a large study, the complication rate of a serious or catastrophic neurologic problem after anterior surgery was 1 in 300.[6]

Prognosis

Symptoms occur in so many people and increase with age, so that symptomatic cure is an unrealistic goal. Most patients understand this and do well over time. Patients involved in litigation or patients with significant psychological or emotional problems are in a poor prognostic category. In patients who continue to be very symptomatic, a thorough investigation for the reasons of persistent symptoms should be undertaken. In the absence of clear neurologic loss, spinal instability, iatrogenic or spontaneous infection, or fracture, the repetitive surgical approach to patients with persistent pain is not appropriate. Caution and prudence must be exercised in managing those difficult cases, and the clinician must recognize his or her own limitations in pursuing expensive, debilitating, or hazardous treatment options.

RHEUMATOID DISEASE OF THE CERVICAL SPINE

The general considerations of diagnosis and management of rheumatoid arthritis (RA) are given in Chapters 3 and 25. This section deals primarily with the effects on the spine and RA. The adult spine is primarily affected at the cervical and occipitocervical levels by RA. As with other joints, the inflammatory synovitis associated with RA can cause an expanding destructive process within and around the joint. In addition to the joint itself, the surrounding capsule ligaments and bone may be eroded by the destructive process. Although in other anatomic locations the pannus may be quite large without affecting vital structures, in the spine, encroachment of the pannus into the spinal canal or through the foramen magnum can have significant neurologic complications. Stretching or destruction of the ligaments may result in instability anywhere along the cervical spine.

Subluxations of the cervical spine are the main clinical problem in RA. The degree of cervical subluxation mirrors the involvement of peripheral joints. The more severe and aggressive the disease in the hands, the greater the likelihood that cervical spine subluxations exist. In addition, a history of glucocorticoid use, seropositivity, and presence of subcutaneous rheumatoid nodules have been shown to correlate with the progression of subluxations in the cervical region. Finally, men appear to be more prone to symptomatic subluxations than women.

Types of Subluxations

Three main patterns of cervical subluxation are seen in patients with RA: (1) atlantoaxial subluxation, (2) atlantoaxial impaction or so-called basilar impaction, and (3) subaxial subluxation (meaning below the C2 vertebrae). The first of these, atlantoaxial subluxation, is by far the most common (see Chapter 3). Erosion of the ligaments and joints between the C1 and C2 vertebrae may allow the subluxation of the odontoid in a posterior direction, which would compress the area available for the spinal cord. This variety of subluxation is found in more than half of patients with severe peripheral joint disease, although only 50% of the patients with subluxation had any signs or symptoms of cervical instability. The C1–C2 segment may also be unstable in rotation, shifting either to the right or to the left. This instability is seen as a lateral mass subluxation on anteroposterior radiographs. More than 2 mm of subluxation on this view is considered pathologic. In addition, the subluxation may be posterior; however, this is rarely associated with neurologic problems.

Atlantoaxial or basilar impaction may be visualized as a settling of the cranium and foramen magnum on progressively eroded elements of C1. As this settling progresses, there is a relative extension of the odontoid into the foramen magnum and against the brain stem. It is primarily the loss of joint space between the occiput and C1 and between the facets of C1 and C2 that allows this vertical migration of the odontoid. Different series have reported this finding in 5% to 30% of RA patients.

Subaxial cervical subluxation may be seen in varying degrees in 10% to 20% of patients. It can be discriminated from the more common osteoarthritic changes of the cervical spine by the lack of osteophytes, a cascading or stepladder appearance of the subluxations (see Chapter 4), and a tendency to involve the higher cervical segments from C2 to C4. The nerve roots or the spinal cord may be involved, irritated, or damaged by the abnormal motion or by extension of the synovitis and rheumatoid pannus against the nerves directly.

Natural History

The data on the natural history of rheumatoid changes of the cervical spine are confusing. The beginning and end points in different series are difficult to compare, and the prevalence in different subpopulations is most likely different.[7–11] In the general rheumatoid population, the presence of some subluxation in the cervical spine does not change the life expectancy of the patients compared to others with RA. The mortality rate for RA patients is roughly 17% at 5 years follow-up, but 10% higher than an age-matched nonrheumatoid population.

The presence of rheumatoid subluxations of the cervical spine has been noted to develop within about 2 years of the diagnosis of the disease. New subluxations at varying levels are reported in patients followed over time. Neurologic progression occurs in 2% to 36% of the patients with subluxations. In patients with clear cervical myelopathy, progressive neurologic impairment and death are possible outcomes if the spinal cord is not decompressed and the spine stabilized. Premature death in rheumatoid patients with myelopathy appears to be mainly due to the associative debilitating effects of progressive quadriparesis (infection, pulmonary problems with immobility, decubiti) and not directly due to the spinal cord injury. Fewer than 25% of rheumatoid patients with myelopathy have any recovery once the myelopathy begins.

Clinical Presentation

Many patients with RA have posterior head and neck pain. Not all of these patients have a subluxation of the spine. Conversely, many patients with cervical instability have no primary complaints of pain or neurologic signs. The neurologic examination in patients with severe peripheral RA may be challenging. In particular, spinal cord compression can be missed in the presence of significant contractures or joint destruction that limits the ability to detect spasticity on reflex testing. Also, foot deformities may obscure a Babinski sign. Nonetheless, a low threshold of consideration should be maintained in patients whose functional capacities are deteriorating.

Upper extremity symptoms such as radicular pain should alert the clinician to the possibility of cervical involvement, as should the complaint of paresthesias in the hands. This pain may be confused with carpal tunnel compression or cubital tunnel compression, and an electromyelogram may be helpful in determining the level of neurologic involvement. A *L'hermitte* sign may be present, in which the patient has an electrical shock sensation to the arms, back, and legs with movements of the head or neck. Although initially described with multiple sclerosis, it is not uncommonly seen in patients with cervical spinal cord compression. Despite careful neurologic examination, only 10% to 30% of patients with cervical instability resulting from RA have clear neurologic signs on examination.

Radiographic Evaluation

Despite advances in CT and MRI, plain radiographs still play a key role in evaluation of rheumatoid cervical spine instability. There is a wealth of prognostic data that can be taken on the plain radiographs. In addition to the standard anteroposterior and lateral x-rays, lateral views of flexion and extension should be taken, unless the patient is seen to be manifesting signs of progressive spinal cord injury.

Several measurements made on plain radiographs are standard reference points for cervical instability. The most common subluxation, anterior atlantoaxial, is schematically depicted on Figure 20–2 (also, see Chapter 4). The distance between the anterior arch of C1 and the dens, depicted as line *a* on the schematic, should be less than 3.5 mm in adults. Flexion/extension views may show that, when the posterior ligament holding the odontoid in place is stretched, eroded, or both, the dens migrates 10 mm or more posteriorly with flexion of the head in severe cases of C1–C2 instability. The posterior atlantodental interval (line *b* on the schematic) has been shown to have a high sensitivity in predicting paralysis. This interval posterior to the dens indicates the maximal amount of space available for the spinal cord as it passes from the foramen magnum to the spinal canal. The posterior atlantodental interval when measuring less than 14 mm correlates well with the future spinal cord compression. As can be seen on Figure 20–1, however, the pannus, which is not seen on plain radiographs, may occupy varying amounts of canal and can be assessed only on MRI or myelography. The radiographic measurements for atlantoaxial impaction are complicated and not appropriate for discussion in a pri-

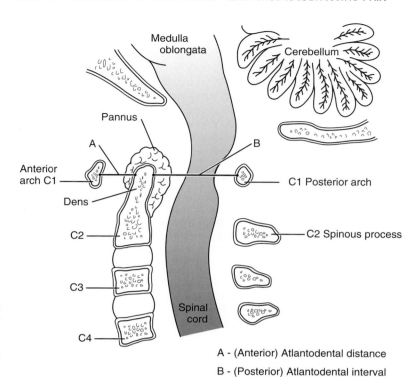

Figure 20–2. Anterior C1–C2 subluxation.

A - (Anterior) Atlantodental distance

B - (Posterior) Atlantodental interval

mary care text. When any form of subluxation is noted, referral to an orthopaedist or neurosurgeon should be carried out soon.

Plain radiographs have significant limitations in the evaluation of the rheumatoid spine. Osteopenia may make the reference points difficult to measure. The overlap of structures at the base of the skull often obscures the foramen magnum and hard pallet for assessment, and the tip of the odontoid may be extremely osteopenic or replaced by pannus, leading the clinician to underestimate the upper extent of compression. For these reasons, if significant instability is found on flexion/extension radiographs or suggestion of basilar impaction is seen, further evaluation with MRI should be undertaken. This scanning clearly identifies the brain stem as it exits the foramen magnum into the spinal canal and depicts the dens and pannus about the C1–C2 region. It also gives an impression of the spinal canal in the subaxial region. MRI sequences with the neck in flexion and extension are sometimes done to account for dynamic instability and compression.

CT is especially helpful when surgery is planned because it gives excellent bony detail that is superior to MRI. It is less helpful, particularly without myelography, in depicting spinal cord compression or the extent of pannus. With myelography, however, dynamic flexion and extension x-rays can be taken that may indicate the spinal cord compression not seen on static films.

Treatment

When RA patients have cervical spine symptoms and the investigation depicts no significant cervical instability and the neurologic examination is normal, medical management for peripheral synovitis is contin-

ued. There is some indication that measures that successfully decrease the disease activity peripherally also decrease the progression of destruction in the cervical spine. For patients with cervical instability, the primary treatment should be surgical. Cervical collars often decrease pain but do not protect against subluxation or neurologic injury. In addition, some collars may maintain the patient in a more flexed position of comfort, which is actually a position of greater spinal cord compression in atlantoaxial instability.

Indications for surgical management in the absence of progressive neurologic loss depend on the clinical and radiographic investigations. Basilar impaction, clear radiographic C1–C2 instability, and radiographic subaxial instability have been well documented to indicate an impending neurologic deficit. As a group, these patients appear to do better with surgery. Particularly, patients at risk for myelopathic progression appear to do better if operated on before severe neurologic losses incurred.

The most common instability, isolated anterior C1–C2 subluxation, occurs most frequently in patients who are doing well in other respects. In most cases, the subluxation is reducible with posture, and the patient can undergo a posterior C1–C2, fusion in a relatively straightforward manner. However, the situation is not always this straightforward. Not uncommonly the surgeon is faced with a patient with marked debilitation resulting from chronic RA. The cervical deformity may be rigid or completely fixed in position. The patient may be severely malnourished and have a limited rehabilitation potential regardless of treatment. Often the previous injudicious use of glucocorticoids has produced severe osteopenia complicating any surgical attempt at fixation. The ongoing use of cytotoxic agents in controlling the RA may seriously decrease the fusion potential postoperatively. For these reasons, surgical management of these cases requires thoughtful preoperative consideration and involvement of the rheumatologist.

Prognosis

After cervical fusion of an area of instability, a possibility remains for the development of further instability at other levels with time. This possibility is particularly true when an occipital cervical fusion has been done to C2 or C3. The increased forces on the subaxial spine are significant, and the clinician must be alert to further deterioration over time.

WHIPLASH SYNDROME

The complaint of neck pain after motor vehicle accidents is quite common and a particularly difficult management problem for most clinicians. This is a field in which there are many strongly held beliefs and relatively little good science to back them. The presence of legal claims as a result of these accidents can make assessment difficult.

The generally accepted mechanism of injury in whiplash syndromes is a rapid acceleration and deceleration of the head on the cervical spine. Work with selective and differential anesthetic blocks has shown that at least in some subgroups the pain may originate from the zygapophyseal joints (facet joints) in the midcervical region.[7, 8] Some patients may have undetected fractures along the facet joints or unrecognized subluxations or dislocations of the midcervical segments. Other studies have shown that patients with significant ongoing pain may have disc pathology as a contributing factor. Because the injury, usually in a motor vehicle accident, has so many variables, including speed; direction of impact; size and weight of the relative vehicles; position of the occupants; and size, weight, and strength of the occupants, it is not surprising that there is a wide range of clinical presentations. The common thread in most incidents is that the forced extension of the neck during acceleration causes a compressive-type injury to the posterior aspects of the spine and sometimes a traction-type injury anteriorly. There is a lesser degree of flexion at the start of the impact and again after the forced extension.

Clinical Presentation

The range of patient complaints is wide. Some patients may be involved in severe accidents and have relatively little complaint of neck or head pain. Others may be involved in trivial-appearing accidents and have disabling symptoms. The most common complaints are neck pain, occipital headache, shoulder pain, low back pain and interscapular pain, arm and hand pain, vertigo, and hearing and visual problems. It is important in the history to ascertain the sequence of events, the patient's position during the accident, whether there was closed head injury from hitting the dash or windscreen, and whether an appropriately placed head rest was in place.

Because many of these cases involve litigation, it is important for the clinician to get a detailed history of events. It is also important to understand the patient. Previous neck and back injuries, previous litigation, and previous worker's compensation claims should be inquired about directly and in a straightforward manner. The treating physician may be asked to provide medical reports giving opinions regarding causation of the patient's complaints. If the patient has had similar complaints in the past or has had similar accidents previously, it is often worthwhile to review those records before a definitive opinion is rendered.

It is incumbent on the primary care physician evaluating the patient to be sure no serious injury has been missed. Indications in the history that more serious trauma to the neck had occurred include difficulty swallowing after the accident. This difficulty may indicate a prevertebral hematoma. Neurologic symptoms, such as persistent dysesthesias or electric shock–type pain with neck motion into the extremities, should prompt further investigation. A commonly encountered complaint is the impairment of cognitive function after these accidents.

Physical Examination

Physical findings are most often nonspecific. There may be a decreased range of motion of the neck. Care should be taken in the examination to assess thoroughly the neurologic function in both the cranial nerves and the upper and lower extremities. As previously mentioned, the failure to examine the lower extremities in neck injuries is a common but serious omission. One should not fail to recognize long track signs for spasticity while focusing on a neck injury.

Imaging Studies

Depending on the severity of complaints or the mechanism of injury, some investigation may be required. Typically, plain radiographs of the neck, including flexion/extension, are taken. If these are unhelpful and the patient continues to have significant pain, it is probably worthwhile ruling out the presence of fractures along the lateral masses and facets. The presence of fracture can be evaluated with a CT scan or special oblique views of the cervical spine. MRI examination in patients with neurologic complaints is appropriate. It must be explained to the patient that degenerative changes are often seen in asymptomatic or minimally symptomatic individuals and impressed on the patient that one is looking for serious pathology or evidence of neurologic injury.

Natural History

It is a common feature of whiplash injuries that the patient may not complain of the pain immediately. Most patients develop difficulties over the first 2 days, but some patients indicate that symptoms, which they relate to the accident, develop a week or more afterward. In large series, 90% of patients continue to work and function well. Most patients recover within 3 weeks, and some patients may continue to report improving symptoms for 1 or 2 years. In some studies, more than 40% of the patients continue to have neck pain at long-term follow-up. In other studies, there were no differences found in the prevalence in neck pain in patients after whiplash injuries compared to the general population. It has been suggested that the presence of litigation or perhaps social conditioning to associate neck pain with these types of accidents has a significant impact on the prevalence and severity of whiplash complaints after accidents. In an effort to test this hypothesis, a study was done in Lithuania shortly after the dissolution of the Soviet Union.[1] In this country, where litigation, compensation issues, and Western ideas about how one should feel after motor vehicle accidents, were largely unknown, people involved in car accidents were evaluated at long-term follow-up. When compared against age-matched and sex-matched controls, there was no increase in chronic neck pain, headache, low back pain, or cognitive and psychological troubles on review. It is difficult to reconcile these data with the 40% or more serious persistent symptoms found in patients in other studies in which compensation issues loom large in the clinical context.

Treatment

The natural history indicates that patients improve spontaneously. It is likely that early mobilization is better than rest and collar immobilization. Some studies have shown that home therapy is as effective as prolonged outpatient physical therapy. Some centers offer aggressive rehabilitation programs after whiplash injury. Theoretical reasons support this in some cases, but formal testing of this expensive and time-consuming practice has not been done. In addition, there is an implicit message to the patient that he or she must be badly injured because such intensive treatment is required. This message may have an unintended deleterious impact on the patient's sense of his or her injury.

A common regimen recommended is topical ice and rest for the first 24 hours followed by a progressive neck mobilization program begun the next day. Initially, this program begins with passive range of motion, and over the second and third day this progresses to active neck range of motion. As the pain improves, isometric resisted exercises are added. In patients without neurologic signs or symptoms, with no evidence of bony or ligamentous damage on imaging studies, a relatively rapid return to full activities should be encouraged. Although no firm guidelines exist, return to full duties in about 3 weeks or sooner should be the goal. If this goal is not met, the patient needs to be reassessed. Care must be taken in this ambiguous setting regarding the prescription of opioid narcotics, muscle relaxants, or sedative-hypnotic drugs. For patients having difficulty sleeping, low doses of tricyclic antidepressants help both sleep and pain.

In the patient with significant continuing complaints after several weeks, it may be necessary to repeat the initial work-up and add further imaging studies, including possibly a bone scan, MRI scan, or CT imaging. This work-up is intended to identify occult fractures, clear clinical instability, or other serious occult processes. The finding, for instance, of a degenerative disc at C5–C6 should not be interpreted as the definite source of the patient's problem. Biomechanical studies have shown that it is unlikely that a normal disc would have been injured in a typical whiplash injury without serious ligamentous and bone damage as well. The degenerative disc seen on this sort of evaluation likely existed before the injury and may or may not have anything to do with the patient's pain. In most instances, the finding of some minor degenerative changes on MRI should be frankly discussed with the patient as changes consistent only with their age and that no specific cause of their pain has been found. To suggest otherwise is disingenuous. Some patients often focus on a degenerative disc or mildly arthritic facet area, and the road becomes paved to continue the disability and possibly unwarranted surgery.

In the absence of firm objective evidence of spinal instability, fracture, or disc herniation with neurologic radiculopathy or myelopathy, surgery in whiplash disorders is rarely indicated. Cervical discography remains controversial, and consistently good results after fusion of discographically positive discs has not been found. Patients with pain diagnosed as coming from the cervical facet joints on diagnostic anesthetic blocks have been treated with local nerve oblation. There is some indication that this treatment may give long-term relief in selective patients, but confirmatory studies are still pending.

REFERENCES

1. Macnab I: The "whiplash syndrome." Orthop Clin North Am 2:389–403, 1971.
2. Davis SJ, Teresi LM, Bradley WB Jr, et al: Cervical spine hyperextension injuries: MR findings. Radiology 180:245–251, 1991.
3. Flynn T: Neurologic complications after anterior cervical interbody fusion. Spine 7:536–539, 1982.
4. Barnsley L, Lord S, Wallis B, et al: The prevalence of chronic cervical zygapophysial joint pain after whiplash. Spine 20:20–26, 1995.
5. Nurick S: The natural history of and the results of surgical treatment of the spinal cord disorder associated with cervical spondylosis. Brain 95:101–108, 1972.
6. Boden S, Dodge L, Bohlman H, et al: Rheumatoid arthritis of the cervical spine: A long-term analysis with predictors of paralysis and recovery. J Bone Joint Surg Am 75:1282–1297, 1993.
7. Barnsley L, Lord S, Bogduk N: Whiplash injury. Pain 58:283–307, 1994.
8. Barnsley L, Lord S, Wallis B, et al: Lack of effect of intraarticular corticosteroids for chronic pain in the cervical zygapophyseal joints. N Engl J Med 330:1047–1050, 1994.
9. Dwyer A, Aprill C, Bogduk N: Cervical zygapophyseal joint pain patterns. I: A study of normal volunteers. Spine 15:453–454, 1990.
10. Lee F, Turner J: The natural history and prognosis of cervical spondylosis. BMJ 2:1607–1610, 1963.
11. Okada K, Shirasaki N, Hayashi H, et al: Treatment of cervical spondylotic myelopathy by enlargement of the spinal canal anteriorly, followed by arthrodesis. J Bone Joint Surg Am 73:352–364, 1991.

Chapter 21

The Painful Foot and Ankle—Viewpoints From Orthopaedics and Podiatry

Loretta B. Chou ▪ Lawrence M. Oloff ▪ Alan P. Bocko

There are two sections to this chapter, one written by an orthopaedic surgeon who specializes in diseases of the foot and ankle and another by two academically oriented podiatrists. The editors realize that there may be overlap in content and presentation that is generated by this format but believe that the primary care physi-cian can benefit from the approaches to diagnosis and therapy by both of these specialists. It is recommended that the primary care physician use the talents of the podiatrist and surgeon as a team of collaborative con-sultants in managing the often perplexing and refrac-tory problems that foot and ankle pain generate.

FOOT AND ANKLE PAIN

Loretta B. Chou

Humans have the unique ability to engage in bipedal motion. The foot and ankle are anatomically designed for weight-bearing activities; the multiple bones and joints are balanced to allow one to transmit body weight through the foot and ankle to walk, run, climb stairs, dance, and jump. The foot and ankle can have patho-logic disorders, such as neuromas, bunions, tendinitis, and arthritis. Also, abnormalities in the foot and ankle can be magnified with weight-bearing activities. Pain and swelling are the most common complaints. Shoes play an important role in a patient's symptoms. Ill-fit-ting shoes are a common cause of foot complaints, and simple shoewear modification can help alleviate many problems or prevent chronic deformities.

ANATOMY AND BIOMECHANICS OF THE FOOT AND ANKLE

The ankle joint is composed of the distal tibia, fibula, and the talus, and its primary function is dorsi-flexion and plantar flexion with walking and running.

These activities are complex and require participation of all motion segments of the body, including the hip and knee. The joints in the foot include the subtalar (talocal-caneal), talonavicular, calcaneocuboid, tarsometatarsal, and metatarsophalangeal joints. These are also involved with locomotion. The gait cycle of one foot in stance be-gins with heel strike and progresses to foot flat, mid-stance, heel rise, and toe-off. There is a period of double weight-bearing in which both feet are on the ground. After toe-off, the foot goes into the swing phase of the gait cycle. This phase is made of acceleration, toe clear-ance, and deceleration. The stance phase makes up 62% and the swing phase 38% of the cycle.[1] If there is any ab-normality of the bones, joints, ligaments, nerves, or ex-trinsic or intrinsic muscles of the foot and ankle, it may be manifested in the function of gait.

DIAGNOSIS

As with other evaluations, the foot and ankle eval-uation begins with the history. The age, sex, injury, time of onset, type of pain, and localization of the pain are noted. Relief of pain with rest and aggravation with weight bearing indicate a mechancial problem. Associated symptoms, such as redness, swelling, and radiation, can occur. The patient's occupation, sports activities, and shoewear are included in the history.

The second part of the evaluation is the physical examination.[2] Both lower extremities are undressed and evaluated with standing, gait, and sitting with the legs dangling. The foot and ankle are inspected for color, swelling, deformities, and other abnormalities. The joints are examined for range of motion, and the symmetry is noted. The pulses are palpated, and the sensory examination is completed. Palpation of the areas of complaint or deformity usually help the physician pinpoint the anatomic site of the disorder. Rarely, abnormalities of the spine, hip, or knee may be the cause of symptoms of the foot and ankle. A careful history and examination should help with the diagnosis.

Diagnostic Studies

Laboratory studies can be helpful in diagnosing infection, inflammatory arthritis, or tumor. A white blood cell count with a differential cell count and an erythrocyte sedimentation rate are generally used to help diagnose an infection and are reviewed in Chapter 5.

Musculoskeletal Imaging

Radiographic examinations are the most commonly used diagnostic tool in evaluation of the foot and ankle. Except in the case of an acute injury, weight-bearing studies provide the most functional information. Anteroposterior, oblique, and lateral views are taken of the foot. Similarly, anteroposterior, mortise, and lateral views are taken of the ankle. At times, a three-phase bone scan can be helpful for the diagnosis of an infection, stress fracture, or tumor that is not seen on a radiograph. A magnetic resonance imaging (MRI) scan delineates soft tissue structures as well as bony ones and can be helpful with the diagnosis of tendinitis, tendon rupture, stress reaction of bone, infection, and tumor. A computed tomography (CT) scan can be used to supplement bone detail in a fracture or deformity.

DISEASES OF THE FOOT AND ANKLE

Bunions

A bunion is the medial prominence of the base of the hallux and is also known as a *hallux valgus deformity*. There is a genetic predisposition, but the primary cause is ill-fitting shoes.[3] A possible cause of valgus deformity is muscle imbalance related to excessive pronation. It is more frequently seen in women

than in men (ratio $\geq 9:1$).[4] Populations that rarely wear shoes have a low incidence of bunions.

The hallux metatarsophalangeal joint is unique because it has the sesamoid mechanism, with intrinsic and extrinsic muscular structures that play an important role in the development of this deformity. Pes planus, or flatfoot, can be a contributing factor to this deformity. Also, if there is an increase in the angle between the first and second metatarsals, metatarsus primus varus, the patient may be predisposed to develop a bunion.

Radiographs show deviation of the proximal phalanx on the first metatarsal head, with or without dorsal subluxation of the joint.

The patient's most common complaint is pain over the bunion. The physical examination should be performed with the patient standing and sitting because the deformity is worse with weight bearing. The prominent medial eminence of the first metatarsophalangeal joint and lateral deviation of the hallux is seen. There may be inflammation of the bursa manifested by erythema and swelling. There can be redness and swelling of the prominence, breakdown of the skin, painful calluses under the second metatarsal head, or deformities of the lesser toes. Shoe fitting is difficult with the symptomatic bump. Radiographs show deviation of the proximal phalanx on the first metatarsal head, with or without dorsal subluxation of the joint.

In many patients, symptoms can be reduced by removing the pressure over the medial eminence. Proper footwear involves sufficient cushioning and a wide toe box to allow for the toes to spread. The patient should avoid a high-heel shoe with a narrow toe box. The shoe upper should be made of a soft material without a seam overlying the prominence. Sometimes, padding the painful area can be helpful. If nonoperative measures fail, the patient may consider surgical repair. Surgery consists of removing the bony medial eminence with or without an osteotomy to correct the hallux valgus deformity. In cases of hallux valgus deformities with degenerative joint disease, a fusion of the first metatarsophalangeal joint is indicated. After the surgery, some patients, approximately one third, continue to have limits for the type of shoe they can wear.[4]

Achilles Tendinitis

Achilles tendinitis is caused by overuse and is seen predominantly in runners. It can occur with other sports, such as cycling, tennis, basketball, or even walking. Patients present with pain and swelling of the posterior heel and ankle. Tendinitis can also occur in a middle-aged patient as a result of degeneration from repetitive stress.

The examination reveals localized swelling or thickening of the Achilles tendon. There is tenderness with palpation over the involved area. There can be loss of dorsal flexion strength or discomfort with resisted motion. Peritendinitis can be distinguished from Achilles tendinitis by the painful arc sign: Peritendinitis involves the tendon sheath, and as the foot is moved through dorsiflexion to plantar flexion, the area of tenderness is unchanged, whereas with tendinitis, the area of tenderness moves with the foot.

Treatment begins by having the patient avoid the precipitating or aggravating activities. A heel lift decreases the stress on the tendon. This device can be purchased by the patient; it is a 0.5-inch felt heel pad or a viscoelastic gel heel pad. A nonsteroidal anti-inflammatory drug can be added to the treatment plan to decrease the inflammatory response. Occasionally a short course of cast immobilization provides relief in symptoms. If this course is necessary, a removable walking cast can be used, which allows the patient to bathe and perform gentle active range-of-motion exercises. Once the symptoms begin to resolve, the patient can be taught heel cord stretching exercises. For these, the patient leans onto a wall with the feet turned in or stands on a tilted board. The activities then can gradually be increased as tolerated; brisk walks can be attempted and, eventually, short segments of jogging several weeks later.

Except with an acute rupture of the Achilles tendon, it is rare that a patient requires surgical intervention. Failure of conservative treatment, even up to 6 months, may be an indication for surgical débridement of the diseased tendon sheath. The tendon itself can have areas of degenerative tissue with thickening that can be débrided.

Pes Planus

Flexible pes planus is also known as flatfoot. It is commonly seen in children and is caused by ligamentous laxity. It is considered as a variation of normal. The medial longitudinal arch is determined by age and heritable traits; it develops with age as ligamentous laxity present at birth resolves.

Patients may complain of pain around the medial arch. If the deformity is severe, they can have symptoms on the lateral aspect of the hindfoot. This is called *impingement*, and it is the result of the calcaneus, in valgus, abutting the lateral malleolus. The patient may also have the feeling of tired feet or weakness. There often is a family history of flatfeet. As the patient stands, the physician sees loss of the medial longitudinal arch. Some of the arch may be present in a sitting position. There is usually generalized ligamentous laxity of the joints throughout the feet. There may be an associated equinus contracture or tightness of the Achilles tendon.

The treatment for symptomatic flatfeet is conservative. In a child, the treatment is simply observation. The natural history of flexible flatfeet is not changed by corrective shoes, orthotic devices, or exercise. Some parents may observe a functional improvement with the use of a supportive medial arch. In the symptomatic adult patient, heel cord stretching and activity modification can be used initially. A soft medial arch can provide support and help prevent hyperpronation. A simple, inexpensive felt pad can be applied to the shoe. Alternatively a custom total contact orthotic device can be prescribed. This latter treatment is more costly and

may be no more effective than the use of the soft felt pad. In prescribing a medial arch, it is important not to attempt to overcorrect the deformity, and it should be written as "total contact orthosis from firm materials, with added support in the medial heel and arch."[5] The patient may not tolerate a large support in the shoe. It is important to follow-up on the symptoms and treatment. The pain may resolve, then the arch support can be discontinued.

Surgery is rarely performed in patients with flexible pes planus. If the problem is caused by an associated equinus contracture, lengthening the Achilles tendon provides improvement. With severe or chronic deformities, sometimes a salvage operation is required to treat the symptoms, such as a triple arthrodesis. This procedure removes the degenerative joint disease and allows for some correction of the deformity but is rarely needed.

Rheumatoid Arthritis

Rheumatoid arthritis is reviewed in detail in Chapter 25. It involves the feet in about 89% of cases.[6] The forefoot is the most common site involvement followed by the hindfoot then the ankle. As with the hands, both feet are affected. The initial involvement is synovitis, which leads to forefoot deformities, such as hallux valgus with dislocation and cock-up deformities of the lesser metatarsophalangeal joints. As the hindfoot and midfoot become involved, there is collapse of the longitudinal arch. It is important to treat foot and ankle problems in the rheumatoid patient because they often have other joint involvement that further compromises function.

Patients complain of pain and deformity. With severe cases, patients can have difficulty wearing a shoe. They have pain with weight-bearing activities and state they feel like they are walking on bones or marbles from the plantar prominence of the metatarsal heads. The physician should examine both lower extremities to determine other joint involvement. On standing, the deformity is more apparent. In most cases, the hallux is in lateral or medial deviation, and there are lesser toe deformities. The plantar fat pad is atrophied and pulled distally, which accentuates the prominence of the metatarsal heads. The hindfoot can be in valgus with loss of the medial longitudinal arch. With chronic disease, these deformities are fixed. There may be skin ulcerations over the bony deformities. Radiographic examinations show diffuse osteopenia with joint involvement of the hindfoot, midfoot, or forefoot. The clinical examination must be correlated to the x-ray findings to determine treatment.

Many patients with rheumatoid foot and ankle involvement can be treated conservatively. Principles of treatment include relief of pain, prevention of deformity, and improvement of function. Physical therapy with range-of-motion and strengthening exercises should be started. An extra-depth shoe with a wide toe box accommodates the forefoot deformities. A severe hindfoot and midfoot deformity may require an ankle-foot orthosis to provide support for ambulation.

Patients with rheumatoid arthritis benefit from surgical treatment if their symptoms persist and deformities are developing. A synovectomy can help decrease pain and swelling and may delay further development of deformity. In progressive, destructive synovitis, forefoot reconstruction that fuses the first metatarsophalangeal joint and resects the lesser metatarsal heads to decompress the joints can provide significant relief. The pes planovalgus from hindfoot and midfoot disease can be corrected with a triple arthrodesis.

Gout

A frequent presentation of gout is in the foot; most cases involve the first metatarsophalangeal joint, and it is called *podagra*. The ankle joint can also be affected although less commonly. The keys to management are recognizing that the patient has gout, and then instituting diet and drug therapy to normalize serum urate concentrations. A full discussion of gout and other crystalline arthropathies can be found in Chapter 30.

Heel Pain Syndrome (Plantar Fasciitis)

Heel pain syndrome is also known as *plantar fasciitis*. It is one of the most common disorders of the foot, and it is difficult to treat. The average duration of symptoms is 1 year, leading to much frustration for the patient as well as the physician. The plantar fascia is one of the primary supporting structures of the arch in the plantar foot. It is subjected to repetitive forces with weight-bearing activities. There is an association with obesity, abnormal biomechanics of the foot, middle age, and repetitive stress (such as walking and running).[7] Other causes of heel pain include stress fractures of the calcaneus, acute tears of the plantar fascia, nerve entrapment of the nerve to the abductor digiti quinti minimi, infection, and tumor.

The diagnosis usually can be made by a careful history and physical examination. The patient localizes the pain to the plantar heel at the medial calcaneal tuberosity. This location differentiates heel pain from disorders of the Achilles tendon that are focused at the posterior heel. The pain can be sharp, dull, or burning in nature. Patients complain of pain with the first few steps in the morning or after prolonged sitting. The symptoms may subside until prolonged walking or standing aggravates the pain. Rest, slight elevation of the heel, and analgesics provide some relief. The examination shows localized tenderness at the medial calcaneal tuberosity on the plantar aspect. The patient may have a tight heel cord. Radiographs of the foot are not required, unless a fracture, infection, or tumor is suspected. The bone spur that may be seen on the radiograph is an incidental finding and is not associated with the symptoms.

There are many types of treatment, but there is no panacea. The patient should avoid repetitive stress activities. Initial treatment includes stretching, a heel cup, and a nonsteroidal anti-inflammatory drug. The patient is taught to stretch the heel cord by leaning against a wall, feet flat and turned in slightly for 30 seconds, with multiple repetitions. This stretch should be done several times a day. Many patients find this to be helpful in relieving pain and stiffness. The heel cup or pad (such as a viscoelastic polymer) absorbs weight-bearing forces and elevates the heel. An orthotic device may be beneficial, especially if there is an anatomic or biomechanical abnormality to be corrected.

Injections into the affected area have been used with variable success. A combination of an anesthetic (e.g., lidocaine) and glucocorticoid can provide temporary relief. The anesthetic and glucocorticoid placed with a 22-gauge needle into the medial calcaneal tuberosity area after preparing the skin from the lateral side of the foot. Multiple injections can increase the chance of rupture of the plantar fascia and should be avoided. In patients with severe and persistent discomfort, a course of cast immobilization helps break the chronic pain cycle. Most patients have complete relief of pain, although some have a flare-up of discomfort once the cast is removed after 6 to 8 weeks. The American Orthopaedic Foot and Ankle Society recommends that 6 to 12 months of nonoperative treatment be used before considering an operative procedure. More than 90% of patients respond to nonsurgical treatment within 6 to 10 months. If surgery is planned, a partial plantar fascia release is performed with or without decompression of the nerve to the abductor digiti minimi.

Morton's Neuroma

Morton's neuroma is also called an *interdigital neuroma* or *interspace neuroma*. The cause is entrapment of the nerve by perineural fibrosis from repetitive trauma. It most commonly affects the third interspace, followed by the second. The patient complains of pain between the metatarsal heads of the third or second interspace on the plantar aspect. The pain is sharp, tingling, burning, or radiating, with or without numbness of the involved toes. If the patient removes the shoe and rubs the foot, the pain lessens. Examination shows reproduction of the symptoms with compression of the metatarsal heads and palpation of the interspace. A radiographic series helps distinguish Morton's neuroma from a bone cause, such as a stress fracture.

The treatment begins with relieving the area of pressure. The toe box of the shoe should be wide enough to allow the toes to spread. Avoiding a high heel decreases the weight placed on the forefoot. The metatarsal area can be elevated with a metatarsal felt pad placed proximal to the neuroma. At times, a glucocorticoid injection into the involved nerve may provide relief of pain, but this is usually temporary. A short-acting glucocorticoid and lidocaine are placed in the point of maximal tenderness between the metatarsal head. A small needle is used (e.g., 25 gauge), and the injection is placed from the dorsal aspect, of the foot. Patients often experience immediate relief. Some have some temporary discomfort from the volume injected into the area, but this usually resolves after the first day. If conservative measures fail, the patient may elect to have the neuroma excised, but even after excision, some patients may continue to experience some symptoms.

SUMMARY

The foot and ankle have the unique function of locomotion. An injury, deformity, or manifestation of a systemic disease causes disability along with pain. Most diagnoses can be made with a careful history and physical examination. The most commonly used imaging study is weight-bearing radiographs of the foot and ankle to accentuate abnormalities.

Most foot and ankle problems are caused or worsened by improper footwear. Women should avoid shoes with a narrow toe box and high heels. Shoes should be tried on at the end of the day when the foot is the largest from swelling. Because most people have one foot that is longer than the other, the shoe should fit the longer foot. Shoe sizes vary by different manufacturers

and one should not purchase a shoe only by its size. A good shoe is larger than the foot, having an extra 0.5 inch at the end of the shoe to the longest toe (first or second toe). One should not expect the shoe to stretch out to fit the foot, and the shoe should be made of a soft upper material, such as leather. Close collaboration of the primary care physician with an experienced and creative podiatrist is useful. The podiatrists' contribution to diagnosis and therapy are developed in the next section of this chapter.

REFERENCES

1. Sarrafian SK: Anatomy of the Foot and Ankle, 2nd ed. Philadelphia, JB Lippincott, 1993.
2. Hoppenfeld S: Physical Examination of the Spine and Extremities. Norwalk, CT, Appleton-Century-Crofts, 1976.
3. Coughlin MJ: Hallux valgus. J Bone Joint Surg Am 78:932–966, 1996.
4. Mann RA: Hallux valgus. In Mann RA, Coughlin MJ, ed: Surgery of the Foot and Ankle, 6th ed. St. Louis, Mosby-Year Book, 1993, pp 167–296.
5. Janisse D: Pedorthics. Foot Ankle Int 18:526–527, 1997.
6. Abdo RV, Iorio LJ: Rheumatoid arthritis of the foot and ankle. J Am Acad Orthop Surg 2:326–332, 1994.
7. Gill LH: Plantar fasciitis: Diagnosis and conservative management. J Am Acad Orthop Surg 5:109–117, 1997.

MANAGEMENT OF COMMON FOOT PROBLEMS

Lawrence M. Oloff ■ Alan P. Bocko

The multispecialty approach to rheumatologic disease is the most effective way to manage focused systemic diseases that manifest in the foot and ankle. The podiatrist is an integral specialist in the diagnosis and treatment of foot and ankle pathology and hence plays an important team role. This section presents to the primary care physician the appropriate clinical management of common foot and ankle musculoskeletal disorders. To treat these patients properly, it is imperative that an accurate diagnosis be made; otherwise, any therapy is doomed to failure. The proper timing of certain treatments is emphasized. Examples of surgical intervention when clinical management of some musculoskeletal disorders fail are presented.

NERVE ENTRAPMENT DISORDERS OF THE LOWER EXTREMITY

Cutaneous Nerve Entrapment

EXAMINATION

Typically, nerve pathology in the lower extremities is the result of an inflammatory process on local injury to the nerve or structures adjacent to the nerve. Injuries may be the result of a single episode or cumulative trauma. Early damage to the peripheral nerves is usually exhibited as sensory abnormalities as opposed to muscular dysfunction. Many times, the outward physical signs of entrapment are few until the process becomes more chronic. For this reason, it is extremely important to obtain an accurate history of the patient's local pain course, duration, type of sensation, alleviating and aggravating factors, location, and previous treatment instituted.[1]

Patients generally perceive entrapment neuropathy pain as *pins and needles, burning, shocking,* or *stinging,* with or without radiation of the symptoms. Musculoskeletal pain is more often described as dull, achy, or sharp in nature. Pain originating in a nerve is often difficult to localize and may exist over the entire distribution of the nerve. In contrast to musculoskeletal discomfort, entrapment neuritis is more likely to be painful when the patient is not weight bearing and tends to be worse at night. The onset of symptoms many times corresponds with a history of prior trauma or surgery at the site. Neurologic pain also tends to start gradually, and as it intensifies, patients report it as unrelenting or constant in nature. The degree of continuously of the pain as well as the severity is helpful in accessing improvement or worsening of symptoms once therapy is instituted.

When entrapment neuropathy is suspected, the lower extremity physical examination should focus on the specific distributions of the involved nerve. It is also helpful to allow the patient to outline specifically with a ballpoint pen the involved area directly on the foot or ankle. Many describe the distribution of specific peripheral nerves or dermatomes in the lower extremity (Fig. 21–1).[1] A dermatomal distribution can indicate that the pain is radiating from the spinal cord and is therefore radicular in origin. Direct visualization of the extremity may reveal a prominence, scar, trauma, deformity, or anatomic location that may be associated with a site of previous nerve injury. In the later stages of nerve degeneration, muscle atrophy or trophic changes (vasospasm, color change, hyperhydrosis, or hypohydrosis) may be apparent as well. Once a specific nerve is identified as the primary source of discomfort, palpation or percussion may elicit radiation distal or proximal to the site of entrapment in the form of paresthesias. Distal radiation (Tinel's sign) may replicate symptoms the patient has been experiencing away from the site of actual impingement. Deep tendon reflexes (patellar—L3, L4, Achilles—S1, S2) can help indicate whether the process is an upper versus lower motor neuron pathology. Finally, it is imperative that all the aforementioned findings be compared with the opposite or uninjured extremity.

DIAGNOSIS

Further information may be obtained by electrophysiologic assessment. When performed by a physiatrist or neurologist, nerve conduction velocities and electromyogram can give insight as to the level of pathology and degree of degeneration of the involved nerve. Once the level of the entrapment is determined, confirmation of the diagnosis and subsequent treatment may be achieved in many ways. First, local diagnostic and therapeutic blocks with local anesthetic with or

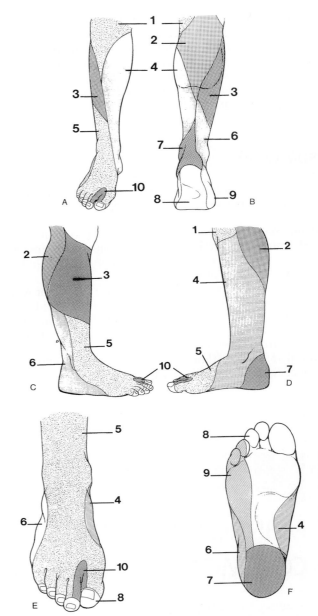

Figure 21–1. Anatomic sensory distribution of peripheral nerves. *A,* Anterior. *B,* Posterior. *C,* Lateral. *D,* Medial. *E,* Dorsal. *F,* Plantar. 1, Medial and intermediate femoral cutaneous nerves (L2, 3). 2, Posterior femoral cutaneous nerve (S1, 2, 3). 3, Lateral sural cutaneous nerve (L5; S1, 2). 4, Saphenous nerve (L3, 4). 5, Superficial peroneal nerve (L4, 5; S1). 6, Sural nerve (L5; S1, 2). 7, Medial calcaneal nerve branch (S1, 2). 8, Medial plantar nerve (L4, 5). 9, Lateral plantar nerve (S1, 2). 10, Deep peroneal nerve (L4, 5). (From Oloff LM: Musculoskeletal Disorders of the Lower Extremities. Philadelphia, WB Saunders, 1994, pp 686–687.)

without glucocorticoids should be considered. Specifically, blocking the nerve above the level of the entrapment can help confirm the diagnosis. When there is relative certainty that a specific nerve is the cause, a short-acting glucocorticoid (such as dexamethasone phosphate) may be included for injection at the site of entrapment with the hopes of reducing inflammation or scar tissue at the site. The short-acting, highly soluble glucocorticoids are used to minimize the risk of skin or soft tissue atrophy and hypopigmentation.

Radiographs sometimes reveal bony prominences, periarticular osteophytic proliferation, or expansile bone lesions that may be applying underlying pressure to cutaneous nerves.[2] MRI can elicit evidence of masses, fluid collections, or other space-occupying soft tissue or bone lesions causing impingement as well. Some of these conditions require referral to a foot and ankle specialist for excision or release of the nerve; however, most cutaneous nerve entrapments can be treated well in the office setting.

TREATMENT

The initial treatment of nerve entrapments should be conservative, especially if the symptoms are indicative of early, reversible damage. Most should be initially managed in two ways: anti-inflammatory medication and removal of any source of potential irritation or pressure stimuli to the involved nerve. Resting or off-weighting the area can be accomplished in many ways. Placing simple padding around a prominence, changing shoes to avoid pressure, and attempting mechanical control of a foot (over-the-counter orthoses) are often of significant benefit. If the patient's symptoms seem to improve slowly with these steps, the entrapment is most likely a reversible inflammatory process. If symptoms do not resolve the likelihood of in situ scar tissue formation or more substantial nerve injury is high. Injection therapy should be considered (see Chapter 6) as well as physical therapy modalities for reduction of surrounding scar or inflammation.

Care must taken by the physical therapist not to manipulate aggressively an already irritated nerve. Drugs, such as gabapentin (Neurontin), that are useful in neuropathies may be helpful[3]; used usually as an anticonvulsant, gabapentin has been found to correct the polarity of peripheral nerves and reduce certain entrapment pains. When conservative modalities fail or the nerve exhibits significant decrease in function, with definite source of impingement, consultation by a foot and ankle specialist is warranted.

Common Forms of Entrapment Neuropathy

The most frequently encountered entrapment neuropathy is *Morton's neuroma*. One primarily relies on the clinical examination for diagnosis. A positive Mulder's sign is useful for diagnosis. When the physician applies medial-to-lateral compression of the forefoot while pushing in a plantar direction on the area of suspected neuroma, a palpable click is appreciated. This maneuver also replicates the patient's symptoms. Glucocorticoid injections, off-weighting the neuroma by pads or orthoses, and surgical removal are treatment alternatives.

Tarsal tunnel syndrome is classically described as an entrapment neuropathy of the tibial nerve as it crosses inferior to the medial malleolus. The flexor reti-

naculum in this location (also called the *laciniate ligament*) may cause entrapment, especially if there is trauma to the site or if an expansile process exists within this fibro-osseous tunnel. As the tibial nerve branches into the foot, it courses beneath the abductor hallucis muscle belly (porta pedis), another potential site of entrapment. Traversing in close proximity with the nerve are two veins and the posterior tibial artery. Varicosities within the tarsal tunnel, another potential cause of pressure, may be alleviated with the simple use of compressive stockings.[4] Any source of fluid or mass effect on the nerve has the potential to cause permanent damage. Early symptoms of neuropraxia typically occur first, and these are treatable. Surgical release for tarsal tunnel syndrome is less successful than for carpal tunnel syndrome, so conservative therapy should be tried vigorously.

Other specific areas in the foot and ankle are more amenable to treatment and permanent relief of symptoms. Entrapment of the superficial and deep peroneal nerves has been called *anterior tarsal tunnel syndrome*. There is a soft tissue tunnel on the front of the ankle where the deep peroneal nerve courses on its way to the first intermetatarsal space (between the hallux and second toes). Certain foot types are predisposed to developing an exostosis over the first or second metatarsocuneiform articulation directly under the deep peroneal nerve as well.[5] The superficial peroneal nerve arises through a fascial tunnel and the interosseous membrane on the anterolateral leg; both are known areas of entrapment. Also, it travels in close proximity to the anterior ankle joint and is commonly irritated with inversion ankle injuries. Laterally the sural nerve originates superficially running along the course of the lesser saphenous vein, posterior to the lateral malleolus and out to the lateral side of the foot. Although it has not been described in a compression syndrome, the sural nerve is prone to traumatic entrapment, especially in patients who have had a peroneal tendon injury or calcaneal fracture.

In the foot and ankle all cutaneous nerves are anatomically adjacent to musculoskeletal structures. Therefore, synovitis, tendinitis, and arthritis can be the primary causes of any nerve entrapment syndrome for that reason. Treatment of the primary inflammatory process is the logical initial step in the management of peripheral entrapment neuropathies in these types of clinical settings.

SOFT TISSUE ABNORMALITIES

Tendon Disorders

Of all the soft tissue abnormalities in the lower extremity, tendon disorders have the greatest potential for causing severe dysfunction, pain, and deformity. Local pathology, both acute and cumulative injuries, is common. Tendon injuries have classically been divided into two main categories—acute and chronic. Although acute total or partial tendon rupture can be a devastating injury, it is not common and is treated surgically on an emergent basis.

ANATOMY AND PATHOPHYSIOLOGY OF TENDINITIS

Tendons are unique connective tissue structures composed primarily of type I collagen oriented in a longitudinal fashion. The internal structure of a tendon contains two structures, the endotenon and the epitenon, which serve specialized functions in the reparative process of this tissue.[6] Externally, tendons are surrounded by two different structures depending on their course from muscle to bone insertion. The paratenon is an areolar tissue that surrounds the tendon when it courses a straight path. Synovial-lined tendon sheaths cover the tendon as it changes directions along its course. Both play a primary role in facilitating tendon glide in normal function.[7] Tendons are susceptible to injury where they bend around corners. In the foot and ankle, the posterior tibial, peroneus longus, peroneus brevis, and flexor hallucis longus tendons are the most susceptible to injury.

There are two main mechanisms for tendon repair. Intrinsic repair of tendons occurs when fibroblasts within the tendon synthesize new collagen. This process reconstitutes normal tissue. The other mechanism is extrinsic repair when structures that surround the tendon contribute to the reparative process.[8] Adhesions that can limit tendon function and cause pain occur often during the extrinsic repair process.[9] When normal passive motion of a tendon is slowly started during the reparative process, intrinsic repair seems to be induced, reducing the potential of painful adhesions. Tendons that become chronically painful generally have suffered minor injury or inflammation that leads to fibrous adhesions to surrounding tissue during the extrinsic reparative process. This process weakens the structure of the tendon and a higher probability of rupture.

There are three forms of chronic tendon injury.[10] *Peritendinitis crepitans* is a process that occurs more at the musculotendinous junction and is the result of repetitive strain or motion. Crepitations noted on palpation or on auscultation of the painful site are almost pathognomonic for this process. *Chronic tendinitis* occurs around and within the tendon sheath. This process is the result of repetitive stress or trauma and is usually diagnosed as pain with passive motion of the tendon. Multiple sites of chronic tenosynovitis should alert the clinician that a systemic process may be present. Both of the aforementioned processes are generally treated conservatively by removing the source of repetitive stress and using anti-inflammatory measures. *Stenosing tenosynovitis* is a more dire condition because it tends to be refractory to conservative treatment. It develops after trauma or as an evolution of chronic tendinitis. Stenosing tenosynovitis prevents the normal gliding action of a tendon because adhesions form to surrounding structures along the tendon course. With restricted motion, fibrosis of the tendon progresses. Eventually, tendon deterioration or rupture can occur.[11]

DIAGNOSIS AND TREATMENT

Accurate clinical examination is essential, including observation, palpation, and, if necessary, diagnostic studies. MRI is the gold standard albeit expensive, for confirmation of tendon pathology. MRI is generally reserved for patients who do not respond favorably to standard conservative protocol or when rupture is suspect. Not only does MRI reveal discontinuity or scar tissue replacement within a tendon, but also chronic or acute inflammation is readily apparent (Fig. 21–2).[12] Limitations to MRI are the cost of the study and the difficulty in diagnosing stenosing tenosynovitis. Contrast radiography in the form of tenogram is a much more accurate way of diagnosing stenosing tenosynovitis and may be therapeutic as well. Hydrostatic pressure increased by the infusion of fluid within a tendon sheath can free adhesions. Follow-up with injection of short-acting corticosteroids reduces inflammation and discourages additional fibrosis. Ultrasonography of tendon pathology is a growing field with equipment becoming more sensitive with better resolution. Its cost-effectiveness and safety are unmatched, but it is technician dependent. Plain radiographs and CT are useful in the examination for potential extra tendinous osseous causes.

Treatment of early tenosynovitis should focus on anti-inflammatory treatments and elimination of mechanical stresses to the particular tendon.[11] Immobilization is definitely effective, although it can potentially accelerate the formation of restrictive tendon adhe-

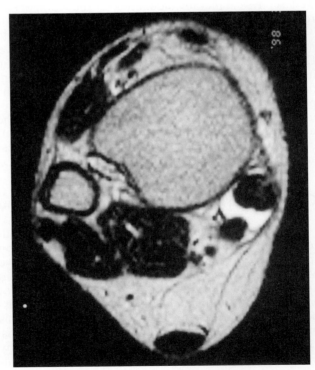

Figure 21–2. Magnetic resonance imaging of the ankle in a patient with rheumatoid arthritis demonstrates inflammation around a markedly thickened posterior tibial tendon. This inflammation is evidenced by increased signal (white) around the tendon within its sheath. The heterogenous appearance is consistent with a partial tear and scar tissue replacement within the tendon substance.

sions.[6] A better choice is to provide a removable form of immobilization, such as an ankle brace or weight-bearing cast boot. This form of immobilization allows intermittent physical therapy in the form of gentle strengthening and range-of-motion exercises. Also, orthoses or over-the-counter arch supports can help in controlling abnormal motion in the foot when this is thought to play a role in the genesis of the tendinitis. A case in point is the common occurrence of posterior tibial tendinitis with flatfoot deformity. It is specifically important to control posterior tibial tendinitis because of the inherently poor vascular supply of this tendon making it prone to spontaneous rupture. When rupture occurs, collapse of the medial longitudinal arch soon follows.

Nonsteroidal anti-inflammatory drugs should be a staple of early therapy. Control of any underlying systemic inflammatory process is always essential as mentioned earlier. If the aforementioned treatments fail, contrast material is infused into the tendon sheath (a tenogram) for both diagnostic and therapeutic reasons. Glucocorticoids must be used judiciously because of the potential risk of tendon rupture[10] induced by these compounds. When conservative treatment fails to relieve symptoms in a reasonable amount of time or diagnostic studies reveal irreversible damage or stenosing tenosynovitis of the tendon, referral to an orthopaedic surgeon for surgical intervention is warranted. Examples include weakness, dysfunction, and changes in structural integrity and gross flattening of the foot because of posterior tibial tendon pathology. Without early surgical intervention of this tendon disorder, a patient may develop severe arthritis requiring fusion of the rearfoot because of chronic malposition and gait abnormalities.

Rheumatologic Soft Tissue Masses

GOUTY TOPHI

Gout has long been known as *the great imitator.* The stereotypical clinical appearance of this monarthropathy as a red, hot, painful, swollen joint is often confused with infection or trauma in an office or emergency department setting. Patients with chronic tophaceous gout (see Chapter 30) can present with a mass causing shoe irritation and, perhaps, ulceration if they have been neglected. These subcutaneous masses are crystalline deposits of sodium monourate crystals that usually occur around the small joints of the foot (first metatarsophalangeal joint is most common).[14] They may also present as fusiform swelling of the Achilles tendon or retro-Achilles bursa near its insertion. Rarely, associated tendon ruptures are reported in long-standing cases.[15] With the development of allopurinol that effectively and safely controls hyperuricemia in most patients, severe tophaceous gout is much less common than it was 30 years ago.[16]

RHEUMATOID NODULES

Nodules are the most common subcutaneous manifestation of rheumatoid arthritis. They occur over areas of bony prominence or as peritendinous lesions. They are not invasive.[17] Nodules tend to occur in patients with more active and aggressive forms of rheumatoid arthritis and those with high titers of rheumatoid factor (see Chapter 25). These typically rubbery mobile masses are asymptomatic and nontender. If they become large enough, they can cause impingement or irritation of surrounding structures. Surgical excision is warranted in certain cases, especially when tendinitis and nerve entrapment are a secondary finding unless the underlying disease is controlled, recurrence of rheumatoid nodules is high.

GANGLION CYSTS AND BURSITIS

Ganglionic cysts develop from synovial-lined structures, such as joint capsules and tendon sheaths. Histologically, ganglions are a form of myxoid degeneration of these connective tissues that results in a herniation of the synovial lining.[18] Typical ganglia follow a path of least resistance in the foot or ankle coursing along a tendon or in subcutaneous tissue around a joint. Even though they are benign fluid-filled lesions, ganglia can proliferate to involve surrounding structures many centimeters away from their point of origin. Palpation may reveal either a soft or a hard mass as ganglia tend to fluctuate in size and firmness. Changes in size or symptome can be related to activity or can correlate with the activity of a systemic disease process. As with other masses in the foot and ankle, ganglions may cause irritation of nerve, tendon, or overlying cutaneous structures.

Although there are many anatomic locations where bursae are common, they can form as a result of repetitive pressure over a prominence as well. They do not communicate with a joint or tendon sheath but may become inflamed usually as a result of repetitive stress or strain. Common locations around the foot or ankle include the Achilles tendon insertion, the plantar aspect of the calcaneus or metatarsals, and on the dorsum of the foot under any hyperkeratotic lesion. Treatment is generally the same as with ganglion cysts.

As with most lesions in the foot, removal of the aggravating force is essential along with the use of anti-inflammatory measures. Diagnosis of ganglia or inflamed bursae and their cause may be obtained in many ways. Plain radiographs may show a bony prominence underlying a lesion. MRI is especially helpful in determining the extent of a lesion for planned surgical excision. Simple aspiration of a suspected ganglion or bursa is confirmatory and therapeutic as well. On aspiration, the fluid of a bursa is thin, with a cell count proportional to the degree of inflammation. Ganglia usually contain thicker, more viscous, almost gelatinous contents. A short-acting glucocorticoid may be injected at the same site to reduce the size of the lesion. Pressure over the area of aspiration should be mandatory for several weeks to help prevent rapid reformation of a ganglion. Patients who present with pain associated with ganglia that are recalcitrant to conservative treatment may need further study to rule out an associated entrapment neuropathy necessitating surgical excision of the lesion.

ARTICULAR AND OSSEOUS DISORDERS

Mechanical Instability

Chronic inflammation in and around joints is the hallmark of most systemic rheumatologic diseases and may have devastating clinical ramifications in lower extremities. Inflammation of the supporting architecture of pedal joints can also arise as a result of poor foot mechanics. The course of the latter is usually less fulminant.

LESSER METATARSOPHALANGEAL JOINTS

During active rheumatoid arthritis, the joint capsule, ligaments, and tendons become susceptible to injury, which, in turn, leads to instability and subsequent deformity. In the foot, the metatarsophalangeal joints are most often affected. The primary complaint is pain on the plantar aspect of the lesser metatarsophalangeal joints. The second metatarsophalangeal joint is usually the first to exhibit signs of instability or deformity for two reasons. Anatomically the second metatarsal is the longest and therefore accepts the majority of force during normal gait. Also, many patients exhibit some hypermobility at the level of the metatarsocuneiform joint, which transfers most of the forefoot weight bearing laterally. The authors often see patients referred with suspected second intermetatarsal neuromas when, in fact, the problem lies in the joint and not the adjacent nerve. It is not unheard of to have a second interspace neuroma in the setting of active inflammatory joint disease; however, entrapment of this nerve is uncommon in comparison with the adjacent third intermetatarsal space in the general population.

Some simple clinical examination techniques may differentiate between nerve and joint pain in this setting. Instability is often seen grossly as subtle malalignment of the toe in any plane. Typically the toe is slightly dorsally displaced and has medial deviation toward the hallux at the metatarsophalangeal joint. This is primarily due to the loss of integrity of the collateral ligaments or insufficiency of the flexor (plantar) plate apparatus.[19] This type of instability leads to further mechanical deformity of the digit in the form of hammertoes. Palpation of the distal aspect of the metatarsal head reveals significant discomfort relative to the adjacent intermetatarsal space. Sagittal plane instability may be assessed with the modified Lachman's test (Fig. 21–3).[19] This test may reveal marked plantar pain confirming either chronic inflammation or even disruption of the flexor plate apparatus. In the case of neuromas, a positive Mulder's sign is seen, as previously mentioned in the nerve entrapment section. Subtle findings may be confirmed with the aid of intra-articular diagnostic injection. After sterile preparation of the skin, injection of the joint with lidocaine can produce immediate pain relief. Glucocorticoid injection is recommended in this setting as a last resort, once all other conservative treatment has failed, because further weakening and instability of the joint may occur as a side effect.[20]

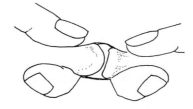

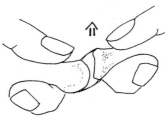

Figure 21–3. Modified Lachman's test of the metatarsophalangeal (MTP) joint. Dorsally dislocating the proximal phalangeal base out to the MTP joint is a positive result. It indicates loss of integrity of the *intrinsic ligaments,* which results in instability of the MTP joint. (From Oloff LM: Musculoskeletal Disease of the Lower Extremities. Philadelphia, WB Saunders, 1994, p 488.)

Early treatment of the underlying synovitis, if present, is crucial to avoid progressive deformity. Local therapy involves off-weighting the painful area with padding, orthoses, or both and splinting of the toe into a rectus, plantar flexed position. Also, all aggravating activities should be curtailed in favor of non–weight-bearing activities. If the initial therapy is unsuccessful, formal physical therapy should be considered. Once the acute inflammatory stage is controlled, long-term maintenance of the instability should focus on prevention. This is primarily in the form of orthoses, in-shoe padding, and gradual return to activity as tolerated.

Failure of conservative therapy typically results for two reasons: Inflammation progresses to rupture of periarticular structures, or recalcitrant plantar forefoot pain occurs because of deformity. Realistically the deformity and instability should be surgically managed at this time to avoid progression. Surgical correction of the instability is achieved with straightening of the digital contracture (usually by fusing the proximal interphalangeal joint) and metatarsophalangeal joint release dorsally (release of the extensor tendons or dorsal joint capsule) with proximal translocation of the flexor tendon at the level of the proximal phalanx. This procedure serves to correct both the toe position and the mechanical instability. In a joint that is not arthritic, this is a highly successful procedure.

HALLUX VALGUS

One of the most common deformities seen in the foot is hallux valgus, or bunion deformity. In most patients without rheumatologic disease, the cause is muscle imbalance of the long tendons of the hallux that overpower the short flexors and ligaments, which are meant to stabilize the first metatarsophalangeal joint. This imbalance usually occurs because of excessive pronation of the foot during the stance portion of the gait cycle. In inflammatory joint disease, the cause of hallux valgus is multifactorial. Poor-fitting shoes play a large role in development of this lesion. Besides the mechanical causes mentioned, chronic inflammation of ligamentous and capsular structures leads to instability similar to lesser metatarsophalangeal pathology. Also, the existence of these additional factors translates to accelerated formation of deformity. In erosive rheumatoid arthritis, joint capsule distinction leads to significant subluxation and pain (Fig. 21–4). In some cases, the abnormal position of the hallux imposes its deviated position on the lesser toes with resultant lesser metatarsophalangeal joint deformities as well.

Treatment of hallux valgus in the office setting is typically palliative in nature. Padding may be applied medially at the prominence of the first metatarsal. Dorsal medial cutaneous nerve entrapment can occur in this location, which may warrant glucocorticoid injection. Changes in footwear are necessary in most cases because of widening of the foot and the medial prominence of the great toe. Splinting of the hallux into a corrected position has been attempted in the past, even with elaborate devices, but usually proves ineffective as a long-term solution. Functional orthoses are used in many cases in an attempt to control the abnormal biomechanics leading to hallux valgus formation. Although the aforementioned therapies are sometimes effective in the short term, the instability present, whether of mechanical or inflammatory origin, is difficult to address conservatively. To reduce the possibility of joint degeneration, surgery is recommended for realignment of the hallux as a more long-term solution. The procedures for hallux valgus have quite a high success rate. Without control of abnormal biomechanics (usually with or-

thoses) and effective treatment of inflammatory disease postoperatively, however, recurrence is a definite possibility.

STRUCTURAL DEFORMITIES AND ARTHRITIS

In the face of rheumatologic disease, arthritis of the foot and ankle is not only painful, but also deforming and debilitating. In rheumatoid arthritis, invasive synovitis at the level of the metatarsophalangeal joints can cause severe deformity. Marked fibular deviation of the toes and sagittal plane contractures cause severe retrograde forces on the metatarsals (see Fig. 21–4A). These bones, combined with cartilage erosion and wasting or displacement of the forefoot adipose padding, cause crippling pain. Local management should focus on accommodation of prominent forefoot deformities. In the elderly or less active patient, custom-molded shoes with accommodative soft insoles are extremely effective. More active, youthful patients are sometimes not amenable to wearing such devices. Also their activity level is such that these conservative measures are insufficient. For this select patient population, referral to a foot and ankle surgeon for reconstruction is often needed. With severe forefoot deformity, the pan metatarsal head resection and first metatarsophalangeal joint arthrodesis offers a good solution (see Fig. 21–4B). This has been found to be one of the most satisfying procedures in these patients with intractable, debilitating pain.

HALLUX RIGIDUS

Hallux rigidus is a common disorder of the first metatarsophalangeal joint, best described as decreased range of motion of the hallux on the first metatarsal. For *normal* gait, the hallux is said to require 65 to 75 degrees

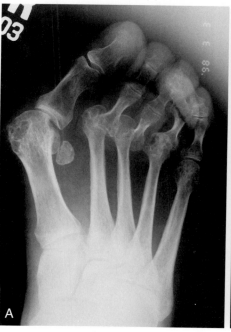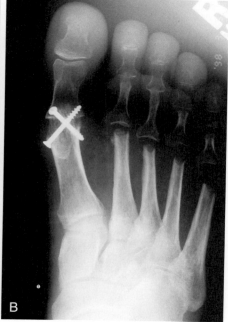

Figure 21–4. *A,* Dorsoplantar radiograph of a 44-year-old woman with rheumatoid arthritis causing marked joint instability and resultant forefoot deformity with severe hallux valgus causing marked pain *B,* The same patient 10 weeks after undergoing pan metatarsal head resection, digital corrections, and arthrodesis of the first metatarsophalangeal joint.

Approach to the Patient with Musculoskeletal Pain

of dorsiflexion. Limited motion may be the result of trauma, poor anatomic biomechanics, or degenerative or inflammatory joint disease. No matter what the causative factors are, the process results in progressive arthritis. Dorsal first metatarsophalangeal joint pain and joint stiffness are the predominant symptoms, and radiographic changes are obvious in most cases (Fig. 21–5A).

Conservative therapy is the same as with any degenerative joint process, starting with anti-inflammatory measures, and acetaminophen for pain. Intra-articular cortisone injection may provide temporary relief. Hallux rigidus is also amenable to accommodative insoles, specifically those that limit motion in a painful first metatarsophalangeal joint. In custom orthoses, this modification is called *Morton's extension*. Relief of symptoms as a result of conservative treatment is often short-lived. The surgical treatment of hallux rigidus depends on the primary complaints. If the symptoms are limited to dorsal osteophyte pain, related to shoe pressure, simple removal of the prominence may suffice. This is referred to as a *cheilectomy*. If there are additional articular complaints, attention needs to be directed to either improving joint mechanics or more radical procedures. Mechanical issues may be addressed with an osteotomy if ample cartilage remains for joint function (see Fig. 21–5). For end-stage arthritis, arthrodesis, joint replacement, and joint arthroplasty are the only options. Active patients do well with a fusion of the first metatarsophalangeal joint. Total, nonconstrained, two-component implants for this joint are used as well (Fig. 21–6).

REARFOOT AND ANKLE ARTHRITIS

Inflammatory arthritis can also be responsible for rearfoot and ankle pain and deformity. Direct causes result from pannus formation in and around joints causing early erosion of the articular surfaces. Even minor trauma in such joints accelerates degenerative processes. Pain in the rearfoot and ankle tends to perpetuate deformity when peroneal spasticity pulls the foot into an abducted and everted position. Peroneal spastic flatfoot is a well-known response to rearfoot pain seems to resolve only with absence of arthralgia. Indirectly, tendinopathy (posterior tibial is the most worrisome) may significantly increase the morbidity from the past. Aside from surgical arthrodesis of ankle, subtalar, or midtarsal joints, many bracing techniques are available to immobilize painful or dysfunctional situations externally. Early arthritis responds well to functional orthotic therapy when modifications such as a flat rearfoot post are applied to reduce motion in the subtalar joint. Ankle-foot orthosis, a custom posterior splint fixed to the lower leg, can serve to reduce painful motion at rearfoot, midfoot, and ankle joints. Both of the aforementioned modifications provide a partially concealed apparatus that may be cosmetically pleasing. With more advanced arthritis, patellar-tendon weight-bearing braces may serve to transfer all weight away from the lower extremity. Problems that exist with patellar-tendon weight-bearing braces are the bulkiness of the devices and transference of stress to the knee. Short-term relief may also be obtained with intra-articular injections of glucocorticoids, especially for end-stage arthritic disease when one is not as fearful of the deleterious side effects of the treatment.

A surgical therapy not often discussed in the treatment of arthritic joints is arthroscopy. It is well accepted that removal of peripheral osteophytes, intra-articular scar tissue, and chronic synovitis is extremely effective in temporary relief of the symptoms of mild-to-moderate degenerative joint disease.[21] The authors have had great success at prolonging the activity of these pa-

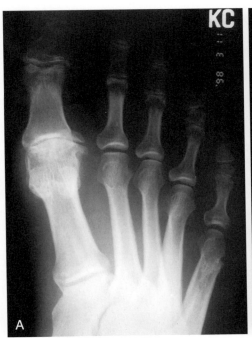
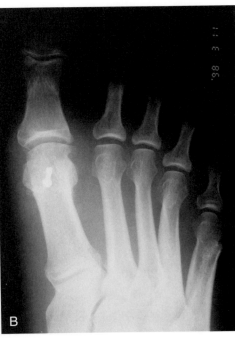

Figure 21–5. *A,* Dorsoplantar radiograph of a 48-year-old man with moderate degenerative changes resulting from hallux rigidus. *B,* The same patient 10 weeks after undergoing an osteotomy for correction of poor first ray mechanics. The patient had adequate remaining cartilage to avoid joint destruction. Joint space is increased after the procedure.

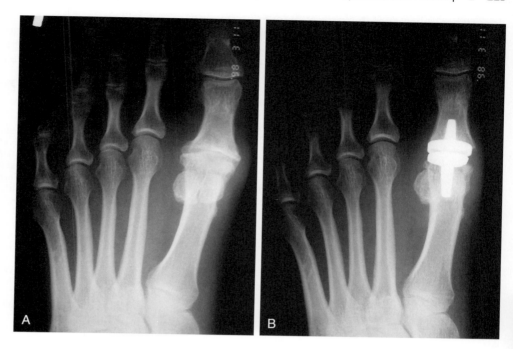

Figure 21–6. *A,* A 50-year-old woman with end-stage arthritis of the first metatarsophalangeal joint as a result hallux rigidus. *B,* The same patient after implantation of a two-component implant for replacement of the joint.

tients by maintaining joint motion and reducing inflammatory tissue in the ankle and subtalar joints for months to years; however, patients are to be cautioned that their disease process is progressive, and they will likely need a definitive procedure in the future. Permanent solutions for severe and progressive arthritis require surgical arthrodesis. Success is seen in patients who have isolated fusions of a severely arthritic joint, provided that the surrounding joints are not sources of pain (Fig. 21–7). In the foot and ankle, these joints are in close proximity to one another and the joint that is primarily responsible for pain may be difficult to identify. Sequential, intra-

articular diagnostic injections with lidocaine are quite useful in these situations.

Local Complications of Glucocorticoid Use

It is of great importance to discuss and consider two potential osseous complications that occur with long-term use of local or systemic glucocorticoids. Osteoporosis is a well-known side effect of this therapy in the management of articular pain.[20] The loss of bone

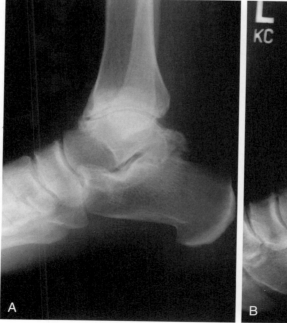
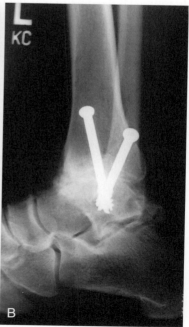

Figure 21–7. *A,* Radiograph of a 46-year-old man with seronegative arthritis primarily involving the ankle joint. *B,* Three months after arthroscopic arthrodesis of the ankle joint with crossed percutaneous screw fixation and, clinically, complete resolution of symptoms.

density not only makes this patient population susceptible to stress fractures, but also slows healing of these injuries. It is not uncommon to see stress fractures of the metatarsals in these patients that do not heal in 6 to 8 weeks. Protected weight bearing in these cases is essential but may be insufficient in the face of osteoporosis.

Tarsal bone stress fractures may present a diagnostic dilemma because it may take 2 to 4 weeks to see these injuries on plain radiographs. Even then, it is difficult for radiologists to see such subtle injuries. Consider the following examples: In a patient with a calcaneal stress injury, the injury is treated as a plantar fasciitis; a navicular stress fracture is treated as dorsal tendinitis or anterior ankle pain; or a stress fracture of the cuboid or cuneiform bones is treated as midtarsal joint sprain. Because non–weight-bearing is the staple treatment in these cases and delays can lead to potential delayed union or nonunion of bone, other diagnostic modalities should be considered early in this patient population. A three-phase bone scan is useful, although quite nonspecific and may be confusing in the face of overlying soft tissue inflammation. MRI is confirmatory of bone stress injuries and may rule out a superimposed soft tissue cause. CT scan is a less costly alternative but does not have the sensitivity of MRI or scintigraphy. As mentioned earlier, non–weight bearing or protected weight bearing is essential in these cases. Resolution of symptoms and evidence of bony callus on plain radiograph are good indicators of healing. In situations in which delayed healing is suspected, bone stimulation devices are a viable option.

Avascular or aseptic necrosis has been reported as a spontaneous finding in patients on long-term glucocorticoids.[22] Minor trauma may precipitate avascular necrosis, which typically presents as pain or joint stiffness with surrounding inflammation. This condition may occur in any bone in the foot or ankle but has been reported most often in the talus, perhaps because of the fragile vascular supply to this bone. Diagnosis is a dilemma. Hints of avascular necrosis may be present on plain radiographs as sclerosis or increase in density. Bone scan is helpful but is nonspecific. MRI may be the diagnostic modality of choice in the face of avascular necrosis, presenting as decreased signal of both T1 and T2 images when the disease is acute. If suspected or confirmed, treatment for avascular necrosis is strict non–weight bearing of the limb until there is radiographic evidence of revascularization. On x-ray, this presents in the talus as a line of lucency immediately deep to the subchondral bone (Hawkin's sign). Electrical stimulation of bone growth is also a treatment alternative in these cases. If revascularization does not occur, arthritis may be inevitable because of collapse of weakened avascular bone. In these cases, surgical fusion of the adjacent joint may prove necessary.

Early and accurate recognition has been stressed in this chapter many times and is nowhere more important than with avascular necrosis, in which delays in conservative therapy may have devastating consequences.

REFERENCES

1. Downey MS: Surgical treatment of peripheral nerve entrapment syndromes. In Oloff LM, ed: Musculoskeletal Disorders of the Lower Extremities. Philadelphia, WB Saunders, 1994, pp 685–717.
2. Downey MS: MRI of tarsal tunnel pathology. In Ruch JA, Vickers NS, eds: Reconstructive Surgery of the Foot and Leg: Update '92. Tucker, GA, Podiatry Institute, 1992, pp 104–110.
3. Rosenberg JM, et al: The effect of gabapentin on neuropathic pain. Clin J Pain 13:251–255, 1997.
4. Gould N, Alvarez R: Bilateral tarsal tunnel syndrome caused by varicosities. Foot Ankle 3:290–292, 1983.
5. Tobin R, Krych S, Harkless LB: First metatarsal-cuneiform dorsal exostosis: Its anatomical relation with the medial dorsal cutaneous nerve. J Foot Surg 28:442–444, 1989.
6. Mattews P, Richards H: The repair potential of digital flexor tendons. J Bone Joint Surg Br 56: 618–624, 1974.
7. Miller SJ: Principles of muscle tendon surgery and tendon transfers. In McGlamry ED, ed: Comprehensive Textbook of Foot Surgery. Baltimore, Williams & Wilkins, 1987.
8. Strickland JW: Flexor tendon injuries: I. Anatomy, physiology, biomechanics, healing, adhesion formation around a repaired tendon. Orthop Rev 15:632–645, 1986.
9. Peacock EE Jr: Biologic principles in the healing of long tendons. Surg Clin North Am 45:461–476, 1965.
10. Trevino S, Gould N, Korson R: Surgical treatment of stenosing tenosynovitis at the ankle. Foot Ankle 2:37–45, 1981.
11. Gilula LA, Oloff L, Caputi R, et al: Ankle tenography: A key to unexplained symptomatology: Part 2. Radiology 151:581–587, 1984.
12. Sartoris DJ, Resnick D: Magnetic resonance imaging of tendons in the foot and ankle. J Foot Surg 28:370–377, 1989.
13. Wyngaarden JB: Gout. In Wyngaarden JB, Smith LH, Bennett JC, eds: Cecil Textbook of Medicine, 19th ed. Philadelphia, WB Saunders, 1992, pp 1107–1115.
14. Addante A, Paicos P: Tophaceous gout involving the fourth toes bilaterally. J Am Podiatr Med Assoc 78:599–603, 1988.
15. Patel D, Stavosky J: Crystalline deposition disease. In Oloff LM, ed: Musculoskeletal Disorders of the Lower Extremities. Philadelphia, WB Saunders, 1994, pp 141–151.
16. McCarthy GM, Barthlelemy CR, Veum JA, et al: Influence of antihyperuricemic therapy on the clinical and radiographic progression of gout. Arthritis Rheum 34: 1489–1494, 1991.
17. Davis JA: Rheumatology, In Zier BG, ed: Essentials of Internal Medicine in Clinical Podiatry. Philadelphia, WB Saunders, 1990, pp 135–177.
18. O'Keefe RG: Surgical management of soft tissue tumors. In Oloff LM, ed: Musculoskeletal Disorders of the Lower Extremities. Philadelphia, WB Saunders, 1994. pp 626–638.
19. Thompson FM, Hamilton WG: Problems of the second metatarsophalangeal joint. Orthopedics 10:83, 1987.
20. Fitzgerald RH: Intrasynovial injection of steroids: Uses and abuses. Mayo Clin Proc 51:655, 1976.
21. Lundeen RO: Role of arthroscopy in the treatment of arthritic ankle disorders. In Oloff LM, ed: Musculoskeletal Disorders of the Lower Extremities. Philadelphia, WB Saunders, 1994, pp 612–625.
22. Perlman MD, Gold ML, Schor AD: Usage of long-term steroid therapy. J Foot Surg 26:233, 1987.

Chapter 22

Pain in the Jaw Joint: Diagnosis and Treatment

Andrew E. Turk ■ Stephen A. Schendel

The causes of jaw pain, in addition to masticatory dysfunction, myofascial pain syndromes, and atypical facial pain, are temporomandibular joint (TMJ) abnormalities, which can make diagnosis and treatment difficult in this group of patients. Differential diagnosis of pain resulting from vascular, neuralgic, neuritic, and temporomandibular origin complicates the management even further in these patients. This chapter focuses on jaw pain resulting from myofascial disease and TMJ abnormalities.

ANATOMY

The mandible is a unique bone that allows for rotational and translational movement through the TMJ. The blood supply to the mandible is through the inferior alveolar artery and the muscle and gingival attachments.[1] The myohyoid muscle, which elevates the tongue, attaches to the medial surface of the mandible. The geniohyoid muscles insert onto the genial tubercles and, with the anterior belly of the digastric muscle, depress and retract the mandible (Fig. 22–1).

The muscles that elevate or protrude the mandible are the masseter, temporalis, medial, and lateral pterygoid muscles (Fig. 22–2). The inferior portion of the lateral pterygoid muscle inserts onto the neck of the condyle, helping to protrude the mandible when contracting. The superior portion of the lateral pterygoid muscle inserts on the fibrous capsule and meniscus of the TMJ, to stabilize the meniscus during the movement of the mandible. The TMJ articular surfaces are lined with fibrocartilage, differing from other synovial joints that are lined with hyaline cartilage. The articular disc is a dense fibrous connective tissue structure that separates the joint into two spaces.[2] Hinge movement of the mandible is completed in the inferior space (ginglymus), and translation is followed in the superior space (arthrodial). The retrodiskal pad is an area of highly vascularized and innervated loose connective tissue. It is believed to be the origin of pain in TMJ dysfunction. If there are abnormal loading forces on the joint surfaces as a result of disc disease, this can lead to TMJ disorders.[3, 4] The interface of the mandibular condyle and temporal articular area is the joint surface. The condyles are elliptical measuring 20 mm medial to lateral and 10 mm anteroposterior. The fibrous joint capsule attaches to the condyle inferiorly and the zygomatic arch superiorly.[3] It is reinforced anteriorly and laterally by the temporomandibular ligament (Fig. 22–3).

The blood supply comes from the superficial temporal vessels and branches of the masseteric artery. The auriculotemporal, masseteric, and deep temporal branches of the trigeminal nerve supply innervation to the TMJ.[1]

TEMPOROMANDIBULAR JOINT MOTION

The mechanics of TMJ function are important in the diagnosis and management of TMJ disease. The masticatory and suprahyoid muscles are involved with TMJ motion. The mandible functions in chewing food and speech. During initiation of oral excursion or opening of the jaw, hinge motion of the joint achieves an initial 20 to 25 mm of interincisor distance. The following 15 to 20 mm of interincisor opening is due to the translatory motion of the mandible anteriorly along the articular eminence.[4–6] This combination of hinge and translation movement in the mandible allows TMJ protrusion, retrusion, and lateral excursion.

PATIENT EVALUATION

History

A patient may describe the pain originating from the TMJ, preauricular area, or surrounding masticatory muscles. Additionally the discomfort may radiate from the ear, teeth, or neck area. Often the onset of pain originating in the morning is due to nocturnal bruxism, grinding of teeth, in which constant pain after jaw function suggests intracapsular joint pathology. Patients with TMJ dysfunction relate a triad of preauricular pain, clicking or grinding noises from the TMJ, and poor mandibular movement.[6]

Some patients may describe noises in the joint associated with daily jaw movement. Such clicking may be

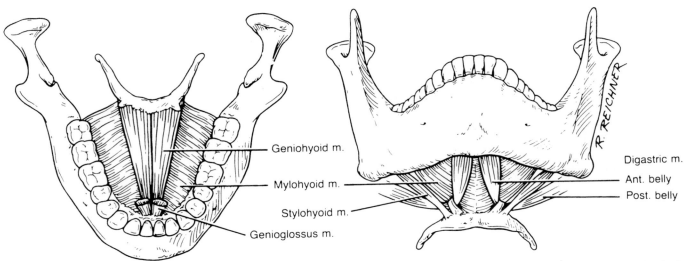

Figure 22–1. Muscles of the floor of the mouth and suprahyoid region: depressors of the anterior mandible. (From Georgrade G, ed: Textbook of Plastic Maxillofacial Surgery, 2nd ed. Baltimore, Williams & Wilkins, 1992.)

benign solitary clicks, which occur in 40% of the normal population. When there is anterior subluxation of the disc with jaw opening, condylar contact results in a click. A reciprocal click occurs as the disc subluxes when the condyle repositions into the glenoid fossa. The abnormal joint surfaces lead to a grinding or crepitus from the joint. *Closed lock* is a sudden irreducible anterior subluxation of the disc, limiting mandibular motion. Other reasons for limited excursion of the jaw may be due to local mus-cular dysfunction, bony or fibrous ankylosis of the joint, and blocking of the coronoid process by the zygoma.

Physical Examination

GENERAL EXAMINATION

Before the oral evaluation, a complete physical ex-amination is required. The examination of the patient

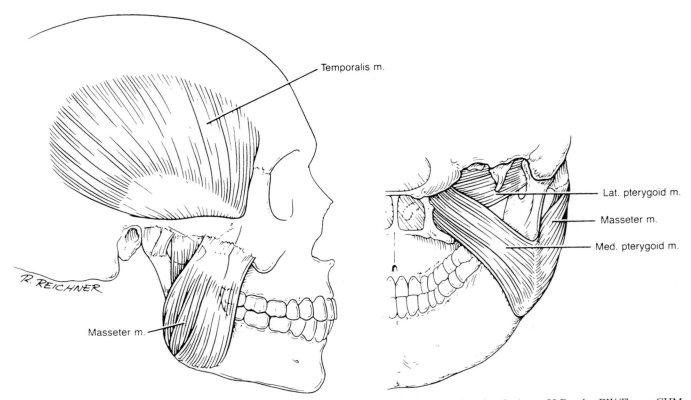

Figure 22–2. Muscles of mastication. (From Bessette RW, Jacobs JS: Temporomandibular joint dysfunction. In Aston SJ, Beasley RW, Thorne CHM, eds: Grabb and Smith's Plastic Surgery Philadelphia, Lippincott-Raven Publishers, 1997).

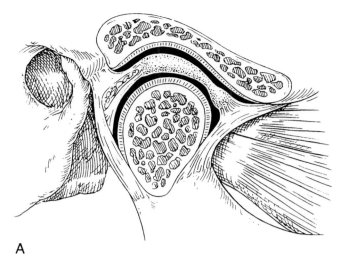

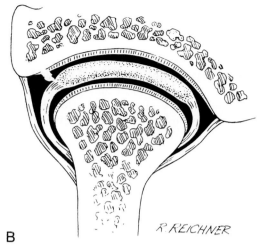

A

B

R. KEICHNER

Figure 22–3. *A,* Temporomandibular joint in sagittal section demonstrates the concave configuration of the articular disc, bilaminar posterior attachment, and insertion of the external pterygoid on the disc and the condylar head. *B,* Temporomandibular joint in coronal section demonstrates the position of the disc over the convexity of the condylar head and the separate attachments of the disc on the condyle in distinction from the capsule. (From Bessette RW, Jacobs JS: Temporomandibular joint dysfunction. In Aston SJ, Beasley RW, Thorne CHM, eds: Grabb and Smith's Plastic Surgery. Philadelphia, Lippincott-Raven Publishers, 1997.)

with TMJ pain centers on the head, neck, and TMJ. The facial examination includes any soft tissue asymmetry or skeletal deformities. Examination of the cranial nerves I through XII is performed to exclude any central nervous system disorders. The ear canals and tympanic membrane are examined to rule out primary benign or malignant diseases. Similarly the oral tissues are evaluated for mucosal lesions, swellings, periodontal disease, alveolar process abnormalities, and evidence of cheek or lip biting.

ORAL EXAMINATION

The teeth are examined for caries, mobility of teeth, absent teeth, prosthetics, molar impactions, supra-erupted teeth, malocclusion, and displacement of the mandible during contact of the teeth. The incisor relationship is important to delineate overbite, overjet, or open bite, all of which can contribute to the TMJ symptoms. Palpation of the area of the TMJ can detect clicking or crepitus. Joint sounds must be determined as popping, clicking (reciprocal or nonreciprocal), or crepitations.

Palpation of the TMJ can detect swelling, the presence of tenderness, and joint sounds. Auscultation can be more sensitive in determining the type of joint sounds. The masticatory and cervical muscles must also be excluded as areas of tenderness or spasm. The presence or absence of pain, intensity of pain, location of pain, and referred pain must be documented.

The TMJ range of motion should be measured. Any pain or deviation to the left or right on opening is noted. The normal interincisor opening distance is 40 to 50 mm. The lateral jaw movement is at least 10 mm on each side of the incisor midline. Any restriction of interincisal range of motion at opening, lateral restriction, deviation on opening, and development of new anterior open bite can be indicators of the degree of joint involvement. At this point, diagnostic imaging is required.

DIAGNOSTIC IMAGING

The most common conventional radiography is the *transcranial projection*, depicting the TMJ with the glenoid fossa, articular tubercle, and condyle. *Tomography* provides sectional images in the sagittal or coronal views. This modality demonstrates bone pathology and range of condylar motion but provides no information on soft tissue disease. One study showed that up to 85% with TMJ disease patients had normal tomography.[7]

The evaluation of the TMJ soft tissue and disc has traditionally been with *contrast arthrography*. Arthrography can be performed either as single-contrast lower compartment[8] or as dual-space contrast arthrotomography.[9] The information from TMJ arthrography is highly reliable in determining disc disease. Magnetic resonance imaging (MRI) provides similar information to these techniques. MRI visualizes soft tissue directly and is noninvasive.[10]

With abnormal findings, MRI commonly detects anterior, anterior medial, and anterior lateral displacement of the disc. In sagittal images, the disc is located anteriorly to the condyle in the closed mouth position. Furthermore, the MRI may provide insight into the bone marrow abnormalities of the condyle. If the central area of the condyle has a low signal, this may suggest a pathologic condyle consistent with avascular necrosis.

Computed tomography (CT) scanning is useful to evaluate bone abnormalities, bony ankylosis, and acute traumatic injuries to the head and neck areas. Otherwise, CT of the disc is difficult. The advantages of MRI over CT include absence of ionizing radiation, fewer artifacts from dense bone and metal clips, imaging in multiple planes, and good detail of the soft tissues.

The first step in imaging a patient with TMJ pain and dysfunction is a plain film or tomography. The next

Approach to the Patient with Musculoskeletal Pain

modality should be arthrography or MRI, focusing on the soft tissue and disc. For postsurgical imaging, MRI is the best choice.[11]

MYOFASCIAL PAIN AND DYSFUNCTION

The masticatory muscles are usually the primary source of this complaint. Myofascial pain and dysfunction (MPD) were first described by Laskin[12] and is characterized by a limited range of motion, aching pain, and severe tenderness on palpation of the muscles. Certain trigger points within the masticatory muscles refer the pain. The masseter muscle, producing an ache in the jaw, is most common. Next most common is pain in the temporalis muscle, producing pain in the side of the head. The lateral pterygoid muscle can generate an earache or pain behind the eye. Medial pterygoid involvement causes pain on swallowing or *stuffiness* in the ear.[13]

The limitation of mandibular movement in MPD usually correlates with the amount of pain. The cause of MPD can be due to overclosure, occlusal prematurity, bruxism, and severe anxiety. Each of these leads to spasms of the masticatory muscles focusing pain around the TMJ.

The key to management is to break the cycle of spasm. Occlusal splint therapy can guide the dental occlusion to relax the muscular system. Other treatment includes drug therapy, such as nonsteroidal anti-inflammatory drugs, muscle relaxants, antidepressants, and local anesthetics for diagnostic blocks.[14] Physical therapy using modalities of heat, massage, diathermy, ultrasound, and biofeedback is also indicated in these patients. Any question regarding disc disease warrants MRI in these patients.

ARTHRITIS

Osteoarthritis

Osteoarthritis is a chronic noninflammatory disease that characteristically affects the articular cartilage of synovial joints and is associated with remodeling of the underlying subchondral bone and development of a secondary synovitis. It is the most common disease affecting the TMJ. It has a gradual onset. Usually, only one side is affected. The radiographic change is subchondral bone sclerosis in the condyle. Severe stages of this disease can cause a bone cyst within the condyle.[16] Treatment frequently involves drug therapy, occlusal appliance therapy, physical therapy, and, when most severe, surgery.

Rheumatoid Arthritis

Rheumatoid arthritis is a chronic inflammatory disease that primarily affects the periarticular structures, such as the synovial membrane, capsule, tendons, and ligaments. More than 50% of patients with rheumatoid arthritis have involvement of the TMJ during the course of their disease.[15,16] When the TMJ is involved, patients relate a dull aching pain in the preauricular area, muscle tenderness, poor range of jaw motion, clicking, and TMJ stiffness in the morning. Progression of the disease includes condylar resorption and fibrous and bony ankylosis. The classic malocclusion is caused by loss of height of the condyles. Juvenile rheumatoid arthritis affects patients before the age of 16 years. Up to 40% of children with juvenile rheumatoid arthritis involvement of the TMJ.[17] Defective development of the mandible leads to micrognathia. MR imaging can delineate disc destruction, condylar bone erosion, and cartilaginous thinning. The radiographs of the TMJ include loss of joint space and condylar resorption with anterior subluxation of the condyle.

The treatment goals in rheumatoid arthritis are pain relief, reduction of inflammation, maintainance of function, and prevention of further deformity. This treatment may include drug therapy, occlusal appliance, physical therapy, and dental and surgical procedures of the TMJ and mandible. Most surgery is reserved for correction of joint ankylosis and severe malocclusion.

INTERNAL DERANGEMENT OF THE JOINT

The existence of a natural progression of internal derangement of the TMJ is well documented.[18] In patients with early stage I derangement, the patient complains of clicking in opening and closing of the jaw (Fig. 22–4, Table 22–1). The problem is secondary to anterior disc displacement. The oral excursion and lateral movements of the jaw should be within the normal range.

In stage II, the patient begins to complain of intermittent limitation of jaw movement. Internal derangement is due to anterior disc displacement with reduction and intermittent locking. Pain is common at this stage and localized over the TMJ. In stage III, the patient has a chronic limitation of opening less than 25 to 30 mm. The mandible deviates to the affected side on opening and with protrusive movements. The internal derangement is without disc reduction or *acute closed lock*.

Chronic internal derangement without disc reduction (stage IV) results in injury to the retrodiscal tissue. Pain may diminish because of fibrous changes occurring in the retrodiscal tissue.[19] In stage V, remodeling of the temporal and condylar bone components occurs. The management of stage I or II is nonoperative. Such treatment includes occlusal splint therapy, allowing the normal disc condylar relationships to be reestablished. Those with later-stage disease require aggressive intervention; the surgical alternatives are discussed subsequently with TMJ arthrotomy and reconstruction of the joint.

MEDICAL OCCLUSAL MANAGEMENT

When the probable diagnosis of TMJ dysfunction or arthritis is made, it is appropriate for the primary care physician to ask for consultation by specialists in

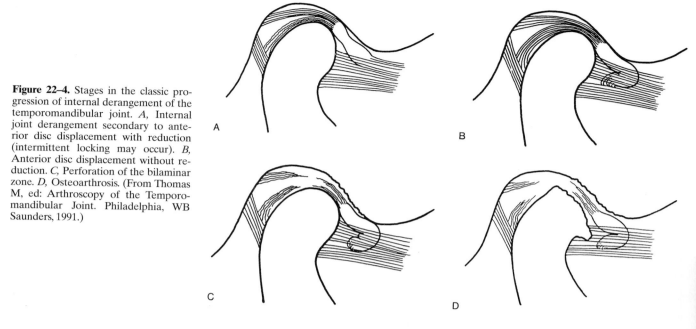

Figure 22–4. Stages in the classic progression of internal derangement of the temporomandibular joint. *A,* Internal joint derangement secondary to anterior disc displacement with reduction (intermittent locking may occur). *B,* Anterior disc displacement without reduction. *C,* Perforation of the bilaminar zone. *D,* Osteoarthrosis. (From Thomas M, ed: Arthroscopy of the Temporomandibular Joint. Philadelphia, WB Saunders, 1991.)

the area. The goal of medical management is to break the cycle of pain and anxiety in MPD. The common area to begin is the dental occlusion. With a fabricated occlusal splint, the mandible can be guided along a path to relax the neuromuscular system that is strained during premature contact of the teeth. With occlusal therapy, resolution of myofascial pain and dysfunction is a realistic goal. If pain is exacerbated by splinting, however, internal derangement of the disc should be ruled out with an MRI.

Many factors can affect the success of occlusal appliance therapy. The insertion and adjustment of the appliance and patient compliance are examples. The various types of occlusal splints are the muscle relaxation appliance, the anterior bite plate, and the soft appliance.

The choice of the splint depends on the patient's history, physical examination, needs, and the cause of the MPD.

SURGICAL MANAGEMENT

Primary care physicians should be aware of the possibilities for surgical management.

Temporomandibular Joint Arthroscopy

The arthroscope enables the surgeon to perform endoscopic joint examination, biopsy, and lavage.

Table 22–1. STAGING OF INTERNAL DERANGEMENT OF TEMPOROMANDIBULAR JOINT

Stage	Clinical	Imaging	Surgical
I Early	Painless clicking No restricted motion	Slightly forward disc Normal osseous contours	Normal disc form Slight anterior displacement Passive incoordination (clicking)
II Early/intermediate	Occasional painful clicking Intermittent locking Headaches	Slightly forward disc Early disc deformity Normal osseous contours	Anterior disc displacement Thickened disc
III Intermediate	Frequent pain Joint tenderness, headaches Locking Restricted motion Painful chewing	Anterior disc displacement Moderate-to-marked disc thickening Normal osseous contours	Disc deformed and displaced anteriorly Variable adhesions No bone changes
IV Intermediate/late	Chronic pain, headache Restricted motion	Anterior disc displacement Marked disc thicking Abnormal bone contours	Degenerative remodeling of bone surfaces Osseophytes Adhesions, deformed disc without perforation
V Late	Variable pain Joint crepitus Painful function	Anterior disc displacement with disc perforation and gross deformity Degenerative osseous changes	Gross degenerative changes of disc and hard tissues; disc perforation Multiple adhesions

From Wilkes CH: Internal derangements of the temporomandibular joint: Pathological variations. Arch Otolaryngol Head Neck Surg 115:469, 1989.

McCain et al.[20] found more than 90% of patients with internal derangement treated through arthroscopy had reduced symptoms and improved jaw function.

Open Arthrotomy

Open arthotomy allows an open view and examination of the joint, is highly specialized, and should be performed only by experienced surgeons.[21–23]

Reconstruction

ANKYLOSIS

The type of ankylosis can be intra-articular or extra-articular. The fusion at the articular level may be fibrous or bony in nature.[24] Patients with ankylosis develop poor oral hygiene, dental caries, and abscesses. In juvenile rheumatoid arthritis, mandibular growth and facial development are reduced, sometimes requiring surgery to correct the dentofacial deformities.

Extra-articular ankylosis may be due to the muscles of mastication, the facial nerve, or the coronoid process being enlarged. The common causes of intra-articular ankylosis are trauma, infection, and juvenile rheumatoid arthritis. These lead to the deterioration of disc and bony elements. A fibrous union narrows the joint space leading to a bony fusion. The diagnostic modalities for ankylosis of the TMJ include tomography and CT scanning. These studies can delineate types of ankylosis and allow the physician to choose the optimal therapy.

Surgical treatment of the common ankyloses includes several areas: (1) condylectomy, (2) gap arthroplasty, and (3) interpositional arthroplasty. For cases of early ankylosis, condylectomy is performed. It is technically difficult to release the fused elements of the condylar head at the joint space delineating the glenoid fossa, thereby losing favor as treatment.[6, 11]

A gap arthoplasty involves removal of bone at or below the joint level without interposition of any material. Often, there is high recurrence of the ankylosis as well as producing an open bite deformity.[25] In severe cases, placement of alloplastic or autogenous materials after resection of the condyle is the favored surgical approach. The interposition of materials is used to maintain vertical height and create a functional joint. A commonly used alloplast has been silicone rubber[26] to produce a pseudoarticulation.

The use of autogenous replacement of the resected condyle includes dermis, fat, fascia lata, and muscle. The costochondral graft harvested from the contralateral sixth rib is the optimal approach to reconstruction.[27] The patient needs aggressive physical therapy to maintain motion of the reconstructed joint space.[28]

AVASCULAR NECROSIS

Avasular necrosis is rare. The causes include trauma and complications of TMJ surgery. The classic symptoms include severe pain and decreased range of motion of the jaw. MRI is an important imaging modality for detecting devascularization of the condyle. The management of severe cases, is surgical débridement of the necrotic condyle and reconstruction using autogenous tissue.

DISLOCATIONS

Acute dislocations result from the condyle extending anteriorly beyond the articular eminence. If spontaneous reduction does not occur, manual reduction with a muscle relaxant or anesthesia is often needed. The surgeon places downward force along the inferior border of the mandible while moving the jaw posterior to slide the condyle into the fossa.

REFERENCES

1. Boyer CC, Williams TW, Stevens FH: Blood supply of the temporomandibular joint. J Dent Res 43:224, 1964.
2. Dixon AD: Structure and functional significance of the intraarticular disc in the human temporomandibular joint. J Oral Surg 15:48, 1962.
3. Chonkas NC, Sicher H: Structure of the temporomandibular joint. Oral Surg Oral Med Oral Pathol 13:1203, 1960.
4. Bell WH: Surgical Correction of Dentofacial Deformities: New Concepts. Philadelphia, WB Saunders, 1985.
5. Dautrey J, Pepersack J: Functional surgery of the temporomandibular joint. Clin Plast Surg 9:591, 1981.
6. Bessette RW, Jacobs JS: Temporomandibular joint dysfunction. In Aston SJ, Beasley RW, Thorne CHM, eds: Grabb and Smith's Plastic Surgery. Philadelphia, Lippincott-Raven Publishers, 1997.
7. Stanson AW, Baker HL: Routine tomography of the temporomandibular joint. Radiol Clin North Am 14:105, 1976.
8. Farrar WB, McCarty WL Jr: Inferior joint space arthrography and characteristics of condylar paths in internal derangements of the TMJ. J Prosthet Dent 41:548–555, 1979.
9. Westesson PL: Double-contrast arthrotomography of the temporomandibular joint: Introduction of an arthrographic technique for visualization of the disc and articular surfaces. J Oral Maxillofac Surg 41:163–172, 1983.
10. Schellhas KP, Wilkes CH, Fritts HM, et al: Temporomandibular joint: MR imaging internal derangements and postoperative changes. AJNR Am J Neuroradiol 8:1093, 1987.
11. Greenberg SA, Jacobs JS, Bessette RW: Temporomandibular joint dysfunction: Evaluation and treatment. Clin Plast Surg 16:707, 1989.
12. Laskin DM: Etiology of the pain-dysfunction syndrome. J Am Dent Assoc 79:147, 1969.
13. Laskin DM: Diagnosis and etiology of myofascial pain and dysfunction. Oral Maxillofac Surg Clin North Am 7:73, 1995.
14. Syrop SB: Pharmacologic management of myofascial pain and dysfunction. Oral Maxillofac Surg Clin North Am 7:87, 1995.
15. Laskin DM: Diagnosis of pathology of the temporomandibular joint: Clinical and imaging prospectives. Radiol Clin North Am 31:135, 1993.
16. Akerman S, Kopp S, Nilner M, et al: Relationship between clinical and radiologic findings of the temporomandibular joint in rheumatoid arthritis. Oral Surg Oral Med Oral Pathol 66:639, 1988.
17. Larheim TA, Hoyeraal HM, Starbrun AE, et al: The temporomandibular joint in juvenile rheumatoid arthritis: Radiographic changes related to clinical and laboratory parameters in 100 children. Scand J Rheumatol 11:5, 1982.
18. Friction J, et al: Joint disorders: Derangement and degeneration. In Friction J, Kroening R, Hathaway K, eds: Joint Disorders. St. Louis, Ishiyaku Euro America, 1988, pp 87–89.
19. Scapino R: Histopathology associated with malposition of the human temporomandibular joint disc. Oral Surg 55:382–397, 1983.
20. McCain JP, Sanders B, Koslin MG, et al: Temporomandibular joint arthroscopy. J Oral Maxillofac Surg 50:926, 1992.
21. Kreutziger KL: Surgery of the temporomandibular joint: I.

Surgical anatomy and surgical incisions. Oral Surg Oral Med Oral Pathol 58:637, 1984.

22. Eriksson L, Westesson PL: Long term evaluation of meniscectomy of the temporomandibular joint. J Oral Surg 43:263, 1985.
23. Smith RM, Goldwasser MS, Sabol SR: Erosion of Teflon Proplast implant into the middle cranial fossa. J Maxillofac Surg 51:1268, 1993.
24. Freedus M, Zitoc W, Doyle P: Principles of treatment for temporomandibular ankylosis. J Oral Surg 33:757, 1975.
25. Topazian RG: Comparison of gap and interposition arthroplasty in the treatment of temporomandibular ankylosis. J Oral Surg 24:405, 1966.
26. Gallagher DM, Wolford LM: Comparison of Silastic and Proplast implants in the temporomandibular joint after condylectomy for osteoarthritis. J Oral Maxillofac Surg 40:627, 1982.
27. Munro IR, Chen YR, Park BY: Simultaneous total correction of temporomandibular ankylosis and facial asymmetry. Plast Reconstr Surg 77:517, 1986.
28. Murray JE, Kaban LB, Mulliken JB: Analysis and treatment of hemifacial microsomia. Plast Reconstr Surg 74:186, 1984.

Approach to the Patient with Musculoskeletal Pain

Chapter 23

Hand and Wrist Pain

Edward Damore ▪ Amy L. Ladd

The human hand allows us to experience the environment and is capable of performing precise delicate movements, such as painting an intricate miniature, to simple powerful movements, such as walking on our hands. Seemingly minor hand injuries can become disabling. The main goal in treating hand problems is to restore function of the hand. Restoring function usually requires restoring anatomy, although this may not always be possible depending on the disorder affecting the hand.

HAND TERMINOLOGY AND ANATOMY

The back of the hand is referred to as the *dorsum*, and the palm side is referred to as *volar* or *palmar* (Figs. 23–1 and 23–2). Each of the fingers has three joints: the metacarpophalangeal (MCP), the proximal interphalangeal (PIP), and the distal interphalangeal (DIP). The thumb has two joints: the MCP and the interphalangeal (IP). *Supination* and *pronation* involve rotating the forearm so that the palm is up and down. *Abduction* separates the fingers, and *adduction* brings the fingers together. *Ulnar* or *radial* deviation is the bending of the hand toward the ulna or the radius.

COMMON ABNORMALITIES AFFECTING THE HANDS

Ganglions

Ganglia are mucinous-filled structures, clear jelly in appearance, that account for more than 50% of the masses in the hand. (See Chapter 21 for a discussion of ganglia in the foot and ankle.) They are found attached to the joint capsules, tendon sheaths, or tendons. They are more frequent in women and usually occur between the teens and 30s. The cause of ganglia is unproven, but theories include trauma, synovial herniation, and mucoid degeneration. The dorsal wrist ganglion is the most common, but others include volar wrist ganglion; flexor tendon sheath ganglion; and mucous cyst, which is a ganglion of the DIP joint caused by arthritis.[1]

Patients usually present with pain over the ganglion, which can range from an achy discomfort to more intense pain associated with joint motion. Flexor tendon sheath ganglions may produce a painful clicking with finger motion, which causes weakness. Patients can present with an asymptomatic ganglion; they are concerned about the lump and simply need reassurance as to the benign nature of the lesion. On examination, the ganglion can range from a firm, pea-sized mass in the flexor sheath to a soft circular mass several centimeters wide on the dorsum of the hand. These masses have minimal mobility and transluminate. Radiographs are typically unremarkable.

TREATMENT

Treatment for asymptomatic lesions is reassurance. Aspiration confirms the diagnosis and decreases the size, but the ganglion is likely to recur. Aspiration requires a sterile preparation before making a skin wheal with a 27-gauge needle using 1% lidocaine. An 18-gauge needle is introduced, large enough to aspirate the tenacious fluid of the ganglion, followed by multiple punctures to the ganglion wall to help discourage recurrence. Surgical excision is recommended for the recurrent, persistently painful ganglion.

SPECIFIC GANGLIA

VOLAR WRIST GANGLIA. Volar wrist ganglions are the second most common ganglion in the hand and are located just proximal to the wrist crease over the radial artery. Because this ganglion is intimately entwined with the radial artery, aspiration is less commonly performed.

FLEXOR TENDON SHEATH GANGLION. Flexor tendon sheath ganglia are firm, pea-sized masses located along the flexor sheath just proximal to the MCP joint. After aspiration, these ganglia tend to have a lower recurrence rate; therefore several attempts at aspiration are recommended. The neurovascular bundles lie close to the tendon sheath, so the clinician must be familiar with the anatomy.

MUCOUS CYST. Mucous cysts occur in people in their 50s to 60s and are located on the dorsal aspect of the DIP joint. They are associated with Heberden's nodes and osteophytes of the DIP joint. Aspiration is not recommended without surgical removal of the bony spur because recurrence is inevitable.

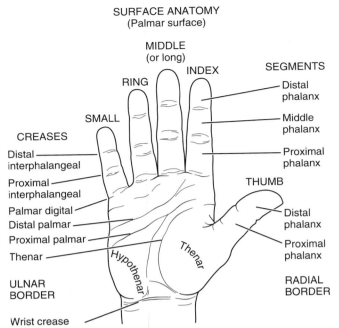

Figure 23–1. Surface anatomy of the hand. (From American Society of the Surgery of the Hand: The Hand: Examination and Diagnosis, 2nd ed. New York, Churchill Livingstone, 1983.)

Tenosynovitis

Tenosynovitis is an inflammatory condition of tendons. Causes may include repetitive trauma and underlying diseases, such as gout, rheumatoid arthritis, and diabetes. Treatment begins with simple measures, such as rest, splinting, and nonsteroidal anti-inflammatory drugs (NSAIDs), but glucocorticoid injections and surgery may be required. Choices of glucocorticoids for injection are reviewed in Chapter 6.

TRIGGER FINGER AND THUMB

The patient complains of painful clicking and popping when the finger or thumb is extended. Although the clicking appears to occur at the PIP joint, it actually involves a nodule at the MCP joint on the flexor tendon that during flexion is pulled underneath a tight tunnel, a *pulley*. With finger extension, the nodule is pulled free, and the patient senses a click. In rheumatoid arthritis, the triggering may originate more distally at the proximal phalanx causing triggering in flexion rather than in attempts at extension. On physical examination, pain localizes to the volar aspect of the MCP joint. The triggering may be subtle and appreciated as a simple give of the tendon or dramatic with actual locking of the finger in flexion.

Nonoperative treatment ranges from splinting, NSAIDs, and glucocorticoid injections. Glucocorticoid injections into the tendon sheath, which provide relief for a variable period of time, involve placing the needle bevel side up into the proximal crease at the MCP joint angling the needle proximally. The needle is inserted until resistance from the flexor tendon is appreciated. The needle is then withdrawn, applying gentle pressure on the plunger. The glucocorticoid is released when the resistance in the plunger decreases, correlating with the needle tip being located at the tendon but still inside the sheath (Fig. 23–3). After two injections without relief of symptoms, surgical release of the proximal *pulley* system is indicated. It is important not to inject glucocorticoids into the tendon itself because atrophy and rupture can occur subsequently.

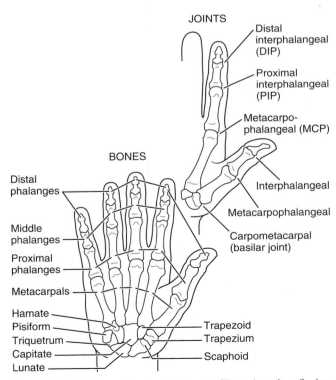

Figure 23–2. Skeleton of the hand and wrist. (From American Society of the Surgery of the Hand: The Hand: Examination and Diagnosis, 2nd ed. New York, Churchill Livingstone, 1983.)

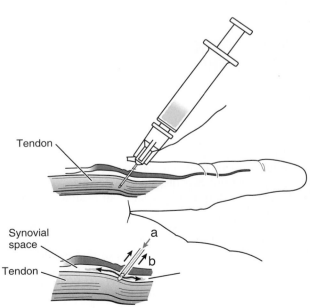

Figure 23–3. Injection of a trigger finger. (From American Society of the Surgery of the Hand: Regional Review Course in Hand Surgery. 1994.)

deQUERVAIN'S DISEASE

Stenosing tenosynovitis of the first dorsal compartment is a common cause of wrist and thumb pain in women aged 30 to 50 years. Patients complain of insidious onset of pain localized to the radial styloid over several weeks to months, often associated with a history of repetitive use of the thumb. On physical examination, one finds a painful enlargement of the first extensor compartment over the radial styloid. The patient demonstrates a positive Finkelstein test (ulnar flexion of the wrist while the fingers encircle and grasp the thumb) when the examiner performs ulnar deviation of the wrist and flexes the thumb (see Chapter 3). This condition can be easily confused with osteoarthritis of the basal joint of the thumb, a condition that frequently coexists with de Quervain's disease.

Nonoperative treatment includes NSAIDs, a splint that partially or totally immobilizes the thumb for activities that exacerbate the pain, and a glucocorticoid injection. The glucocorticoid is injected into the first dorsal compartment by inserting the needle 1.5 cm proximal to the radial styloid, aiming distally. This technique allows the substance to diffuse into the possible multiple tunnels of the first compartment. The injection is repeated once if necessary, and if symptoms still persist, surgical release of the first compartment is indicated.

Compression Neuropathy

Compression neuropathies are nerve injuries that occur in predictable areas of the upper extremity (Table 23–1). The pathology is probably caused by localized ischemia of the nerve by mechanical pressure.

CARPAL TUNNEL SYNDROME

CAUSES AND SYMPTOMS. Compression of the median nerve within the carpal tunnel is the most common upper extremity compressive neuropathy. A nonspecific tenosynovitis in otherwise healthy individuals is thought to cause carpal tunnel syndrome (CTS).[2] CTS occurs more commonly in women and frequently accompanies pregnancy and menopause. Other associated conditions include rheumatoid arthritis, traumatic disorders of the wrist, scleroderma, lupus, myxedema, diabetes mellitus, amyloidosis, benign tumors, and gout. It is unclear whether occupational activity alone can cause

Table 23–1. COMPRESSION NEUROPATHIES

Median nerve
  Carpal tunnel
  Anterior interosseous syndrome
  Pronator syndrome
Ulnar nerve
  Cubital tunnel
  Guyon's canal
Radial nerve
  Posterior interosseous nerve
  Radial tunnel
  Superficial radial nerve

CTS, although many workers' compensation claims involve treatment for CTS.

Most patients complain of numbness or pain that awakens them at night. The thumb, index, and middle finger are most commonly involved, but the whole hand may be numb. Activities that flex the wrists, such as driving, reading the paper, or holding a telephone receiver, may also cause numbness. Clumsiness and pain radiating up the arm to the shoulder are also common complaints. The differential diagnosis includes cervical radiculopathy, diabetic neuropathy, and compression of the median nerve at other locations, such as pronator syndrome and anterior interosseous syndrome.

EVALUATION. Provocative tests to increase paresthesia can be done. Phalen's maneuver is performed by resting the elbows on the examination table while the wrists are passively flexed. The test is positive if the paresthesias increase within 60 seconds. Tinel's sign is performed by tapping the median nerve just proximal to the wrist crease and is considered positive if the patient describes electric sensations radiating to the thumb, index, or middle finger. A Tinel's sign is less sensitive than Phalen's maneuver but more specific, with only a 6% false-positive rate.[3]

Decreased sensibility occurs in patients with more advanced CTS. Thenar atrophy is a sign of long-standing compression. Tests such as the Semmes-Weinstein monofilaments and vibrometry are more diagnostic than two-point discrimination. Electrodiagnostic tests are not routinely necessary but are helpful to evaluate the presence of a possible peripheral neuropathy or radiculopathy and to provide a baseline set of measurements in a patient with previous peripheral nerve surgery who has recurrent or persistent symptoms. A positive test is often required before workers' compensation approves surgery. Sensory nerve conduction velocities are more likely to show abnormalities earlier than motor conduction velocity because the median nerve is composed of 90% sensory fibers at the level of the wrist.[2]

TREATMENT. Conservative measures include NSAIDs, prefabricated volar splints that hold the wrist in a neutral position, and glucocorticoid injections. The volar splints are to be worn at night and during activities that exacerbate the symptoms. To inject the glucocorticoid, the needle is inserted at the wrist crease just ulnar to the palmaris longus, angulated distally at 45 degrees. The needle is passed through the transverse carpal ligament, a process meeting with some resistance. If the patient is complaining of tingling to the fingers, the needle should be partially withdrawn. Nonoperative treatment is less likely to work in patients who are more than 50 years old or have a duration of symptoms greater than 12 months or constant paresthesias[4]. Surgery is indicated when nonoperative measures do not sufficiently control the numbness and paresthesia and when these symptoms interfere with activities of daily living.

CUBITAL TUNNEL SYNDROME

Cubital tunnel syndrome is the second most common compression neuropathy in the upper extremity involving compression of the ulnar nerve around the elbow.

CAUSES AND SYMPTOMS. Causes include direct or repetitive trauma, fractures about the elbow, arthritis, abnormal muscles, recurrent dislocation of the nerve, swelling, and rarely a space-occupying lesion such as a ganglion. Patients most often complain of tingling and coolness in the ring and little fingers, which may be aggravated by flexion of the elbow. A vague complaint of pain around the elbow may be noted. In more severe cases, patients may complain of weakness, clumsiness, and loss of dexterity.[5] Pain with activities such as turning the key in the ignition or turning a doorknob may be a prominent complaint. Sensory findings are more common and occur earlier than motor findings. The differential diagnosis includes thoracic outlet syndrome, C8–T1 root compression, and compression at Guyon's canal, which is located in the palm.

EVALUATION. Tinel's sign at the cubital tunnel is often positive, but studies have shown up to one fourth of normal volunteers can have a positive Tinel's sign.[6] The elbow flexion test is a provocative maneuver performed by fully flexing the elbow for 60 seconds, a maneuver likely to reproduce the symptoms. Weakness of finger abduction is present only in severe cases. Making the diagnosis of cubital tunnel syndrome can be difficult in patients who have pain around the elbow and have minimal physical findings. In these situations, electrodiagnostic tests can help confirm the diagnosis and clarify the level of entrapment. Normal electrodiagnostic tests do not rule out cubital tunnel syndrome.

TREATMENT. Conservative treatment includes patient education to modify work and sleep habits and an elbow pad for protection as well as to serve as a night splint preventing significant flexion of the elbow. Glucocorticoid injections are not commonly used in cubital tunnel syndrome primarily because of the vulnerability of the ulnar nerve. Surgery is indicated when conservative measures do not sufficiently control the symptoms and these symptoms interfere with activities of daily living. Surgery entails decompressing the nerve and possibly transposing it into a more protected bed of tissue.

Dupuytren's Disease

Dupuytren's disease is common in men of Northern European heritage and involves proliferation of the palmar fascia of the hand leading to the development of thickening known as *nodules* and *cords*. As the disease progresses, flexion contractures of the MCP joint, as well as the PIP joint (but rarely the DIP joint) can occur. The pathophysiology is unclear, but proliferation of fibroblasts with excessive collagen production is the likely abnormality.

CAUSE

Dupuytren's disease is inherited as an autosomal dominant trait with variable penetrance and is uncommon in Greece, Asia, Africa, and the Middle East. Dupuytren's disease is associated with alcohol con-

sumption, diabetes, epilepsy, and cigarette smoking, although the precise links are unclear. Even less clear is its occasional association with a single traumatic episode.

A Dupuytren's *diathesis*, or a spectrum of findings, is a more aggressive form of the disease. These patients present earlier in life, often in their 20s to 30s; have a positive family history; and have bilateral hand involvement, including the radial side of the hand, which is rare in most individuals with Dupuytren's disease. Additional physical findings can include prominent *knuckle pads* on the dorsum of the PIP joint, penile fascial involvement (Peyronie's disease), and plantar fibromatosis (Ledderhose's disease).[7]

CLINICAL FEATURES

Dupuytren's disease is usually seen in men between the ages of 40 and 60 years. Patients often present with a tender nodule or a progressively thickening cord in their palm. The ring and little finger are most commonly involved.

EVALUATION AND TREATMENT

Progression of Dupuytren's disease is unpredictable. Nonoperative treatment, such as vitamin E, glucocorticoid injections, creams, and physical therapy, has uncertain value. Although surgical excision does not cure the disease, it may avert or delay progression. The main indications for surgery are progressive joint contracture when the PIP joints are contracted greater than 30 degrees. The surgery involves excision of the diseased fascia with possible skin grafts over the severely involved skin. In routine follow-up, the deformities need to be accurately recorded. The patient needs to realize that complete surgical correction becomes less likely as the disease becomes more severe.

Infections

Infections are uncommon in the hand because of its abundant blood supply. When an infection is present, however, especially bacterial infections, it needs to be treated aggressively to prevent disabling problems. Diabetes, renal failure, human immunodeficiency virus (HIV) infection, malnutrition, and advanced age increase the likelihood of infection. Local factors, such as ischemia, necrotic tissue, and presence of a foreign body, also play a role. The infecting organism can often be indicated from the history (Table 23–2), but proof by culture is essential. Localized pain, especially with joint movement, as well as erythema, swelling, fluctuation, drainage, and pain can all be found. Swelling may be diffuse; an infection in the palmar side of the hand may be swollen dorsally because of extension of inflammation through the loose connective tissue located in the dorsum of the hand.

Cellulitis, or diffusely infected tissue, may be treated with elevation, immobilization, and antibiotics. If an abscess (an infection in a closed space) forms, it

Table 23–2. HAND INFECTIONS AND OCCUPATION

Clinical History	Infection
Medical personnel	Herpetic whitlow
Gardeners	Sporotrichosis
Working in water	Chronic paronychia
Marine environment	*Mycobacterium marinum*
Human bite	*Eikenella corrodens*
Dog or cat bite	*Pasteurella multocida*

must be surgically drained. Examples of closed spaces in the hand include the joints, tendon sheaths, and palmar spaces.

ACUTE PARONYCHIA

The eponychium is the fold of skin that borders the nail known as the *cuticle*. Any break in the border between the nail fold and the nail plate from activities, such as nail biting, pulling out hangnails, or manicures may act as a portal for bacteria. An acute paronychia is an infection of the space surrounding the nail fold and is most commonly caused by *Staphylococcus aureus*.

EVALUATION AND TREATMENT. Early in the course of acute paronychia, the patient presents with erythema and swelling around the nail fold. Treatment includes warm soaks and oral antibiotics. Once a collection of pus has formed, drainage is required. A digital block is sufficient anesthesia. For simple cases involving one side of the nail, a hemostat or a no. 11 blade is placed into the nail sulcus. The nail fold is elevated to decompress the abscess. Warm soaks are continued to encourage drainage. A longitudinal incision parallel to the nail plate, which can lead to skin bridge necrosis and deformation of the nail sulcus, should be avoided. In more complicated cases that involve both sides of the nail fold or lead to accumulation of pus under the nail plate, the nail should be removed.[8]

CHRONIC PARONYCHIA

Chronic paronychial infections are most commonly caused by *Candida albicans*. They usually occur in people whose hands are exposed to frequent moisture, such as bartenders and dishwashers, or in immunocompromised patients. Redness and pain typically are mild but long-standing. Swelling and inflammation of the eponychial space is found. There is often a cheese-like material under the eponychium. Avoidance of moisture and antifungal medications may not be successful in achieving permanent cure, and surgical débridement by a method called *eponychial marsupialization* is recommended.

FELON

A felon is an infection in the closed space in the pulp of the fingertip. There is often a history of a puncture wound. Patients present with marked, throbbing pain and swelling of the entire pulp. *S. aureus* is the most

frequently involved causative agent. Treatment requires surgical decompression of the pulp. Untreated felons can lead to skin necrosis, osteomyelitis, and pyogenic flexor tenosynovitis.

PYOGENIC FLEXOR TENOSYNOVITIS

Pyogenic flexor tenosynovitis is an infection of the flexor tendon sheath. Penetrating trauma is usually the source. Anatomically the flexor tendon sheaths start midpalm and end just proximal to the DIP joints. The four cardinal signs of acute pyogenic tenosynovitis include (1) uniform swelling of the digit, (2) flexed position of the digit, (3) tenderness along the entire flexor sheath, and (4) marked pain along the entire flexor sheath on passive extension of the digit.[9] The condition requires immediate referral. If the patient is seen within the first 48 hours, a trial of intravenous antibiotics and arm elevation are attempted. If no improvement is seen within 24 hours, surgical débridement is required.

SEPTIC ARTHRITIS

Joint infections in the hand or wrist usually occur from direct inoculation, such as a bite from a tooth, but can also arise from spread of an adjacent infection. Hematogenous seeding may occur in an immunocompromised patient. On examination, the joint is usually red, swollen, and associated with severe pain on passive range of motion. Immediate referral for surgical drainage and débridement is imperative to prevent extensive joint destruction. Joint sepsis is discussed in detail in Chapter 33.

HUMAN BITES

Human bites occur most often during a fight when a clenched fist strikes the opponent's tooth; these are especially prone to penetrating the MCP joint. These wounds initially appear benign, only to have the patient return later with a septic MCP joint. The most common organism is *S. aureus,* but the antibiotic used must also cover the gram-negative rod *Eikenella corrodens*.

These wounds require irrigation with possible extension of the wound for adequate débridement and are left open. If the injury is seen early, and the wound is relatively benign, it is reasonable to try a 24-hour trial of oral penicillin with expanded coverage such as amoxicillin and clavulanate (Augmentin). If the wound appears worse after 24 hours, intravenous antibiotics should be started and surgical débridement of the wounds considered.

DOG AND CAT BITES

Dog bites are more common than cat bites, but cat bites tend to be more serious. Cats tend to cause puncture wounds, whereas dogs tend to cause lacerations in the skin. The small puncture wounds of cats inoculate the deep tissues and therefore render it a more serious infection. The most common organism is *S. aureus,* but the antibiotic must also cover the gram-negative rod

Pasteurella multocida. These wounds are treated similarly to human bites with irrigation and a penicillin with expanded coverage such as Augmentin.

HERPETIC WHITLOW

Herpes simplex is a viral infection spread by orotracheal secretions that can involve the fingertips. Medical and dental personnel and immunocompromised patients are at increased risk. The incubation period is 2 to 14 days. The patient presents with prodome of throbbing pain in the fingertip followed by grouped vesicles surrounded by erythema. Fluid in the vesicles is usually clear. Because the patient may present at a later time with scabs, it may be difficult to distinguish this infection from a bacterial infection. The diagnosis can be confirmed by a Tzanck smear, culturing the vesicular fluid, or antiherpes antibody if fluid is present. Herpetic whitlow is a self-limiting infection lasting approximately 3 weeks. Treatment with acyclovir 200 mg three times a day for 10 days given early may shorten its course. The same dosage given in its prodromal stage also helps to shorten the duration of the infection.[10] Patients who have contact with others may return to activity when their scabs are dry and there is no more drainage. Incision of the vesicles is contraindicated and may lead to viral encephalitis.

ATYPICAL MYCOBACTERIAL INFECTIONS

Mycobacterium marinum presents as a chronically inflamed finger after puncture by marine life, whereas *Mycobacterium kansasii* results from skin abrasions in farm workers. A biopsy specimen requires a Löwenstein-Jensen medium at 30 to 32°C instead of 37°C. Treatment involves a combination of isoniazid, rifampin, pyrazinamide, and ethambutol for 6 to 9 months and possible irrigation and débridement.

Vascular Disorders

VASCULAR ANATOMY

The ulnar and radial arteries supply the hand. Arterial arches in the palm permit redundant circulation that may protect from ischemia to the hand with either a radial or ulnar artery injury.

EVALUATION OF VASCULAR DISORDERS

Patients with vascular disorders can present with ulcerations and pain from ischemia, cold intolerance, a mass, and color changes in the skin. The Allen test may indicate an abnormality. This test, an assessment of collateral flow of the radial and ulnar arteries through the palmar arches, is performed by the examiner compressing both the ulnar and the radial arteries, then having the patient make a fist several times to exsanguinate the hand. The examiner releases the ulnar artery, then repeats the test releasing the radial artery. A delay in the appearance of a capillary flush reveals poor perfusion.

Further noninvasive diagnostic studies may provide additional information and include Doppler scans to evaluate flow; plethysmography, which uses limb or digit volume changes to measure flow indirectly; and cold stress testing to evaluate the effect of cold on arterial spasm. Invasive diagnostic studies include arteriography and radionuclide scans.

ULNAR ARTERY THROMBOSIS

Hypothenar hammer syndrome describes thrombosis of the ulnar artery in the palm, found mostly in men whose hands are subjected to blunt trauma. These patients may complain of pain and cold intolerance in the hypothenar area of the hand or ulnar fingers and may also have diminished sensation to the ring and little fingers because of secondary compression of the ulnar nerve. The Allen test reveals ulnar ischemia, and angiography is confirmatory. Treatment involves surgical resection of the thrombosis with either reanastomosis or interpositional vein graft.

ARTERIAL LINE PLACEMENT INJURIES

Cannulation of the radial artery that commonly occurs in the intensive care unit setting can lead to ischemia of the radial digits in patients who do not have communication between the ulnar and radial arteries in the palm. Careful vascular evaluation using the Allen test before line placement is important. These complications are rare.

RAYNAUD'S PHENOMENON AND DISEASE

Raynaud's phenomenon is pallor of the digits typically with cyanosis on exposure to cold. *Raynaud's disease* occurs without a demonstrable or causative process. Raynaud's disease usually presents in women younger than 40 years old and progresses slowly. They infrequently get ulcers on the tips of their fingers, and laboratory tests are normal. *Raynaud's syndrome* is the name given when the phenomenon is associated with, or caused by, a disease such as scleroderma, systemic lupus erythematosus, or hematologic abnormalities.[11] Raynaud's phenomenon is rare to absent in definite rheumatoid arthritis. Fingertip ulcerations occur in patients with more ischemic changes.

Treatment is the same for both Raynaud's disease and Raynaud's syndrome. Conservative treatment includes avoidance of cold, wearing of mittens to keep hands warm, biofeedback, exhortation to quit smoking, and treatment of systemic disorders. The most effective current medical therapy is calcium channel blockers. Nifedipine 10 to 20 mg three times per day given for short periods may be useful in treating painful ischemic ulcers. A surgical digital sympathectomy for persistent ulcers or debilitating disease, which involves stripping the adventitia off the common digital artery over a short segment, may improve circulation.

Hand Trauma

GENERAL EVALUATION

Trauma to the hand requires prompt attention, particularly with open injuries. For closed injuries, the examiner assesses for local tenderness, swelling, rotational or angular deformity, neurovascular status, and joint range of motion. Radiographs are necessary for specific bone tenderness. Posteroanterior and true lateral views are obtained for fingers and neutral posteroanterior and true lateral views for the wrist. Special views may be required to evaluate the scaphoid (posteroanterior in ulnar deviation) and ligament instability of the wrist (posteroanterior of clenched fist). Table 23–3 lists common terminology to describe the fracture. Rotation of the fracture is a clinical and not a radiographic diagnosis.

An injured hand requires splinting or casting. A basic principle is to immobilize a joint above and a joint below the fracture. The universal splinting position of the hand is the so-called position of safety: MCP joints, 70 degrees flexed; PIP joints, 20 degrees flexed; and DIP joints, 10 degrees flexed. Follow-up radiographs are obtained in 1 to 2 weeks to verify that the position of the fracture or dislocation has not changed.

NAIL BED INJURIES

The common fingertip injury often masks an underlying nail bed injury. A nail bed laceration often accompanies a distal phalanx fracture. A subungual hematoma of less than 50% may be evacuated if it is painful. This evacuation can be done by burning a hole into the nail plate over the hematoma using a hot paperclip sterilized by matches or by drilling a hole into the nail plate using an 18-gauge needle. When the subungual hematoma is greater than 50%, it is preferable to remove the nail plate and suture the nail bed with a fine absorbable suture (e.g., 6-0 chromic). This approach minimizes future nail plate irregularities. A nail is removed after performing a digital block by placing a blunt probe such as a hemostat under to elevate and remove the nail plate. Either the nail is replaced or a dressing is placed under the nail fold for 2 weeks to prevent scarring of the eponychium and future nail plate irregularities.

Table 23–3. DESCRIPTION OF FRACTURES

Bone involved
Location within bone
  Base, shaft, neck
Displaced/nondisplaced
Closed/open
Intra-articular/extra-articular
Angulation
  Dorsal/volar
  Radial/ulnar
Stable/unstable
Associated injuries
Children's fractures
  Salter-Harris classification
Avulsion fracture

DISTAL PHALANX FRACTURES

Distal phalanx fracture is the most common fracture in the hand. Because the nail bed is adherent to the distal phalanx, displaced fractures often create nail bed lacerations. The nail plate may need removal and repair of the nail bed, depending on the presence of a subungual hematoma (see earlier). Treatment involves splinting the distal phalanx and the DIP joint for 3 to 4 weeks. Pin fixation may be required for marked fracture displacement. The fingertip tends to be sensitive for many months after these injuries.

MALLET FINGER

Mallet finger is a fingertip droop resulting from disruption of the terminal extensor tendon. This injury occurs from a flexion force while the finger is extended, such as catching a ball with a fingertip. Treatment involves uninterrupted splinting of the DIP in slight hyperextension for 8 weeks. If residual drooping of the DIP joint is noted, an additional 4 weeks of splinting are required. After 8 weeks, gradual motion is started with a splint worn at night and progressive range of motion for several more weeks. Aluminum splints with taping, although cumbersome, provide superior immobilization compared with prefabricated splints, which often fit poorly.

BONY MALLET

A bony mallet involves an avulsion fracture from the dorsal lip of the distal phalanx at the DIP joint. A bony mallet is treated similarly to the soft tissue mallet with splinting for 8 weeks, but surgical intervention may be required if the main articular portion of the distal phalanx is displaced in a volar direction.

PROXIMAL INTERPHALANGEAL JOINT INJURY

Injury of the PIP joint, which commonly occurs as a *jammed finger* during sporting activities, ranges from a partial to a complete tear and dislocation. The severity of this injury may go unrecognized because many are reduced spontaneously or are pulled back into place by the athlete or trainer. The history provides valuable information regarding the mechanism of injury; a hyperextended finger injury requires different treatment than one in which the finger is flexed. The direction of the dislocation is based on the direction of the middle phalanx in reference to the proximal phalanx. If the patient can fully actively extend the PIP joint and the joint is most tender on the volar surface, the presumptive diagnosis is dorsal dislocation from hyperextension. In a volar dislocation, the patient is not able to extend the PIP joint actively and fully, and the joint is most tender dorsally over the central slip. A true lateral radiograph is important to determine the congruency of the joint.

DORSAL DISLOCATION. A dorsal dislocation is more common than a volar dislocation. The ligament on the volar side of the PIP joint, the *volar plate,* is usually torn off the middle phalanx and may include a small fragment of bone. Treatment is based on the stability assessed by a true postreduction lateral radiograph. For a stable reduction, the PIP joint is dorsally splinted in 15 degrees of flexion for 3 to 5 days, then buddy taped to the adjacent finger for 4 weeks. Incomplete reductions may require surgical intervention. Flexion of the DIP joint while in the splint should be encouraged.

DORSAL FRACTURE DISLOCATION. A dorsal fracture dislocation involves a fracture of the volar lip of the middle phalanx producing a potentially more inherently unstable injury than does a simple dorsal dislocation. Stable reductions are treated by splinting dorsally the PIP joint in 15 degrees of flexion for 3 to 5 days, then buddy taping for 4 weeks. Incomplete reductions may require surgical intervention.

VOLAR DISLOCATION. A volar dislocation involves rupture of the central slip from the middle phalanx, which can lead to a boutonnière deformity over several months if untreated. Treatment consists of dorsal splinting in full extension for 6 to 8 weeks. A large avulsion fracture off the dorsal top of the middle phalanx may need surgical fixation.

PROXIMAL INTERPHALANGEAL JOINT SPRAIN. PIP joint sprains are treated with buddy tape for several weeks until comfortable. Motion of the fingers is encouraged. Avulsions of a small fragment off the volar lip of the proximal fragment without a dislocation are treated as a sprain with buddy tape for several weeks.

PROXIMAL AND MIDDLE PHALANX FRACTURES

Angulation of the fracture fragments is based on the direction or mechanism of injury and the tendon forces inserting on the bone. Malrotation is the deformity most overlooked. Malrotation is especially evident when the fingers are flexed. Undisplaced stable fractures require buddy taping for 4 weeks. Displaced fractures that are stable to reduction are placed in a splint or cast with the finger in a position of safety. Displaced fractures that are unstable to reduction or demonstrate malrotation require surgical repair with hardware fixation. These fractures are followed weekly with radiographs to check for fracture displacement.

METACARPAL FRACTURES

Metacarpal fractures are classified by their location.

METACARPAL HEAD FRACTURES. Metacarpal head fractures involve the articular surface. Nondisplaced fractures may be treated with a splint or cast with the hand in the position of safety for 4 weeks. Displaced fractures require surgical evaluation.

METACARPAL NECK FRACTURES. The fifth metacarpal neck is the most commonly fractured. It is also known as a boxer's fracture often resulting from a blow to a wall or other unyielding object. The compression on impact displaces the head into a flexed position.

An acceptable reduction is up to 40 degrees of flexion of the ring and little finger, given the increased mobility of the carpometacarpal joint at the base of the metacarpal. Treatment involves closed reduction and splinting or casting for 4 weeks, the deformity that usually remains is manifested as a loss of the knuckle prominence but without functional loss. Indications for surgical pinning include severe displacement and rotation.

METACARPAL SHAFT FRACTURES. Given that the middle and ring metacarpals are stabilized by the intermetacarpal ligament, they are less likely to shorten, angulate, and rotate when fractured as compared with the index and little metacarpals. Stable isolated metacarpal fractures can be treated with a cast or splint immobilization for 4 weeks. The cast should include the MCP joint flexed to 70 degrees, leaving the fingers free if they are sufficiently stable.

THUMB METACARPAL FRACTURES

Most fractures of the thumb metacarpal occur at or near the base, and three patterns are frequently seen.

BENNETT'S FRACTURE. A Bennett's fracture is an intra-articular fracture in which the volar ligament holds the small radial fragment in place while the thumb abductor displaces the shaft proximally and radially. Although nondisplaced fractures may be treated in a cast that incorporates the thumb for 4 weeks, displaced fractures require surgical treatment.

ROLANDO'S FRACTURE. A Rolando's fracture is a comminuted fracture of the articular base of the metacarpal. Cast or surgical treatment depends on the severity of the fracture.

EXTRA-ARTICULAR FRACTURES. Extra-articular fractures are the least common but the easiest to treat. Because the thumb has great mobility, significant angulation may be accepted without a functional loss and treated with a cast incorporating the thumb. Surgery rarely is indicated.

THUMB METACARPOPHALANGEAL JOINT

The most common injury to the thumb MCP joint is called a *gamekeeper's* or *skier's thumb* occurring with a valgus stress that tears the ulnar collateral ligament (UCL). When the UCL tears from the proximal phalanx, a Stener lesion may occur; this is when the adductor tendon becomes interposed between the bone and the torn ligament preventing the UCL from reattaching to the bone. A Stener lesion occurs in approximately 65% of complete tears. Chronic laxity of the thumb MCP joint makes tasks such as picking up a large heavy jar painful and renders the joint vulnerable to arthritis because of a change in the force patterns of an unstable joint.

The patient presents with localized pain over the UCL and weakness with pinch. A complete tear is detected by the following test: The MCP joint is radially stressed approximately in 30 degrees of flexion and compared with the other side. Opening greater than 30 degrees from the opposite thumb is consistent with a completely torn ligament.[12] Cast immobilization suffices for incomplete tears, whereas a complete disruption requires surgical repair.

Wrist Injuries

The precise motion between each of the eight carpal bones and their interrelationship with the distal radius and ulna collectively forms a complex pattern of motion. Injuries that disrupt this pattern predispose the patient to traumatic arthritis because of the alteration in forces. The clinician must therefore perform a careful evaluation and have a high index of suspicion when seeing a patient with an injured wrist.

WRIST SPRAINS AND INSTABILITY

Injuries to the wrist ligaments, similar to all ligaments, include the minor sprains to completely disrupted ligaments or dislocations. Patients usually present complaining of pain in their wrist after a fall on an outstretched hand. Wrist motion may be limited by pain, or there may be little pain except at the extremes of motion. A complete series of radiographs includes a neutral posteroanterior, a true lateral, and possibly a posteroanterior with the wrist in ulnar and radial deviation and a clenched fist. One of the more common and serious injuries includes a disruption between the scaphoid and lunate, which may show a gap of 3 mm or more between the scaphoid and lunate on the clenched first view. Wrist sprains can be persistently symptomatic and can take several months to heal.[13] Minor sprains may be treated with splinting, whereas serious ligament disruptions between the scaphoid and lunate require surgical treatment.

SCAPHOID FRACTURES

The scaphoid is a unique carpal bone. Mostly articular, it links the proximal row of four carpal bones with the distal four carpal bones, depending on the position of the wrist. The scaphoid is also the most vulnerable to fracture, particularly as the result of a fall on an outstretched hand in a young man. Tenderness in the snuffbox is a common clinical finding, and in this setting, radiographs are mandatory. Casting for nondisplaced scaphoid fracture varies from 6 weeks for a tuberosity fracture to many months for a proximal pole fracture; the unique vascularity of the scaphoid accounts for the variability. Displaced fractures require surgical reduction and fixation. Even if the initial radiographs are negative but there is snuff-box tenderness, the patient should be treated with casting that includes the thumb followed by repeat radiographs in 2 weeks. In this instance, the scaphoid fracture becomes more apparent on subsequent radiographs because of the fracture edges resorbing and new bone (callus) formation. If the repeat radiographs at 2 weeks are negative but the patient still complains of pain, the patient needs to be evaluated for a (scaphoid) lunate dissociation before the diagnosis of a wrist sprain can be given.[14]

Hand Arthritis

Osteoarthritis and rheumatoid arthritis constitute most arthritic hand conditions, but several other arthritic conditions may result in hand deformities: Psoriatic arthritis may present with fusiform swelling of the digits and involvement of the DIP joint, systemic lupus erythematosus involves ligament laxity rather than joint destruction, and arthritis mutilans results in severe bone loss with collapse and shortening of the digits.[15] The goals of treatment in order of priority are to alleviate pain, improve function, slow disease progression, lessen deformity, and improve appearance.

RHEUMATOID ARTHRITIS

The inflammatory component of rheumatoid arthritis, a systemic autoimmune disease, affects periarticular tissue and joints. A common presentation of the advanced deformities in the rheumatoid hand is the wrist in radial deviation, the MCP joints flexed and ulnarly deviated, and the fingers in either a boutonnière or swan-neck deformity (Fig. 23–4). The synovitis can also lead to de Quervain's disease, CTS, trigger finger or thumb, and tendon rupture. Aggressive medical management helps to lessen the destructive synovial proliferation and preserve function. Resting and functional splints often improve hand function. Many patients benefit from a consultation with a hand or occupational therapist for splinting and adaptive devices. As pointed out in Chapter 25, it is important to ask for consultation from hand surgeons earlier rather than later in rheumatoid arthritis.

In individuals with progressive disease despite appropriate medical management, surgery is effective for many patients to maintain function and minimize pain. There are several options for the rheumatoid hand depending on the level of involvement (Table 23–4). Reconstructive surgery is most predictable and successful when done early before fixed deformity or tendon

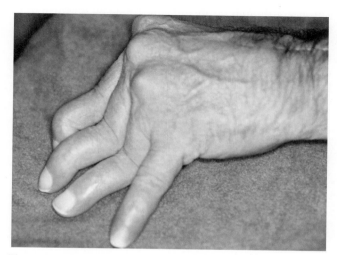

Figure 23–4. Rheumatoid arthritis of the hand. This patient has the typical presentation with radial deviation of the wrist, flexion and ulnar deviation of the metacarpophalangeal joints, and swan-neck deformity of the digits.

Table 23–4. SURGICAL TREATMENT OPTIONS FOR RHEUMATOID ARTHRITIS
Preventive/palliative
Tenosynovectomy
Synovectomy
Corrective
Tendon transfer
Nerve decompression
Soft tissue reconstruction
Salvage
Joint replacement
Fusion

rupture occurs. Close involvement with a hand surgeon early in the course of the disease allows the patient to be a candidate for function-preserving procedures rather than salvage procedures, such as fusions, which only partially restore function.[16]

OSTEOARTHRITIS

Osteoarthritis or *wear-and-tear arthritis* affects most elderly individuals and many starting in the 40s. Degeneration of articular cartilage, erosion and thickening of subchondral bone, and reactive osteophyte production are the hallmark of osteoarthritis (see Chapter 31). Patients typically present with pain, deformity, and limitation of motion in the affected joints. Risk factors for developing osteoarthritis are being a woman, being elderly, and having a positive family history. The most frequently involved joints in the hand are the DIP joints and the thumb MCP joints and less commonly the PIP joints. Most patients can be treated with NSAIDs, splinting, and activity modification. Radiographs are helpful to confirm the diagnosis and assess bone loss and deformity. The primary indication for surgery is pain unresponsive to nonoperative treatment.

DISTAL INTERPHALANGEAL JOINTS. The bony enlargement from the osteophytic spurs around the DIP joint are referred to as *Heberden's nodes*. Often a mucous cyst accompanies osteophyte formation. Surgery, although rarely indicated, may be performed to débride spurs or fuse the joint.

THUMB METACARPOPHALANGEAL JOINT. Patients usually complain of pain over the thenar eminence. The grind test, which is axial compression of the thumb MCP joint with a circumduction motion, reproduces the pain. Radiographs may demonstrate subluxation, narrowed joint space, sclerosing, and osteophytes of the thumb MCP joint. Injection with glucocorticoid at the MCP joint may provide temporary relief. For continued pain, arthroplasty or arthrodesis depending on the demand of the patient provides predictable relief.[16]

PROXIMAL INTERPHALANGEAL JOINTS. The bony enlargement from the osteophytic spurs around the PIP joint are referred to as *Bouchard's nodes*. For pain unresponsive to conservative treatment, surgical options include arthroplasty or arthrodesis.

SUMMARY

There are many potential sources for hand and wrist pain. A thorough history and an understanding of the pathoanatomy of the hand and wrist help the clinician make the proper diagnosis. The urgency and aggressiveness of the treatment for each problem vary, but the main goal of the treatment is to restore the function of the hand.

REFERENCES

1. Carl L, Nelson C.L, Sawmiller S, et al: Ganglions of the wrist and hand. J Bone Joint Surg Am 54:1459–1464, 1972.
2. Omer G: Median nerve compression at the wrist. Hand Clin 8:317–324, 1992.
3. Gellman H, Gelberman RH, Tan AM, et al: Carpal tunnel syndrome: An evaluation of the provocative diagnostic tests. J Bone Joint Surg Am 68:735, 1986.
4. Kaplan SJ, Glickel SZ, Eaton RG: Predictive factors in nonsurgical treatment of carpal tunnel syndrome. J Hand Surg [Br] 15:107, 1990.
5. Adelaar RS, Foster WC, McDowell C: The treatment of cubital tunnel syndrome. J Hand Surg [Am] 9:90–95, 1984.
6. Rayan G: Proximal ulnar nerve compression—cubital tunnel syndrome. Hand Clin 8:325–336, 1992.
7. Benson LS, Williams CS, Marjorie K: Dupuytren's contracture. J Am Acad Orthop Surg 6:24–35, 1998.
8. Canales FL, Newmeyer WL, Kilger ES: The treatment of felons and paronychias. Hand Clin 5:515–523, 1989.
9. Linscheid RL, Dobyns JH: Common and uncommon infections of the hand. Orthop Clin North Am 6:1063–1104, 1975.
10. Diest WL, Dightman L, Dwarkin MS, et al: Pinning down skin infection: Diagnosis, treatment, and prevention in wrestlers. Physician Sportsmed 25:45–56, 1997.
11. Miller LM, Morgan RF: Vasospastic disorders: Etiology, recognition, and treatment. Hand Clin 9:171–187, 1993.
12. Green PG, Rowland SA: Fractures and dislocations in the hand. In Rockwood CA, Green DP, Bucholz RW, eds: Fractures in Adults. Philadelphia, JB Lippincott, 1991, pp 441–561.
13. Linscheid RL, Dobyns JH, Beckenbaugh RD, Cooney WP: Instability patterns of the wrist. J Hand Surg 8:682–686, 1983.
14. Gelberman RH, Wolock BS, Siegal DB: Current concepts review: Fractures and nonunion of the carpal scaphoid. J Bone Joint Surg Am 71:1560, 1989.
15. Schumacher HR: Primer on Rheumatic Diseases, 10th ed. Atlanta, Arthritis Foundation, 1993, pp 86–181.
16. Wilson RL: Rheumatoid arthritis of the hand. Orthop Clin North Am 17:313–343, 1986.
17. Pellegrini VD: Osteoarthritis at the base of the thumb. Orthop Clin North Am 23:83–102, 1992.

Chapter 24

Musculoskeletal Pain and Emotional Disorders

Eugene J. Carragee

This chapter examines how musculoskeletal pain syndromes in many instances may be primarily related to the patient's psychological, social, or emotional circumstances and outlines some practical approaches to the diagnosis and management of musculoskeletal pain syndromes.

CASE PRESENTATION

A 49-year-old woman had a long history of lower back discomfort. By her report, several times since her teenage years she had been completely disabled with back pain. She complained of back, buttock, and thigh pain with no radiation below the knee. She had not worked in 16 years and was cared for by her husband and daughter. She was seen in the clinic in 1992 and at that time had been unable to leave her bed for 16 weeks. She was taking 8 to 10 Percodan (oxycodone) each day, and she complained that physical therapy had increased her symptoms, not relieved them. She also reported headaches, palpitations, epigastric pain, upper extremity tingling, and multiple drug allergies. She had undergone a hysterectomy and appendectomy for pelvic pain, laparoscopic cholecystectomy for epigastric pain and gallstones, and bilateral carpal tunnel releases. None of these procedures resulted in lasting relief, although each helped transiently. She had recently been seen in an emergency department because she "could not move her legs," although thorough evaluations had revealed only degenerative changes in the lower back consistent with her age. She had undergone epidural, facet, and root injections, all without lasting effect. No structural reason for her severe illness and pain behavior was found. A diagnosis of somatization disorder was considered and referral for treatment offered. This was refused, and the patient left dissatisfied with her care.

In 1995, she returned with similar complaints in her back and legs. Since her prior visit, she had undergone a computed tomography–discogram, which showed a normal L3–L4 disc and degenerative and fissured L4–L5 and L5–S1 discs. A severe pain response was noted at L4–L5 and L5–S1 on injection of the discs. The patient felt both injections reproduced her usual discomfort in her back and legs. Apparently an anterior and posterior L4–S1 fusion was then done and provided some relief for 3 months, but then her pain returned more severely than preoperatively, and she was contemplating having the screws and rods removed because she felt these were

causing her pain. Radiographs showed a solid anterior fusion at 16 months postoperatively.

The hardware was removed a year later by another surgeon. The posterior fusion appeared solid. Again short-term relief after surgery was followed by return of her usual symptoms. She was seen back in the clinic in 1997 with similar complaints as to those 5 years earlier and pain around her incision areas and bone graft sites. At this visit, she related all of her symptoms to her spinal operations.

Most physicians enter medicine with the ideal of treating and, it is hoped, curing disease, yet there are many patients whose severe illness does not seem to be proportionate to the pathology encountered. The records of the patient in the case presentation indicate that she had seen 16 physicians, including many specialists, for her spine problem alone. Only her family physician 20 years ago had suggested her illness was more psychological than physical.

The post–world War II medical idioms of the 1950s and 1960s influenced the way society thinks about *fighting* disease and winning the *war* on cancer, poverty, crime, and drugs. The construct implies that there is a known enemy to fight. The reality discovered in medical practice is that, at times, the patient's nature, temperament, or personality seems to be what physicians are fighting, not well-defined, organic problems. This situation is vividly seen in the diverse approaches to treatment of patients with chronic musculoskeletal pain in whom no identifiable serious pathology is discovered. This group of patients can be divided into those who require little support and for whom the pain is incidental to the business of their lives and those who are euphemistically called *pain patients*. The lack of response to usual treatments and the physician's failure to find serious *real disease* frustrates both the patient and the physician. The physician is often labeled as uncaring and unhelpful, and the patient is referred to as difficult or malingering. In an effort to be more helpful, physicians may aggressively pursue the treatment of minor anatomic or physiologic pathology. Degenerative processes of the bones, joints, and spine are commonly seen in these cases, but treating these abnormalities is rarely helpful.

Fundamental to understanding the treatment of pain is the understanding that life is painful. The nature of human relations involves separation and loss. Family and social circumstances vary, but no one is exempted from the hardships and heartaches of life. With aging, physical impairments inexorably mount, and the loss of vitality and strength may be painful and disheartening. Although physicians may hope to ameliorate some symptoms, a goal of restoring a patient to a pain-free state is often without a basis in reality. The traditional axiom, "*Life* is trouble, only death is no trouble," is applicable across time, culture, and circumstance. It is clear that some individuals are poorly prepared emotionally, socially, or psychologically to deal with the vicissitudes of life. Recognizing the individual with this problem is critical to making a reasonable diagnosis and managing the pain.

EMOTIONS, SOCIAL CONTEXT, AND PAIN

Acute Pain

The complaint of pain is always influenced by circumstance and psychology. Although the protestations of an 8-year-old with a stomachache on an examination day may be transparent, life becomes more complex with time. Soldiers in battle with serious wounds often carry on with little complaint and on reflection insist that their wounds did not hurt terribly much during combat. Experience from the Korean War has shown that pain medication requirements by combat casualties correlated closely with the expectation of returning to a forward area. Soldiers with similar wounds requested more pain medicine if it was understood that they would not be further evacuated but would return to their units and be exposed to combat again.

CASE PRESENTATION

A 22-year-old motorcycle rider was admitted with a femoral shaft fracture after a collision with a parked car. There was a history of alcohol abuse, and the patient's blood alcohol level was 0.05. Despite the application of a traction splint in the field, the patient was seen in the emergency department writhing in pain. He received 28 mg of morphine and 0.25 mg of fentanyl within the first hour after the injury, and although somewhat somnolent, he still complained bitterly of pain. A closed rodding of the femur was performed under general anesthesia, but postoperatively the patient denied satisfactory analgesic effect despite the use of patient-controlled analgesia at a high rate. A thorough reevaluation failed to find a cause for his disproportionate pain. He complained that the medication was "not working," that the physical therapist rebroke his leg getting him up, and that the bed had reinjured him by jerking into the upright position. Escalated doses of narcotics were unhelpful, and on the seventh postoperative day he was found difficult to arouse with an oxygen saturation of 75%. This was reversed with naloxone (Narcan). He was discharged home on day 12 still ambulating only minimally, and 8 months later, he had not returned to normal activities.

Acute trauma always has a context and sometimes an important context is one's cultural expectations. I and co-workers[1] studied 25 patients with femoral shaft fractures treated in the United States and compared these with a matched group from three urban hospitals in Vietnam (two in Hanoi and one in Ho Chi Minh City [Saigon]). Ages and sex were not significantly different. The mean weight of the Vietnamese group was significantly less than that of the American group (58 kg versus 81 kg). Over the first 14 days after injury, the Vietnamese group was given a mean of 0.9 mg morphine/kg/day versus 30.2 mg morphine/kg/day for the Americans. Despite 20 to 30 times more narcotic usage in the Americans, most believed they had been *undermedicated*, whereas fewer than 10% of the Vietnamese group believed similarly. Fewer than 10% of the Americans, compared with 30% of the Vietnamese group, believed they had received *too much* pain medication. Mean heart rates over the first 5 days after surgery were not significantly different in the two groups, implying similar physiologic distress. The expectations of pain were found to be widely different in the American and Vietnamese groups. Only 4% of the American group believed they had an accurate impression of how much a femur fracture would hurt before the injury, whereas 76% of Vietnamese patients responded that they imagined such an injury would be approximately as painful as it was. Results were similar for preconceptions of pain because of surgery and in the postoperative period. More than 50% of patients from the American group believed there must be some explanation other than the femur fracture to explain the severity of their pain (infection, missed injury, hardware failure, inappropriate medical care).

Chronic Pain

More commonly, pain complaints are of a more chronic nature. Psychological problems confound the evaluation of these complaints. Chronic pelvic pain, atypical chest pain, temporal mandibular joint pain, low back pain, persistent headaches, and foot and ankle pain are all clinical conditions in which psychological and social factors are notorious for influencing the nature of the illness. In these and similar conditions, it is imperative that the clinician clearly distinguish the illness (what patients feel and how they are affected by a condition) from disease (the pathoanatomic or pathophysiologic process causing dysfunction).

As a clinical model, the low back pain syndrome is used to illustrate the interaction of psychological and social elements in clinical practice. Low back pain syndromes are similar to other chronic musculoskeletal pain syndromes in the following ways: (1) mainly degenerative pathologic features, (2) a benign clinical course in a majority of patients, and (3) a small subset of severely affected patients without additional pathologic findings. Low back pain syndromes have the advantage in this discussion of having been closely studied from psychological, social, and epidemiologic standpoints. Many of the features may be expanded to chronic pain syndromes of the neck, wrist, pelvis, temporomandibular joint area, and other regions of the musculoskeletal system.

LOW BACK PAIN SYNDROMES

The evaluation-associated, treatment-associated, and disability-associated losses make low back complaints the most expensive medical problem involving working-age people (see Chapter 19). Low back problems are the second most common reason a physician is seen in the United States after upper respiratory infections. The costs are enormous—more than $100 billion per year including indirect expenses in the United States. The surgical management of these problems results in more than 250,000 operations per year, almost one each minute. The number of nonsurgical invasive procedures, such as epidural injections, intradiscal steroid instillation, and percutaneous annular thermocoagulation, among others, is unknown but certainly greater than the operative case rate. Low back–related disability doubles every 8 to 10 years. Tumors, infections, fractures, deformity, and other serious diseases account for a minuscule number of these cases. However, except for a herniated intervertebral disc causing sciatica, the underlying cause is unconfirmed. The diagnosis is usually considered to be *degenerative* or *discogenic* low back pain.[2–4]

Low back pain, similar to musculoskeletal pain referable to other sites, is a nearly universal, intermittent, and recurring human predicament.[5] Most people do not seek medical care when their back hurts; they automatically adjust certain aspects of their lives, accept some pain, and continue on. Of those seeking professional care, 80% to 90% are better in 6 weeks without specific treatment. Individuals with chronic disabling low back pain often have psychological problems.[6] Depression and anxiety have been reported as more prevalent in patients with chronic back pain.[5–7] Early researchers found psychometric testing to show characteristic abnormalities in patients with chronic back pain,[8] and abnormal psychometric evaluation (Minnesota Multiphasic Personality Inventory [MMPI]) appears to predict failure with some treatments.[9]

In the industrial setting, the existence of a workers' compensation claim in a low back pain case is a poor prognostic event. Regardless of the anatomic pathology, the social context of the painful complaint appears to determine the course of the illness. A comprehensive prospective evaluation of back injuries reported in 3020 aircraft manufacturing employees showed that certain patient qualities evidently precede the *work injury* and correlate with long-term back disability.[10, 11] Comprehensive physical examinations, education and medical histories, cardiovascular fitness, and demographic and psychosocial data were prospectively collected on the workers, and they were followed for 4 years. A history of low back troubles predicted future problems. Younger employees (with fewer degenerative changes) were more likely to report work injuries than older ones. Patients who sought medical attention in the past for pain problems of any kind were more likely to report work-related back troubles. Physical variables

such as strength, flexibility, and fitness did not predict future back troubles, although a positive smoking history did. The strongest predictors of future back problems were psychosocial factors and work perceptions. Low job enjoyment, emotional distress, and somatic complaints on the MMPI all predicted future low back problems.

In a nonindustrial setting, similar results have been reported. In a study of 300 acute low back pain patients, data collected during the first week could accurately predict 88% of those who would go on to have chronic severe problems.[12] The most predictive variables included a *fear-avoidance* pattern of behavior with other painful episodes in life. Patients with a history of functioning well despite common medical problems, such as headache or minor trauma, were unlikely to develop chronic low back troubles. Persons rating the discomfort from previous common conditions (e.g., toothache, headache, cut finger) as very painful were more likely to experience severe low back conditions.

In another study, 250 patients with low back pain seen in a primary care setting were given a battery of psychosocial tests as well as the usual medical evaluation. The psychosocial variables predicted 76% of those who would not recover in short order. Previous and current coping strategies for pain and somatization perceptions were the most powerful indicators that a patient would not recover.[7]

Mannion and colleagues[13] reported on 403 volunteers without a history of *serious* low back pain. Although a history of any previous low back pain predicted future *serious* pain, those individuals with high initial somatization and depression scores were 2.7 times more likely to develop serious low back pain than those with normal scores. Most scores did not change significantly despite continued pain. That is, patients with abnormal scores and low back pain had abnormal scores that preceded the development of chronic back troubles. In these instances, it appears that the psychological profiles often seen in chronic pain were present, before the onset of the pain and were not, in fact, the result of the back troubles themselves. These and other studies therefore indicate that psychological and social factors may predispose to development of chronic low back pain. Previous low back pain, passive pain-coping strategies, economic disincentives, and social and cultural motivation all appear to contribute.

EVALUATION OF THE PSYCHOLOGICAL ASPECTS IN A PATIENT WITH MUSCULOSKELETAL PAIN

The first step in the practical evaluation of a patient with pain problems of a musculoskeletal nature is to rule out serious underlying disease. A 30-year-old individual with low back complaints for 3 weeks is unlikely to have a serious anatomic problem. Even if the pain is severe and the individual is distraught, in the absence of additional symptoms suggesting malignancy, infection, or fracture, testing is likely to show only degenerative changes. If the patient leaves the encounter believing the clinician thinks there is a serious pathologic cause of the complaint, a negative test result would mean only more tests need to be done to find the problem.[5]

A highly stressed executive may have chest pain that is not likely cardiac angina by history. He can be told that he probably has chest wall pain, but a treadmill and thallium scan would be done to *confirm* the clinician's suspicion that he does *not* have coronary disease. The negative work-up is greeted with relief and an openness to stress reduction. In another instance, a worker may be seen with low back pain, clearly disliking his job and his boss. If he believes the radiographs and magnetic resonance imaging (MRI) are being done to discover why he feels so sick, he is not likely to understand why the testing is negative for serious problems because he *does* feel badly. The clinician should explain that his pain is likely not a serious physical condition and that the work-up is being done to be sure this is the case. This concept is often given little attention in clinical practice. Consequently, MRI findings of a lumbar *disc bulge,* loss of disc signal in the cervical spine, degenerative meniscus changes in the knee, and minor nerve conduction abnormalities are often interpreted as diagnoses of serious import by a poorly informed patient.[15, 16]

HISTORY

The history in cases of serious emotional trouble contributing to a pain process is usually not subtle. However, it usually is not sought by the physician. It is disconcerting to find a patient out of work for months, taking large amounts of narcotics, and appearing despondent who has never been asked about his job, home, marriage, or emotional state. This sort of inquiry should be done on the first visit or when the usual recovery in days or weeks is not seen. A comprehensive history takes time, effort, tact, and sensitivity, and it is poorly reimbursed. Red flags that should alert the clinician to possible serious psychological amplification of painful conditions include the following:

1. Current or previous drug or alcohol problems
2. History of other poorly defined pain syndromes (headaches, spastic bowel disease, pelvic pain, carpal tunnel or thoracic outlet syndrome, chronic fatigue syndrome, fibromyalgia)
3. History of many previous treatments for this and other problems having been ineffective
4. Multiple analgesic drug allergies
5. Unstable or chaotic work or home life
6. Perceived childhood neglect or abuse

The concept of a *parallel history* is important. A parallel history refers to life events occurring concurrently with the development or exacerbation of a painful condition.[5] These events may include a change of job, divorce, death in the family, and social or professional reversals. These life stresses have been shown to predict a poor low back pain prognosis.[12] Eliciting them provides insight into the patient's emotional resources for recovery.

EXAMINATION

Several signs on physical examination suggest emotional problems that complicate a physical complaint. In the examination of the low back, the Waddell's sign and others (detailed in Chapters 3 and 19) describe reactions to simple physical tests that cannot be explained by pathologic impairment alone. For example, severe low back pain with head percussion is not seen in fractures, infections, or tumors but is often seen in persons with significant psychological troubles. Collapsing weakness on manual testing does not have a neurologic basis and usually is not seen in serious painful destructive processes.

Bizarre behavior, weeping, outbursts of anger, or dramatic appeals for the clinician to *do something* should be thoughtfully assessed. The experienced clinician resists the temptation to become the latest white knight in the disturbed patient's epic treatment quest. That sort of projection on the clinician is usually not helpful, and the clinician eventually disappoints the patient by not meeting expectations. Although one occasionally may make the previously unsuspected diagnosis of porphyria or cervical syringomyelia, usually the missing diagnosis is not found because it does not exist as a discrete pathologic finding.

DIAGNOSTIC TESTING

Degenerative Discs in Spine

The finding of degenerative discs on plain radiographs and computed tomography scanning is common.[14, 15] The more sensitive the study, the more common the finding will be. With magnetic resonance imaging, the prevalence of degenerative findings increases with age until nearly all elderly patients have disc changes. In asymptomatic individuals with no history of low back troubles, 40% to 70% have these changes. The common mistake is to attribute nonspecific low back complaints to these findings. The more serious mistake is to attribute serious disabling pain in an emotionally troubled person to these findings, as in the case introducing this chapter. Once this implication has been made, it is all but impossible to rectify. The patient will continue to believe that the fault is in his or her spine and not in their psyche.

Provocative Testing

Distinguishing anatomic changes that are without significant symptoms from those causing severe pain and functional loss has led investigators to apply *provocative* testing in an effort to elicit the patient's usual pain by stimulating or anesthetizing certain spinal structures. Provocative tests are used for suspected spinal disc and facet, shoulder, wrist, and sacroiliac problems. All claim an objective result that relies on the patient's subjective response to provocative stimulation or anesthetic block of a supposed painful site. In many cases, this response is reliable, but the reliability is notably lacking in patients with disturbed emotional or psychosocial profiles.

The specificity of pain reproduction by stimulating an anatomic site has not been proven. In the presence of chronic pain, there is a known increased responsiveness to normally innocuous stimuli as well as a hyperalgesia of uninjured tissue surrounding an area of injury.[16] It is also known that stimulation of structures proximal to a lesion may mimic the quality and affective component of the patient's usual pain[17,18] Even primarily psychogenic pain may be simulated by specific anatomic stimulation.[17,18] Parallel work on anesthetic blocks used in diagnosing pain location has also proven problematic. Studies have shown that anesthetic blocks applied to areas of referred pain (i.e., not the true pain generator) can provide significant pain relief.[16,19] Even central pain resulting from central nervous system lesions can be sometimes relieved by peripheral local anesthetic action in the distal location of perceived pain.[20]

Discography is an example of a provocative test that has serious flaws, particularly in the patient with significant psychological problems.[21–24] The test is performed by inserting a needle into an intervertebral disc, injecting a contrast agent, and asking the patient if this is painful and whether the pain simulates the usual pain for which he or she sought treatment. In some centers, it is accepted that a patient with chronic back pain, no other clearly identifiable spinal or regional pathology, and positive pain reproduction on discography is suffering primarily from an illness caused by the disc pathology. Specifically, it is degenerative or traumatic fissuring through the innervated outer anulus that is the perceived significant pathology.[25,26]

Recent work has shown that discographic injections in subjects *without low back pain* are frequently positive in subjects with chronic pain states and in patients with abnormal psychometric testing for somatization disorder or depression. Disc stimulation in subjects without low back pain and with normal psychological profiles rarely is painful.[23] In subjects with chronic pain but no low back pain, disc injection often caused pain (40% of subjects). Finally, in subjects with somatization disorders despite an absence of low back pain history, disc injection caused pain in 83%. It appears that in some cases discography may be testing for the emotional disorder and not the anatomic pathology. These spurious results may distract the clinician from more serious problems at hand, such as social issues, work-related problems, and depression.

Psychometric Screening

A number of psychometric tests are available for office screening. None of these is foolproof. They need to be used in conjunction with a thorough history, physical examination, and review of records. The most useful psychometric test is the record review. If records are available back to the patient's adolescent years, a pattern of illnesses and pain behavior is often clear. School health

records and military service records often reveal the cycle of illness extending back, illustrating how being ill has become established as a strategy for getting along in life.[5] More formal psychometric tests, including the MMPI, the Zung Depression Scale, Beck Depression Index, Modified Somatization Perceptions Questionnaire, Pain Drawings, and others are widely used.

A good approach is for the physician to speak with the psychologist or psychiatrist who is a consultant for the practice. The psychologist or psychiatrist may suggest one or two short forms to be used as a screening test and reserve more involved testing for use in consultation. These tests do not make diagnoses and do not determine treatment. However, the use of psychometric screening tests is useful in supporting a clinical impression or alerting to a possibly missed emotional element to a patient's problem.

APPROACH TO THE PATIENT WITH EMOTIONAL PROBLEMS COMPLICATING A PHYSICAL CONDITION

There are always situations in which a clinician believes that most or a significant part of a patient's illness is due to psychosocial factors. Even when this belief is recognized at some level, it is not regularly acted on. There are compelling reasons why this is so:

1. The issue is difficult to address. The discussion cannot usually be brief, and time is limited. The writing of a prescription or a consultation request is the traditional signal that the medical encounter is over. These cases do not have such an easy end point.

2. The medicolegal implications in personal injury or workers' compensation cases may be daunting. The legal system of advocacy pits opposing blameless camps against each other. A realistic assessment of the complexity of an illness is not welcomed by either party.

3. Many patients have poor insight into their situation. In fact, the lack of insight is often related to how things have gone so badly for so long. Responding to the knee-jerk accusation, "so you're saying it's all in my head..." is difficult at best and can be dangerous. It is easier simply to avoid the issue.

4. Consultants often feel professionally compelled to make diagnoses only in their narrow field. Ego and income may also be tied to the aggressive treatment of the patient others could not treat.

TREATMENT AND CONCLUSIONS

It is surprising how little treatment is sometimes required once the basic underlying problem is identified. Some patients quickly agree with the assessment that, for instance, their back arthritis is relatively mild, but it is true that they hate their job and probably should address that problem first. For other patients, however, the art of physician-patient relations is taxed by these encounters. Several points should be kept in mind:

1. *Early recognition:* The sooner the subject is broached in the investigation of suspicious complaints, the better. Patients complaining of months of extreme fatigue, aches, and pains very likely have an emotional component to their illness. This component should be discussed as the investigation into other possibilities is begun. If the patient is found to have Addison's disease, he or she will need little convincing that this is the true diagnosis. If nothing physical is found, bringing up emotional problems after 6 months of searching seems disingenuous. Finally, if the patient has been told that the reason he or she has been unable to work for 23 years was a minor back strain at age 25, the physician has virtually no chance of addressing the emotional issues decades later.

2. *Identifying obstacles:* The psychological and social reasons why a patient is not improving may not be as obscure as sometimes assumed. The physician should take the time to explore the background.

3. *Functional-oriented goals:* As mentioned earlier, a goal of the obliteration of the subjective feeling of pain and suffering in chronic degenerative conditions is unrealistic. In patients without serious underlying disease and chronic pain, the focus should be turned to function and away from passive pain control.

4. *Treatment of depression:* Depression can be the source of or complicate a patient's musculoskeletal complaints. It should be treated directly. Sedative and opioid drugs used to treat the *pain problem* can exacerbate depression.

5. *Consultation:* The emotionally troubled patient requires a lot of work and time. The physician's diagnosis may be correct but appear as a weak voice in the wilderness of quick fixes. It pays to cultivate relationships with therapists who have experience in this field. Often, more or less formal combined treatment plans can be developed.

6. *Accepting the limits of physicians' skills:* The physician should be clear with patients that most of the burden of getting well is their own. The responsibility to follow directions, comply with rehabilitation regimens, establish limits on medication refills, and limit antisocial behavior ultimately rests on the patient, not on health-care professionals.

REFERENCES

1. Carragee EJ, Vittum D, Truong TP, Burton D: Pain control and cultural norms and expectations after closed femoral shaft fractures. Am J Orthop 28:97–102, 1999.
2. Carragee EJ: The prevalence and clinical features of internal disk disruption in patients with low back pain [letter]. Spine 21:776, 1996.
3. Schwarzer A, Aprill C, Derby R, et al: The prevalence and clinical features of internal disc disruption in patients with chronic LBP. Spine 20:1878–1883, 1995.
4. Schwarzer A, Bogduk N: The prevalence and clinical features of internal disk disruption in patients with low back pain [letter]. Spine 21:776, 1996.
5. Barbour A: Caring for Patients: A Critique of the Medical Model. Stanford, Stanford University Press, 1995.
6. Burton A: Spine update: Back injury and work loss: Biomechanical and psychosocial influences. Spine 22:2575–2580, 1997.
7. Burton A, Tillotson K, Main C, Hollis S: Psychosocial predictors of outcome in acute and subacute low back trouble. Spine 20:722–728, 1995.
8. Main C, Wood P, Hollis S, et al: The distress and risk assessment method (DRAM): A simple patient classification to identify distress and evaluate the risk of a poor outcome. Spine 17:42–52, 1992.
9. Wiltse L, Rocchio P: Pre-operative psychological tests as predictors of success of chemonucleolysis in the treatment of low back pain. J Bone Joint Surg Am 57:478–483, 1975.
10. Bigos S, Battie, M Spengler, D, et al: A prospective study of work perceptions and psychosocial factors affecting the report of back injury. Spine 16:1–6, 1991.
11. Bigos S, Battie M, Spengler D, et al: A longitudinal, prospective study of industrial back injury reporting. Clin Orthop 279:21–34, 1992.
12. Klenerman L, Slade P, Stanley I, et al: The prediction of chronicity in patients with acute attack of low back pain in a general practice setting. Spine 20:478–484, 1995.
13. Mannion A, Dolan P, Adams M: Psychological questionnaires: Do "abnormal" scores precede or follow first-time low back pain? Spine 21:2603–2611, 1996.
14. Boden S, Davis D, Dina T, et al: Abnormal magnetic resonance scans of the lumbar spine in asymptomatic subjects: A prospective investigation. J Bone Joint Surg Am 72:403–408, 1990.
15. Jensen M, Brant-Zawadzki M, Obuchowski N, et al: Magnetic resonance imaging of the lumbar spine in people without back pain. N Engl J Med 331:69–73, 1994.
16. Siddle P, Cousins M: Spinal pain mechanisms. Spine 22:98–104, 1997.
17. Lenz F, Gracely R, Hope E, et al: The sensation of angina can be evoked by stimulation of the human thalamus. Pain 59:119–125, 1994.
18. Lenz F, Gracely R, Romanoski A, et al: Stimulation in the somatosensory thalamus can reproduce both the affective and sensory dimensions of previously experienced pain. Nat Med 1:910–913, 1995.
19. North R, Kidd D, Zahurak M, Piantadosi S: Specificity of diagnostic nerve blocks: A prospective, randomized study of sciatica due to lumbosacral spine disease. Pain 65:77–85, 1996.
20. Kibler R, Nathan P: Relief of pain and paraesthesiae by nerve block distal to a lesion. J Neurol Neurosurg Psychiatry 23:91–98, 1960.
21. Block A, Vanharanta H, Ohnmeiss D, Guyer R: Discographic pain report: Influence of psychological factors. Spine 21:334–338, 1996.
22. Carragee EJ, et al: Positive provocative discography as a misleading finding in the evaluation of low back pain. North American Spine Society, Proceedings, New Orleans, 1997, p 388.
23. Carragee EJ et al: False positive lumbar discography in select patients without low back complaints. Spine (in press).
24. Nachemson A: Lumbar discography—where are we today? Spine 14:555–657, 1989.
25. Moneta G, Videman T, Kaivanto K, et al: Reported pain during lumbar discography as a function of anular ruptures and disc degeneration: A reanalysis of 833 discograms. Spine 19:1968–1974, 1994.
26. Schwarzer A, Aprill C, Derby R, et al: The prevalence and clinical features of internal disc disruption in patients with chronic low back pain. Spine 20:1878–1883, 1995.

Part III

RECOGNITION AND MANAGEMENT OF PATIENTS WITH SPECIFIC RHEUMATOLOGIC PROBLEMS

Rheumatoid Arthritis and Lyme Disease

Edward D. Harris, Jr.

Most patients who develop chronic and persistent inflammation of multiple peripheral joints have rheumatoid arthritis (RA). When patients first present with polyarthritis, the differential diagnosis is broad (see Chapter 18). In this chapter, discussion focuses only on RA and Lyme disease. The latter is added because the synovitis in this process caused by a spirochete is virtually identical to that seen in RA. The lessons learned from study of Lyme disease at a molecular level may have relevance to RA, although the treatment of the two processes is quite different.

In the best circumstances, management of a patient with RA is handled by a team of physicians and allied health professionals:[1] a primary care physician who has first recognized the process; a rheumatologist consulted to outline appropriate therapy; a team of nurse, physical therapist, and occupational therapist to be involved in joint protection; and a group of orthopaedic and hand surgeons who can recommend appropriate surgical intervention at the right time. This group is best equipped to provide expert, prospective (rather than reactive) care. In particular, the primary care physician and rheumatologist should work closely to initiate, carry out, and change management strategies. The primary care physician should take advantage of each patient with RA to expand his or her knowledge about the basic processes, the range of diagnostic techniques, and the spectrum of therapy (as well as the side effects of those therapies).

The pathophysiologic mechanisms that produce RA are described because an understanding of them is helpful in appreciating what therapies are appropriate. This discussion is followed by a clinical description of the disease, guidelines for predicting the course of RA, and a long discussion of therapy.

PATHOPHYSIOLOGY OF RHEUMATOID ARTHRITIS AND ITS RELATIONSHIP TO CLINICAL FINDINGS

RA has four stages (Table 25–1).

Stage 1

CLINICAL FINDINGS

Patients with stage 1 RA are seen early in the disease, within *a few weeks or 1 or 2 months* of onset of symptoms. Morning stiffness and fatigue are often dominant. Joint pain and swelling are variable but usually affect metacarpophalangeal proximal interphalangeal, wrist, and metatarsophalangeal joints. Knees, elbows, and shoulders can be involved, but hips are asymptomatic. On examination, the hands and wrists may be puffy, or individual joints may be swollen (Fig. 25–1). Veins are prominent on the dorsum of wrists and hands. The patient moves slowly and is anxious. No deformity is present. The joints are often tender, but definite synovial proliferation or joint fluid is difficult to define. Subcutaneous nodules are not found. Laboratory abnormalities classically include a slightly high white blood cell count (WBC), slight thrombocytosis, an erythrocyte sedimentation rate (ESR) of 20 to 30 mm/h, and a low normal hemoglobin. In these early stages, tests for rheumatoid factor (RF) are often negative. Radiographs (not needed) are normal.

BIOPATHOLOGY

Biopsy specimens of synovium in the early stages of RA have revealed some edema in the subsynovial layer and presence of new capillaries, perivascular lymphocytes, and mononuclear cells. Within the synovium, antigen presenting cells (APC) are in contact with lymphocytes (Fig. 25–2). In most patients, the HLA antigens on the APC surface are DR4 alleles that have a specific *shared epitope* that binds peptides and presents them to the T-cell receptors.[2] These are CD4$^+$/Th1 cells that generate interleukin (IL)-2, γ-interferon, and cytokines such as IL-15 and tumor necrosis factor (TNF)α. The antigen that is being presented to T cells is unknown but could be a heat-shock protein from common bacteria or a superantigen or an endogenous autoantigen. It is likely that there is activation of multiple T-cell clones as the cellular immune response becomes less specific. Cytokines (e.g., IL-1 and TNFα) activate endothelial cells

Recognition and Management of Patients with Specific Rheumatologic Problems

Table 25–1. FOUR STAGES OF RHEUMATOID ARTHRITIS

	Duration	Symptoms	Signs	Pathology
Stage 1	Few weeks–2 months	Morning stiffness, fatigue, joint pain	Mild puffiness in hand/wrist, individual joint swelling *Lab:* ↑ WBC, ESR 20–30, RF: negative	Synovial biopsy reveals edema, new capillaries, and perivascular lymphocytes and monocyte.
Stage 2	6 weeks–6 months	Fatigue, weakness, joint pain, stiffness	Synovitis, effusion, ↓ ROM, warmth *Lab:* ↑ WBC, Hgb 10–20 g/dL, ESR 30–60 mm/hr, RF: ⊕ 70% *X-ray:* periarticular osteopenia	Synovial biopsy reveals organized inflammation. Abundant proliferation of many cell types.
Stage 3	≥ 6 months	Fatigue, weakness, stiffness, joint pain, loss of function	Synovitis, effusion, ↓ ROM, soft tissue contracture, rheumatoid nodule formation, extra-articular manifestations *Lab:* ↑ WBC, ESR 30–60, ↓Albumin *X-ray:* ⊕ erosion	Synovial biopsy reveals organized and proliferating synovium with degradation of cartilage and bone.
Stage 4	2 years, but usually significantly longer	Fatigue, weakness, joint pain, possible symptoms related to extra-articular manifestations	Deviation, deformity, ↓ ROM, extra-articular manifestations, possible vasculitis *X-ray:* erosion, ankylosis, subluxation, loss of joint space	Synovial biopsy reveals cellular proliferation subsides and is replaced by atrophy and fibrosis.

Lab, laboratory tests; WBC, white blood count; ESR, erythrocyte sedimentaiton rate; RF, rheumatoid factor; ROM, range of motion; Hgb, hemoglobin.

on synovial capillaries to express vascular adhesion molecules; these serve as receptors for ligands on neutrophils and mononuclear cells in the circulation, enabling them to gain access to the synovium and to the synovial fluid.[3]

Stage 2

CLINICAL FINDINGS

Patients with stage 2 RA have had symptoms from 6 weeks to 6 months. The diagnosis of RA has been established. Fatigue and weakness are prominent symptoms as well as joint pain and stiffness. By now, 70% have a significant titer of RF. The proliferative synovium in involved joints is palpable and can be differ-

entiated from synovial fluid. Some joints may lack full active motion because of pain. Additional joints not previously involved (e.g., temporomandibular, ankle) may have become symptomatic. Aspiration of joint fluid reveals many neutrophils (e.g., 5000 to 20,000/mm³), no crystals, and negative cultures. The ESR in uncontrolled cases increases, often to as high as 45 to 60 mm/h. An anemia of chronic disease may have developed (rarely < 10 g/dL), and the WBC and platelets remain elevated (see Chapter 5). Radiographs can show early diffuse demineralization of the bones immediately adjacent to involved joints, but the joint spaces are normal, and there is no evidence of erosions (see Chapter 4).

BIOPATHOLOGY

Synovial biopsy specimens reveal a much more organized inflammation, with a well-demarcated lining of plump synovial cells, lymphoid follicles around multiple capillaries that are lined with tall endothelial cells, and subsynovial proliferation of new connective tissue (Fig. 25–3). The dominant histologic feature is abundant proliferation of many different types of cells, with evidence that cytokines produced by one type of cell are stimulating activation of other types of cells. Evidence suggests that among the many cytokines, TNFα is a principal one (Fig. 25–4)[4]; it stimulates proliferation of synovial lining cells, helps drive the immune response, and triggers synthesis of other cytokines, including IL-1. T-cell proliferation becomes even more polyclonal, suggesting that there is an immune response to *bystander* antigens that may include epitopes on host tissues, such as type II collagen in cartilage. T-cell help leads to activation and proliferation of B cells that produce RFs (antibodies against immunoglobulin G [IgG]) that then form immune complexes sufficiently large to activate the complement system. In the synovial fluid, polymorphonuclear leukocytes are activated by multiple stimuli and release prostaglandins, leukotrienes, proteases, and

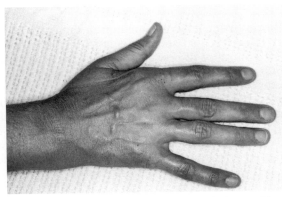

Figure 25–1. Hand of a young man several weeks into an illness that was diagnosed 2 months later as definite rheumatoid arthritis. His principal symptom was morning stiffness in the hands. The only objective abnormalities were a mild diffuse swelling of the dorsum of the hand, prominent veins, and slight swelling of the fourth proximal interphalangeal and second metacarpophalangeal joints. (From Harris ED Jr: Rheumatoid Arthritis. Philadelphia, WB Saunders; 1997, p 217.)

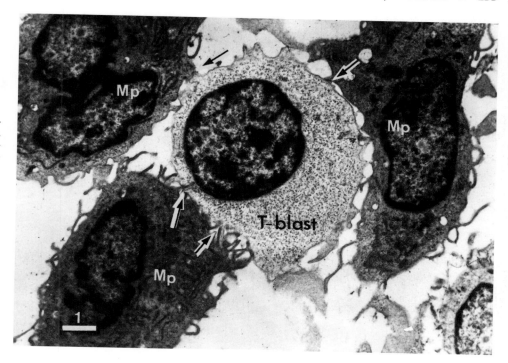

Figure 25–2. Electron photomicrograph of cells in rheumatoid synovium. The center cell with speckled cytoplasm represents a lymphocyte. Contacts with macrophages (Mp) are shown by arrows. (Courtesy of Dr. Morris Ziff, University of Texas Southwestern Medical College, Dallas, Texas; from Harris ED Jr: Rheumatoid Arthritis. Philadelphia, WB Saunders, 1997, p 53.)

oxygen-derived free radicals. All the pathology and biochemistry at this stage suggest that despite the lack of clinical evidence for joint destruction, there are proliferating and activated cells sufficient in the synovium and synovial fluid to begin sustained aggressive erosion of bone and loss of cartilage.

Stage 3

CLINICAL FINDINGS

If the synovitis has not been suppressed by therapy or spontaneous remission (a rare phenomenon), patients who progress to stage 3 RA begin to lose function from pain and loss of cartilage and bone. Soft tissue contractures can limit motion of joints. Effusions in large joints are painful, producing flexion contractures. Synovial proliferation in extensor tendon sheaths of the fingers can erode tendons leading to rupture. Rheumatoid nodules develop frequently in patients with high titers of RF. These can appear in the lung or rarely in the heart as well as in subcutaneous areas over bony prominences. The systemic effects of chronic, active RA become evident: These patients lose weight; have significant anemia of chronic disease; have hypoalbuminemia; and can develop localized vasculitis of medium-sized blood vessels in skin, in the gastrointestinal tract, along peripheral nerves, or in several other organs. At this stage, irreversible destruction of joints occurs (Fig. 25–5). Once the glycosaminoglycans are depleted from cartilage matrix, this tissue loses its resilience and is further degraded by normal mechanical forces.

BIOPATHOLOGY

At this stage, the organized and proliferating synovium begins to degrade cartilage and bone (Fig. 25–6). The erosive process is a centripetal one; the process invades from the periphery to the center of the joint. It is probable that deposits of RF/IgG or IgG/collagen com-

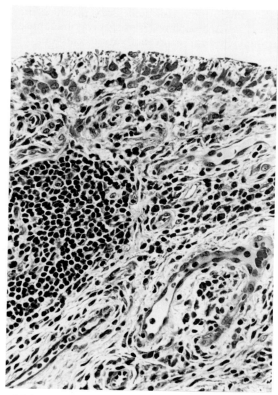

Figure 25–3. Light photomicrograph of rheumatoid synovial tissue showing hyperplastic synovial lining cells and lymphocyte aggregations in the sublining cell layer. (Hematoxylin and eosin stain ×165.) (Courtesy of Dr. Yasunori Okada; from Harris ED Jr: Rheumatoid Arthritis. Philadelphia, WB Saunders, 1997, p 136.)

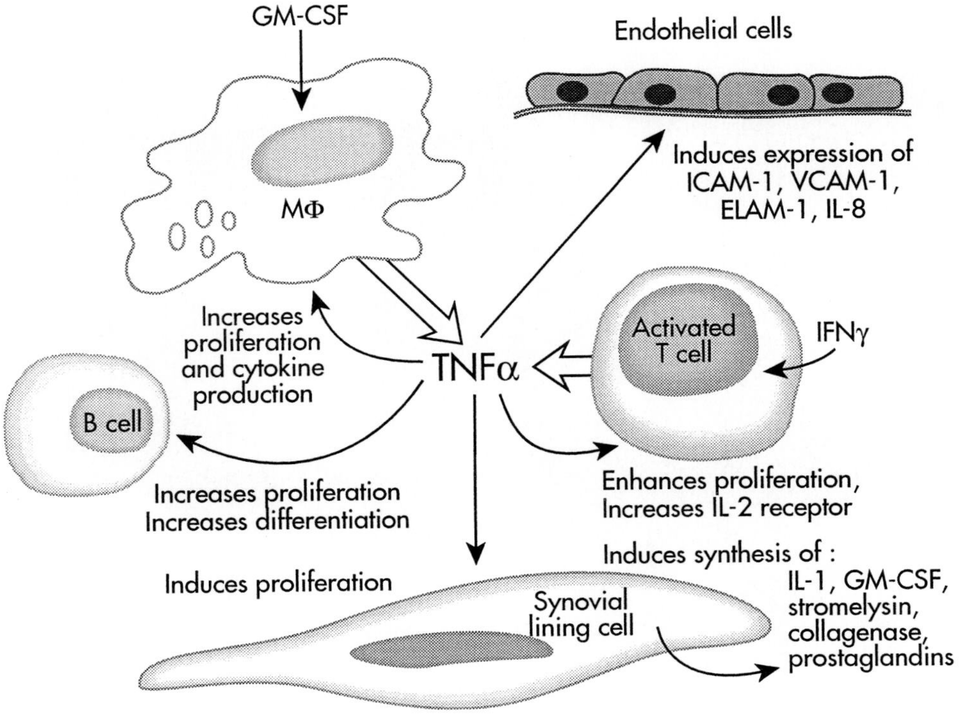

GM-CSF

Endothelial cells

MΦ

Induces expression of
ICAM-1, VCAM-1,
ELAM-1, IL-8

Increases
proliferation
and cytokine
production

TNFα

Activated
T cell

IFNγ

B cell

Increases proliferation
Increases differentiation

Enhances proliferation,
Increases IL-2 receptor

Induces proliferation

Synovial
lining cell

Induces synthesis of :
IL-1, GM-CSF,
stromelysin,
collagenase,
prostaglandins

Figure 25–4. Tumor necrosis factor (TNF)α is a cytokine with multiple potentials for driving many engines of the inflammatory/proliferative processes in rheumatoid arthritis. It appears that both activated macrophages and T cells produce TNFα, which, in turn, can act back on these cells as well as on the synovial lining cells, endothelium, and B cells. All of the major activity of TNFα in model systems can be inferred to be proinflammatory. The fact that active TNFα enhances interleukin (IL)-1 production by cells is additional evidence for its primacy in generating and sustaining rheumatoid synovitis. (From Harris ED Jr: Rheumatoid Arthritis. Philadelphia, WB Saunders, 1997, p 110.)

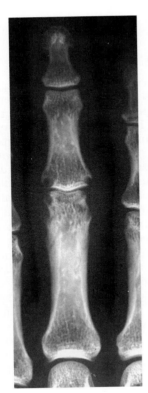

Figure 25–5. Radiograph of the long finger in a 42-year-old woman with rheumatoid arthritis. Periarticular soft tissue swelling is present at the proximal interphalangeal joint, with bony erosions on both sides of the joint. There is associated narrowing of the cartilage space, whereas the cartilage spaces at the metacarpophalangeal and distal interphalangeal joints are normal. (Courtesy of A. Gabrielle Bergman, M.D., Stanford University Medical Center; from Harris ED Jr: Rheumatoid Arthritis. Philadelphia, WB Saunders, 1997, p 267.)

plexes, along with activated complement, in the superficial layers of collagen act as chemoattractants for the invasive tissue (Fig. 25–7). The cells that degrade cartilage, bone, and tendon are synovial lining cells activated by TNFα and other cytokines. They produce metalloproteases in proenzyme forms, procollagenase and prostromelysin that after activation can degrade all of the collagen and glycosaminoglycans in cartilage and tendon. Mineral in bone is depleted by activated bone cells releasing hydrogen ions at marrow-bone interfaces. Mononuclear cell proliferation in splenic tissue can generate Felty's syndrome (to be discussed later) and in salivary tissue can initiate Sjögren's syndrome.

Stage 4

CLINICAL FINDINGS

Stage 4 is the end stage of RA. For reasons still unclear, perhaps explained by lack of motion or cartilage-containing immune complexes, once a given joint is destroyed, the synovitis in that joint becomes less active. Beginning in stage 3 and continuing into stage 4, there is an increasing role for orthopaedic surgery, including total joint replacement. The osteopenic bones of patients at this stage make successful joint replacement a true challenge. These patients—often weakened by excessive catabolism and poor nutrition—are particularly susceptible to side effects of medications, including gastrointestinal bleeding and renal insufficiency. Those who have had active disease for more than 15 years may develop amyloidosis. Many patients are immobilized to bed and chair, unable to care for themselves. Mortality

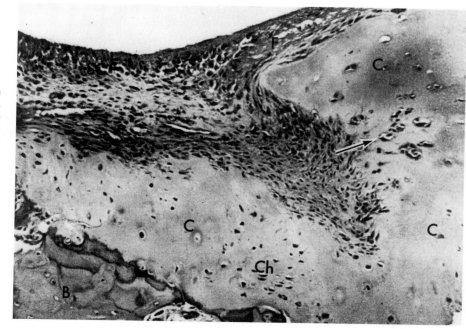

Figure 25–6. Photomicrograph showing the initial process of cartilage (C) destruction in rheumatoid arthritis. The mesenchymal cells proliferate and penetrate the lateral borders of articular cartilage near the chondral-bone (B) interface. Chondrocytes (Ch) are activated as well and tend to proliferate within lacunae as well as to release proteases into the surrounding matrix. The arrow indicates the direction of the synovial invasion into the cartilage. (Courtesy of Kingsley Mills; from Harris ED Jr; Rheumatoid Arthritis. Philadelphia, WB Saunders, 1975, p 128.)

may be as high in these individuals as it is for many patients with cancer.

BIOPATHOLOGY

At this stage of the disease, cellular proliferation subsides and is replaced by atrophy and fibrosis. The catabolic effects of the disease dominate. Granulomas in bone are additive with osteoclast-mediated bone loss, leading to fractures from minimal trauma. Immune complexes of IgG and RF are capable of initiating vasculitis in multiple organs.

COURSE AND COMPLICATIONS OF RHEUMATOID ARTHRITIS

The primary care physician who cares for a patient with RA should consult with a rheumatologist who can help plan a therapeutic regimen and with whom the primary care manager can discuss unforeseen complications and setbacks. The physician must recognize the potential dysfunction and complications that can develop in these patients and be ready to respond appropriately. Special problems that can affect particular joints are outlined here.

Complications of Joint Disease

CERVICAL SPINE

Subluxation of the atlanto-occipital joint can have serious neurologic associations and sequelae. (See Chapter 20 for a detailed discussion of the cervical spine in rheumatoid arthritis.) The most common presenting symptom is pain radiating from the neck into

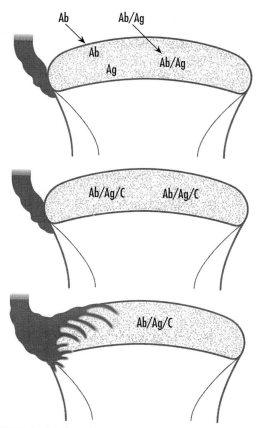

Figure 25–7. Is the deposition of antigen (Ag), antibody (Ab), and complement (C) within superficial layers of articular cartilage an attractant for the invasive synovial pannus in rheumatoid arthritis? Another possible attractant is an autoimmune response against some chondrocyte membrane component. (From Harris ED Jr: Rheumatoid Arthritis. Philadelphia, WB Saunders, 1997, p 166.)

the occiput. More rare are slowly progressive quadriparesis, paresthesias in the shoulders or arms when the neck is flexed, transient medullary dysfunction, drop attacks, or loss of sphincter control.[5] When any of these symptoms appear in a patient who has significant destruction of peripheral joints, consultation with a skilled radiologist is essential to obtain the most appropriate imaging to examine this area. Initially, flexion/extension x-rays of the cervical spine may be obtained. A worrisome finding is atlanto-occipital subluxation as evidenced by a gap of 8 mm or more between the odontoid and atlas. Magnetic resonance imaging (MRI) can be particularly useful because the spinal cord as well as bone can be visualized. Operative stabilization can be considered if symptoms are progressive.

TEMPOROMANDIBULAR JOINTS

As many as 75% of RA patients have radiographic evidence for structural alterations of these joints, and about half of RA patients have jaw symptoms at some time in the course of their disease. Material in Chapter 22 outlines the evaluation and management of this complication.

CRICOARYTENOID JOINTS

The cricoarytenoid joints are lined by synovium. As many as 30% of RA patients complain of hoarseness, and these patients have a minimal but definite risk of developing stridor or even asymptomatic aspiration of pharyngeal contents into the lungs. Computed tomography (CT) scans have detected abnormalities on these joints in half of RA patients with moderately severe peripheral joint disease.

STERNOCLAVICULAR JOINTS

Involvement of these joints can produce local pain in patients while sleeping on their side and during shoulder motion.

SHOULDER

Rheumatoid damage to the rotator cuff apparatus leading to superior subluxation of the humerus and impingement on the acromion is one of the most common causes of shoulder pain and dysfunction in these patients. Sudden tears in the inflamed rotator cuff can cause such pain as to suggest sepsis. Proliferative shoulder synovitis can produce rupture of one or both biceps tendons, diagnosed clinically by a bunching of part of the biceps muscle down near the elbow during forearm flexion. As with other complex joint involvement, skilled orthopaedic consultation is often essential for coordinated management (see Chapters 3 and 18).

ELBOW

Because the shoulder and wrist can compensate for a loss of elbow motion, loss of full extension may be asymptomatic. Loss of elbow extension may become a concern only when pronation and supination become painful.

HAND AND WRIST

The many joints of the hand and wrist are the most important for upper extremity function and the most frequently involved of all joints by RA. The primary care physician should pay particular attention to chronic swelling in the tendon sheaths of the finger extensor muscles as they course along the dorsum of the wrist; they are particularly susceptible to rupture by the invasive synovium, something that can be repaired by hand surgeons if alerted quickly. The primary care physician should also be concerned about loss of wrist extension in RA patients, arranging for wrist splints through occupational therapists to help maintain at least a neutral position for the wrist at rest. On the volar surface of the wrist, proliferative synovium can compress the median nerve, producing the carpal tunnel syndrome with numbness, pain, and eventually weakness of the thumb and second and third fingers.

The primary care physician should focus on function more than form in analysis of the patient's hands. If a patient has strong grip and good dexterity, it is not indicated to refer a patient to hand surgery for an early swan-neck or boutonnière deformity. Deformity is not necessarily associated with loss of function in the hands (Fig. 25–8). In contrast, substantial ulnar deviation at the metacarpophalangeal joints can lead to a weakened grip, and corrective surgery may alleviate this. Severe active and chronic synovitis of the finger joints can lead to resorptive arthropathy presenting as *accordion* fingers and a *pencil in cup* appearance on radiographs.

A treatable cause of inability to flex or straighten a digit, particularly at the proximal interphalangeal joint, can be the development of a flexor tendon nodule that effectively *locks* the finger in place. These can often be palpated as they move under the examiner's palpating finger during passive motion of the joint involved (Fig. 25–9). *De Quervain's tenosynovitis* is tenosynovitis of thumb extensors that produces severe pain at the base of the thumb during ulnar flexion of this digit (see Chapters 18 and 23). Distal interphalangeal joints have only a small amount of synovium; it follows therefore that they are much less involved in RA than the proximal interphalangeal and metacarpophalangeal joints. A significant contribution to hand weakness can be atrophy and fibrosis in and around intrinsic muscles of the hand, complications that lead to flexion deformity (particularly at the metacarpophalangeal joints) (Fig. 25–10).

HIP

The hip is one of the last joints to become symptomatic in adults with RA, whereas it is a common early involved joint in children. Preexisting osteoarthritis is accelerated when RA develops in the same person. Remodeling of the acetabulum results in *protrusio acetabuli*, as the femoral head works its way deeper into the

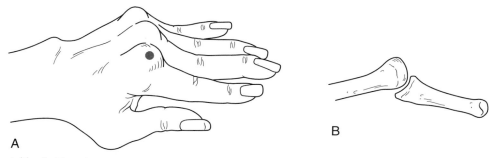

Figure 25–8. Rheumatoid arthritis and metacarpophalangeal subluxation. *A,* Appearance of the hand. There also is an early swan-neck deformity. *B,* A sketch of the alignment of the second metacarpal and phalanx. The prominence felt at the black dot is actually the cartilaginous surface of the metacarpal bone. The phalanx, because of stretching of the joint capsule secondary to inflammatory synovitis, has slipped (subluxed) in a palmar direction. This patient, despite the subluxation, had good grip strength.

pelvis (Fig. 25–11). Total hip replacement in RA patients is rarely as useful as it is in patients with pure osteoarthritis because the bone structure is porotic and weak.

KNEE

Inflammation of synovium in the knee leads almost immediately to reflex atrophy of the quadriceps mechanism, which, in turn, feeds back to put more stress on the knee joint. Preexisting *genu varum* or *genu valgum* is accelerated. Flexion contractures develop and often are secondary to large effusions. Popliteal cysts develop as synovial fluid, under pressure during weight bearing in flexion, collects in the popliteal space. Also known as *Baker's cysts,* they can mimic chronic thrombophlebitis by restricting venous and lymphatic return or can rupture into the calf, mimicking acute thrombophlebitis. As in the hip, synovial inflammation can accelerate osteoarthritis that is a preexisting condition; the same enzymes that degrade articular cartilage destroy the fibrocartilage in the menisci of the knee.

FOOT AND ANKLE

Involvement of the multiple joints here is not dissimilar to that noted in disease of the hand and wrist. The ankle and foot, similar to the hand and wrist, function in coordinate fashion. Early in active RA, pain in

the ankle and forefoot prevents any effective pushing off the toes during gait. The result of this is a tendency for the foot to be everted and inverted so that the patient pushes off the broad inferomedial portion of the foot as he or she walks. This tendency may be accentuated by painful metatarsal subluxation caused by distention of the joint capsule from the proliferative syn-

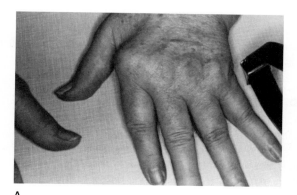

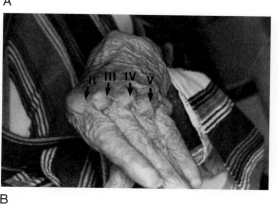

Figure 25–10. *A,* Early ulnar deviation of the metacarpophalangeal joints without subluxation. Extensor tendons have slipped to the ulnar side. The fifth finger, in particular, is compromised with weak flexion, causing loss of power grip. *B,* Complete subluxation with marked ulnar deviation at the metacarpophalangeal joints of a 90-year-old woman with rheumatoid arthritis. Arrows mark the heads of the metacarpals, now in direct contact with the joint capsule instead of the proximal phalanges. (Courtesy of James L. McGuire, M.D.; from Harris ED Jr: Clinical features of rheumatoid arthritis. In Kelley WN, Harris ED Jr, Ruddy S, Sledge CB, eds: Textbook of Rheumatology, 4th ed. Philadelphia, WB Saunders, 1993, pp 874–911.)

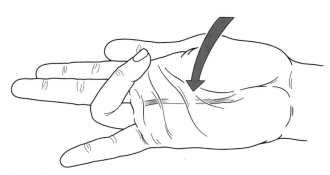

Figure 25–9. The arrow points to a flexor tendon nodule in the hand of a rheumatoid patient that obstructs full extension of the fourth digit, *locking* it in a flexed position. These nodules, even when not blocking motion, can be felt by an examiner's fingers.

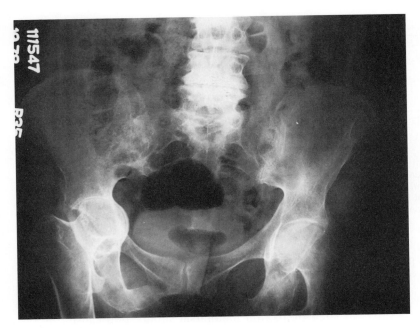

Figure 25–11. Right hip of a 57-year-old rheumatoid patient. This radiograph shows a remodeled, serviceable hip joint that developed largely because, it is posited, she was bearing no weight over the previous 8 years. (From Harris ED Jr: Rheumatoid Arthritis. Philadelphia, WB Saunders, 1997, p 263.)

ovitis. As the metatarsal heads are depressed inferiorly, the proximal interphalangeal joints point superiorly, producing hammertoe deformities that can be extremely painful for the patient wearing standard shoes (Fig. 25–12).

Complications of Extra-Articular Disease

SKELETON

Cytokines generated by rheumatoid synovial tissue have a substantial effect on bone, leading to periarticular osteopenia, which is accentuated by glucocorticoid therapy. Acute leg pain, particularly in elderly patients,

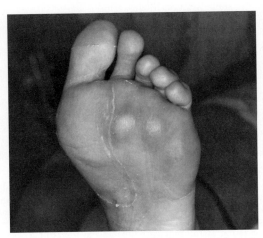

Figure 25–12. In this plantar view of a rheumatoid foot, the shiny, thickened calluses over the depressed and subluxed metatarsal heads of the second, fourth, and (to a lesser extent) fifth metatarsal are apparent. The toes are in a *cock-up* deformity. (Courtesy of James L. McGuire, M.D.; from Harris ED Jr: Rheumatoid Arthritis. Philadelphia, WB Saunders, 1997, p 239.)

can be a sign of a stress fracture; the fibula is the most common site of bone fracture.[6]

MUSCLE

Clinical weakness is caused both by reflex inhibition of muscles around inflamed joints and, in patients with severe active disease, by a mild inflammatory *myositis*. Some of the lymphocytic infiltrates can be shown to be producing RF.

SKIN

Manifestations of hypersensitivity angiitis in RA are unusual, but in some patients with active disease palpable purpura may be found. Rarely, patients with severe active disease have developed *pyoderma gangrenosum*, deep skin ulcers with heaped-up edges.

EYE

Perhaps related to the large amounts of collagen found in eye structures, *scleritis* and *episcleritis* are found in RA, although in fewer than 1% of patients. The development of a rheumatoid nodule in the sclera can lead, rarely, to actual perforation of the globe of the eye, a complication known as *scleromalacia perforans*. At the first sign of a red painful eye in an RA patient, ophthalmologic consultation is essential (Fig. 25–13).

RHEUMATOID NODULES

Although most frequently found in the subcutaneous areas over pressure points in patients with substantial titers of RF, these granulomas can occur in heart, lung, and the central nervous system. On clinical examination, they can be confused with granuloma annulare, xanthomatosis, tophi of gout, and other rare le-

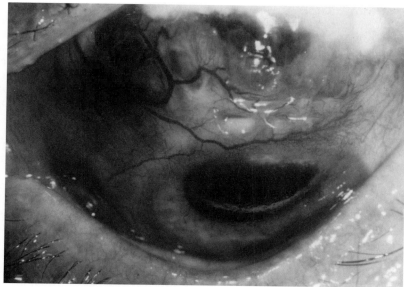

Figure 25–13. Manifestations of increased reactivity of mesenchymal tissue in rheumatoid arthritis appearing within the sclera of the eye. The eye lesion represents scleral perforation associated with a granulomatous scleral reaction. Treatment was placement of a scleral patch graft. Note the increase in vascularity of the sclera. The dark areas represent scleral thinning with exposure of uveal pigment. (Eye patient of Drs. S. Arthur Bouchoff and G. N. Fouhls; photograph courtesy of Marty Schener; from Harris ED Jr: Clinical features of rheumatoid arthritis. In Kelley WN, Harris Ed Jr, Ruddy S, Sledge CB, eds: Textbook of Rheumatology, 4th ed. Philadelphia, WB Saunders, 1993, pp 874–911.)

sions. Patients with both rheumatoid nodules and high titers of RF are more likely to have erosive disease and vasculitis than those without.

ANEMIA

Patients with RA frequently have a mixed anemia. The anemia of chronic disease can be correlated with the ESR and C-reactive protein. This form of anemia is probably generated by cytokines.[7] Many RA patients have blood loss from the gastrointestinal tract related to nonsteroidal anti-inflammatory drug (NSAID) use. Rarely a red cell aplasia develops, generated by drug toxicity or a suppressive cytokine generated by a rogue T-cell clone.

VASCULITIS

There are five principal expressions of vasculitis seen in RA: (1) digital arteritis (ranging from splinter hemorrhages to gangrene), (2) cutaneous ulceration (including pyoderma gangrenosum), (3) peripheral neuropathy, (4) arteritis of viscera, and (5) palpable purpura. Rheumatoid vasculitis is a panarteritis.[8] All of the layers of vessels are infiltrated with mononuclear cells. Immune complex deposits have been found in small vessels in digits as well as in larger vessels in which the pathology resembles polyarteritis nodosa. Vasculitis is unusual; it occurs only in the sickest of patients, representing no more than 5% of RA patients. The neurovascular disease may be the hardest to diagnose, with presenting symptoms ranging from a mild distal sensory neuropathy to mononeuritis multiplex and footdrop.

KIDNEY

Indirect compromise of renal function is the principal way in which kidneys are affected. Some examples are given in Box 25–1.

LUNGS

There are five principal types of pulmonary pathology in RA, listed in descending order of frequency:

- *Pleural disease*: As many as 20% of RA patients have symptomatic or radiographically demonstrable pleural effusions. The pleural fluid is exudative, often with a low glucose concentration, and fewer than 3500 mononuclear cells/mm³.

Box 25–1. RENAL FUNCTION COMPROMISE IN RHEUMATOID ARTHRITIS

Pathology	Cause
Amyloidosis	Long-standing and active rheumatoid arthritis
Renal papillary necrosis	Phenacetin abuse
Acute ischemic renal insufficiency	NSAID use in patients with a low circulating blood volume dependent on prostaglandins to maintain adequate renal perfusion. This is a particular danger in the elderly[9]
Acute interstitial nephritis	NSAIDs. This is a rare occurrence (occurring in <1 : 5000 patients)
Analgesic nephropathy	NSAIDs are the most common drug-induced cause of chronic renal failure, particularly in elderly patients. Cyclosporine also causes a decrease in glomerular function
Membraneous nephritis	D-Penicillamine

- *Airways disease*: Airways disease is defined by a reduced maximal midexpiratory flow rate and may be present in 25% of patients.
- *Interstitial fibrosis*: Before dyspnea develops, radiographs can demonstrate a diffuse reticular (interstitial) or reticulonodular pattern at the bases of both lungs and can progress to a characteristic honeycomb appearance on radiographs. High-resolution CT scans can be useful in early diagnosis.[10] Early in the process, the carbon monoxide diffusion test may be the only abnormality, but this can progress to respiratory insufficiency. Pulmonary function tests, including measurements of diffusion, can be helpful serial measurements.
- *Nodular lung disease*: Nodular lung disease appears in patients with significant titers of RF and can mimic lung cancer or infection. Histologically, these pulmonary nodules are identical to rheumatoid nodules found subcutaneously. They can cavitate and produce bronchopleural fistulas.
- *Bronchiolitis*: Bronchiolitis is a rare process that begins as an interstitial pneumonitis and can progress to bronchiolitis obliterans. Occasionally an arteritis is found on biopsy.

HEART

Pericarditis is found in up to 50% of patients in autopsy series and in up to 30% of patients examined by careful echocardiographic techniques. Tamponade has occurred but is rare. Myocarditis occurs as a granulomatous process or as interstitial myocarditis in rare patients. Direct granulomatous involvement of the conduction system is also rare but when present can cause heart block. Coronary vasculitis has caused myocardial infarction. Rheumatoid nodules can develop on heart valves.[11]

FELTY'S SYNDROME

Felty's syndrome occurs in about 1% of seropositive patients. The principal sign is neutropenia, sometimes severe, occasionally accompanied by anemia or thrombocytopenia. Splenomegaly is usually present. Two thirds of patients with Felty's syndrome are women, and most are older than 50 years. Morbidity and increased mortality are associated with neutrophil counts less than $500/mm^3$ when infections develop. Bone marrow examination shows myeloid hyperplasia, suggesting a maturation arrest. Two thirds of Felty's syndrome patients have positive fluorescent antinuclear antibody tests, elevated serum IgG concentrations, and antineutrophil cytoplasmic antibodies directed against lactoferrin.

The management of Felty's syndrome, in addition to therapy aimed at the disease itself, is based on the need to limit infection. Ninety percent of patients respond for at least a brief period to splenectomy. Lithium salts and granulocyte colony-stimulating factor have been used also.[12] The best therapy is suppressing the active RA.

A subset of RA patients have the *large granular lymphocyte syndrome*. These cells, found in rare patients, are believed to be cytotoxic T cells or natural killer cells. Up to 14% can progress to leukemia (Fig. 25–14). The fact that this syndrome is associated with neutropenia and recurrent infections has led investigators to link the large granular lymphocyte syndrome with Felty's syndrome.[13]

SJÖGREN'S SYNDROME

There are primary and secondary forms of Sjögren's syndrome; only the secondary form is associated with RA. The diagnostic criteria are stringent and require, in addition to the presence of active RA, objective evidence for keratoconjunctivitis sicca and objective evidence for diminished salivary gland flow.

Other findings are often enlarged or tender salivary glands (Fig. 25–15) and hyperglobulinemia. These patients are not as at risk for malignant degeneration at the same high rate as are patients with primary Sjögren's syndrome. This process is best described as an ex-

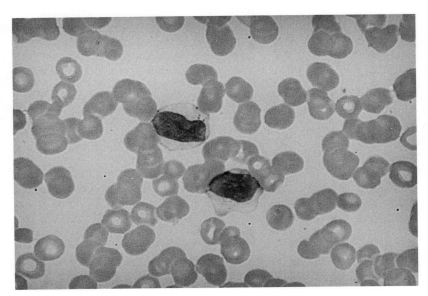

Figure 25–14. Peripheral blood smear with large granular lymphocytes. (From Pinals RS: Felty's syndrome. In Kelley WN, Harris ED Jr, Ruddy S, Sledge CB, eds: Textbook of Rheumatology, 5th ed. Philadelphia, WB Saunders, 1997, p 951.)

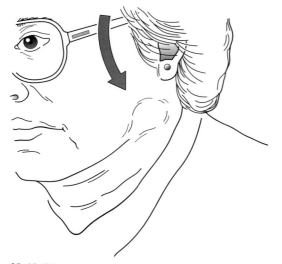

Figure 25–15. Sjögren's syndrome. The arrow points to an often subtle preauricular prominence of the parotid gland of this woman with rheumatoid arthritis who complains of a gritty, sandy feeling in her eyes and a dry mouth ("like I've got cotton in it"). This sicca syndrome can be mild or severe.

ocrinopathy. In addition to dry mouth and eyes, these patients can develop

Tenacious lung secretions, pleurisy, and interstitial fibrosis
Gastrointestinal symptoms (dysphagia and atrophic gastritis)
Dyspareunia from vaginal dryness
Autoimmune thyroiditis (often asymptomatic)
Renal tubular acidosis
Hypergammaglobulinemia, occasionally with cryoglobulinemia or purpura

This secondary form of Sjögren's syndrome rarely has central nervous system manifestations, pseudolymphoma, or lymphomatous degeneration—all of which are complications of primary Sjögren's syndrome. The primary care physician should urge Sjögren's syndrome patients to seek frequent dental care to preserve teeth.[14] Oral pilocarpine is available to increase salivary secretions.

EVALUATION, ASSESSMENT, AND PROGNOSIS OF RHEUMATOID ARTHRITIS

Diagnostic Imaging

A primary care physician should rarely need imaging studies in RA, principally because once the diagnosis is made, the need for imaging specific joints is usually related to complications of the erosive disease (described previously, joint by joint), which are most appropriately managed in concert with rheumatologists and orthopaedic surgeons (see Chapter 4). Once a firm diagnosis of RA has been made, it is wise to obtain two radiographs: one posteroanterior of both hands and wrists on the same film and one standing radiograph of

both feet on the same film. This short series serves as a useful baseline against which to monitor progression of the disease after a year or so or when clinical trials with different medications are started. The sequence of change, as noted in the earlier part of this chapter, is

- *First:* Periarticular osteopenia, secondary to activation of prostaglandin synthesis and release from synovial cells, bone cells, and polymorphonuclear neutrophil leukocytes in synovial fluid.
- *Second:* Narrowing of the apparent joint space, related to superficial destruction of articular cartilage, and erosions of bone at the synovial-bone interface. Larger joints, such as the knee, may be clinically symptomatic, yet have few early radiographic changes.
- *Third:* Subluxation and deformity. These changes are rarely seen before there is evidence for either joint space narrowing or erosion of bone.

Once baseline films are obtained, there is little need for follow-up films at intervals of less than 6 months in active disease and at yearly or more intervals in mild disease. During the first 2 years, the rate of joint destruction is most aggressive. Therefore, it is appropriate that the most aggressive evaluation and therapy occur during this crucial 2-year interval. After 2 years, the interval between images can be dictated by the need for orthopaedic consultations. The exceptions to this are (1) patients with synovial effusions in the knee who have acute calf pain, suggesting that a popliteal cyst has ruptured into muscles below the knee; (2) patients with neck disease who have severe occipital headaches or paresthesias in the arms, suggesting the possibility of atlanto-occipital subluxation (see Chapter 20); and (3) patients taking methotrexate who have fever, cough, or dyspnea, in whom it is important to rule out a pneumonitis related to this drug (see Chapter 9). Even in cases when joint sepsis is suspected, there is no acute indication for radiographs; the joint fluid analysis gives an accurate assessment of the degree of inflammation and existence of bacteria.

Laboratory Assessment

As outlined in Chapter 5, there are relatively few useful laboratory tests for diagnosis, evaluation, assessment, or prognosis in RA. Nevertheless, those available and tested can be helpful in assessing the progress, or lack of it, of individual patients. It is rare for patients who have had positive tests for RF to test negative later for this antibody to gamma globulin. The exception is a small group of individuals who have mild-to-moderate disease originally, then go into a sustained remission from symptoms. Therefore, there is little indication for repeat testing in any patient. Titers rarely change in a rhythm coincident with clinical symptoms and thus are not helpful for serial assessment of disease activity.

The most useful assays of activity in RA are the acute-phase reactants. Although the ESR is an established test, it is an indirect assay and subject to aberrations related to changes in plasma proteins that may have no link to the arthritis. For example, a patient with mild RA and an unrelated nephrotic syndrome has a low serum albumin and a high globulin, a combination that generates a high ESR. A similar change is associated with cirrhosis of the liver. Many clinical laboratories now offer assays of C-reactive protein. The C-reactive protein is produced by liver cells in response to inflammation. It is reproducible, sensitive, and accurate from 0.5 mg/dL (normal levels) through 10 to 15 mg/dL (severe inflammation).[15]

As patients respond to therapy, the following parameters change in addition to acute-phase reactants:

- Hemoglobin rises toward normal, assuming there is not an associated iron deficiency.
- Total WBC falls from elevated levels.
- Eosinophilia and thrombophilia—often present in severe cases of active disease—fall toward normal.

The only other assay that is useful as a marker of inflammation is the WBC in synovial fluid (see Chapters 5, 6 and 18). Counts greater than 25,000 mm^3 are found in active disease and when present are indications for intensifying therapy. The primary care physician should be sensitive to a patient's complaint of one joint becoming acutely and severely symptomatic while others remain about the same as before; a joint tap to rule out bacterial infection is necessary.

Functional Assessment

Self-report questionnaires have been shown to correlate strongly with joint counts, radiographic scores, and laboratory tests. They can be especially useful because they take little professional time and cost virtually nothing. One useful form is a simple functional assessment.[16] It assesses the following eight functions, each prefaced by: "How often is it *painful* for you to . . ."

1. Dress yourself?
2. Get in and out of bed?
3. Lift a cup or glass to your lips?
4. Walk outdoors on flat ground?
5. Wash and dry your entire body?
6. Bend down to pick up clothing from the floor?
7. Turn faucets on or off?
8. Get in and out of a car?

The four choices for each of these are *never*, *sometimes*, *most of the time*, and *always*. The last question is a visual analogue scale with the question, "How much pain have you had in the *past week*?" with zero being *no pain* and 100 being *pain as bad as it can be*.

A 15-minute return visit to the primary care physician of an RA patient should consist of the following:

- Subjective assessment—review of modified health assessment questionnaire (see earlier)
- Questions about possible side effects of medications
- Brief examination of joints for swelling, tenderness, and range of motion
- Other relevant *complaint-directed* physical examination

- Review of medications, functional issues, need for referral, imaging studies

One of the best physician extenders is the well-trained nurse-practitioner or physician's assistant who can become part of a practice, learn the basics of chronic disease management, and be able to spend more time with the patient than the primary care physician can. Someone must be available to discuss the subtle aspects of function (e.g., bladder, bowel, sexual function, life's relationships, job problems—these cannot be neglected simply because of the pressures of managed care).

Prognosis of Patients With Rheumatoid Arthritis

Every patient with chronic disease feels a strong need to know of his or her future. Will I be crippled? How much longer have I to live? These are reasonable questions. The therapy of RA has increased in effectiveness to the point that prognostic guidelines of 10 years ago no longer are relevant. For individual patients, there are some clinical predictors of more severe disease in those with definite RA of recent onset:

- Persistent swelling of the proximal interphalangeal joints
- Flexor tenosynovitis of the hands
- A high C-reactive protein or ESR
- A large number of swollen joints
- High RF titer

Immunogenetic studies, too expensive for routine studies, are used increasingly in clinical trials in attempts to identify subpopulations of RA patients who are at risk for relatively rapid erosive destruction of joints. Patients carrying the *04/04* combination of HLA-DRB1 chains are particularly at risk to require joint surgery, to have rheumatoid nodules, and to have extra-articular organ disease.[2]

Although most rheumatologists are optimistic about the capability of the therapeutic regimens described here to suppress disease and restore patients to good function, there are insufficient data to support this optimism. Particularly disturbing are the mortality rates that indicate an overall mortality ratio of 2.3 for women and 2.1 for men. It is apparent that ". . . it is not merely having rheumatoid arthritis that is bad, but it is the progressive burden of disability, decrepitude, pain, treatment, and treatment side effects, operating over time, that increasingly leads to death in rheumatoid arthritis patients."[17]

THERAPY OF RHEUMATOID ARTHRITIS

The challenge for treating RA is to begin early with therapy likely to down-regulate the disease process, without causing morbidity or death from side effects of treatment. The goal is to alter, by treatment, the slope of the curve of destruction of joints (Fig. 25–16).

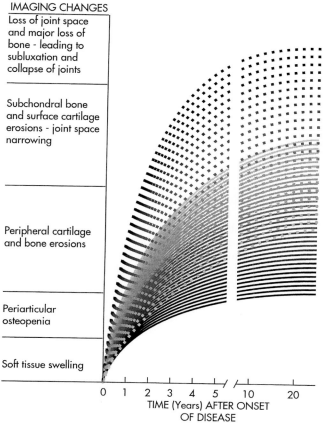

IMAGING CHANGES

Loss of joint space and major loss of bone - leading to subluxation and collapse of joints

Subchondral bone and surface cartilage erosions - joint space narrowing

Peripheral cartilage and bone erosions

Periarticular osteopenia

Soft tissue swelling

TIME (Years) AFTER ONSET OF DISEASE

Figure 25–16. The progression over time of imaging changes of rheumatoid arthritis. This figure emphasizes two major points about rheumatoid arthritis. (1) There is great variation in the degree of joint destruction among patients. Some (*solid black lines*) never develop more than periarticular osteopenia. Others, with sustained and aggressive disease, go on to destruction of cartilage, bone, and tendon (*dotted lines*). Others (*dotted/solid mix*) have erosions without complete joint destruction. (2) The rate of destruction is greater in the first 2 years of disease than in later years. For this reason, it is essential that effective therapy be instituted early in hopes of altering the slope of the curves. Measurable determinants of the rate of progression include the mean erythrocyte sedimentation rate, joint count, Health Assessment Questionnaire results, pain, and a positive rheumatoid factor test. (Modified from Wolfe F, Sharp JT: Long term radiographic outcome of patients seen in the course of rheumatoid arthritis [abstract no. 1056]. Arthritis Rheum 38 [suppl 9], 1995.)

Stage 1

Even before the diagnosis is made in a patient with polyarthritis, therapy can begin. It is appropriate to find a formulation and dosage of anti-inflammatory medication that the patient can tolerate and is effective. The initial choice is between one of the many NSAIDs and various formulations of salicylates (see Chapter 9). Enteric-coated aspirin (e.g., Ecotrin-R) may be, for some patients, easier on the stomach than the classic nonsteroidal compounds. Similarly, nonacetylated salicylates, such as salsalate (Disalcid), have antinflammatory effects but have minimal inhibitory activity on cyclooxygenase. Patients with *Helicobacter pylori* infection determined by the breath test should have this organism eradicated with triple therapy because NSAIDs

and *H. pylori* are independent risk factors for gastro-duodenal mucosal erosive disease. In addition, misoprostol in doses of 100 to 200 μg two to four times daily is often sufficient to alleviate dyspeptic symptoms without causing diarrhea. The use of proton-pump inhibitors and possibly high doses of H$_2$ blockers are an expensive but probably equally effective alternative to misoprostol. Other dangers of NSAIDs are reviewed in Chapter 9.

A frequently asked question is which NSAID should be used? The answer is as many as it takes to find one that the patient tolerates and that provides some symptomatic relief of pain and swelling. As noted in Chapter 9, the dosage schedule is one of the major differences among these, as is the variable effect of the drugs on the gastric mucosa and the kidneys. A drug with a long half-life can be given once daily; the downside of single daily dosage is the lack of flexibility and the likelihood that if side effects develop, they last longer because it takes longer to clear the drug from the tissues and circulation. Cost is an additional factor. Starting with a less expensive NSAID that can be administered on a twice-daily basis is a reasonable approach. The physician should not hesitate to switch from one to the other in maximal doses in search of one that fits the patient and alleviates symptoms. There are convincing data to show that there is a subset of patients (probably < 30%) with RA who have a response to NSAIDs that is more than symptomatic; these individuals manifest decreasing C-reactive protein, granulocyte counts in blood, and IgM RF along with decreased evidence of synovitis.[18]

One selective *cyclooxygenase-2 (COX-2) inhibitor (celecoxib)* is approved for use by the Food and Drug Administration for use in rheumatoid and osteoarthritis, and another (rofecoxib) should soon be approved. The background behind their development was the discovery that although COX-1 is a constitutively active enzyme in gastric mucosa, kidneys, and platelets, COX-2 is found in large quantities only in areas of inflammation and is induced by the cytokines (e.g., IL-1 and TNFα) that are propelling the synovial inflammation. In RA, celecoxib, in doses of 100 or 200 mg twice a day, has been shown to be comparable to naproxen (500 mg twice a day)[19] and to diclofenac SR 75 mg twice a day.[20] Fewer patients taking celecoxib withdrew from studies because of gastrointestinal adverse effects, and the frequency of endoscopic ulcers in patients taking celecoxib in short-term studies was equivalent to that found in patients receiving placebos. At present, the COX-2 inhibitors should be useful for patients at high risk for peptic disease, but their high cost dictates that if patients have efficacy and no significant toxicity from the standard NSAIDs, there is no reason to switch to the more expensive ones.

Along with a baseline of anti-inflammatory therapy, patients must have a foundation of teaching about joint protection. Keeping muscle strength intact without inducing pain is important, as is learning how to use joints in ways that minimize impact loading or stress across the joint. Proper instruction in these efforts can be done most effectively by physical therapists and occupational therapists. During this period, patients can be educated about RA, what is known about its causes, natural history, response to therapy, and prognosis. Emphasis on compliance must be stressed, and—most important—a relationship of trust with the physician must be developed.

Supplemental therapy may include doxycycline (100 mg/day) or minocycline (100 mg twice a day); these tetracycline derivatives have been helpful and are believed to act by inhibition of metalloproteases that are released by synovial cells and have capacity to degrade cartilage, tendon, and bone.[21] Another form of supplemental therapy is local injection of especially involved joints with long-acting glucocorticoids. Triamcinolone hexacetonide is particularly useful in the following doses (see Chapter 6):

Knee, 40 mg
Shoulder, ankle, elbow, 20 mg
Wrist, sternoclavicular joint, proximal interphalangeal joints, and metacarpophalangeal joints (and corresponding joints in the feet, 5 to 10 mg

Joint fluid, before injection, should always be sent for Gram stain, cell count, and culture. An individual joint should not be injected more often than once every 3 to 4 months for fear of inducing damage to articular cartilage. Care must be taken not to inject these glucocorticoids into tendon, joint capsule, or skin to prevent atrophy of these tissues in response to high concentrations of the material.

Stage 2

At stage 2, more than 6 weeks into sustained synovitis, the diagnosis of RA accepted, and a baseline of nonsteroidal therapy installed, it is appropriate that more aggressive treatment be instituted. There are two alternative approaches to this. One is to add the least toxic of second-line therapies and then, if that fails to control the process, add another or replace the first with a second, and so on. The problem with this approach is that the physician and therapy may always be two steps behind the progression of disease and joint destruction. A more sound approach, although one with a higher risk of side effects, is to treat the patient, with early continuous and symptomatic disease, with whatever it takes to down-regulate and suppress the process. As these decisions are being made, consultation with an experienced rheumatologist is appropriate. This consultation reassures the patient that all that is appropriate is being done and helps get the patient involved in the decision-making processes of therapy as he or she weighs potential benefits against toxicities.

A useful therapeutic strategy at this stage is as follows:

- Add hydroxychloroquine, 200 mg twice a day, to the baseline therapy. This drug has less toxicity than most and reasonable efficacy, and the concerns that evolved from use of chloroquine that led to retinal deposits of the drug with visual disturbances have not appeared with hydroxychloroquine.[22]

- Four to 6 weeks later, if a decrease in symptoms and signs (including laboratory parameters) is not apparent, add methotrexate beginning at 7.5 mg each week by mouth, with plans to increase the dose by 2.5 mg every 4 weeks if sustained improvement is not noted up to a dose of 20 mg per week.[23] When doses of up to 30 mg are needed, methotrexate can be given subcutaneously. Folic acid (1 mg/day) is generally given to minimize mucosal toxicity.

Methotrexate is not appropriate for every patient. It is contraindicated in those with liver disease or progressive pulmonary fibrosis or respiratory insufficiency from other causes. It is wise, in every patient, to draw blood for tests to rule out hepatitis A, B, or C infection because the use and then cessation of methotrexate in such individuals may precipitate active aggressive hepatitis. Alternatives to methotrexate in patients in whom this drug is contraindicated at these relatively early stages of RA include the following medications, each of which *except* azathioprine can be given in addition to methotrexate.

- *Auranofin* (3 to 6 mg/day): This oral gold compound has less toxicity than the gold salts (e.g., gold sodium thiomalate) administered by intramuscular injection but is less effective than the latter preparations.

- *Prednisone* (5 to 7.5 mg/day): The glucocorticoids are truly double-edged swords in this disease. They never should be used at this stage except as bridge therapy and the clearly defined objective established of tapering the dose to less than 2 mg/day within several months as other forms of therapy down-regulate the synovitis.[24] Bone-protective agents, including 1500 mg elemental calcium and 400 IU vitamin D each day, should be given at the start of glucocorticoid therapy. Preparations that have long half-lives (e.g., dexamethasone) should be avoided; they produce more side effects at doses that are clinically equally effective. If glucocorticoids must be used in patients with established osteoporosis, inhibitors of resorption, such as the bisphosphonates, should be considered.

- *Sulfasalazine* (1.0 to 3.0 g/day). This drug, better tolerated in the enteric-coated preparation, can be used in place of, or in addition to, hydroxychloroquine and has been proven effective as a component of triple therapy (methotrexate, hydroxychloroquine, and sulfasalazine) in active and resistant disease.[25]

- *Azathioprine* (1.5 to 2.5 mg/kg/day): This purine analogue has more toxicity than methotrexate and should not be used in addition to methotrexate because this combination has been associated with an acute febrile toxic reaction characterized by fever, leukocytosis, and cutaneous leukocytoclastic vasculitis in as many as 8% of patients given the combination. Azathioprine is not effective in doses less than 1.0 mg/kg, and monitoring of granulocyte counts is essential if it is used.

In stage 2 disease, if methotrexate, alone or in combination with hydroxychloroquine and sulfasalazine, has not produced a marked drop in joint swelling and pain, it is appropriate to consider more aggressive therapy. Three additional drugs have been shown to provide added benefit when combined with methotrexate: leflunomide, TNF blockers, and cyclosporine.

Leflunomide is a pyrimidine synthesis inhibitor and has antiproliferative activity. There are no pharmacokinetic interactions between leflunomide and methotrexate, but coadministration might increase the risk of hepatotoxicity. The accepted dosage is 100 mg daily for 3 days and then maintenance with 20 mg daily. Doses higher than 20 mg/day are not recommended. Leflunomide appears to be equivalent in efficacy to methotrexate and can be used either alone or in combination with methotrexate when the latter drug has been only partially effective in achieving the therapeutic goals. As for toxicity, liver function abnormalities and diarrhea have been notable but not excessive; the former must be assayed as would be those of patients on methotrexate.

Etanercept is a genetically engineered fusion protein consisting of two identical chains of the recombinant human TNF receptor p75 monomer fused with the Fc domain of human IgG$_1$. Having a dimer of the receptor ensures better binding of TNFα, and the Fc portion gives a longer half-life in vivo while ensuring clearance of the immune complex by the reticuloendothelial system. Administered subcutaneously (like insulin) at 25 mg twice weekly, etanercept has substantial efficacy. In one study, the addition of etanercept to methotrexate (15–25 mg/week) compared with methotrexate/placebo combination resulted in sustained and rapid improvement.[26] Thirty-nine percent of the patients receiving etanercept plus methotrexate and 3% of those receiving placebo plus methotrexate met the ACR 50% criteria (for a 50% improvement). These data were equaled in another study of etanercept given with only low-dose prednisone (<10 mg/day) and NSAIDs.[27] At 6 months, 40% of the etanercept cohort achieved an ACR 50% response, whereas only 5% of the placebo group did. In this study, the group given 10 mg twice weekly did almost as well as those receiving 25 mg twice weekly. Mild injection-site reactions were the only adverse side effect acutely; in the long term, the possibility of immune reactions against the Fc chains must be monitored. Why should not every rheumatoid patient receive etanercept? One major obstacle is cost. The average wholesale price for 6 months' treatment is about $3600, whereas the cost to the pharmacist for 6 months of an equivalent of therapy with leflunomide is about $1600.

Infliximab is a chimeric human/mouse anti-TNF monoclonal antibody. A single 5 mg/kg infusion of infliximab has a half-life of about 10 days. Monthly injections of 10 mg/kg have led to an improvement in most patients.[28] The need for intravenous infusions has resulted in more side effects, it seems, than does the subcutaneous administration of receptor blockers. Hypersensitivity reactions, including fever, chills, urticaria, dyspnea, and hypotension, have occurred, and human antichimeric antibodies have been produced by recipients of the antibody. The cost of three doses of 3 mg/kg would be approximately $4,000.

Cyclosporine, which inhibits the activation of T-helper/inducer lymphocytes by blocking IL-2 produc-

tion, has been shown to be of use when used alone[29] or in combination with methotrexate.[30] Its use should be supervised by someone who is experienced with administration of the drug, because the toxicities are multiple and include hypertension, renal insufficiency, hyperuricemia, hirsutism, and liver dysfunction. Not permitting the creatinine level to exceed 30% of baseline by lowering the dose is important, and 2.5 mg/kg is the best beginning dose.

It is important to note that there are many other touted and newer therapies for RA. Each must be evaluated for efficacy, toxicity, and costs in double-blind trials. Some have efficacy, but not as much as etanercept, and they cost more; an example of this is Prosorba, the immunoabsorption column. The standard set by etanercept of a high degree of meeting the 50% improvement by ACR criteria must be the one others should match if they are to be used in place of this anti-TNF compound, especially when the dollar cost for many is so high.

Stage 3

At stage 3, the patient has active synovitis despite a base of therapy including NSAIDs; low-dose daily prednisone, plaquenil, sulfasalazine; plus methotrexate (and in some patients, all three). It is best that further interventions be prescribed by rheumatologists, although it is appropriate that patients be managed on a daily basis by the primary care physicians (see Chapter 9). Patients resistant to complex therapy outlined previously should have a complete reevaluation. Do they have insufficient sleep? Is there a component of fibromyalgia superimposed on the RA because of stress in their lives or inadequate sleep? Do they have insufficient rest during the days? Are they truly compliant with medications? Is some of the apparent failure of therapy related to side effects or drug-drug interactions? Often a change in therapy is appropriate as well as a change in lifestyle that includes more rest during each day and reassessment of physical therapy modalities. A revisit to the consulting orthopaedic surgeon may help isolate a particular joint that would benefit from synovectomy or replacement, synovium in a tendon sheath that needs debulking, or painful feet that need more appropriate orthoses.

At this stage of disease, specific complications of the rheumatoid process can produce discomfort. Gritty eyes and a dry mouth may mean development of Sjögren's syndrome, and painful red eyes can herald the onset of scleritis or episcleritis. Occipital headache can indicate symptomatic atlanto-occipital subluxation. Pain and numbness in the thumb and first two fingers of a hand are signs of carpal tunnel syndrome. Hoarseness is a symptom of cricoarytenoid arthritis. Inspiratory chest pain could possibly mean the appearance of symptomatic pleurisy or pericarditis. Skin or pulmonary infections can be associated with leukopenia from Felty's syndrome or drug toxicity. Time spent with a psychologist or social service worker may be beneficial in turning up problems with spousal relationships, sexual inadequacy, depression, or feelings of worthlessness, all problems that can arise in patients with chronic disease.

At this stage, a reassessment of medications is essential. If pain in a joint is related to destruction of bone and cartilage by synovial invasion, escalating therapy is not beneficial, but if symptoms are related to boggy and proliferative synovitis, it is worth considering the benefit-to-cost ratio of new treatment. In patients with severe systemic disease, the benefit of increasing the daily dose of prednisone may be indicated. In some patients, *pulse* therapy of *methylprednisolone* (e.g., 200 mg intravenously on 3 successive days) may produce temporary alleviation of symptoms. FK-506, an immunosuppressive drug with a mechanism of action similar to that of cyclosporine, is being used in severe disease. There is little evidence that total lymphoid irradiation or cyclophosphamide has an acceptable benefit-to-cost ratio. D-*Penicillamine* has efficacy in this disease but is associated with many side effects, including the onset of variable presentations of autoimmune syndromes, membranous glomerulitis, and bone marrow suppression.

LYME DISEASE

The rationale for including Lyme disease with RA is the similarity of the histopathologic samples of synovitis of the two disease, particularly when Lyme disease settles chronically within one joint. Approximately 90,000 cases have been reported to the Centers for Disease Control and Prevention since 1982. During the years of 1992 through 1994, Lyme disease was the ninth most common notifiable infectious disease in the United States, after gonorrhea, primary and secondary syphilis, acquired immunodeficiency syndrome (AIDS), salmonellosis, tuberculosis, hepatitis A, hepatitis B, and shigellosis.[31] Physicians must remember that although sporadic cases have been reported in 47 states, the life cycle (involving a mouse, deer, and tick) has been described in only 19 states. The primary foci are in the coastal states between Massachusetts and Maryland, in the Midwest (Wisconsin and Minnesota), and in northern California and Oregon. The diagnosis should be made only if rigid criteria are met in patients from any other geographic location.

Joint manifestations are only a part of this complex multisystem illness caused by the tick-borne spirochete *Borrelia burgdorferi*. Phase I of Lyme disease begins, in a majority of cases, with an annular skin lesion, *erythema chronicum migrans*, that surrounds a tick bite site with a pink halo, expanding peripherally. Organisms can be detected in the skin lesion. It is accompanied often by nonspecific symptoms of a flu-like illness, including migratory arthralgias that subside within several weeks. Secondary lesions can develop on the skin in other sites that are similar to the primary skin lesion.

Approximately 15% of patients develop neurologic signs several weeks later (phase II); these include facial nerve palsy (that can be bilateral), motor and sensory radiculitis, meningitis, minor encephalopathic signs, or combinations of these plus peripheral neuropathies.

The cerebrospinal fluid contains lymphocytes and an elevated protein. Rarely, a chronic encephalopathy develops. Fewer than 10% of patients have cardiac involvement, beginning at about the same time as the neurologic changes. Conduction abnormalities (first-, second-, and third-degree block) are most common.

As part of phase III of Lyme disease, frank arthritis may develop months after the initial symptoms have subsided. Arthritis can occur in up to 60% of untreated patients and begins approximately 6 months after the appearance of the initial skin lesion.[32] In contrast to RA, the joint disease is usually brief but recurring attacks of monarthritis or oligoarthritis involving large joints, especially the knee, may be troublesome. If untreated, the attacks may recur for longer periods and even become a chronic proliferative invasive synovitis identical to RA in the involved joints. The synovial cells produce the same cytokines and metalloproteases as do rheumatoid cells. The difference is that although the driving force of Lyme disease is the spirochete, the cause of RA has not yet been identified. In addition, chronic and disabling neurologic symptoms (e.g., a subtle encephalopathy or axonal polyneuropathy) can appear during the late stages of the process.

The diagnosis is made most efficiently by first obtaining an enzyme-linked immunosorbent assay and following that with the less sensitive but highly specific Western blot analysis. Fibromyalgia is the most common diagnosis confused with Lyme disease.

Although Lyme disease is endemic in southern Connecticut, Long Island, Cape Cod, and parts of Wisconsin and Michigan, it is sporadic in other parts of the United States. Thus it should be a minor consideration in differential diagnoses in these latter places. In patients who live in endemic areas or have a history of hiking in woods in other areas and present with a large joint monoarthritis or oligoarthritis, enzyme-linked immunosorbent assay antibody test to *B. burgdorferi* should be requested, perhaps on immediate return from trips. If this test is positive, Western blot confirmation is essential because there are numerous false-positive results. Diagnosis can often be a clinical one when the characteristic skin lesion is present. After 4 weeks of active infection, almost all patients have an elevated IgG response to the spirochete.

Treatment of cases diagnosed early[33] consists of doxycycline (100 mg twice a day) for 10 to 30 days or amoxicillin (500 mg four times daily for the same period) and is usually effective. Cefuroxime (500 mg four times daily) is useful in those with penicillin allergies. Parenteral therapy (ceftriaxone 2 g intravenously daily for 30 days) may be indicated in patients with objective neurologic abnormalities. Oral regimens of up to 30 days can be effective in patients with arthritis, but resistant cases should be treated with the intravenous regimen. When the synovitis becomes chronic, it may be resistant to antibiotics and should be treated as would oligoarticular RA; rarely, erosive disease develops, and synovectomy is appropriate therapy.

The primary care physician must emphasize prevention of Lyme disease. Using long trousers tucked into socks, frequent tick checks, and insecticides containing DEET (*N,N*-diethylmetatoluamide) are effective deterrents. There is growing of optimism that a vaccine against Lyme disease may soon be available.[34]

See Appendix to this chapter for algorithms and tables addressing diagnosis and management of several inflammatory disorders and musculoskeletal pain syndromes.

REFERENCES

1. Harris ED Jr: Rheumatoid Arthritis. Philadelphia, WB Saunders, 1997.
2. Weyand CM, McCarthy TG, and Goronzy JJ: Correlation between disease phenotype and genetic heterogeneity in rheumatoid arthritis. J Clin Invest 95:2120, 1995.
3. Szekanecz A, Szegedi G, Koch AE: Cellular adhesion molecules in rheumatoid arthritis: Regulation by cytokines and possible clinical importance. J Invest Med 44:124, 1996.
4. Koch AE, Kunkel SL, Strieter RM: Cytokines in rheumatoid arthritis. J Invest Med 43:28, 1995.
5. Henderson FC, Geddes JF, Crockard HA: Neuropathy of the brainstem and spinal cord in end stage rheumatoid arthritis: Implications for treatment. Ann Rheum Dis 52:629, 1993.
6. Lingg GM, Stoltesz I, Kessler S, et al: Insufficiency and stress fractures of the long bones occurring in patients with rheumatoid arthritis and other inflammatory diseases, with a contribution on the possibilities of computed tomography. Eur J Radiol 26:54, 1997.
7. Davis D, Charles PJ, Potter A, et al: Anaemia of chronic disease in rheumatoid arthritis: In vivo effects of tumour necrosis factor alpha blockade. Br J. Rheumatol 36:950, 1997.
8. Danning CL, Illei, GG, Boumpas DT: Vasculitis associated with primary rheumatologic diseases. Curr Opin Rheumatol 10:58, 1998.
9. Ailabouni W, Eknoyan G: Nonsteroidal anti-inflammatory drugs and acute renal failure in the elderly: A risk-benefit assessment. Drugs Aging 9:341, 1996.
10. Perez T, Remy-Jardin M, Cortet B: Airways involvement in rheumatoid arthritis: Clinical, functional, and HRCT findings. Am J Respir Crit Care Med 157:1658, 1998.
11. Mounet FS, Soula P, Concina, P, et al: A rare case of embolizing cardiac tumor: Rheumatoid nodule of the mitral valve. J Heart Valve Dis 6:77, 1997.
12. Starkebaum G: Use of colony-stimulating factors in the treatment of neutropenia associated with collagen vascular disease. Curr Opin Hematol 4:196, 1997.
13. Starkebaum G, Loughran TP Jr, Gaur LK, et al: Immunogenetic similarities between patients with Felty's syndrome and those with clonal expansions of large granular lymphocytes in rheumatoid arthritis. Arthritis Rheum. 40:624, 1997.
14. Fox PC, Brennan M, Pillemer S, et al: Sjögren's syndrome: A model for dental care in the 21st century. J Am Dent Assoc 129:719, 1998.
15. Kushner I: C-reactive protein in rheumatology. Arthritis Rheum 34:1065, 1991.
16. Callahan LF, Brooks RH, Summey JA, et al: Care of rheumatoid arthritis patients, using a pain scale based on activities of daily living and a visual analog pain scale. Arthritis Rheum 30:630, 1987.
17. Wolfe F, Mitchell DM, Sibley JT, et al: The mortality of rheumatoid arthritis. Arthritis Rheum 37:481, 1994.
18. Cush JJ, Lipsky PE, Postlethwaite AE, et al: Correlation of serologic indicators of inflammation with effectiveness of nonsteroidal antiinflammatory drug therapy in rheumatoid arthritis. Arthritis Rheum 33:19, 1990.
19. Geis GS, Hubbard R, Callison D, et al: Safety and efficacy of celecoxib, a specific COX-2 inhibitor, in patients with rheumatoid arthritis. Arthritis Rheum 41:S364, 1998.
20. Lanza FL, Simon T, Quan H, et al: Selective inhibition of COX-2 with MK-0966 (250 mg qd) is associated with less gastroduodenal damage than aspirin 650 mg qid or ibuprofen 800mg tid. Gastroenterology 112:A194, 1997.
21. Tilley B, Alarcon G, Heyse S, et al: Minocycline in rheumatoid arthritis: A 48-week, double-blind, placebo-controlled trial. Ann Intern Med 122:81, 1995.
22. Morand EF, McCloud PI, Littlejohn GO: Continuation of long term treatment with hydroxychloroquine in systemic lupus erythematosus and rheumatoid arthritis. Ann Rheum Dis 51:1318, 1992.
23. Weinblatt ME, Kaplan H, Germain BF, et al: Methotrexate in rheumatoid arthritis. Arthritis Rheum 37:1492, 1994.
24. Furst DE: Rational disease-modifying anti-rheumatic drug (DMARD) therapy: Is it possible? Br J Rheumatol 35:707, 1996.
25. O'Dell JR, Haire CE, Erikson N, et al: Treatment of rheumatoid arthritis with methotrexate alone, sulfasalazine and hydroxychloroquine, or a combination of all three medications. N Engl J Med 334:1287, 1996.
26. Weinblatt ME, Kremer JM, Bankhurst AD, et al: A trial of etanercept, a recombinant tumor necrosis factor receptor: Fc fusion protein in patients with rheumatoid arthritis receiving methotrexate. N Eng J Med 340:253, 1999.
27. Moreland LW, Schiff MH, Baumgartner SW, et al: Etanercept therapy in rheumatoid arthritis. Ann Intern Med 130:478, 1990.
28. Elliott MTJ, Maini RN, Fellmann M: Randomized double-blind comparison of chimeric monoclonal antibody to tumor necrosis factor alpha (cA2) versus placebo in rheumatoid arthritis. Lancet 344:1105, 1994.
29. Tugwell P, Bombardier C, Gent M, et al: Low-dose cyclosporine versus placebo in patients with rheumatoid arthritis. Lancet 335:1051, 1990.
30. Tugwell P, Pincus T, Yocum D, et al: Combination therapy with cyclosporine and methotrexate in severe rheumatoid arthritis. N Eng J Med 333:137, 1995.
31. Niskar AS, Koo D: Differences in notifiable infectious disease morbidity among adult women—United States, 1992–1994. J Womens Health 7:451, 1998.
32. Sigal LH: Musculoskeletal manifestations of Lyme arthritis. Rheum Dis Clin North Am 24:323, 1998.
33. Rahn DW, Felz MW: Lyme disease update: Current approach to early, disseminated, and late disease. Postgrad Med 103:51, 1998.
34. Marwick C: Guarded endorsement for Lyme disease vaccine. JAMA 279:1937, 1998.

E Algorithm E: Acute Inflammatory Mono/Oligoarthritis

If the condition is acute inflammatory mono/oligoarthritis, the provider should determine whether infection is present, whether crystal-induced arthritis (gout or pseudogout) is present, or whether further investigation is necessary.

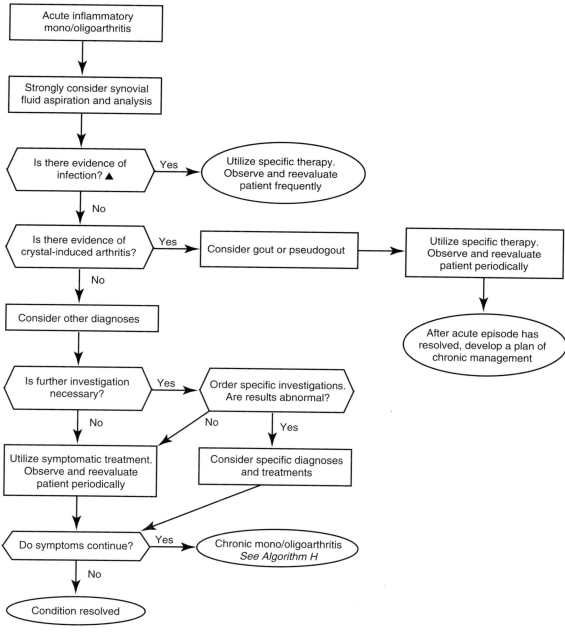

Modified from Lipsky PE: Algorithms for the diagnosis and management of musculoskeletal complaints. Am J Med 103(6A): 56S, 1997.

Recognition and Management of Patients with Specific Rheumatologic Problems

F Algorithm F: Acute Inflammatory Polyarthritis

If the condition is acute inflammatory polyarthritis, the provider should determine whether infection is present or whether further investigation is necessary.

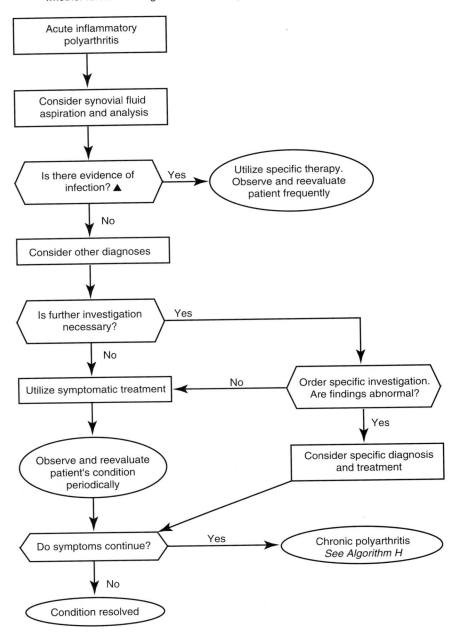

Modified from Lipsky PE: Algorithms for the diagnosis and management of musculoskeletal complaints. Am J Med 103(6A): 57S, 1997.

Algorithm H: Chronic Inflammatory Arthritis

If the condition is chronic and-inflammatory, the provider should determine whether mono/oligoarthritis or polyarthritis is present. If mono/oligoarthritis, the provider should determine whether infection is present or further investigation is necessary. If polyarthritis, the provider should determine whether the condition is a spondyloarthropathy, RA, or if further evaluation is necessary.

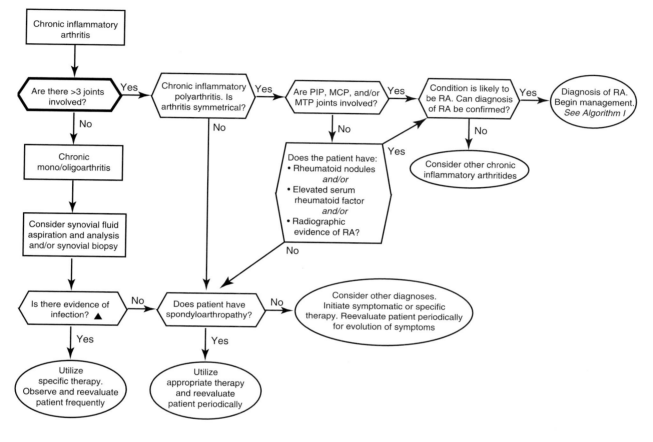

Algorithm I: Management of Rheumatoid Arthritis

The provider should determine whether RA is slowly progressive or aggressive, develop a plan of clinical management, assess outcomes, and modify therapy as needed.

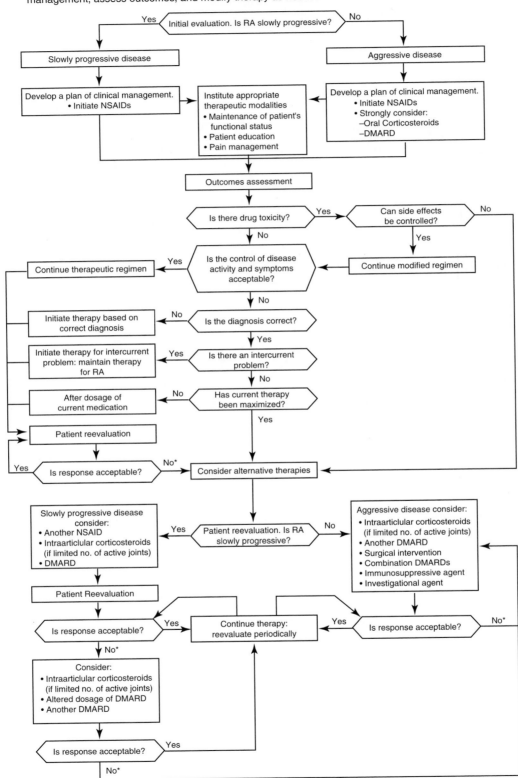

* Unacceptable = continued pain and/or inflammation, progressive disability, progressive joint damage, drug toxicity.

Modified from Lipsky PE: Algorithms for the diagnosis and management of musculoskeletal complaints. Am J Med 103(6A): 60S, 1997.

Table 25A–1. CHRONIC INFLAMMATORY POLYARTHRITIS: DIAGNOSIS

Diagnosis	Joint Manifestations	Extra-articular Manifestations	Laboratory Findings
Rheumatoid Arthritis	• Symmetric polyarthritis involving typical joints	• Rheumatoid nodules, vasculitis, ocular, pulmonary lesions	• Elevated rheumatoid factor level in ≥80% of patients
Spondyloarthropathy	• Asymmetric oligoarthritis • Inflammatory back pain • Sacroiliitis	• Typical skin rash • Ocular involvement • Genitourinary tract inflammation • Bowel inflammation	• Radiographic findings of sacroiliitis • HLA-B27
Psoriatic Arthritis	• Asymmetric oligoarthritis • Erosive peripheral arthritis involving DIP and/or PIP joints • Spondylitis	• Psoriatic skin lesions • Nail changes	• Normal rheurmatoid factor level in 80% of patients
Gout	• Episodic mono/oligoarthritis • Rarely symmetric chronic arthritis	• Tophi	• Intracellular monsodium urate crystals in synovial fluid • Serum urate level elevated at some time in >90% of patients with chronic disease
Pseudogout	• Episodic mono/oligoarthritis	• Associated endocrinopathy	• Calcium pyrophosphate crystals in synovial fluid
Systemic Lupus Erythematosus	• Nondeforming inflammatory arthritis	• Criteria for systemic lupus erythematosus	• Antinuclear antibodies, or autoantibodies • Rheumatoid factor usually not elevated
Other Connective Tissue Diseases	• Intermittent nondeforming inflammatory arthritis	• Classic features of individual disease	• Relevant autoantibodies or laboratory alnormatities

Modified from Lipsky PE: Algorithms for the diagnosis and management of musculoskeletal complaints. Am J Med 103(6A): 73S, 1997.

Table 25A–2. CONFIRMING A DIAGNOSIS OF RHEUMATOID ARTHRITIS

1. RA often begins insidiously with vague constitutional and musculoskeletal symptoms that may last for weeks or months before synovitis becomes apparent.
2. During the first 6 mo of RA, <50% of patients will be RF-positive and the sensitivity of the 1987 ACR criteria is reduced.
3. A variety of less common chronic inflammatory seronegative articular conditions may clinically resemble early RA. It may be necessary to observe and evaluate the patient repeatedly for evolution of the disorder and manifestation of features that will distinguish them from RA. The following disorders can mimic RA:

Diagnosis	Sex	Age	Laboratory Tests	Comments
Undifferentiated seronegative polyarthritis	F > M	35–85	10–15% RF+	Chronic seronegative inflammatory polyarthritis, atypical of RA or fails to meet classification criteria for RA. Up to 20% of cases may evolve into RA and nearly 50% will go into remission.
Psoriatic arthritis	M = F	30–55	<20% RF+	10% of those with psoriatic arthritis will have an RA-like distribution (MCPs, PIPs, wrists) Cutaneous psoriasis will be evident in the vast majority of cases.
Tophaceous gout	M > F	Male 25–70 Female > 45	95% RF− >95% ↑ serum urate	Intermittent inflammatory arthritis during the onset, with evolution of tophi and chronic inflammatory polyarthritis. Elevated serum urate and tophi help distinguish from RA.
Erosive inflammatory OA	F > M	>60	RF− (or normal for age)	Chronic polyarthritis with intermittent or sustained inflammation affecting PIP and DIP joints. Radiographs demonstrate distinctive erosions and evidence of OA.
Pseudogout	F = M	>60	5–10% RF+	5% of patients will have "rheumatoid-like" inflammatory arthritis with stiffness, fatigue, synovitis, and elevated ESR, often lasting 4 wk to several mo.
Reiter's syndrome	M > F	16–50	95% RF− 50–80% HLA-B27+	See criteria for spondyloarthropathies. Often associated with low back pain, ocular, genitourinary, or gastrointestinal (GI) symptomatology and enthesitis (heel pain).
Enteropathic arthritis	M = F	All age groups	95% RF−	20% of patients with Crohn's disease or ulcerative colitis will develop peripheral arthritis. Diagnosis may be difficult until GI involvement becomes apparent. Associated with oral ulcerations, GI symptoms, or other features of spondyloarthropathy.
SLE	F > M	15–40	10–15% RF+ Usually ANA+	Chronic nondeforming inflammatory polyarthritis associated with ANA positively and other features of SLE.
Polymyositis/ dermatomyositis	F > M	30–60	95% RF− 50% ANA+ 70% ↑ CPK	Chronic inflammatory arthritis uncommonly occurs early in course of PM/DM. Features of proximal muscle

Table 25A–2. CONFIRMING A DIAGNOSIS OF RHEUMATOID ARTHRITIS

Diagnosis	Sex	Age	Laboratory Tests	Comments
				weakness, bulbar dysphagia, muscle enzyme elevation or skin involvement (ie, Gottron's papules) should be sought.
Scleroderma	F > M	30–50	95% RF− >90% ANA+	Chronic inflammatory polyarthritis may predominate over skin changes early in the disease. Associated with Raynaud's phenomenon, sclerodactyly, dysphagia, hypertension, or renal abnormalities.
Sarcoid arthritis	F > M	20–40	25% RF+	15% of patients with sarcoidosis will develop arthritis. Early in the disease a chronic inflammatory oligo- or polyarthritis lasting weeks to months may develop and typically involves the ankles and knees. Other features of sarcoidosis (i.e, erythema nodosum, hillar adenopathy) are usually apparent.
Parvovirus B19–associated arthritis	F > M	Any age	<10% RF+ >80% anti-B19 lgM antibodies (acutely)	Adults manifest a flu-like picture, seldom develop the "slapped-cheek" rash and arthralgias are more common than arthritis. Arthritis is an acute inflammatory polyarthritis with an RA-like distribution lasting 2 wk. <10% develop a chronic inflammatory arthritis.
Polymyalgia rheumatica	F > M	>50	90% RF− >95% ↑↑ ESR	Proximal girdle pain and stiffness without synovitis.

Modified from Lipsky PE: Algorithms for the diagnosis and management of musculoskeletal complaints. Am J Med 103(6A): 76S, 1997.

Table 25A–3. THERAPY OF RHEUMATOID ARTHRITIS: MONITORING FOR TOXICITY

Agent	Frequency of follow-up[1] (wk)	CBC	Creatinine	Glucose	LFTs	Urinalysis[2]	Occult GI Blood Loss[3]	Ophthalmologic Exam	Liver Biopsy
NSAIDs	4[4]	✓	✓		✓		✓		
Oral corticosteroids	4–12			✓		✓ (glucose)			
DMARDs Hydroxychloroquine	4–12	[5]						baseline, then 1 yr.	
Sulfasalazine	4–8	✓[5]				✓ (protein)			
Auranofin	4–8	✓				✓ (protein)			
Parenteral gold	1–4	✓							
Methotrexate	4–8	✓	✓[6]		✓	✓ (protein)			✓[7]
D-penicillamine	4–8	✓			✓				
Azathioprine	2–4	✓			✓				
Cyclosporine	2–4	✓	✓						
Cyclophosphamide	2–4	✓	✓[6]			✓ (RBC)			
Leflunomide	4–8	✓			✓				

[1] Determined by consensus.
[2] Urinalysis to determine glycosuria, proteinuria, or hematuria.
[3] Examination of stool for occult blood loss is an insensitive measure of gastrointestinal (GI) bleeding. If GI symptoms persist or anemia develops, further investigation should be considered. Persons at increased risk for NSAID-induced GI ulceration, including the elderly, those with a previous history of peptic ulcer disease or GI blood, those with a serious comorbid disease, and those receiving concomitant therapy with corticosteroids should be considered for prophylaxis with misoprostol.
[4] During the first 6 months, the patient should be evaluated every 4 to 8 weeks. After 6 months, the patient may be seen less frequently (e.g., every 6 months), depending upon age and comorbid conditions.
[5] Consider analysis for glucose-6-phosphate dehydrogenase deficiency.
[6] To adjust dosage.
[7] Indications include persistently abnormal LFTs, and a need after 3 to 4 years on methotrexate to increase doses. Hepatitis C serology should be checked before starting methotrexate.
Modified from Lipsky PE: Algorithms for the diagnosis and management of musculoskeletal complaints. Am J Med 103(6A):79S, 1997.

Chapter 26

Seronegative Spondyloarthropathies

Michael M. Ward

The group of conditions known as the *seronegative spondyloarthropathies* includes ankylosing spondylitis, psoriatic arthritis, reactive arthritis (including the subtype Reiter's syndrome), and arthritis associated with inflammatory bowel disease. These conditions are linked by several common features, including inflammatory low back pain, sacroiliitis, enthesitis (or inflammation at ligamentous and tendinous insertions on bone), and a predilection to occur in people who carry the HLA-B27 marker.[1] Not all of these features are present in every patient with these conditions, and the frequency with which they occur differs somewhat among these conditions (Table 26–1). However, these features overlap to a sufficient degree to allow the grouping of these conditions as the seronegative spondyloarthropathies. The term *seronegative* indicates that serum rheumatoid factor is not present in patients with these conditions. This chapter focuses on inflammatory back pain. A full discussion of noninflammatory causes of back pain (e.g., disc disease, osteoarthritis of spine) is found in Chapters 19 and 32.

CLINICAL FEATURES COMMON TO SERONEGATIVE SPONDYLOARTHROPATHIES

Inflammatory low back pain is a hallmark of the seronegative spondyloarthropathies. It is important to distinguish inflammatory low back pain from mechanical low back pain, a more common problem in both young and older patients. Inflammatory low back pain typically improves with activity or exercise and is not relieved by rest, often forcing the patient out of bed at night. The converse associations usually hold in mechanical low back pain (see Chapter 32). Inflammatory low back pain is also associated with morning stiffness of greater than 30 minutes or with stiffness after periods of inactivity. It usually has a gradual onset and lasts more than 3 months. Mechanical low back pain, particularly in young adults, is often acute in onset and of shorter duration. Both inflammatory and mechanical low back pain can be diffuse and can radiate to the buttocks or posterior thigh, but inflammatory low back pain is not associated with neurologic deficits.

Low back pain in patients with seronegative spondyloarthropathies results from inflammation in the sacroiliac joints and intervertebral joints. The sacroiliac joint has two parts, an inferior part with cartilage and synovial tissue, and a superior ligamentous part. Inflammation occurs in both the synovial and the ligamentous parts. Initially, inflammation in the synovial part of the joint results in erosions of the surrounding bone, but later new bone proliferates and begins to bridge both the synovial and the ligamentous parts, eventually resulting in fusion or ankylosis of the sacroiliac joint. A similar process of inflammation, erosion, bone proliferation, and fusion occurs at the junction between the vertebral bodies and the intervertebral discs and at the vertebral facet joints, leading to spinal fusion and restricted lumbar motion. Over time, higher levels of the vertebral column often become involved.[2]

Enthesitis, or inflammation at sites of ligamentous insertions on bone, occurs not only in the sacroiliac joints and the spine, but also at the Achilles' tendon insertion, the plantar fascial insertion on the calcaneus, the pelvic ligaments, the ischial tuberosity, the greater trochanter of the femur, and the iliac crest, each of which can be a site of pain. Similar changes can be seen at the symphysis pubis and the manubriosternal joint, highlighting the involvement of the axial skeleton in these conditions.

It is not known how HLA-B27 predisposes patients to sacroiliitis and enthesitis, but each of the seronegative spondyloarthropathies is related to this marker. Among whites, 90% or more of patients with ankylosing spondylitis have HLA-B27, as do 75% of patients with reactive arthritis. Among Africans and African-Americans, 50% or fewer patients with these conditions have HLA-B27. In patients with psoriatic arthritis and arthritis associated with inflammatory bowel diseases, HLA-B27 is present in about 50% of patients with the spondylitic subtypes of these conditions but is not increased in patients who have peripheral arthritis only. Patients with a seronegative spondyloarthropathy who do not have HLA-B27 may have an HLA marker closely related to B27, such as B7, B22, or B42. There is little clinical difference between patients who have and do not have HLA-B27, but some evidence suggests that patients who do not have HLA-B27 have the onset of

Table 26–1. COMMON FEATURES OF THE SERONEGATIVE SPONDYLOARTHROPATHIES

	Ankylosing Spondylitis	Arthritis Associated With Inflammatory Bowel Disease	Psoriatic Arthritis	Reactive Arthritis (and Reiter's Syndrome)
Age at onset	Adolescent or young adult	Young adult or middle age	Young adult or middle age	Young adult
Male:female ratio	4:1	1:1	1:1	5:1 (GU) 1:1(GI)
Inflammatory low back pain	100%	10–20%	15%	40–50%
Sacroiliitis	100%	10–20%	40%	10–20%
Symmetry of sacroiliitis	Symmetric	Symmetric	Asymmetric	Asymmetric
Peripheral arthritis	25%	10–20%	80–90%	80–90%
Peripheral enthesitis	Uncommon	Uncommon	Common	Common
HLA-B27[*]	90%	50%	50%	75%

[*] Among whites. Proportions in inflammatory bowel disease and psoriatic arthritis represent only the subgroup with spondylitis.
GU, genitourinary; GI, gastrointestinal.

disease at a later age, are less likely to have affected relatives, and have less severe radiographic changes.

ANKYLOSING SPONDYLITIS

Ankylosing spondylitis is the prototypic seronegative spondyloarthropathy because inflammatory low back pain, sacroiliitis, enthesitis, and HLA-B27 are almost universally present.[3] The prevalence of ankylosing spondylitis among whites is estimated to be about 0.2%. The diagnosis is based on the presence of both clinical and radiographic features (Table 26–2). Onset is usually in late adolescence or young adulthood, and males are affected three to four times more commonly than females. There is often a family history of ankylosing spondylitis.

Clinical Features

The main clinical feature of ankylosing spondylitis is arthritis in the axial skeleton. Typically the onset of in-

Table 26–2. MODIFIED NEW YORK CRITERIA FOR THE DIAGNOSIS OF ANKYLOSING SPONDYLITIS

Clinical criteria
  Low back pain of at least 3 months' duration improved by exercise and not relieved by rest
  Limitation of lumbar spine motion in sagittal and frontal planes
  Limitation in chest expansion relative to normal for age and sex
Radiologic criteria
  Sacroiliitis of grade 2 (minimal), 3 (moderate), or 4 (complete ankylosis)
Definite ankylosing spondylitis is considered present in patients with
  Any clinical criterion and bilateral sacroiliitis of grade 2 or higher
    or
  Any clinical criterion and unilateral sacroiliitis of grade 3 or higher

flammatory low back pain is gradual and can be intermittent but later becomes persistent. Lumbar paravertebral muscle spasm contributes to low back pain, and patients can complain of buttock pain. Stiffness, fatigue, and sleep disturbance are common. Over time, inflammation progresses to involve higher levels of the spine, usually in a continuous fashion so that the entire vertebral column eventually becomes fused. This process proceeds slowly and can take 30 years or more. With involvement of the thoracic spine and the costovertebral joints, the rib cage becomes fixed, chest expansion is limited, and breathing becomes diaphragmatic. Thoracic kyphosis is exaggerated. Cervical spine involvement can lead to neck fusion, limitation in neck extension and rotation, and a stooped posture so severe that the patient cannot see the horizon. Loss of segmental motion in the fused spine and vertebral osteopenia greatly increase the risk of spine fracture with even minor trauma. However, progression is not universal. Occasionally, symptoms and limited motion are restricted to the lumbar spine, even after decades of disease.

Approximately 25% of patients have peripheral joint arthritis in addition to axial arthritis. Although any peripheral joint can be involved, large joints of the lower extremities are most often affected. Rarely, ankylosing spondylitis can present as a peripheral monarthritis or oligoarthritis, with back symptoms and signs developing only later. Pain and inflammation can also occur at the costochondral junctions, manubriosternal joint, sternoclavicular joint, and heels.

Extra-Articular Manifestations

Ankylosing spondylitis can affect organ systems other than the spine and peripheral joints. Acute anterior uveitis, with pain, blurred vision, and photophobia, occurs in 20% to 40% of patients and can precede the onset of back symptoms. It usually is unilateral and tends to respond well to local treatment but can recur. Inflammation in the ascending aorta can lead to dilation of the aortic root and aortic valve insufficiency. Inflammation can extend into the interventricular septum, causing cardiac arrhythmias. These problems are more common late in the disease. Aortic insufficiency can affect up to 10% of patients with durations of ankylosing spondylitis of 30 years or more. Lung fibrosis, typically affecting the upper lobes, can also occur after decades of ankylosing spondylitis. More commonly, patients have restrictive defects in pulmonary function resulting from chest wall immobility. Cauda equina syndrome, with urinary or fecal incontinence, saddle anesthesia, and weakness or pain in the legs, and renal disease resulting from amyloidosis are two other rare complications of ankylosing spondylitis.

Although women are less likely to have ankylosing spondylitis than men, there are few clinical differences between women and men with this condition. Women may experience a longer delay in diagnosis because the diagnosis is less often considered and because radiographic changes in the sacroiliac joints and spine can be less striking in women than in men. Women also more commonly have spondylitis in discontiguous segments of the spine, for example, having neck and lumbar involvement without thoracic involvement.

Physical Examination

The physical examination of patients with inflammatory low back pain from ankylosing spondylitis often reveals loss of the normal lumbar lordosis, and palpation over the sacroiliac joints elicits tenderness. Pain from sacroiliitis can also be detected by putting downward pressure on the pelvis while the patient lies on his or her side. Decreased lumbar mobility is also a feature of ankylosing spondylitis. Forward flexion, lateral flexion, and rotation of the lumbar spine are reduced. The Schober test (Box 26–1) is commonly used to quantify the limitation of lumbar forward flexion. This test measures the increase in length with full forward flexion of a 10-cm segment marked on the patient's low back (with its inferior border at the level of the posterior-superior iliac spines). Normally, this length should increase by 5 cm or more with flexion, and patients with ankylosing spondylitis typically have an increase of less than 5 cm. Limitation in chest expansion can be assessed by the difference in chest circumference between full inspiration and full expiration, measured at the nipple line. Normal chest expansion is greater than 5 cm. The degree of thoracic kyphosis and flexion deformity of the neck can be quantified by measuring the distance from the patient's occiput to the wall as the patient

stands against a wall. Serial monitoring of these measurements can provide an indication of the progression of ankylosing spondylitis and a patient's response to treatment.

Radiographic and Laboratory Features

The radiographic features of early ankylosing spondylitis include erosions at the sacroiliac joints, with surrounding reactive sclerosis of bone (Fig. 26–1; also see Chapter 4). Sacroiliitis is bilateral and symmetric in ankylosing spondylitis, points that help differentiate it from other seronegative spondyloarthropathies. In the spine, sclerosis can also be present at the junction of the vertebral body and intervertebral disc, which on lateral views gives the *shiny corner* sign. It is important to recognize that sacroiliitis and lumbar spondylitis may not be evident on radiographs obtained early in the course of disease. Typical radiographic changes may sometimes not be evident even after 5 or more years of symptoms. If radiographs are normal, bone scanning or computed tomography or magnetic resonance imaging of the sacroiliac joints can be helpful in establishing the diagnosis early in the course of disease.

As the disease progresses, fusion of the sacroiliac joints occurs so that the joint space is no longer detectable. The ligaments of the annulus fibrosis surrounding the intervertebral discs ossify and appear as dense lines of calcification extending from the edges of the vertebral bodies eventually bridging the disc space (Fig. 26–2). These calcifications, known as *syndesmophytes*, encircle the disc space. The classic radiographic appearance of the *bamboo spine* occurs when the entire spine is joined by these syndesmophytes.

There are no laboratory markers unique to anky-

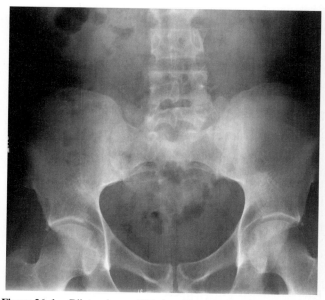

Figure 26–1. Bilateral sacroiliitis in a 29-year-old man with a 9-year history of ankylosing spondylitis. The margins of both sacroiliac joints are irregular and blurred because of bone erosions. The bone adjacent to the erosions is also sclerotic.

Box 26–1. PHYSICAL MEASUREMENTS TO ASSESS ANKYLOSING SPONDYLITIS

Schober test
Chest circumference, inspiration and expiration
Distance of occiput to wall

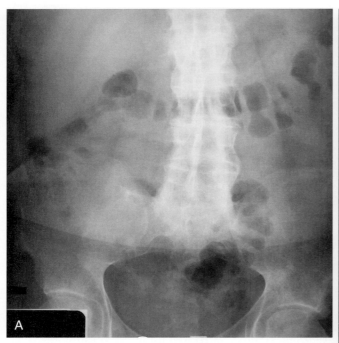

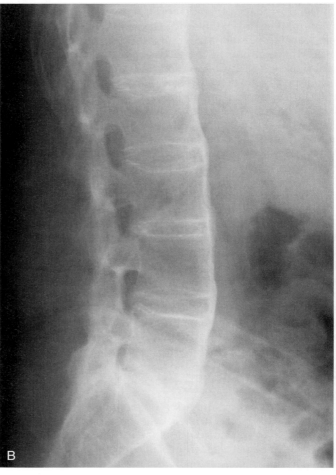

Figure 26–2. Ankylosis of the sacroiliac joints and lumbar spine in a 37-year-old man with a 19-year history of ankylosing spondylitis. *A,* The sacroiliac joints are completely fused by bone bridging and are no longer visible. Thin, vertically oriented syndesmophytes also bridge the intervertebral disc spaces, best seen on the lateral view (*B*), and lead to fusion of the spine.

losing spondylitis. Acute-phase reactants, such as the erythrocyte sedimentation rate, can be elevated. Synovial fluid from peripheral joints typically shows inflammatory changes, but white blood cell counts in these fluids are rarely higher than 50,000/mm^3. Although 90% of patients with ankylosing spondylitis have HLA-B27, testing for this marker *should not* be routinely performed. HLA-B27 is a common marker, present in about 10% of whites. Because only 0.2% of the population has ankylosing spondylitis, the vast majority of people who have HLA-B27 do not have ankylosing spondylitis, and HLA-B27 is much more often a false-positive test for ankylosing spondylitis than a true-positive test. The proportion of patients with HLA-B27 who have ankylosing spondylitis (the positive predictive value of the test) is less than 1%. The only patients in whom determination of HLA-B27 is indicated are those with atypical back pain or spine/sacroiliac radiographs with features both for and against ankylosing spondylitis in whom a positive or negative B27 test could justify tipping the balance for aggressive therapy.

Differential Diagnosis

Ankylosing spondylitis can be distinguished from other seronegative spondyloarthropathies by the pre-

dominance of spinal arthritis over peripheral arthritis and by the absence of psoriasis, inflammatory bowel disease, or a history of infectious enteritis or urethritis. A patient with a family history of ankylosing spondylitis is much more likely to have ankylosing spondylitis than another type of spondyloarthropathy. Radiographically, ankylosing spondylitis can be differentiated from psoriatic arthritis and reactive arthritis by the presence of bilateral sacroiliitis and by thin, vertically oriented syndesmophytes in the spine, as opposed to unilateral sacroiliitis and bulky syndesmophytes characteristic of the latter two conditions. Sacroiliac joints can become infected, but this is almost always unilateral. Young patients presenting with inflammatory arthritis in one or a few peripheral joints should be questioned about low back pain because ankylosing spondylitis can rarely present in this way and must be differentiated from infectious arthritis, crystal-induced arthritis, and rheumatoid arthritis. Arthrocentesis and testing for serum rheumatoid factor can help in these settings. Older patients with diffuse idiopathic skeletal hyperostosis have radiographic changes that can be confused with ankylosing spondylitis. In diffuse idiopathic skeletal hyperostosis (DISH), calcification occurs in the anterior longitudinal ligament of the thoracic and cervical spine, particularly on the right side, and a lucent space between this ligament and the anterior surface of the vertebral bodies distinguishes this condition from the syndesmophytes of ankylosing spondylitis (see Fig. 4–5). Patients with DISH can also have spinal pain and restricted motion, but this condition is noninflammatory, begins in late middle age, and is not associated with sacroiliitis. If there is uncertainty about the correct diagnosis, the patient should be referred to a rheumatologist.

Course and Outcomes

The course of ankylosing spondylitis varies from a mild self-limited disease to a progressive debilitating chronic condition.[4] Many patients experience intermittent flares, with increased pain and stiffness, even after decades. It is important to recognize that the maxim that pain remits in spinal regions that have fused and that pain disappears when spinal fusion is complete does not hold for many patients. Most studies of the quality of life of patients with ankylosing spondylitis find that functional ability is often well preserved. Most functional difficulties arise late in the course from restriction in neck motion. Driving can be particularly difficult for such patients. More than 80% of patients remain employed after 20 years of disease. Those working in physically demanding jobs are at greater risk of work disability than those in less physically demanding jobs. Premature mortality can result from complications of spinal fractures, aortic insufficiency, respiratory failure, or treatment-related side effects.

Treatment

Effective treatment of patients with ankylosing spondylitis relies heavily on exercise to maintain upright posture and spinal flexibility.[5] Patients must be educated in back stretching and strengthening exercises, preferably by a physical therapist skilled in working with patients with spondyloarthropathies. Patients should be repeatedly encouraged to do these exercises daily. Attention to posture is also important, and patients should avoid activities that promote a kyphotic posture. Recreational physical activity should also be encouraged. Water exercises and swimming have traditionally been recommended, but any recreational activity is likely to be beneficial. Smoking cessation is essential to prevent further compromise of pulmonary function.

Pharmacologic treatments include nonsteroidal anti-inflammatory drugs (NSAIDs), analgesics, glucocorticoids, and second-line medications. NSAIDs are useful to reduce pain and stiffness and thereby permit increased activity. A dose before bedtime can be particularly helpful in reducing pain during the night, allowing uninterrupted sleep and decreasing morning stiffness. Any NSAID can be used, but the maximal dose should be tried for at least 2 weeks before switching to another medication. Once a clinical response is achieved, the dose may be lowered to the minimal effective dose. Many patients receive the most benefit

from indomethacin (150 to 200 mg/day). However, indomethacin is one of the more toxic NSAIDs, with a substantial risk of gastrointestinal bleeding and of renal insufficiency in patients with conditions that result in decreased effective circulatory volume. Indomethacin can also cause headache and, in elderly patients, confusion.

Patients who do not respond to these treatments may benefit from referral to a rheumatologist to explore other treatment options. Phenylbutazone is a potent NSAID that can be effective in ankylosing spondylitis. Because it can cause bone marrow aplasia and requires special monitoring, phenylbutazone should not be prescribed by physicians unfamiliar with this medication. Local glucocorticoid injections into inflamed peripheral joints can be helpful, but systemic glucocorticoids have no role in the treatment of sacroiliitis. Of the second-line medications, sulfasalazine has been demonstrated to alleviate peripheral arthritis in patients with ankylosing spondylitis, but the spinal arthritis does not appear to improve. Methotrexate has been used in rare patients with severe unremitting arthritis, with some reported benefit. No pharmacologic treatment has been demonstrated to induce remission or halt or slow the progression of spinal fusion.

Total hip arthroplasty is effective treatment for patients with severe hip arthritis. Surgery to correct severe kyphotic deformities of the spine is only rarely performed and carries a substantial risk of paraplegia and death.

ARTHRITIS ASSOCIATED WITH INFLAMMATORY BOWEL DISEASES

Spondylitis and inflammation of peripheral joints develops in some patients with Crohn's disease and ulcerative colitis.

Clinical Features

Ten percent to 20% of patients with inflammatory bowel disease have sacroiliitis and spondylitis that is clinically and radiographically indistinguishable from ankylosing spondylitis. These patients have inflammatory low back pain, sacroiliitis, and limitation in spinal flexibility resulting from progressive spinal fusion. The spondylitis can precede the gastrointestinal symptoms by years, particularly in patients with ulcerative colitis, and patients often retain diagnoses of both ankylosing spondylitis and inflammatory bowel disease. The symptoms and progression of the spondylitis are unrelated to the activity of gastrointestinal disease. In contrast to idiopathic ankylosing spondylitis, men and women are equally affected by the spondylitis associated with inflammatory bowel diseases.

Peripheral arthritis occurs in 10% of patients with ulcerative colitis and in up to 20% of patients with Crohn's disease. Typically, one or a few joints become inflamed for several weeks or months before resolving. The knee, ankle, and elbow are most frequently affected. Recurrences are common and often coincide with flares of gastrointestinal disease. Peripheral arthritis develops most often after the gastrointestinal disease has been present for some time and is more likely to develop in patients with other extraintestinal manifestations of inflammatory bowel disease, such as erythema nodosum, uveitis, and pyoderma gangrenosum. Rarely, persistent inflammation in peripheral joints can lead to bone erosion and joint destruction. Enthesopathy, including plantar fasciitis and Achilles' tendinitis, also commonly occurs.

Laboratory Features

Laboratory findings are similar to those of patients with idiopathic ankylosing spondylitis. HLA-B27 is present in approximately 50% of patients with spondylitis associated with inflammatory bowel diseases, but the prevalence of this marker is not increased among those with peripheral arthritis only. Testing for HLA-B27 is of little diagnostic or predictive value because sacroiliitis and spondylitis are often present by the time gastrointestinal symptoms occur.

Treatment

The approach to treatment is generally similar to that of ankylosing spondylitis. NSAIDs can occasionally worsen colitis, and their use can cause diagnostic confusion if gastrointestinal bleeding occurs. Some gastroenterologists recommend that patients not take NSAIDs when bowel disease is active. Peripheral arthritis can improve when systemic glucocorticoids, sulfasalazine, azathioprine, 6-mercaptopurine, or methotrexate is used to treat gastrointestinal disease. Sulfasalazine can improve symptoms in early spondylitis, but second-line medications are not known to slow the progression of spondylitis in these patients. Peripheral arthritis in patients with ulcerative colitis remits after colectomy.

PSORIATIC ARTHRITIS

Five percent to 10% of patients with psoriasis develop an associated inflammatory arthritis or spondylitis.[6] In contrast to the other seronegative spondyloarthropathies, psoriatic arthritis more commonly involves the peripheral joints than the axial skeleton.

Clinical Features

Five patterns of joint involvement have been described in psoriatic arthritis: (1) an asymmetric oligoarthritis involving small joints of the hands or feet or large joints of the legs (50% of cases), (2) arthritis of the distal interphalangeal joints of the hands (5% to 10%), (3) arthritis mutilans with marked bony destruction and resorption of phalanges (5%), (4) symmetric polyarthritis mimicking rheumatoid arthritis (25%),

and (5) a spondylitic form without much peripheral arthritis (15%). Radiographic sacroiliitis and spondylitis can be found in patients with any subtype and can affect up to 40% of patients with psoriatic arthritis, but in many of these patients it is asymptomatic or only minimally symptomatic.

Peripheral arthritis usually develops gradually and can persist for months or years. Men and women are equally affected. Involved joints are swollen by either synovitis or effusions, are tender, and can be warm or erythematous. Morning stiffness is common. Occasionally, inflammation of the tendon sheaths of a finger or toe causes diffuse swelling of the entire digit, resulting in a so-called sausage digit that is typical of psoriatic arthritis. Patients with the spondylitic subtype have inflammatory low back pain, stiffness after inactivity, and limitations in spinal flexibility. In contrast to ankylosing spondylitis, patients with psoriatic spondylitis more commonly have involvement of discontiguous segments of the spine rather than inflammation that ascends progressively up the spine over time. For example, they can have sacroiliitis and cervical spine disease or only limited involvement of a few vertebrae in the lumbar or thoracic spine. Symptoms of pain and stiffness localize to the site of spinal involvement.

Relationship Between Skin and Joint Features

Psoriatic arthritis usually begins several years after the onset of psoriasis. In up to 15% of patients, the arthritis can precede the skin disease. In these cases, patients are often diagnosed as having an inflammatory arthritis (possibly even seronegative rheumatoid arthritis), only to have the diagnosis of psoriatic arthritis arrived at retrospectively when psoriatic skin lesions develop. There is little concordance between the severity of the skin disease and the presence or severity of the arthritis. Patients with arthritis can have only a small patch of psoriasis and may be unaware of its presence if it is located in the scalp, behind the ear, or around the anus. A careful skin examination with inspection of the scalp, intergluteal folds, perianal area, and umbilicus can reveal a patch of psoriasis and lead to the correct diagnosis in a patient with an unclassified inflammatory polyarthritis or oligoarthritis. There is no temporal relationship between flares of psoriasis and flares of arthritis in patients with psoriatic arthritis. Psoriatic nail changes such as onycholysis and pitting are more frequent in patients with arthritis than in those without arthritis and are most common in patients with the subtype of distal interphalangeal joint arthritis.

Radiographic and Laboratory Features

Radiographs of peripheral joints affected by psoriatic arthritis commonly show both bone erosions and bone proliferation in the same joint. The bone erosions typically start at the margins of the joint and progress inward, resulting in a whittled appearance. Proliferation of new bone adjacent to the erosion is distinctive for psoriatic arthritis. Bone erosion can progress to near-complete resorption of the bone. This resorption most commonly occurs in the digits, and the subsequent subluxations result in the mutilans appearance. Resorption of the tufts of the distal phalanges is also characteristic of psoriatic arthritis. Erosions and bone proliferation can also occur at entheses. Calcifications extending from the greater trochanters, iliac crests, ischial tuberosities, and calcaneus are common.

Sacroiliitis in patients with psoriatic arthritis differs from that of patients with ankylosing spondylitis in that it is more often unilateral. When bilateral changes are present, both sacroiliac joints are often not involved to the same extent or may be in different stages. Over time, complete fusion of the sacroiliac joints can occur. In addition to having skip lesions, spine involvement is usually marked by large, bulky syndesmophytes that bridge the intervertebral disc space on one side, rather than the thin vertical circumferential syndesmophytes seen in ankylosing spondylitis. Complete fusion of the spine is rare in psoriatic spondylitis.

There are no specific laboratory markers of psoriatic arthritis. Measurement of acute-phase reactants reflects systemic inflammation. HLA-B27 is present in about 50% of patients with spondylitis (even among those with asymptomatic spondylitis), but the prevalence of HLA-B27 is not increased in patients with peripheral arthritis alone. Testing for HLA-B27 is not indicated.

Differential Diagnosis

The differential diagnosis of psoriatic arthritis includes all other causes of seronegative inflammatory arthritis. Because skin lesions are necessary to establish the diagnosis of psoriatic arthritis, it is not possible to make the diagnosis in the subset of patients in whom the arthritis develops before the skin lesions. Although most patients with psoriatic arthritis do not have serum rheumatoid factor, a small percentage of them are seropositive (as is a small percentage of healthy individuals). This seropositivity can lead to some diagnostic confusion, particularly in patients who have the polyarthritis subtype of psoriatic arthritis. Helpful clues to the diagnosis of psoriatic arthritis in these patients include the presence of sacroiliitis or spondylitis (which can be asymptomatic), radiographs without osteopenia and with bony proliferation, and the absence of extra-articular features of rheumatoid arthritis (e.g., lung disease, subcutaneous nodules). Consultation with a rheumatologist can help establish the correct diagnosis. Patients with psoriasis often have hyperuricemia, and acute episodes of arthritis can be acute gouty arthritis rather than a flare of psoriatic arthritis.

Course and Outcomes

For many patients with psoriatic arthritis, particularly those with oligoarthritis or primarily spondylitis,

long-term outcomes are good, with usually mild functional disability and little risk of work disability. Patients with polyarthritis and persistent joint inflammation have outcomes comparable to those of patients with persistent rheumatoid arthritis. These patients can develop substantial joint deformity and functional disability and are at risk for loss of employment.

Treatment

The treatment of psoriatic arthritis is tailored to the extent and severity of joint involvement. Patients with intermittent oligoarthritis can respond well to NSAIDs and analgesics. If one or two joints are persistently inflamed, intra-articular glucocorticoid injections can help. Patients with the spondylitic subtype are treated similar to patients with ankylosing spondylitis, with reliance on therapeutic exercises for spinal flexibility, NSAIDs, and analgesics. Most patients with polyarthritis are treated similarly to patients with rheumatoid arthritis, with usually a combination of NSAIDs and second-line medications.

Methotrexate is often the preferred second-line medication because it can improve skin lesions as well as the arthritis. Doses of methotrexate needed to control joint inflammation in psoriatic arthritis tend to be higher than those usually effective in rheumatoid arthritis. Doses greater than 25 mg/week can be given subcutaneously or intramuscularly to avoid excessive gastrointestinal side effects. Supplemental folic acid (1 mg/day) protects against some mucocutaneous side effects of methotrexate. Patients with psoriatic arthritis are also more highly predisposed to methotrexate-induced liver damage than patients with rheumatoid arthritis, and close monitoring is required. Periodic liver biopsies to identify hepatic fibrosis are recommended by some dermatologists and rheumatologists. Other second-line medications have been used to treat psoriatic arthritis, with little evidence demonstrating one to be superior. Some dermatologists recommend not using hydroxychloroquine because it can cause an exfoliative skin reaction. Systemic glucocorticoids should also be used with caution because they can cause erythroderma or a flare of skin disease when discontinued or tapered.

As in rheumatoid arthritis, aggressive anti-inflammatory and immunosuppressive treatment is being used for patients with early psoriatic polyarthritis or ongoing oligoarthritis in the belief that suppression of inflammation reduces joint damage and preserves long-term functioning. Aggressive anti-inflammatory treatment is not indicated for patients with late-stage mutilans arthritis. Patients with inadequate clinical responses to NSAID treatment and rehabilitative measures should be referred to a rheumatologist for consideration of treatment with second-line medications.

REACTIVE ARTHRITIS

Reactive arthritis is an inflammatory arthritis that occurs in genetically susceptible individuals in response to a genitourinary or gastrointestinal infection.[7] The most common genitourinary infections associated with reactive arthritis are urethritis, prostatitis, and cervicitis resulting from *Chlamydia trachomatis*. The most common gastrointestinal infections associated with reactive arthritis are gastroenteritis and colitis resulting from *Salmonella, Shigella, Yersinia,* or *Campylobacter*. Reactive arthritis can occur after epidemic outbreaks of gastroenteritis or after sporadic cases. Reactive arthritis associated with gastrointestinal infections can affect persons of any age, and affects men and women equally. In the United States, most cases of reactive arthritis are due to sexually transmitted infections with *C. trachomatis*. Reactive arthritis associated with genitourinary infections occurs primarily in young adults, and men are affected about five times more often than women. Reactive arthritis may be underdiagnosed in women because cervicitis is commonly asymptomatic and may not be detected. Although the history and physical examination usually provide clues to the possible inciting infection, an infectious trigger is not identified in 25% of patients.

Clinical Features

Inflammatory arthritis usually develops within 3 weeks of the inciting infection. The most commonly involved joints are the knees, ankles, and feet, although any joint can be affected. An asymmetric oligoarthritis is typical. Joints usually demonstrate moderate swelling, warmth, and tenderness. Patients can occasionally develop a sausage digit, as occurs in psoriatic arthritis. Patients with reactive arthritis also often have enthesitis, most commonly at the Achilles' tendon insertion and plantar fascial insertion at the heel (Fig. 26–3; also

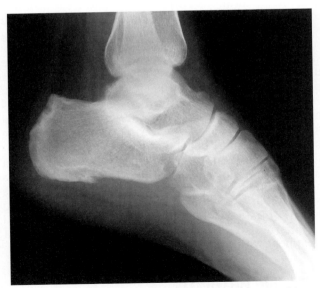

Figure 26–3. Enthesitis at the Achilles tendon insertion in a 34-year-old man with reactive arthritis. Irregular scalloped erosions are present at the superior-posterior aspect of the calcaneus. The plantar spur may also represent a site of enthesitis.

see Fig. 4–6). Other sites of enthesitis include the base of the fifth metatarsal, ligamentous attachments about the pelvis, and the lateral rib cage.

Inflammatory low back pain is common, but its absence does not decrease the likelihood that reactive arthritis is the diagnosis. Radiographs of the sacroiliac joints are normal in the early stages. However, sacroiliitis may be detected on bone scan. Although the back pain is diffuse, the sacroiliitis in reactive arthritis is usually unilateral.

Patients with reactive arthritis can have several characteristic extra-articular manifestations. These occur similarly after genitourinary and gastrointestinal infections. Keratoderma blenorrhagica is a hyperkeratotic skin lesion, identical to pustular psoriasis, that develops in up to 25% of patients. Although it can be present anywhere on the body, it is most often seen on the plantar surfaces of the feet. Circinate balanitis is a painless ulcerative lesion of the glans penis that develops in 10% to 15% of men with reactive arthritis. Urethritis, with dysuria and a mucoid penile discharge and occasionally moderate-to-severe hematuria, can be present in cases in which gastrointestinal or genitourinary infection was the precipitant. Conjunctivitis occurs in 30% to 40% and acute anterior uveitis in 5% to 10%. The triad of arthritis, urethritis, and conjunctivitis constitutes Reiter's syndrome. Because all three manifestations are required for this diagnosis, most patients with reactive arthritis do not have Reiter's syndrome. The frequency of Reiter's syndrome does not vary with the type of inciting infection.

Radiographic and Laboratory Features

Radiographs of peripheral joints in acute reactive arthritis usually demonstrate only soft tissue swelling or joint effusions. In more long-standing disease, radiographic changes similar to those seen in psoriatic arthritis occur, but extensive bone erosion and resorption is not seen. The radiographic appearance of the sacroiliitis and spondylitis of reactive arthritis is indistinguishable from that of psoriatic arthritis.

Although reactive arthritis was once considered a sterile immune-mediated arthritis, investigations have detected bacterial antigens of *Chlamydia, Salmonella,* and *Yersinia* in synovial fluid as well as ribosomal RNA of *Chlamydia* in synovial tissue. Infectious organisms have not yet been cultured from the joints of patients with reactive arthritis, but the presence of chlamydial RNA in synovial tissue suggests that this condition may be a true infectious arthritis. In the laboratory evaluation of patients with suspected reactive arthritis, urethral or cervical swabs should be obtained for testing with a chlamydial DNA probe. This test has excellent sensitivity and specificity. Stool culture for enteric pathogens can identify the triggering infection in cases following a diarrheal illness. Tests of acute-phase reactants generally demonstrate mild-to-moderate systemic inflammation as does synovial fluid analysis. HLA-B27 is present in 75% of patients, even in those without spinal arthritis, and imparts genetic susceptibility to this condition. Testing for HLA-B27 can be useful in the diagnosis of a seronegative inflammatory oligoarthritis or polyarthritis in cases in which the more specific features of enthesitis, low back pain, sacroiliitis, or skin lesions are absent.

Course and Outcomes

Reactive arthritis typically follows one of three courses. A minority of patients ($\leq 10\%$) have a single bout of arthritis and associated illness that lasts several weeks or a few months before resolving. Between 15% and 50% have recurrent episodes of arthritis separated by asymptomatic periods. Episodes can persist for several years but tend to diminish in frequency and intensity over time. Twenty percent to 50% of patients develop a chronic persistent arthritis affecting the peripheral joints or the spine (or both). Factors that determine the course a particular patient will follow have been poorly defined. Patients with HLA-B27 are more likely to have persistent spinal arthritis. Aortitis with aortic valve insufficiency and cardiac conduction disturbances, similar to that which occurs in ankylosing spondylitis, can develop in patients with long-standing reactive arthritis.

Treatment

The treatment of the musculoskeletal manifestations of reactive arthritis follows closely that of the treatment of psoriatic arthritis. In addition, reactive arthritis resulting from *Chlamydia* improves more rapidly in patients treated soon after the onset of symptoms with a 3-month course of tetracycline-based antibiotics. Antibiotic treatment has thus far not been demonstrated to improve the course or outcome of patients with reactive arthritis after gastrointestinal illness or of patients with long-standing arthritis.

UNDIFFERENTIATED SPONDYLOARTHROPATHY

Occasionally a patient presents with certain features of the seronegative spondyloarthropathies, such as with Achilles tendinitis and uveitis, or with inflammatory low back pain and ankle arthritis but not with features that would allow categorization as one of the four above-mentioned conditions.[8] These patients are often diagnosed as having an undifferentiated spondyloarthropathy. This situation arises commonly early in the disease process. Patients can also have a *forme fruste* of one of the more typical spondyloarthropathies or an overlap of the features of two or more spondyloarthropathies. Most patients have inflammatory low back pain and peripheral arthritis, usually monarthritis or oligoarthritis of large joints of the legs. Fifty percent have enthesitis, and 30% have uveitis or sacroiliitis. Over time, approximately 60% evolve to ankylosing

spondylitis, 20% evolve to other conditions, and 20% remain undifferentiated for 10 or more years. Treatment is directed by the clinical manifestations present. For patients with inflammatory low back pain or sacroiliitis, the treatment follows that outlined for ankylosing spondylitis. Peripheral arthritis or enthesitis is treated as outlined for reactive arthritis.

SPONDYLOARTHROPATHY IN CHILDREN

Spondyloarthropathy is one form of juvenile chronic arthritis. Older children and young adolescents are usually affected, and boys far outnumber girls. The joint manifestations usually begin as an oligoarthritis, often of the large joints of the legs, or as an enthesitis. Inflammatory low back and spinal arthritis often develop after 2 or 3 years of peripheral arthritis. Patients may initially be diagnosed with pauciarticular juvenile chronic arthritis and only later reclassified as having spondyloarthropathy when back symptoms develop. Sacroiliitis or spondylitis is present on radiographs in fewer than 25% of patients at disease onset but is evident in most patients after 5 to 10 years of disease. Enthesitis, present in 80% of patients, helps to distinguish early spondyloarthropathy from other forms of juvenile chronic arthritis. Ninety percent of patients have HLA-B27. Spondyloarthropathy in children is rarely associated with psoriasis or inflammatory bowel disease. Treatment includes physical therapy, NSAIDs, and, in patients with persistent arthritis, sulfasalazine or methotrexate.

INDICATIONS FOR REFERRAL

Referral to a rheumatologist should be considered for patients with low back pain that has features of inflammation and that lasts longer than 3 months. Evaluation by a rheumatologist can lead to the correct clinical diagnosis and avoid the expense of computed tomography or magnetic resonance imaging in patients in whom plain radiographs are normal. Patients with an established diagnosis of a seronegative spondyloarthropathy should also be referred to a rheumatologist if they have persistent symptoms despite compliance with an exercise program and NSAID treatment or to determine if an escalation of treatment is needed. Any patient whose peripheral arthritis affects their functioning should also be referred.

All patients with spondylitis should be educated in back stretching and strengthening exercises and posture by a physical therapist experienced in the treatment of spondyloarthropathies. Periodic re-education may be needed. Referral to an orthopedist or hand surgeon is indicated when long-standing joint inflammation results in intractable pain or in an irreversible mechanical limitation that interferes with function.

See Appendix to this chapter for algorithmic tables for the diagnosis and therapy of the spondyloarthropathies.

REFERENCES

1. van der Linden S, van der Heijde DMFM: Ankylosing spondylitis and other B27 related spondyloarthropathies. Bailliere's Clin Rheumatol 9:355, 1995.
2. Resnick D: Ankylosing spondylitis. In Resnick D, ed: Bone and Joint Imaging, 2nd ed. Philadelphia, WB Saunders, 1996, p 246.
3. Ball GV: Ankylosing spondylitis. In McCarty DJ, Koopman WJ, eds: Arthritis and Allied Conditions, 12th ed. Philadelphia, Lea & Febiger, 1993, p 1051.
4. Ward MM: Quality of life in patients with ankylosing spondylitis. Rheum Dis Clin North Am 24:815, 1998.
5. Gall V: Exercise in the spondyloarthropathies. Arthritis Care Res 7:215, 1994.
6. Gladman DD: Natural history of psoriatic arthritis. Bailliere's Clin Rheumatol 8:379, 1994.
7. Toivanen A, Toivanen P: Reactive arthritis. Curr Opin Rheumatol 8:334, 1996.
8. Zeidler H, Mau W, Khan MA: Undifferentiated spondyloarthropathies. Rheum Dis Clin North Am 18:187, 1992.

Table 26A–1. **Diagnosis of the Spondyloarthropathies**

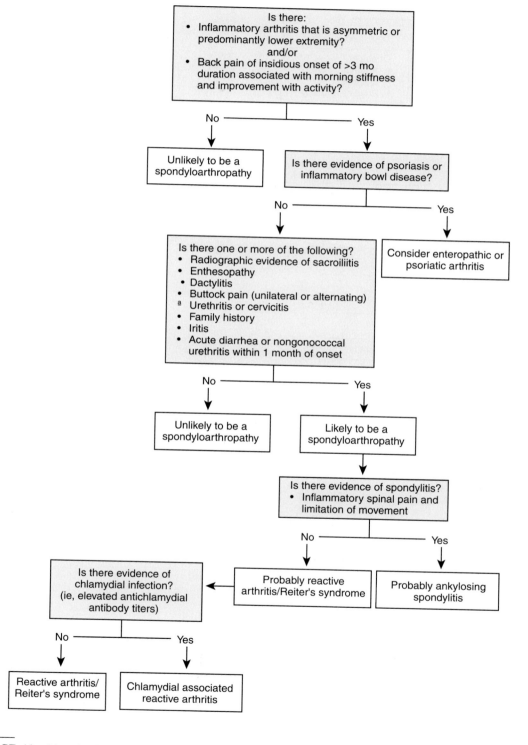

From Lipsky PE: Algorithms for the diagnosis and management of musculoskeletal complaints. Am J Med 103(6A): 74S, 1997.

Table 26A–2. Therapy of the Spondyloarthropathies

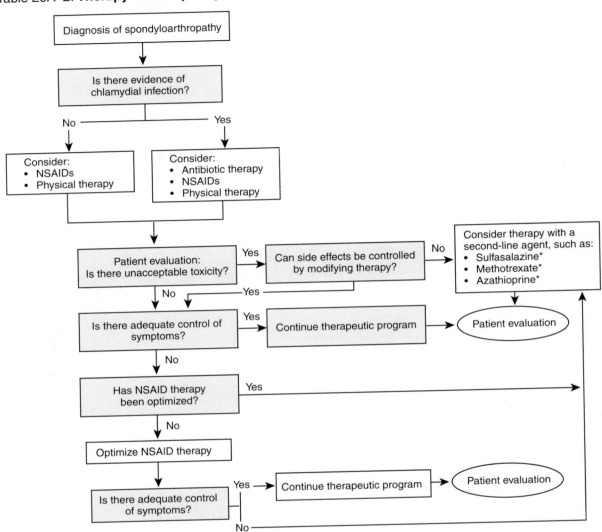

* Not approved by the FDA for treatment of spondyloarthropathies.

From Lipsky PE: Algorithms for the diagnosis and management of musculoskeletal complaints. Am J Med 103(6A): 75S, 1997.

Chapter 27

Systemic Lupus Erythematosus and Systemic Vasculitis

Halsted R. Holman ▪ Mark C. Genovese

Modern understanding of systemic lupus erythematosus (SLE) and systemic vasculitis began in the late 1950s when immunologic studies identified the antinuclear antibodies and the rheumatoid factor as autoantibodies, and when glucocorticoids became widely used in treatment. In the more than 40 years since, clinical sophistication and laboratory knowledge have grown steadily. Three developments concerning rheumatic diseases generally are relevant for a broad understanding by primary care physicians of these processes.

VARIABILITY OF CLINICAL PATTERNS

SLE and vasculitis were first named in the nineteenth century. In those days, only the most severe forms of the disease were recognized as discrete entities. Although the historical classification is still valid, it applies to only a portion of the patients who ultimately fall within the boundaries of the two diseases. Today, many patients come to medical attention in an early and unclassifiable stage of rheumatic disease; a few remain in that unclassifiable stage for months or years. Other patients come to medical attention with clinical manifestations that overlap several classic rheumatic disease diagnoses. An example is mixed connective tissue disease (MCTD), which has attributes of SLE, polymyositis, scleroderma, and rheumatoid arthritis, and may present with synovitis, neuropathy, or vasculitis.

Not only do rheumatic disease patients present with unclassifiable or mixed patterns of clinical disease, but also over time the clinical pattern of a rheumatic disease in an individual can change, often dramatically. Thus, a patient who at one time has rheumatoid arthritis can transform into SLE, or an MCTD patient can transform into typical progressive systemic sclerosis. Also, within a particular diagnosis, such as SLE, the target organs in an individual patient can change, creating quite different clinical patterns. A patient with SLE may have arthritis and rash at one point, thrombocytopenia at another, and nephritis at a third point in time over many years. Modern clinical understanding of the rheumatic diseases recognizes them as pleomorphic, inconstant in clinical characteristics, and often not fitting into traditional diagnostic categories.

The variable and changing character of a rheumatic disease that a patient may experience over time is depicted in Figure 27–1. Using the three-dimensional Venn diagram as a representation of relationships between rheumatic diseases, a patient's clinical attributes may remain stationary within one diagnosis, may change within that diagnosis, or may move between diagnoses. Thus, a patient's course could be characterized by a single point within the diagram or by a line moving over time in different directions with varying speeds.

POOR SPECIFICITY OF DIAGNOSTIC TESTS

Early in the study of autoantibodies in rheumatic diseases, it was thought that particular autoantibodies were associated with specific rheumatic diseases and could be used for accurate diagnosis. Examples are antinuclear antibodies with SLE and the rheumatoid factor with rheumatoid arthritis. It is now clear that such specificity does not exist. Although there is a probabilistic association between particular serologic abnormalities and particular rheumatic diseases, the associations are often not strong enough to establish a diagnosis in an individual case. Just as with clinical manifestations, there is much overlap of serologic reactions and clinical patterns of rheumatic diseases. In addition, many patients who do not meet criteria for any connective tissue disease nevertheless have positive tests for antinuclear antibodies or the rheumatoid factor.

COMMONALITY OF THERAPY

In the early understanding of rheumatic diseases, when the clinical patterns were thought distinct, therapies were also perceived as distinct. Thus, glucocorticoids were used in SLE but not rheumatoid arthritis or scleroderma; methotrexate was used in dermatomyositis but not in other rheumatic diseases. Those views no longer hold. Now the full array of therapies available for rheumatic disease are used in each disease and

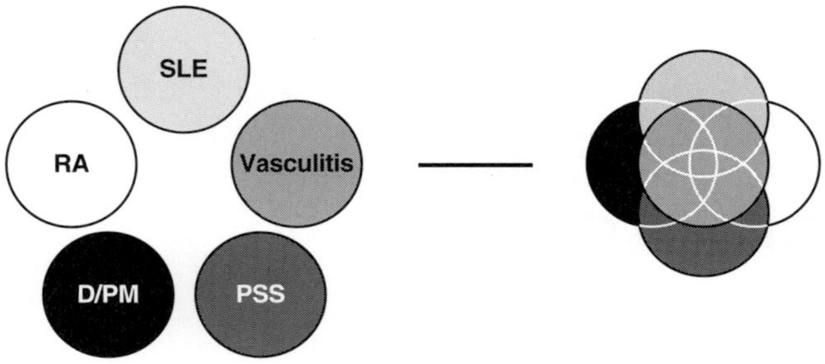

Figure 27–1. Three-dimensional Venn diagram in which each disease can exist as a separate entity and can also overlap with one or more of the others. A few patients, represented by the center, have attributes of all five diseases. Over time, a disease in an individual can evolve as though moving through the representation in different directions at different speeds with resulting changes in disease manifestations. SLE, systemic lupus erythematosus; PSS, progressive systemic sclerosis; D/PM, dermato/polymyositis; RA, rheumatoid arthritis. (From Holman HR: Thought barriers to understanding rheumatic disease. Arthritis Rheum 37:1565–1572, 1994.)

are deployed on the basis of clinical need, not diagnosis. The range of therapies runs from nonsteroidal anti-inflammatory drugs (NSAIDs) through so-called disease-modifying drugs to glucocorticoids, cytotoxic drugs, and experimental biotherapies. A patient with any rheumatic diagnosis whose disease is mild and nonprogressive is given mild medication, whereas involvement of major organs or development of a downward course leads to use of powerful agents. Rheumatic diseases of most types should now be viewed as variable and changing clinical entities whose management depends on an accurate identification of the characteristics of the patient's disease and illness, the trends of those characteristics, and the speed of their movement along the trend lines.

DIAGNOSIS OF RHEUMATIC DISEASE

The first step in the diagnosis of a patient with suggestive rheumatic symptoms, such as musculoskeletal involvement, rash, fatigue, neurologic change, or hematologic abnormality, is to establish the category of disease. Is it a rheumatic disease or something else? (See Chapters 2 and 18.) Alternative disease categories commonly include infection or lymphoma on one hand and fibromyalgia or chronic fatigue syndrome on the other. The distinction between these disease categories is made through a combination of clinical observation and diagnostic studies. The presence of polyarthritis is a strong indicator of a rheumatic disease. However, in other diseases, such as vasculitis, almost any organ system can be affected, just as in infections and lymphomas. Clinical observation may not suffice, and biopsy or other laboratory studies are usually necessary. In the case of vasculitis, biopsy is essential because laboratory studies are often nondiscriminating. Nonetheless, there are clinical and laboratory patterns that are highly suggestive of a particular rheumatic disease, and they are reviewed in relation to SLE and vasculitis.

Fibromyalgia and chronic fatigue syndrome pose a different type of problem because their symptoms overlap almost precisely with symptoms of rheumatic dis-

ease, and there are few distinguishing diagnostic tests. When there is evidence of disease, such as an elevated erythrocyte sedimentation rate, hematologic abnormalities, or positive serologic tests for rheumatic disease, the probability of a rheumatic explanation of symptoms is high. None of the aforementioned laboratory tests, however, is specific for a rheumatic disease. If the test results are only minimally abnormal, firm conclusions cannot be drawn. The distinction is complicated further by the fact that fibromyalgia can coexist with a rheumatic disease. At times, the rheumatic disease may be quiescent with symptoms that may be from what is called *secondary fibromyalgia*. In such situations, careful observation over time is the only way to sort matters out. Further discussion of fibromyalgia and chronic fatigue can be found in Chapter 18.

MANAGEMENT OF RHEUMATIC DISEASE AND ILLNESS

Rheumatic diseases are prototypic chronic diseases. Over years, they undulate in intensity, affect different organs, and rarely respond definitively to therapy. As a result of the disease and its indecisive therapies, the patient may experience many consequences, such as pain, physical dysfunction, disrupted work and social activities, income loss, and emotional distress. In developing an understanding of a patient, it is useful to distinguish between the disease and the illness. The disease is the biologic abnormality, whereas the illness is the disease plus all of its consequences. The disease is that portion of the illness toward which the principal medical management is directed. At times, the biopathology dominates, but at other times, the consequences of the disease are the principal cause of symptoms. For example, disability from physical deconditioning or from damaged joints that are no longer inflamed can be the problem. Depression, which is a common accompaniment of chronic disease, may be responsible for noncompliance with a treatment program. Embarrassment from physical handicap may lead to social isolation and disrupted personal relationships. Situations such as these require specific management; intensifying treatment of the underlying disease can be useless or even harmful. Sometimes the symptoms are a consequence of the medicines used to treat the disease, an outcome readily recognized with long-term glucocorticoid use but also possible with virtually every drug in the rheumatologic armamentarium. *Thus, from the standpoint of clinical care, the issue is not only treating the disease, but also managing the illness.*

Because the course of a patient with a chronic rheumatic disease is often unstable, both disease and illness management depends on an understanding of the trends of each component of the illness and of the tempos along those trends. With rheumatic diseases, accurate reports of symptoms by patients often establish the trend and tempo. Sometimes, when there is an anemia or renal disease, serial laboratory tests may be necessary. Serologic tests, however, are often indecisive or contradictory, as when the sedimentation rate rises without a change in clinical symptoms or physical activity declines from emotional distress despite control of inflammation. Management over time requires knowledge of many trends and responding to those that are influential in determining the patient's state.

The complexity of management of a chronic rheumatic disease places special responsibilities on all involved. The patient becomes a principal caregiver responsible for using medications appropriately, changing behaviors, adjusting life activities, monitoring and reporting illness trends accurately, and participating in management decisions. The physicians must aid the patient to develop those skills. Because continuity of care is essential, the primary care physician who knows the patient best is central to effective management. The specialist serves both the patient and the primary care physician in bringing critical clinical knowledge and interpretations to bear on management decisions. The task of the health care system is to provide the supporting infrastructure for effective discharge of those roles.

SYSTEMIC LUPUS ERYTHEMATOSUS

Clinical Manifestations

SLE is a complex multisystem disease capable of affecting virtually every organ in the body. The underlying cause is not known but thought to be mediated by both environmental and genetic factors. The prevalence of lupus has been reported as approximately 40 cases per 100,000 people.[1] SLE is a disease that predominantly affects women more than men in a ratio of 9:1. It affects African-American women more frequently than white women. The reasons for gender and race bias are not known.

The disease itself is characterized by exacerbations (flares) and remissions. Virtually every organ of the body can be involved, but only rarely does it affect multiple organs at the same time. More commonly, it affects just a few, with different systems being involved as time passes. Cardinal initial symptoms are fatigue, fever, malaise, and some evidence of an inflammatory process or tissue damage. The textbook presentation is fever, facial (malar) rash, synovitis, and serositis, but frequently one or more of those symptoms is absent. The clinician must recognize the extraordinary variability of clinical manifestations (Table 27–1). Table 27–2 shows the most common clinical manifestations of lupus.[3]

Pathogenesis

The pathogenesis of SLE is not known. There appears to be evidence of hyperactivation of B and T cells and notable abnormalities in immunoregulation, including clearance of immune complexes.[4] These are impor-

Table 27–1. REVISED CRITERIA FOR THE CLASSIFICATION OF SYSTEMIC LUPUS ERYTHEMATOSUS (1982)	
Criterion	**Definition**
Malar rash	Fixed erythema, flat or raised, over the eminences, tending to spare the nasolabial folds
Discoid rash	Erythematous raised patches with adherent keratotic scaling and follicular plugging: atrophic scarring may occur in older lesions
Photosensitivity	Skin rash as a result of unusual reaction to sunlight, by patient history or physician observation
Oral ulcers	Oral or nasopharyngeal ulceration, usually painless, observed by a physician
Arthritis	Nonerosive arthritis involving ≥2 peripheral joints, characterized by tenderness, swelling or effusion
Serositis	Pleuritis—convincing history of pleuritic pain or rub heard by a physician or evidence of pleural effusion
	or
	Pericarditis—documented by electrocardiogram or rub or evidence of pericardial effusion
Renal disorder	Persistent proteinuria >0.5 g/day or >3+ if quantification not performed
	or
	Cellular casts—may be red cell, hemoglobin, granular, tubular, or mixed
Neurologic disorder	Seizures—in the absence of offending drugs or known metabolic derangements; e.g., uremia, ketoacidosis, or electrolyte imbalance
	or
	Psychosis—in the absence of offending drugs or known metaboilc derangements, e.g., uremia, ketoacidosis, or electrolyte imbalance
Hematologic disorder	Hemolytic anemia—with reticulocytosis
	or
	Leukopenia—<4000/mm³ total on ≥2 occasions
	or
	Lymphopenia— <1500/mm³ on ≥2 occasions
	or
	Thrombocytopenia—<100,000/mm³ in the absence of offending drugs
Immunologic disorder	Positive lupus erythematosus cell preparation
	or
	Anti-DNA; antibody to native DNA in abnormal titer
	or
	Anti-Sm: presence of antibody to Sm nuclear antigen
	or
	False-positive serologic test for syphilis known to be positive for at least 6 months and confirmed by *Treponema pallidum* immobilization or fluorescent treponemal antibody absorption test
Antinuclear antibody	An abnormal titer of antinuclear antibody by immunofluorescence or an equivalent assay at any point in time and in the absence of drugs known to be associated with *drug-induced lupus* syndrome

From Tan EM, Cohen AS, Fries JF, et al: The 1982 revised criteria for the classification of SLE. Arthritis Rheum 25:1271–1277, 1982.

Table 27–2. CUMULATIVE INCIDENCE OF CLINICAL MANIFESTATIONS IN SYSTEMIC LUPUS ERYTHEMATOSUS	
Clinical Manifestation	**Cumulative Incidence (%)**
Arthritis or arthralgia	53–95
Rash	55–90
Fever	41–86
Proteinuria or abnormal sediment	29–65
Malar rash	10–61
Central nervous system involvement	12–59
Pleuritis	31–57
Pericarditis	6–45
Alopecia	3–45
Raynaud's phenomenon	10–44
Psychosis	5–37
Oral and nasal ulcers	7–36
Nephrotic syndrome	13–26
Seizures	8–26

From Lahita RG: Clinical presentation of systemic lupus erythematosus. In Kelley WN, Harris ED Jr, Ruddy D, Sledge CB, eds: Textbook of Rheumatology, 5th ed. Philadelphia, WB Saunders, 1997 pp 1028–1039.

tant leads that explain some aspects of the disease, but the full mechanisms of tissue damage remain obscure. Significant pathology is created by deposition of immune complexes in tissues. Immune complexes are combinations of antibody and antigen in either soluble or insoluble form. In SLE, there is evidence that complexes of antibody to DNA are localized within the glomerular basement membrane and cause or contribute to lupus glomerulitis. Immune complexes have not been identified in many of the tissues or vessels affected by SLE. In some settings, such as hemolytic anemia or thrombocytopenia, autoantibodies alone may be responsible for tissue damage. The evidence is strong that the disease has an immunologic origin, perhaps with some genetic predisposition. Series have shown that 10% to 15% of patients with SLE have a first- or second-degree relative with SLE, and there is an increase in disease in monozygotic twins when compared with dizygotic twins. Some evidence supports the participation of cytotoxic lymphocytes and of various cytokines released in the process of inflammatory or immunologic reactions. Thus far, the most successful therapies have had anti-inflammatory or immunosuppressive capabilities.

Diagnosis

SLE is a clinical diagnosis. This diagnosis can be supported through biopsy, serology, and laboratory studies. The American College of Rheumatology revised criteria for the classification of SLE are listed in Table 27–1. It provides an important reference point for the primary care physician and the consultant. The criteria were designed to standardize the diagnosis of SLE so that patients could be enrolled in clinical studies. It is required that four individual criteria be met at some time during the illness, but not necessarily be present simultaneously. The criteria were *not* designed for the routine care of patients. Patients can be diagnosed with

SLE while not meeting four of the criteria. In some cases, laboratory or biopsy (skin, renal) results provide enough evidence to make the diagnosis of SLE compelling, despite the absence of four individual criteria. In other cases, patients with fewer than four criteria might be referred to as suffering from a lupus-like syndrome or from undifferentiated connective tissue disease. In either case, these patients should be treated symptomatically and followed longitudinally to detect changes in status.

The most decisive laboratory aid in diagnosis of SLE is the presence of antinuclear antibodies in significant titer found by the fluorescent antinuclear antibody (FANA) test. SLE typically has a positive FANA with diffuse and speckled patterns and is associated with the presence of antibodies to the Sm antigen, double-stranded DNA, or both. Such an antinuclear antibody pattern is essentially unheard of in infections or lymphoma. Some SLE patients (<5%), however, are FANA negative. Those patients are also more likely to have cutaneous manifestations and to have other autoantibodies present, such as anti-Ro/SSA or anti-La/SSB. More frequently, especially in early disease, the FANA can be positive at low or medium titer without either of the antibodies to the Sm antigen or DNA. This pattern is common in many of the different rheumatic diseases, and, although it is helpful in suggesting the presence of a rheumatic disease, it is nondiscriminating among them. Overall, one can expect the FANA to be positive in greater than 95% of patients with SLE, anti–double-stranded DNA antibodies positive in greater than 60% of patients with SLE, and anti-Sm antibodies positive in greater than 30% of cases. Although the FANA is also the most sensitive for SLE, the anti–double-stranded DNA and anti-Sm are significantly more specific (see Chapter 5).

Interpreting the FANA is confounded by other matters. First, antinuclear antibodies are present in normal people, and the cut-off points for a positive test reflect only a quantitative rather than a qualitative departure from normal. Some normal people have positive tests without evidence of disease; this is particularly true of first-degree relatives of patients with rheumatic disease and, to some extent, of the elderly. Second, the FANA may be moderately elevated in other diseases, such as autoimmune thyroid disease, or those with an accompanying polyclonal increase in serum gamma globulin secondary to some chronic infections, liver disease, and occasionally lymphomas. Third, a variety of drugs can induce positive FANA reactions, including some antibiotics (e.g., sulfonamides, isoniazid), many cardiac medications (e.g., procainamide, hydralazine), and some antiepileptic medications (e.g., phenytoin). In interpreting a positive FANA, it is critical to consider the various ways the test can become positive in the absence of SLE. SLE is a clinical diagnosis, and the FANA is used to support the diagnosis.

Additional laboratory parameters assist but are not decisive in the diagnosis of SLE. SLE can manifest as an anemia, a leukopenia, or a thrombocytopenia resulting from either peripheral destruction or a production defect. A general or polyclonal increase in immune globulin is frequent. In the antiphospholipid syndrome, the partial thromboplastin time is elevated, and antibodies to cardiolipin are commonly present. Biopsy can sometimes be helpful, particularly in identifying a lupus skin rash or lupus nephritis. Biopsies of other organs are not helpful because of the paucity of discriminating pathologic changes.

Treatment

The treatment of SLE can be quite difficult and complex. This section is not designed to supplant the advice of the rheumatologist but rather is designed to provide a basic understanding of the treatment options and strategies that can be employed by the primary care physician and the rheumatologist. Treatment of the disease is determined more by the extent of organ involvement than any other factor. SLE can exist in stable mild form, for example, affecting just skin and joints. Alternatively, it can be progressive, unresponsive to therapy, and fatal.

Education of patients is particularly important given the chronic and variable nature of this disease. Because sun exposure can exacerbate the disease, all patients should be advised to avoid prolonged sun exposure, to wear long garments, and to apply sun screen daily. The importance of compliance of patients with therapy must be emphasized strongly.

Patients with the milder forms of the disease may benefit from the use of NSAIDs. These drugs decrease many of the constitutional symptoms, such as fatigue, fever, myalgia, and arthralgia, that plague patients with SLE. Although these agents do not have a direct impact on the disease itself, they help by decreasing pain and increasing function and quality of life. The large number of side effects of NSAIDs are well known; however, in SLE there are some unique issues of concern. Some of the NSAIDs have been associated with the development of aseptic meningitis in patients with SLE. NSAIDs can adversely affect renal function in all patients, but if a patient with SLE has renal involvement, the impairment in renal function can be amplified. Finally, given that patients with SLE occasionally receive at least short courses of glucocorticoids, the physician needs to be aware of the increased risks of NSAID gastropathy in the setting of glucocorticoid use.

An additional agent used frequently in SLE is hydroxychloroquine (Plaquenil). This can be used as a sole agent or in addition to NSAIDs or more potent immunosuppressive agents. Hydroxychloroquine appears particularly useful in the treatment of cutaneous and musculoskeletal involvement. Although it appears to be a relatively weak agent, its use has been shown to lessen the frequency of lupus flares.[5] It is usually dosed at 200 to 400 mg/day, and given that it is slow-acting agent, it takes a period of weeks to months before any significant benefit is achieved. The most frequent side effects associated with hydroxychloroquine are gastrointestinal upset and rash or photosensitivity. These side effects are uncommon, and on the whole, hydroxychloroquine is usually well tolerated. A rare but important side effect is retinal toxicity. Retinal toxicity with deposits that over time can diminish vision has been reported with chloroquine but is rare with hydroxychloroquine. Routine ophthalmologic examinations are recommended for all patients taking this medication; however, the necessity is unclear.

All forms of SLE respond, at least in part, to systemic glucocorticoids in doses of 0.5 to 1.0 mg/kg/day of prednisone. Glucocorticoids are usually reserved for patients who are unresponsive or intolerant to NSAIDs and antimalarials or those suffering with major organ system involvement. The goal is usually to maintain the prednisone dose at less than 10 to 15 mg/day or to use an every-other-day regimen if it is tolerated. Responding patients can sometimes discontinue glucocorticoids once remission has occurred, but recurrences are likely. The dose should be tapered as rapidly as the disease manifestations tolerate. Common side effects of glucocorticoids include weight gain in a characteristic distribution, acne, osteopenia, avascular bone necrosis, cataracts, glaucoma, euphoria, insomnia, tremor, gastropathy, striae, hyperglycemia, hyperlipidemia, and cardiovascular complications.

Some patients respond incompletely to glucocorticoids alone or have severe organ system manifestations (e.g., progressive glomerulonephritis, hemolysis, thrombosis, cytopenia, or central nervous system disease) requiring the addition of cytotoxic drugs, particularly azathioprine or cyclophosphamide, and occasionally methotrexate and cyclosporine. The use of these agents frequently allows the reduction in glucocorticoid dose, and thus they may be used as steroid-sparing agents. These agents all have side effects. They are used when the benefits clearly outweigh the potential risks and should be used only with the guidance of a consulting rheumatologist. Careful follow-up must be maintained when patients are taking these compounds so that severe immunosuppression and opportunistic infections are avoided. In addition, these medications can have adverse effects on the liver, kidneys, and reproductive systems.

One variant of SLE is the antiphospholipid syndrome. It is discussed at greater length in Chapter 14. The antiphospholipid syndrome is often associated with SLE and is an entity characterized by arterial or venous thromboses and spontaneous abortions. Although frequently associated with SLE, the antiphospholipid syndrome can exist separately without other evidence of a rheumatic disease. This syndrome is most effectively treated with anticoagulation rather than immunosuppression, and an algorithm for diagnosis and therapy can be found in Chapter 14.

Modern treatment of SLE is moderately successful in that the majority of patients live well beyond 15 years from diagnosis. The treatment creates a chronic illness, however, consisting of the disease itself, the side effects of therapy, and the many consequences of chronic tissue inflammation. As discussed earlier, proper management enters into many realms of the patient's life. The primary care physician is situated in the center of that management task, working with the specialists to tailor disease treatment and working with the patient and family to minimize the limitations on comfort, physical activity, and independent living.

VASCULITIS

Clinical Manifestations

As an inflammatory disease of blood vessels, vasculitis can affect any organ. All sizes of arteries can be involved from terminal arterioles to the aorta. Sometimes veins are affected as well. The inflammatory change in and around vessel walls leads to vascular necrosis, occlusion of the lumen, and subsequent damage to the vascularized tissues. Conceptually, countless patterns of disease might emerge, but in reality there are dominant clinical patterns. They tend to be associated with the size of the blood vessels that are inflamed. Overall, vasculitis most commonly affects skin, striated muscle, the nervous system, and the kidneys. The skin lesions result in local hemorrhage, whereas the muscle lesions cause pain and occasionally weakness. Neurologic lesions are the result of focal damage from ischemia and can be either central or peripheral. The renal lesions are a form of glomerulitis.

CLASSIFICATION

Historically, particular clinical patterns of vasculitis were given discrete names, often those of the persons who described the pattern (e.g., Churg-Straus, Henoch-Schönlein, Takayasu). *Wegener's granulomatosis,* for instance, was the name given to vasculitis with granuloma formation in the respiratory tract and in the kidney. The term *giant cell arteritis* was applied both to involvement of the temporal artery and to giant cell inflammation of the wall of the aortic arch and its branches. Clinicians still use these terms to describe clinical patterns and to communicate with others in the field concerning a diagnosis. Vasculitis affecting different types of vessels simultaneously and overlapping classic categories are common. For instance, a patient with Wegener's granulomatosis may also have dermal vasculitis and peripheral neuropathy. Table 27–3 provides a framework for conceptualizing the different vasculitic syndromes based on the predominant caliber of vessels that are involved.[6]

Table 27–3. NAMES AND DEFINITIONS OF VASCULITIDES ADOPTED BY THE CHAPEL HILL CONSENSUS CONFERENCE ON THE NOMENCLATURE OF SYSTEM VASCULITIS*

Large vessel vasculitis	
Giant cell (temporal) arteritis	Granulomatous arteritis of the aorta and its major branches, with a predilection for the extracranial branches of the carotid artery. *Often involves the temporal artery. Usually occurs in patients older than 50 and often is associated with polymyalgia rheumatica.*
Takayasu arteritis	Granulomatous inflammation of the aorta and its major branches. *Usually occurs in patients younger than 50.*
Medium-sized vessel vasculitis	
Polyarteritis nodosa[†] (classic polyarteritis nodosa)	Necrotizing inflammation of medium-sized or small arteries without glomerulonephritis or vasculitis in arterioles, capillaries, or venules
Kawasaki disease	Arteritis involving large, medium-sized, and small arteries and associated with mucocutaneous lymph node syndrome. *Coronary arteries are often involved. Aorta and veins may be involved. Usually occurs in children.*
Small vessel vasculitis	
Wegener's granulomatosis[‡]	Granulomatous inflammation involving the respiratory tract and necrotizing vasculitis affecting small to medium-sized vessels (e.g., capillaries, venules, arterioles, and arteries). *Necrotizing glomerulonephritis is common.*
Churg-Strauss syndrome[‡]	Eosinophil-rich and granulomatous inflammation involving the respiratory tract and necrotizing vasculitis affecting small to medium-sized vessels, associated with asthma and eosinophilia.
Microscopic polyangiitis[†] (microscopic polyarteritis)[‡]	Necrotizing vasculitis, with few or no immune deposits, affecting small vessels (i.e., capillaries, venules, or arterioles). *Necrotizing arteritis involving small and medium-sized arteries may be present. Necrotizing glomerulonephritis is common. Pulmonary capillaritis often occurs.*
Henoch-Schönlein purpura	Vasculitis, with IgA-dominant immune deposits, affecting small vessels (i.e., capillaries, venules, or arterioles). *Typically involves skin, gut, and glomeruli and is associated with arthralgias or arthritis.*
Essential cryoglobulinemic vasculitis	Vasculitis, with cryoglobulin immune deposits, affecting small vessels (i.e., capillaries, venules, or arterioles), and associated with cryoglobulins in serum. *Skin and glomeruli are often involved.*
Cutaneous leukocytoclastic angiitis	Isolated cutaneous leukocytoclastic angiitis without systemic vasculitis or glomerulonephritis.

*Large vessel refers to the aorta and the largest branches directed toward major body regions (e.g., to the extremities and the head and neck); medium-sized vessel refers to the main visceral arteries (e.g., renal, hepatic, coronary, and mesenteric arteries); small vessel refers to venules, capillaries, arterioles, and the intraparenchymal distal arterial radicals that connect with arterioles. Some small and large vessel vasculitides may involve medium-sized arteries, but large and medium-sized vessel vasculitides do not involve vessels smaller than arteries. Essential components are represented by normal type; italicized type represents usual, but not essential, components.
†Preferred term.
‡Strongly associated with antineutrophil cytoplasmic autoantibodies.
From Jennette JC, Falk RJ, Andrassy K, et al: Nomenclature of systemic vasculitides: Proposal of an international consensus conference [review]. Arthritis Rheum 37:187–192, 1994.

The Chapel Hill Consensus Conference classification[6] and the American College of Rheumatology 1990 Criteria for the Classification of Vasculitis[7] are criteria that rheumatologists frequently refer to when classifying vasculitis. However, the criteria can be difficult to apply to individual patients because they do not consider the full spectrum of manifestations for each disease. It is important to think of these diseases as a continuum rather than as separate, distinct entities. This lack of distinction is also apparent when considering treatment modalities because glucocorticoids and cytotoxic agents are frequently used for the treatment of vasculitides.

PRESENTATION

The clinical presentation of vasculitis is difficult to summarize. In cases of blindness, stroke, hemoptysis, hematuria, purpura, or footdrop, the first signs are ominous and certainly suggest vaculitis as a potential cause to even the most inexperienced clinician. The presence of hemorrhage or tissue necrosis can provide dramatic and obvious evidence of disease. However, symptoms and signs may be much more subtle and far less specific, such as malaise, arthralgia, headache, sinusitis, or even symptoms of otitis media. These features might easily be dismissed early on.

Progression may be insidious or fulminant, and distinguishing between vasculitis and other systemic diseases is often difficult, time-consuming, and cumbersome. Illnesses that can mimic vasculitis are listed in Box 27–1. Sometimes, physicians may be forced to treat for all contingencies (e.g., infection, atherosclerotic stroke) until a final diagnosis is more clear. The initial evaluation should include a detailed history and physical examination with attention to drug use or abuse (cocaine and amphetamines), exposures to hepatitis B and C, and risk factors for human immunodeficiency virus (HIV). A thorough review of systems needs to be performed looking for evidence that supports the presence of a malignancy; paraneoplastic syndrome; or connective tissue disease, such as SLE, antiphospholipid syndrome, or rheumatoid arthritis. Various chemicals, including pesticides, have also been incriminated.

Characteristic clinical patterns of presentation of vasculitis are helpful in terms of recognizing the disease. The presence of an active urinary sediment with red cell casts, hemoptysis, and sinus inflammation suggests Wegener's granulomatosis. Headache, jaw claudication, visual disturbance, and temporal artery tenderness are all consistent with giant cell arteritis. The majority of cases of vasculitis, however, do not present with all the classic manifestations. A physician is more likely to see a patient with a fever, an active urinary sediment, and a peripheral neuropathy or footdrop. This presentation is sufficient to suggest vaculitis, especially if there is no other evidence of infection, drug reaction, or malignancy. If the patient is already known to be suffering from an established connective tissue disease, such as SLE or rheumatoid arthritis, the patient may have a vasculitis related to the primary disorder.[8]

DIAGNOSIS

Diagnosis of vasculitis can sometimes be made on characteristic clinical symptoms and signs, radiographic findings, and laboratory data. However, the histopathologic features based on tissue biopsy specimens usually are necessary to make a formal diagnosis. Although biopsy specimens of clinically normal tissue are not helpful, tissue from abnormal organs has proven diagnostically useful in greater than 65% of cases.[8] Biopsy results can be subject to error. Patients in early stages of disease may have ambiguous histologic findings. Sampling error may result in an uninvolved area being sampled, especially because vasculitic lesions can occur in a patchy fashion. As well, it is difficult to insure that a single biopsy specimen will contain vessels of various caliber, with larger or smaller vessel involvement going unrecognized.

Alternatively, when biopsy is impractical (e.g., large vessel involvement), angiography can be particularly useful. A characteristic pattern of aneurysm and stenosis in what has been described as a string-of-pearls appearance may be found on angiograms of affected vessels. It is important to keep in mind the following:[8]

Angiography is not capable of detecting involvement of small vessels (capillaries and venules).
Angiographic changes are not as specific as histologic changes.
A disease may be present a long time before gross changes in vessels can be visualized by angiography.
Angiographic lesions do not differentiate among the causes of vasculitis, such as infection (hepatitis B or C, bacteria, fungus), drug use (cocaine and amphetamines), malignancy, or embolic injury.

Laboratory abnormalities characteristic of vasculitis include a high erythrocyte sedimentation rate and C-reactive protein, an elevated fibrinogen level, leu-

---

Box 27–1. ILLNESSES THAT CAN MIMIC VASCULITIS

Infections
    Sepsis
    Subacute bacterial endocarditis
    HIV
    Syphilis
Drug use/abuse
    Antibiotics
    Sulfonamides
    Intravenous drug abuse
    Cocaine
    Amphetamines
    Ergotamine
Malignancy/lymphoma
Antiphospholipid antibody syndrome
Cardiac myxoma
Atheroemboli

kocytosis, eosinophilia, thrombocytosis, and a positive rheumatoid factor test. Serum complement may be reduced, and cryoglobulins may be increased. Although none of these abnormalities are specific, they support a clinical suspicion and strongly direct attention to an appropriate biopsy.

A useful diagnostic test, particularly for Wegener's granulomatosis, is the antineutrophil cytoplasmic antibody (ANCA). Properly conducted, ANCA tests are positive in most forms of necrotizing vasculitis. The ANCA result is typically reported in one of two forms: cytoplasmic (C-ANCA) and perinuclear (P-ANCA). These staining patterns correspond to the presence of certain antibodies. In the case of C-ANCA, the cytoplasmic staining pattern corresponds with antibody binding to an enzyme proteinase 3, whereas P-ANCA corresponds with the binding of antibody to myeloperoxidase. The P-ANCA staining pattern is neither sensitive nor highly specific for any type for vaculits. It may be present in other autoimmune or inflammatory diseases, particularly SLE, but most frequently has been associated with polyarteritis and glomerulonephritis. C-ANCA has a high sensitivity and specificity for Wegener's granulomatosis but does not always distinguish clearly between vasculitic syndromes. In many patients with Wegener's granulomatosis, the C-ANCA is useful to monitor the activity of the disease because the titer can reflect the activity of the disease.

Types of Vasculitis

LARGE VESSEL VASCULITIS

GIANT CELL ARTERITIS. Giant cell arteritis encompasses both involvement of the temporal arteries and giant cell inflammation of the aortic arch vessels. Patients with temporal arteritis are usually older than 50 years of age. The classic symptoms include headache, visual disturbance (tunneling of vision or sudden loss of vision in one eye), jaw claudication, and temporal artery tenderness. Palpation of the temporal arteries can reveal a bounding pulse, absence of pulse, tenderness, or none of these. If temporal arteritis is suspected, the patient should be started on glucocorticoids (prednisone 1 mg/kg/day) immediately to help prevent the loss of vision. Temporal artery biopsy should be performed within a few days. Up to 2 weeks of glucocorticoid therapy does not change the histopathologic findings.[9] Of more concern is a negative biopsy result despite suggestive symptoms or signs. Sampling error can play a role, as can taking too small a sample. If necessary, a second biopsy specimen can be taken from the other side of the head. Markers of disease recurrence include return of symptoms and elevation in acute-phase markers, such as the erythrocyte sedimentation rate or C-reactive protein.

Polymyalgia rheumatica is a poorly understood muscle disease marked by severe myalgia and weakness in the hip and shoulder girdles associated with an increased erythrocyte sedimentation rate or C-reactive proteins, mild anemia, and low-grade fever. No specific muscle lesion has been identified; muscle enzyme levels in the serum are normal as are muscle biopsy specimens. Polymyalgia rheumatica often accompanies temporal arteritis and may be the first indication of an emerging temporal arteritis. It has been reported to occur in 40% to 60% of patients with temporal arteritis. Polymyalgia rheumatica can also occur without definitive evidence of vasculitis. Temporal artery biopsy specimens are positive in approximately 16% of patients with clinical symptoms and signs highly suggestive of polymyalgia rheumatica.[10]

TAKAYASU'S ARTERITIS. Takayasu's arteritis involves the large vessels, including the aorta and its major branches. It typically affects women in their 20s to 30s and presents initially with malaise, arthralgia, and weight loss. As the disease progresses, patients begin to suffer from hypertension, claudication, arm numbness, and fever. They can develop complications such as stroke, myocardial infarction, and peripheral ischemia. On examination, the classic findings include the presence of bruits over affected vessels and a loss of pulses. The diagnosis is typically made based by arteriograms that show evidence of stenosis of major vessels. Laboratory studies are often abnormal with the presence of anemia and an elevated erythrocyte sedimentation rate. In contrast to temporal arteritis, however, these studies can be entirely normal and are neither sensitive nor specific in this illness. Treatment usually involves the use of prednisone at a dose of 1 mg/kg/day and is effective in treating the early stages of disease before permanent structural changes and fibrosis take place. Other agents, including cyclophosphamide and methotrexate, have been tried but are usually reserved for patients having failed glucocorticoids. Surgical intervention and revascularization may be required in situations in which ischemia and stenosis are otherwise irreversible. Antiplatelet drugs, including aspirin, may forestall thrombosis within involved vessels.

MEDIUM VESSEL VASCULITIS

POLYARTERITIS NODOSA. Polyarteritis nodosa predominantly affects medium-sized and small vessels. Polyarteritis nodosa is possibly the most worrisome of all the vasculitides because of the difficulty recognizing the disease and making the diagnosis. It often presents in an insidious fashion with subtle, nondescript features allowing it to go unnoticed. The patient may complain of mild fevers, malaise, myalgia, and arthralgia. These symptoms then can progress to abdominal, chest, or testicular pain; renal involvement; or mononeuritis multiplex with wristdrop or footdrop. Examination often does not reveal particularly striking findings. The exception can be the presence of palpable purpura, livedo reticularis, wristdrop, or footdrop. The diagnosis necessitates a biopsy specimen of an affected area or of sural nerve and gastrocnemius muscle, testicle, bowel, or kidney. The patchy nature of the disease can limit the accuracy of the biopsy. Alternatively an angiogram of the kidneys, bowel, or central nervous system can be helpful. Laboratory studies usually, but not always, show an elevation of acute-phase reactants (erythrocyte sedimentation rate, C-reactive protein). The ANCA is positive in only about 20% of cases. Treatment consists of glucocorticoids (prednisone 1 mg/kg/day) and usually cyclophosphamide. If left untreated, polyarteritis nodosa has a mortality rate of greater than 85% at 5 years.[11] When polyarteritis nodosa is treated with glucocorticoids alone, the 5-year mortality declines to 48%.[12] Combination therapy of glucocorticoids and cyclophosphamide reduces mortality to 20% at 5 years.[12, 13] In the subset of patients with polyarteritis nodosa associated with hepatitis B or C infections, treatment with antiviral agents and possibly plasmapheresis is helpful.

KAWASAKI SYNDROME. Kawasaki syndrome is discussed here because of its association with inflammation of medium-sized vessels; however, it is a disease generally associated with children younger than age 5 and subsequently is not covered in much detail. It is a febrile illness in which infants and children develop mucocutaneous involvement, including conjunctival injection; cracking, fissuring, or bleeding of the lips; strawberry tongue; and diffuse erythema of mucous membranes. Most children also develop a rash on the trunk, erythema of the palms and soles, and desquamation of the fingers and toes. Lymphadenopathy can also commonly be found. The development of myocarditis and aneurysm formation are the most serious consequences of the disease. Treatment usually includes high-dose aspirin and intravenous immunoglobulin.

SMALL TO MEDIUM VESSEL VASCULITIS

WEGENER'S GRANULOMATOSIS. Wegener's granulomatosis is a necrotizing granulomatous vasculitis involving small and medium-sized vessels. The syndrome is classically defined as having involvement of kidney, lungs, and upper respiratory tract (i.e., sinuses). Many other organs can be involved, including the skin, nerves, and joints. Although defined classically as a triad, the disease can exist in a limited fashion with involvement of only the lungs, upper respiratory tract, or kidneys. Sinus inflammation or epistaxis, otitis media in an adult, hemoptysis, and red blood cell casts in the urine are all features suggesting this necrotizing vasculitis. The ANCA test is particularly useful in this disorder to aid in the diagnosis, and occasionally for following disease activity during treatment. Treatment should consist of glucocorticoids and oral cyclophosphamide.

CHURG-STRAUSS SYNDROME. Churg-Strauss syndrome affects primarily small and occasionally medium-sized vessels. The syndrome is characterized as an eosinophilic vasculitis involving the lungs and the gastrointestinal tract. Palpable purpura is common and involvement of peripheral nerves and the kidneys may occur. The hallmark finding in this syndrome is the eosinophilia and the presence of eosinophils in necrotizing arteritis and granulomas. The syndrome is usually preceded by allergic rhinitis and asthma. The treatment is usually glucocorticoids (prednisone 1 mg/kg/day) and, in a minority of cases, cytotoxic agents.

MICROSCOPIC POLYANGIITIS. Microscopic polyangiitis is predominantly a small vessel vasculitis with few or no immune deposits, with involvement most frequently in the kidneys, lungs, skin, and gastrointestinal tract. In many respects, it has a similar pattern of involvement to Wegener's granulomatosis without granulomas, Churg-Strauss syndrome without the eosinophils, and polyarteritis nodosa without aneurysm formation. The treatment of this necrotizing vasculitis is similar to the others: glucocorticoids and the addition of a cytotoxic agent (cyclophosphamide).

HENOCH-SCHÖNLEIN PURPURA. Henoch-Schönlein purpura is another small vessel vasculitis; however, this syndrome is usually localized within postcapillary venules. This disorder predominantly afflicts young children and has been associated with prodromal upper respiratory symptoms with either a bacterial or a viral infection. A possible hypersensitivity component may be responsible for triggering the vasculitis. The hallmark finding in this disease is cutaneous involvement with the development of palpable purpura. The development of arthritis and arthralgia, gastrointestinal involvement (abdominal pain and detectable blood in stools), or renal involvement is quite common. Treatment consists of symptomatic care because the disease is usually self-limited, lasting 1 to 2 weeks. In more serious cases, glucocorticoids are used occasionally as are cytotoxic agents.

VASCULITIS AND CRYOGLOBULINEMIA. Vasculitis and cryoglobulinemia are related to the presence of cryoglobulins. These are immunoglobulins that precipitate when the temperature around them is reduced. The term *essential cryoglobulinemic vasculitis* is used when no underlying or associated condition can be found as the cause. This disorder is characterized by hyperviscosity symptoms or by vasculitis. Patients often suffer from fatigue, arthralgia or arthritis, cutaneous vasculitis or purpura, neuropathy, digital ischemia, and visceral organ involvement (renal or pulmonary). There are three types of cryoglobulins:

Type I: Monoclonal immunoglobulin, either IgG or IgM, and associated with lymphoproliferative disorders (25% of cases).
Type II: Mixed cryoglobulins with a monoclonal component, typically seen in the presence of other connective tissue diseases, infections, or lymphoproliferative disorders. A large number of patients with type II cyroglobulins do not have an identifiable underlying disease (25% of cases).
Type III: Mixed polyclonal cryoglobulin. This disorder can commonly be seen with a variety of illnesses, including connective tissue diseases (SLE and rheumatoid arthritis), bacterial infections, and notably hepatitis B and C infection (50% of cases).

The treatment is usually contingent on the type of cryoglobulin present and the presence or absence of an underlying associated disease. If an underlying disease is present, treatment should uniformly be directed against it. The presence of hepatitis B and C should be searched for and, if present, antiviral regimens implemented. Some symptoms of cryoglobulinemia respond to glucocorticoid therapy. In serious cases, in which there is threat of loss of organ or life, plasmapheresis, cytotoxic agents, and intravenous immunoglobulin have been used with some success.

LEUKOCYTOCLASTIC VASCULITIS (Palpable purpura). Leukocytoclastic vasculitis is the most common type of vasculitis encountered by the primary care physician. Clinically the term *leukocytoclastic vasculitis* is used to describe cutaneous vasculitis, and the typical finding is palpable purpura. The lesions themselves are often described as discrete, red-purple papules that do not blanch on pressure. The lesions are most frequently seen in dependent areas, such as the feet, legs, and buttocks, and they appear in crops, rather than several at a time or all at once. Pathologically the term is used to describe the presence of fibrinoid necrosis of capillary and postcapillary venules and the presence of neutrophils in the vessel and surrounding tissue. A multitude of inciting events can lead to its development. These include infection (e.g., streptococci), hypersensitivity (e.g., drug reactions), malignancy, abnormal proteins (e.g., gammopathies and cryoglobulins), and connective tissue diseases. Treatment should be centered around identifying and treating the underlying cause. Once the offending agent is removed, the cutaneous lesions begin to heal. If an underlying cause cannot be identified, glucocorticoids (0.5 mg/kg/day of prednisone) can be tried; however, glucocorticoids should not be given routinely in patients with leukocytoclastic vasculitis without first excluding the potential underlying causes.

PATHOGENESIS

The underlying cause of most forms of vasculitis is unknown. An important lead to the pathogenesis in vasculitis lies in the immune complex mechanism and the deposition of immune complexes into endothelium causing inflammation and vessel injury. Other pathogenetic mechanisms include direct endothelial infection, antiendothelial antiobodies, antineutrophil cytoplasmic antibody–mediated injury, and T-cell endothelial injury.[14]

As already mentioned, it is known that hepatitis viruses B and C can cause vasculitis in addition to hepatitis. Hepatitis B has been associated with up to 30% of cases of polyarteritis nodosa. Hepatitis C virus is notable for causing vasculitis, cryoglobulinemia, and musculoskeletal symptoms. In patients with hepatitis B or C infections who develop vasculitis, the virus and antibodies to it can be found in the inflammatory lesions of the vessel wall. Some of the patients with hepatitis C vasculitis experience an improvement in the vasculitis when the viremia is reduced with interferon therapy. However, most patients with hepatitis B and C infections do not have vasculitis despite having both antibody and antigen in their circulation, and most cases of vasculitis do not show evidence of immune complex localization in the vessel wall.

Many drugs have been linked to vasculitis. Most notable have been sulfonamides, other antibiotics, antiarrhythmic drugs, and propylthiouracil. The most common type of vasculitis associated with drugs is dermal, but virtually all forms can be found. Small vessel involvement is typical. If recognized early, withdrawal of the offending drug leads to resolution of the vasculitis, although relentless vasculitis has been associated with some drug reactions. Generally the drugs are not antigenic by themselves, but they can become antigenic when combined with plasma or tissue proteins. Whether the drugs attach to a vessel wall and incite reaction, induce an immunologic cross-reactivity, or operate by some other mechanism is unclear.

Treatment

Vasculitis, similar to other rheumatic diseases, exists in forms from mild and transient to relentless and fatal. Occasionally a dermal vasculitis, especially of the lower extremities, waxes and wanes, does not progress to other tissues, is unresponsive to glucocorticoid therapy, and even disappears. Such behavior is rarely the case, however, unless a particular environmental provocateur is identified and removed.

Most forms of vasculitis require treatment, and the staple of treatment is prednisone. Some forms, including palpable purpura and temporal arteritis, respond to glucocorticoid treatment alone. Other forms, such as the granulomatous vasculitis associated with Wegener's disease, respond initially to prednisone alone but usually require a combination of prednisone and cyclophosphamide. Similarly, nervous system and renal vasculitis respond more quickly and better to the combination. Because the possibility of neurologic or renal involvement is present when vasculitis occurs, it is logical to consider treating all but the mildest forms with a combination of glucocorticoid and a cytotoxic agent. As a general rule, necrotizing vasculitis with organ involvement requires therapy with a glucocortiocoid and cyclophosphamide.

The duration and intensity of therapy are determined by the patient's response to and tolerance of the drug. Usually, patients are maintained on a stable glucocorticoid and cytotoxic dose for at least 1 month, at which point the glucocorticoids are slowly tapered or switched to an every-other-day regimen. All patients started on glucocorticoids for more than a month or 6 weeks should be treated with supplemental calcium and vitamin D and perhaps additional bone-protective regimens, such as estrogen replacement, bisphosphonates, or nasal calcitonin (see Chapter 35). The cytotoxic agent is usually continued for a year before adjustments or discontinuation is considered. With suppression of all evidence of the disease as an end point, treatment is often protracted. Evidence has emerged that methotrexate is valuable in treating vasculitis and can serve to reduce the dose of both glucocorticoids and more powerful cytotoxic drugs.

The vasculitis related to hepatitis B and C can fluctuate in relation to the degree of viremia and can be treated with interferon-α and other antiviral agents. However, elimination of the virus is virtually impossible and treatment with glococorticoids and cytotoxic drugs has limited success. Additionally, patients with vasculitis treated with glucocorticoids or combinations of glucocorticoids and cytotoxic agents are at increased risk to develop opportunistic infections and warrant prophylaxis against *Pneumocystis carinii* pneumonia.

REFERENCES

1. Michet CJ, McKenna CH, Elveback LR, et al: Epidemiology of systemic lupus erythematosus and other connective tissue dieases in Rochester, Minnesota, 1950 through 1979. Mayo Clin Proc 60:105, 1985.
2. Tan EM, Cohen AS, Fries JF, et al: The 1982 revised criteria for the classification of SLE. Arthritis Rheum 25:1271–1277, 1982.
3. Lahita RG: Clinical presentation of systemic lupus erythematosus. In Kelley WN, Harris ED Jr, Ruddy D, Sledge CB, eds: Textbook of Rheumatology, 5th ed. Philadelphia, WB Saunders, 1997, pp 1028–1039.
4. Hahn BH: Systemic lupus erythematosus and related syndromes. In Kelley WN, Harris ED Jr, Ruddy D, Sledge CB, eds: Textbook of Rheumatology, 5th ed. Philadelphia, WB Saunders, 1997, pp 1015–1027.
5. Canadian Hydroxychloroquine Study Group: A randomized study of the effect of withdrawing hydroxychloroquine sulfate in system lupus erythematous. N Engl J Med 324:150, 1991.
6. Jennette JC, Falk RJ, Andrassy K, et al: Nomenclature of systemic vasculitides: Proposal of an international consensus conference [review]. Arthritis Rheum 37:187–192, 1994.
7. American College of Rheumatology Subcommittee on Classification of Vasculitis: The American College of Rheumatology 1990 Criteria for the Classification of Vasculitis. Arthritis Rheum 33:1065–1144, 1990.
8. Hoffman GS: Systemic vasculitis, update 28. In Kelley WN, Harris ED Jr, Ruddy D, Sledge CB, eds: Textbook of Rheumatology, 5th ed. Philadelphia, WB Saunders, 1998, pp 1–18.
9. Achkar AA, Lie JT, Hunder GG, et al: How does previous corticosteroid treatment affect the biopsy findings in giant cell (temporal) arteritis? Ann Intern Med 120:987–992, 1994.
10. Salvarani C, Gabriel SE, O'Fallon WM, Hunder GG: Epidemiology of polymyalgia rheumatica in Olmsted County, Minnesota, 1970–1991. Arthritis Rheum 38:369–373, 1995.
11. Frohnert PP, Sheps SG: Long-term follow-up study of polyarteritis nodosa. Am J Med 43:8–14, 1967.
12. Leib ES, Restino C, Paulus HE: Immunosuppressive and corticosteroid therapy of polyarteritis nodosa. Am J Med 67:941–947, 1979.
13. Fauci AS, Katz P, Haynes BF, Wolff SM: Cyclophosphamide therapy of severe systemic necrotizing vasculitis. N Engl J Med 235–238, 1979.
14. Valente RM, Hall S, O'Duffy JD, Conn DL: Vasculitis and related disorders. In Kelley WN, Harris ED Jr, Ruddy D, Sledge CB, eds: Textbook of Rheumatology, 5th ed. Philadelphia, WB Saunders, 1996, pp 1079–1122.

Recognition and Management of Patients with Specific Rheumatologic Problems

Chapter 28

Scleroderma

Edward D. Harris, Jr.

Scleroderma, also known as *systemic sclerosis*, is an autoimmune disorder characterized by thickening and fibrosis of the skin and underlying soft tissue. There also may be involvement of internal organs, such as the lungs, heart, gastrointestinal tract, and kidneys. The disease of systemic sclerosis exists in two forms: limited and diffuse. The limited variant, also known as *CREST* (*c*alcinosis cutis, *R*aynaud's phenomenon, *e*sophageal dysfunction, *s*clerodactyly and *t*elangiectasia) (to be discussed in greater depth later), generally portends a better overall prognosis than does diffuse disease. The two variants can be differentiated on the basis of internal organ involvement and distribution of skin involvement (Table 28–1). Why from the same puffy hands one individual develops an erosive, proliferative synovitis and another progresses to an encasing scleroderma is unknown.

Scleroderma has been linked with the other diffuse connective diseases, such as rheumatoid arthritis (RA) and systemic lupus erythematosus (SLE) because of the frequent association of this disease process with autoimmune phenomena. In addition, each of these processes can begin with a *puffy hand syndrome* characterized by pain, stiffness, and swelling of the hands without much localization to joints. When it evolves into a proliferative synovitis, RA is the most likely diagnosis. When it becomes associated with central nervous system disease, hemolytic anemia, or renal disease, SLE is an appropriate diagnosis. When it is accompanied by Raynaud's phenomenon and gradual loss of motion in finger joints, scleroderma or the mixed connective tissue syndrome is likely to be the final diagnosis.[1]

In its developed, mature, severe form, scleroderma is not likely to be confused with any other disease. Patients have skin fused by fibrosis to the underlying fascia. Subcutaneous tissue is obliterated. Hands are fixed in flexion contracture, and ulcerations at pressure points over knuckles and finger tips are not uncommon. Involvement includes forearms, face, neck, and thorax with remarkable sparing of breasts. The legs and feet are rarely involved to the same degree, but brawny thickening of the thighs and lower legs announces the diagnosis there. From ulceration of the fingerpads, scleroderma can progress to autoamputation of distal fingers. Synovitis is never proliferative or destructive; joints cannot move because the skin is fixed to the underlying fascia.

RAYNAUD'S SYNDROME

Raynaud's syndrome is commonly associated with scleroderma, SLE, and mixed connective tissue disease but not with RA. The symptoms of migraine headaches and irritable bowel are linked with Raynaud's symptoms more often than in the rest of the population. Raynaud's phenomenon is a prototype for peripheral microvascular disease and hyperreactivity to vasoconstrictive stimuli such as cold.[2] *Cold hands* are not a sufficient symptom to make this diagnosis. The triad of blanching of the fingers (and less often the toes), followed by intense pain in the fingers and a subsequent purple suffusion as the vasospasm subsides should be present to generate a definite diagnosis. Raynaud's symptoms and signs in the absence of any other disease are recognized as Raynaud's disease and appear often in women in their 20s and 30s. In addition, there are certain other diseases as well as drugs that can generate the same symptoms. For example, cryoglobulins or other abnormal proteins can generate Raynaud's syndrome by interfering with small vessel blood flow to digits. Endothelial injury by stimuli such as repetitive vibration (e.g., use of a jackhammer on a daily basis), atheroemboli, and vasculo-occlusive disease caused by excessive smoking (Buerger's disease) can present as symptoms of Raynaud's syndrome. Cocaine abuse, amphetamines, and ergotamine generate Raynaud's symptoms.

Every primary care physician should learn to use the +40 lens of the ophthalmoscope to examine the skin at the nail bed for evidence of microvascular disease. The capillaries there, in contrast to any other area of skin, are parallel to the surface of the skin rather than perpendicular to it. Raynaud's patients who are destined to progress to scleroderma or SLE are likely to have dilation of capillary loops in the nailbed and small areas of *dropout* where there are no visible capillaries (Fig. 28–1). The management of Raynaud's signs and symptoms is as follows:

- The patient should be continually monitored for evidence of systemic disease. As long as none is apparent, the patient can be reassured that the problem is underestandably a bothersome one but localized.
- Preventive medicine should be emphasized. Because stress and cold are most often linked to precipitating attacks of digital vasospasm, the patient must make a strong effort to avoid these. Keeping core body tem-

Table 28–1. COMPARISON OF THE TWO FORMS OF SCLERODERMA

	Limited (CREST)	Diffuse (Systemic)
Raynaud's	100%	Majority
Skin/mucous membranes	Involvement of hands and forearms, telangiectasis	Hands, forearms, upper arms, face, chest, back, abdomen, legs, pigmentation change, sicca syndrome
Lungs	Pulmonary hypertension, interstitial fibrosis	Interstitial fibrosis
Heart	Pulmonary hypertension	Myocardial fibrosis, conduction disturbance, pericardial disease
Gastrointestinal	Reflux/dysphagia, esophageal dysmotility, small bowel involvement, primary biliary cirrhosis	Reflux/dysphagia, dysmotility, small and large bowel involvement, bowel obstruction, pseudo-diverticuli
Renal	Rare involvement	Renal crisis, microangiopathic hypertension, hemolysis
Mortality	Low initially (30% at 10 y); later stages increased risk of organ involvement; mortality similar to diffuse disease at later stages	High initially (50% at 10 years); later stages decreased risk of organ involvement
Laboratory tests	Anticentromere	Anti-Scl 70

perature warm, using gloves for cold tasks such as taking bottles out of the refrigerator, managing stress, and exploiting techniques such as biofeedback are all important. Patients with digital ulcers must learn to keep them relatively sterile with weak hydrogen peroxide solutions and protective bandages with topical antibiotics.

• Rheumatologists often titrate smooth muscle relaxation with drugs such as long-acting calcium channel blockers (e.g., nifedipine, diltiazem) and clonidine and use iloprost, a prostacyclin analogue, in severe cases that have early digital ulceration, but data are not optimistic that it provides benefit.[3] Nitroglycerin paste may help generate some peripheral arteriole dilation.

SCLERODERMA

The broad diagnosis of scleroderma (also known as *systemic sclerosis*) has many different expressions. It is

$\frac{1}{10}$ to $\frac{1}{20}$ as common as rheumatoid arthritis, and, similar to rheumatoid arthritis has its highest incidence in late middle age. Women are more often afflicted than men.

Clinically, scleroderma is a fascinating mixture of vascular and fibrotic signs and symptoms. The vascular symptoms include not only Raynaud's syndrome, but also neurovascular disease manifested as diminished esophageal and other gastrointestinal organ motility and demonstrably diminished renal cortical and coronary blood flow in response to cold stimuli. At the same time, virtually every organ in scleroderma except the brain can develop increased deposition of connective tissue that can interfere with function. In the lungs, interstitial fibrosis impairs diffusion of oxygen; within the heart, fibrosis leads to aberrant conduction (including, occasionally, fatal arrhythmias) and diminished cardiac output. The combination of fibrosis and an impaired neurovascular supply can lead to diminished, even absent, motility of the esophagus and small and large intestines.

The pathophysiology of scleroderma, with this in-

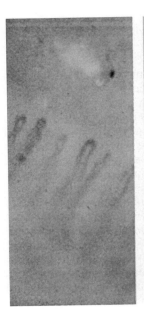
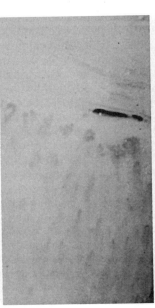
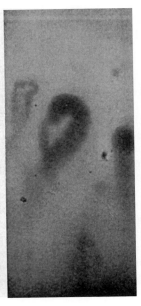

Figure 28–1. Nail fold capillary loop photography. On the left are the delicate and symmetric hairpin loops of normal nail fold circulation. The center photograph reveals tortuosity and redundancy of multiple capillary loops and might be encountered in both systemic sclerosis and other connective tissue disorders. The right photograph reveals disease-specific changes of systemic sclerosis, including a paucity of capillary loops and a single loop with gross dilation of both the venular and arteriolar limbs. (From Dieppe PA, et al: Scleroderma, dermatomyositis and polymyositis. In: Slide Atlas of Rheumatology. London, Gower Medical, 1986. Courtesy of Dr. M. F. R. Martin.)

triguing mixture of microvascular pathology and fibrosis, has led to many hypotheses and both basic and clinical studies to identify the initiating factors. So far, only intriguing hypotheses abound. There is evidence that there are circulating molecules that damage endothelial cells, that fibroblasts from scleroderma generate more collagen per unit of DNA than do normal cells, and that cytokines such as the fibrosis-inducing transforming growth factor-β are produced in excess quantity. One report implicates antiendothalial cell antibodies that induce apoptosis in pathogenesis. The best evidence suggests that scleroderma is *not* related to silicone breast implants.[6] Although it begins most often as puffy hands and Raynaud's syndrome, diffuse cutaneous fibrosis or isolated internal organ involvement can be the presenting symptoms of true scleroderma.

CREST SYNDROME

CREST syndrome is a variant of scleroderma, is also known as *limited cutaneous scleroderma*, and is a syndrome important to recognize.[7] The most important aspect of CREST syndrome is that it has a lower mortality than does diffuse scleroderma, but it carries significant morbidity. The heart, gastrointestinal tract (other than the esophagus), and kidneys are rarely involved. Rather than interstitial fibrosis in the lungs, CREST patients are at risk for development of pulmonary hypertension. Many CREST patients have circulating anticentromere antibodies but do not have the speckled antinuclear antibody pattern and antitopoisomerase I (anti-scl 70) antibodies that are present in diffuse scleroderma. Scleroderma patients also have antinucleolar antibodies directed against RNA polymerases and other large aggregate nuclear proteins. Limited scleroderma (CREST) has a much lower mortality rate than the diffuse variant, at least in the early years of the disease.

OTHER SYNDROMES SIMILAR TO SCLERODERMA

Localized Scleroderma

Localized scleroderma is a rare syndrome that is usually localized to a specific skin site and without diffuse organ involvement and can be recognized by thickened bound-down skin that is similar to what scleroderma would be on multiple sites. In severe cases, appearing in childhood, the fibrosis of the skin can extend down into fascia and muscle, causing hemiatrophy.

Fasciitis With Eosinophilia

Fasciitis with eosinophilia, brought on more than occasionally by vigorous muscular exertion, is characterized by swelling and stiffness of extremities (sometimes asymmetric) related to a combination of subcutaneous inflammation with mononuclear cells and eosinophils, edema, and some fibrosis. The result of this is skin that looks like an orange peel, with dermal rete pegs being held down to the fascia by bounds while the surrounding skin expands from inflammation and edema.[8] Circulating eosinophil counts are high, as is the sedimentation rate. None of the organ fibrosis or microvascular pathology is seen. In contrast to scleroderma, fasciitis with eosinophilia has temporal associations with aplastic anemia and some leukemias and lymphomas. Glucocorticoid therapy usually generates a remission, and methotrexate has been used effectively in several cases.

Epidemic Syndromes Resembling Scleroderma

There have been two syndromes that were caused by ingested toxins in the environment. Both generated an acute febrile syndrome that was followed in many cases by chronic painful neuropathy, scleroderma-like thickening of the skin, and other changes ranging from myalgias to neuropsychiatric symptoms and signs. One was the *toxic oil syndrome* induced in thousands of Spaniards within several weeks early in the 1980s.[9] These people had ingested rapeseed oil containing toxic metabolites of aniline left after inadequate distillation.

The second syndrome was *eosinophilia-myalgia syndrome*. This condition appears to have been caused by a toxin generated during preparation of the amino acid L-tryptophan, which was a popular remedy for insomnia, fatigue, and depression.[10] Although new cases of these toxic reactions are not likely to be found, it is likely that as yet unknown and unanticipated toxins will, in the future, be ingested and cause similar syndromes. Any patient who presents to the primary care physician with a complicated febrile illness that includes myalgias and eosinophilia must be questioned extensively about what he or she has ingested in preceding days and weeks.

DIAGNOSIS OF SCLERODERMA

The diagnosis of scleroderma and its variant syndromes can be a challenge to primary care physicians, in part because therapy is so difficult. Once the diagnosis is made, consultation with an experienced rheumatologist should be made soon and day-to-day management carried out by this team. Patients presenting with Raynaud's phenomenon, the *puffy hand* syndrome, and virtually any undiagnosed polyarthritis should have scleroderma included in the differential diagnosis. Brawny edema of hands and forearms with minimal synovitis makes scleroderma more likely than if the patient has exuberant synovitis with minimal skin involvement. As mentioned previously, the primary care physician should feel comfortable with use of the +40 lens of the ophthalmoscope to examine nail bed capillaries. Listening with the stethoscope over tendon sheaths can, on occasion, reward the physician with the sound of tendon friction rubs.

Changes in the skin usually become apparent first in the fingers and hands. As the skin begins to thicken, the dorsal surface of the fingers begins to look shiny and tight leading to sclerodactyly. There may be loss of hair growth as well as loss of the pulp from the finger pads at the distal ends of the fingers. The skin may further crack and fissure. In some patients, digital infarction and tissue necrosis take place. The skin tightening in the hands usually progresses more proximally to involve the forearms. At this point, the skin manifestations diverge between limited and diffuse systemic sclerosis. With limited disease, skin findings do not progress beyond the forearms. However, in diffuse disease, there can be either rapid or gradual spread of skin thickening to the upper arms, face, torso, abdomen, and legs. Often the progression of skin disease in diffuse scleroderma subsides within the first few years of the disease, and the patient may have some mild improvement. Limited scleroderma, although less diffuse and often less severe, continues to progress slowly over time. Patients often are unable to flex their fingers fully early in the disease or to extend them fully (the *prayer sign*) (Fig. 28–2).

Occasionally, scleroderma is symptomatic first in other organs, hence the synonym, *systemic sclerosis*. The physician should pursue any symptoms or signs in the following organs if the disease is suspected.

Gastrointestinal Tract

Until asked, a narrowing of the mouth aperture is often overlooked by patients (Fig. 28–3). Dysphagia (especially for bulky or dry foods), heartburn, abdominal bloating, constipation, or other changes in bowel function can be an indication that there are neurovascular abnormalities becoming symptomatic. Cine barium swallows or isotope labeling and detection by scanning can demonstrate diminished esophageal motility. Occasionally, dysmotility of the small bowel may be the first manifestation of scleroderma, other than Raynaud's phenomenon. Bowel obstruction with hypoactive rather than hyperactive bowel sounds should be a trigger to put scleroderma in the differential diagnosis. The finding of wide-mouth false diverticula in the large bowel by barium enema is characteristic of this disease.

Cardiopulmonary System

The lungs rarely are involved early in scleroderma. The exceptions to this are a nonproductive cough and pleurisy, an early symptom of pleural inflammation that also is noted in SLE, dermatomyositis and polymyositis, and rheumatoid arthritis. Characteristics of the pleural fluid are those of mild inflammation. Other more insidious symptoms include progressive dyspnea on exertion not related to any cardiac problems. In addition to a routine chest radiograph, rheumatologists may request high-resolution computed tomography in search of the *ground-glass* appearance of alveolar inflammation that precedes fibrosis.[11] In the pulmonary function laboratory, a diminished carbon monoxide diffusion capacity is the first sign of interstitial fibrosis that impedes normal diffusion of oxygen that eventually can lead to hypoxemia, cyanosis, and death. Smoking cessation is mandatory for every patient with scleroderma. Routine use of pulmonary function testing remains an initial tool for evaluation and serial assessment.

Myocardial involvement in scleroderma is a microvascular one, producing occasional arrhythmias and tachycardia. It may progress to patchy then generalized myocardial fibrosis without classic angina pectoris. The electrocardiogram can reveal both supraventricular and ventricular arrhythmias before diminished voltage appears. Although echocardiography can show pericardial fluid and, later, pericardial thickening, these findings are not often symptomatic. In the limited versions of scleroderma (e.g., CREST), pulmonary hypertension

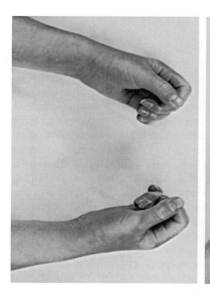
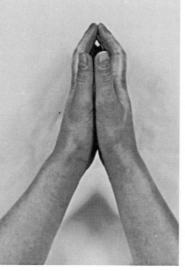

Figure 28–2. The hands of a young woman with several months of rapidly progressive scleroderma. The skin is taut and indurated, and there is limitation of both fist closure and finger extension. (From Seibold JR: Scleroderma. In Kelley WN, Harris ED Jr, Ruddy S, Sledge CB, eds: Textbook of Rheumatology, 5th ed. Philadelphia, WB Saunders, 1997, p 1136.)

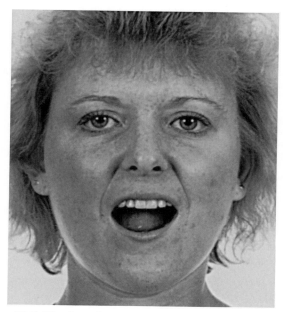

Figure 28–3. The face of a young woman with several months of rapidly progressive scleroderma. The facial skin is taut with an immobile facies and limitation of the oral aperture. (From Seibold JR: Scleroderma. In Kelley WN, Harris ED Jr, Ruddy S, Sledge CB, eds: Textbook of Rheumatology, 5th ed. Philadelphia, WB. Saunders, 1997, p 1136.)

leading to cor pulmonale can complicate the course of disease.

Kidney

The only significant triumph in management of scleroderma came with the aggressive treatment of hypertension in this disease. The pathophysiology appears to be clear: There is intimal proliferation of small renal arterioles that leads to ischemia exacerbated by vasoconstriction associated with Raynaud's phenomenon. This ischemia produces accelerated hypertension fueled by hyperreninemia leading to excess of angiotensin II. Renal failure followed soon in these individuals, and before 1980, there was no effective therapy. The development of angiotensin-converting enzyme inhibitors facilitated control and stability of this process for the first time.[12] The renal failure can be avoided if aggressive therapy is begun before the creatinine levels exceed 4.0 mg/dL. Careful urinalyses and frequent checks of blood pressure are essential for monitoring every scleroderma patient, especially during the first few years of presentation when patients are at the highest risk for developing renal involvement.

Hematoimmunologic Parameters

As with most patients with chronic disease, those with scleroderma have a mild hypochromic microcytic anemia. Erythrocyte sedimentation rates are mildly elevated but not as high as in active SLE, rheumatoid arthritis, or vasculitis. Peripheral blood smears of those with active disease can show fragmented red blood cells, broken by passage through damaged capillaries and arterioles. Scleroderma can be associated with myositis and elevated creatinine kinase levels. Other laboratory values are generally normal.

Most patients with scleroderma have significant titers of antinuclear antibodies. Anti-DNA antibodies are not present. About 20% can have antiribonuclear protein antibodies, rheumatoid factor, or both. Anti-centromere antibodies are positive in most patients with limited scleroderma but in only 10% of those with systemic sclerosis. Of those with systemic disease 20% to 40% have antibodies against DNA topoisomerase I, an intracellular enzyme that helps uncoil supercoiled DNA.

TREATMENT OF SCLERODERMA

Effective therapy in scleroderma is a challenge because no drug or other modality has been shown to reverse the deposition of excessive connective tissue or to repopulate tissue with normal microvasculature.[1, 13] Glucocorticoids, for example, effective in modulating symptoms and signs of SLE, are generally ineffective in scleroderma and may increase the risk of developing renal crisis. Cytotoxic drugs are of limited value except in the early stages of lung disease detected by high-resolution computed tomography scanning when cyclophosphamide can retard progression of the process. Prednisone, cyclophosphamide, azathioprine, apheresis, interferon-γ, and other modalities have not survived close investigations in clinical trials. D-Penicillamine may improve skin involvement, but there is no evidence that it improves vascular and immunologic features of the disease. Management of the hypertensive renal disease has been described in the section on renal disease in these patients.

Perhaps the best help for these patients is the supportive care of their physicians. Patients should be advised to take good care of their skin and hands. Early initiation of hand therapy (range-of-motion, stretching) and avoidance of skin infection may help prolong function and limit the severity of contracture. Paraffin wax treatments usually provide symptomatic benefit for patients. Occasionally the use of static or dynamic splints on the hands, especially at night, may help maintain function. Similar range-of-motion and stretching exercises should be employed for the face so as to limit the loss of oral aperture. H_2 blockers and proton-pump inhibitors can minimize reflux of gastric acid into the esophagus, as can elevating the head of the bed. Early referral to a qualified gastroenterologist can help in management. Broad-spectrum antibiotics can inhibit the blind loop syndrome with bacterial overgrowth that leads to malabsorption. Pulmonary hypertension is now best treated with intravenous infusions of vasodilatory prostaglandins. It is appropriate to enter patients with early pulmonary involvement in therapeutic trials of cytotoxic and other drugs now ongoing at many academic medical centers.

REFERENCES

1. Seibold JR: Scleroderma. In Kelley WN, Harris ED Jr, Ruddy S, Sledge CB, eds: Textbook of Rheumatology, 5th ed. Philadelphia, WB Saunders, 1997, pp 1133–1162.
2. Herrick AL, Clark S: Quantifying digital vascular disease in patients with primary Raynaud's phenomenon and systemic sclerosis. Ann Rheum Dis 57: 70–78, 1998.
3. Wigley FM, Korn JH, Csuka ME, et al: Oral iloprost treatment in patients with Raynaud's phenomenon secondary to systemic sclerosis: A multicenter, placebo-controlled, double-blind study. Arthritis Rheum 41: 670–677, 1998.
4. Bordron A, Dueymes M, Levy Y, et al: The binding of some human antiendothelial cell bodies induces endothelial cell apoptosis. J Clin Invest 101: 2029–2035, 1998.
5. Weinzweig J, Schnur PL, McConnell JP, et al: Silicon analysis of breast and capsular tissue from patients with saline or silicone gel breast implants: II. Correlation with connective-tissue disease. Plast Reconstr Surg 101:1836–1841, 1998.
6. Sergent JS, Fuchs H, Johnson JS: Silicone breast implants and rheumatic diseases. In Kelley WN, Harris ED Jr, Ruddy S, Sledge CB, eds: Textbook of Rheumatology, 5th ed. Philadelphia, WB Saunders, 1997, pp 1169–1176.
7. Steen VD: Clinical manifestations of systemic sclerosis. Semin Cutan Med Surg 17:48–54, 1998.
8. Varga J, Kahari VM: Eosinophilia-myalgia syndrome, eosinophilic fasciitis, and related fibrosing disorders. Curr Opin Rheumatol 9:562–570, 1997.
9. Tabuenca JM: Toxic-allergic syndrome caused by ingestion of rapeseed oil denatured with aniline. Lancet 2:567, 1981.
10. Martin RW, Duffy J, Engel AG, et al: The clinical spectrum of the eosinophilia-myalgia syndrome associated with L-tryptophan ingestion: Clinical features in 20 patients and aspects of pathophysiology. Ann Intern Med 113:124, 1990.
11. Seely JM, Jones LT, Wallace C, et al: Systemic sclerosis: Using high-resolution CT to detect lung disease in children. AJR Am J Roentgenol 170:691–697, 1998.
12. Steen VD: Scleroderma in renal crisis. Rheum Dis Clin North Am 22:861–878, 1996.
13. Pope JE: Treatment of systemic sclerosis. Rheum Dis Clin North Am 22:893–907.

Chapter 29

Inflammatory and Noninflammatory Myopathies: Clinicopathologic Features and Treatment

Ronald F. van Vollenhoven ∎ Nisha J. Manek

Patients presenting with complaints of weakness or muscle pain are common in clinical practice. Patients often present with other nonspecific signs and symptoms, such as fatigue, fever, and malaise, resulting in misdiagnoses and delays in therapy.[1] Because the differential diagnosis of muscle complaints is quite large, a number of disorders should be carefully considered. An appropriate evaluation must include a directed history, physical examination, and laboratory tests. These are described in this chapter with a major focus on the *inflammatory myopathies*, or myositis.

Myositis is a general term indicating muscle inflammation. The cause may be known (viral, bacterial, parasitic, or toxic) or unknown (idiopathic). The idiopathic forms of myositis form a heterogeneous group of subacute and chronic muscle disorders, sharing a common characteristic feature: muscle degeneration mediated by an inflammatory process. Two other conditions commonly presenting to the primary physician with muscle weakness, pain, or both are *polymyalgia rheumatica* and *fibromyalgia*, and these must be differentiated from myositis. These two conditions are covered in more detail in Chapters 18, 19, and 24. The *muscular dystrophies* and *metabolic myopathies* are uncommon conditions that can also cause subacute or chronic muscle weakness and sometimes pain as well.

CLASSIFICATION AND PATHOGENESIS

An inherent difficulty in classifying the inflammatory myopathies is that sharp boundaries do not exist among many of the syndromes that result in muscle weakness, and a number of classification systems have been proposed. The criteria for the diagnosis of polymyositis and dermatomyositis proposed by Bohan and Peter in 1975[2] remain useful today (Table 29–1). After excluding other causes of myopathy, the presence of the following criteria usually establishes a diagnosis of inflammatory myopathy: the findings of proximal muscle weakness, elevated serum levels of sarcoplasmic enzymes, myopathic changes on electromyography, and muscle biopsy specimens showing myofiber degeneration and regeneration with chronic inflammatory infiltrates (and in the case of dermatomyositis, the presence of a typical rash).

Table 29–2 presents the most widely used clinicopathologic classification of myositis. Other rare forms of myositis, such as granulomatous, eosinophilic, ocular, and focal myositis, have also been described.[3] Polymyositis or dermatomyositis in association with other connective tissue diseases is usually characterized by less severe myositis.

The histopathology of the affected muscle provides strong evidence that the inflammatory myopathies have an immune-mediated pathogenesis.[4] In dermatomyositis, the muscle is infiltrated by activated CD4+ T lymphocytes and B lymphocytes. A vasculopathy, but not true vasculitis, is present and results in muscle ischemia and perifascicular atrophy, a diagnostic feature of dermatomyositis (Fig. 29–1).

In polymyositis, the cellular infiltrate is mainly composed of CD8+ T cells and macrophages. Muscle cell degeneration and necrosis are present (Fig. 29–2). The *trigger* for this autoimmune process is unknown, but viruses, including retroviruses, are suspected.

In contrast to the inflammatory myopathies, muscle biopsy specimens in polymyalgia rheumatica and fibromyalgia tend to be normal. The former condition is most likely an inflammatory disorder with some etiologic similarities to rheumatoid arthritis, whereas fibromyalgia is believed by many to be a disorder of pain processing or pain perception. The metabolic myopathies and muscular dystrophies are largely genetically predetermined diseases, although the clinical manifestations may not become apparent until early adulthood. The histopathology reveals diagnostic abnormalities of the muscle fibers in these cases.

Table 29–1. CRITERIA FOR THE DIAGNOSIS OF IDIOPATHIC INFLAMMATORY MYOPATHY[*]

1. Symmetric weakness, usually progressive, of the limb-girdle muscles and anterior neck flexors.
2. Muscle biopsy evidence of myositis:
   Necrosis of type I and type II muscle fibers, phagocytosis, degeneration and regeneration of myofibers with variation in myofiber size. Endomysial, perimysial, or interstitial mononuclear cells.
3. Elevation of serum levels of muscle-associated enzymes:
   Creatine kinase
   Aldolase
   Lactate dehydrogenase
   Transaminases (ALT/SGPT and AST/SGOT)
4. Electromyographic triad of myositis:
   Short, small, low-amplitude polyphasic motor unit potentials
   Fibrillation potentials, even at rest
   Bizarre high-frequency repetitive discharges

[*]In patients in whom all known causes of myopathy have been excluded.
Definite idiopathic inflammatory myopathy = 4 of the above criteria or 4 of the above including the rash for dermatomyositis.
Probable idiopathic inflammatory myopathy = 3 of the above criteria or 3 of the above including the rash for dermatomyositis.
Possible idiopathic inflammatory myopathy = 2 of the above criteria or 2 of the above including the rash for dermatomyositis.
ALT/SGPT, alanine aminotransferase/serum glutamic-pyruvic transaminase; AST/SGOT, aspartate aminotransferase/serum glutamic-oxaloacetic transaminase.
Bohan A, Peter JB: Polymyositis and dermatomyositis (parts 1 and 2). N Engl J Med; 292:344–347, 403–407; 1975.

MYOSITIS: CLINICAL PRESENTATION AND NATURAL COURSE OF THE DISEASE

The onset of inflammatory myopathy can be acute, subacute, or insidious.[5] There is symmetric muscle weakness, which, in contrast to the muscular dystrophies, usually progresses over weeks to months, rather than years. Muscle pain is less prominent than is weakness. Patients may complain of difficulty in rising from a chair or climbing stairs. There is also a predilection for weakness in the neck flexors. Systemic symptoms, such as fatigue, morning stiffness, and anorexia, may accompany the weakness. As the disease progresses, dysphagia may develop, and eventually the respiratory muscles may be affected. Difficulty lifting one's head off the pillow indicates significant neck flexor weakness. Asking the patient to rise from a chair with arms outstretched identifies proximal lower limb muscle weakness. Distal muscle strength is usually preserved. Facial muscles are typically uninvolved. The deep tendon reflexes are maintained. Muscle atrophy may not occur until late in the course of the illness. Frank arthritis should alert one to the possibility of an overlap syndrome.

The *skin* lesions of dermatomyositis are manifest as erythema accompanied by edema of the subcutaneous tissue, particularly in the periorbital, perioral,

Table 29–2. CLINICOPATHOLOGIC CLASSIFICATION OF THE INFLAMMATORY MYOPATHIES

Clinicopathologic Category	Associations and Comments
Primary idiopathic polymyositis	A diagnosis of exclusion—defined by the absence of all the features below; muscle biopsy shows endomysial infiltration, primarily CD8$^+$ cells
Primary idiopathic dermatomyositis	Heliotrope rash or Gottron's papules present; myositis may be clinically absent. Muscle biopsy shows microvascular changes and deposits of the membrane attack complex and prominent perivascular CD4$^+$ T cells and B cells
Myositis associated with another connective tissue disease	Mild myositis, good response to therapy; rheumatoid arthritis, systemis sclerosis, and lupus most common overlaps
Juvenile myositis	Frequent calcifications, gastrointestinal vasculitis
Myositis associated with malignancy	Myositis onset often within 2 years of the diagnosis of cancer
Inclusion body myositis	Occurs mainly in older white men with insidious onset and progression and poor response to therapy; characteristic rimmed vacuoles in myofibers.

Modified from Miller FW: Classification and prognosis of inflammatory muscle disease. Rheum Dis Clin North Am 20:811–826, 1994.

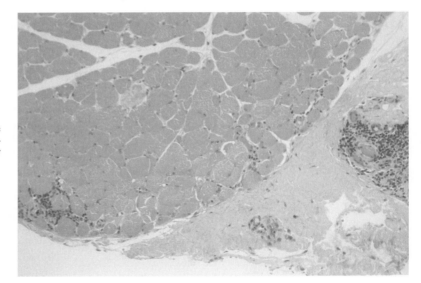

Figure 29–1. Transverse section of a fresh frozen muscle biopsy specimen from a patient with adult dermatomyositis. (H&E, ×420). *Note* the perifascicular atrophy and the area of perivascular infiltrate.

malar, anterior neck, and upper chest regions (V sign), and erythematous, flat, or raised lesions overlying the extensor surfaces of the small joints of the fingers (Gottron's lesions or papules). Additional signs are dilated capillary loops at the base of the fingernails and rough, cracked fingers with dirty irregular lines (*mechanic's hands*).

Myositis ranges in severity from mild to severe and even life-threatening, the last-mentioned in some instances despite appropriate therapy. Serious morbidity and mortality in myositis usually relate to respiratory compromise because of the combined effects of respiratory muscle weakness (decreased volumes and poor clearing of airways), upper esophageal involvement with reflux and aspiration, and interstitial lung disease resulting from the illness itself. Increasingly, treatment-related mortality from opportunistic infections is seen, and iatrogenic morbidity, particularly secondary to the use of corticosteroids, may dominate the clinical picture late in the disease course.

DIFFERENTIAL DIAGNOSIS

The differential diagnosis for muscle pain and weakness is wide (Table 29–3). Certain findings should make one cautious about rendering a diagnosis of inflammatory myopathy; these include evidence for central or peripheral neurologic diseases, such as motor neuron disorders with fasciculations. A family history of muscle disorders or calf enlargement suggests a muscular dystrophy.

The drug-induced causes of myopathy warrant special emphasis because they are often overlooked.[6] Recognition of this possibility is essential because a myopathy that is drug induced usually is cured or significantly improved by discontinuing the offending medication. A salutary lesson was learned from the syndrome characterized by eosinophilia and profound myalgia that emerged in the late 1980s and was found to be due to contaminated batches of the health food supplement L-tryptophan. Even after discontinuation of tryptophan,

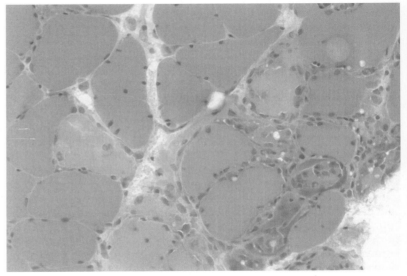

Figure 29–2. Transverse section of a fresh frozen muscle biopsy specimen from a patient with polymyositis. (H&E, ×640) *Note* endomysial inflammation and lymphoid cells surrounding or beginning to invade healthy muscle cells.

Table 29–3. DIFFERENTIAL DIAGNOSIS OF INFLAMMATORY MYOPATHY

Toxic Myopathies

Alcohol (ethanol)
Chloroquine
Cholesterol-lowering agents
Cimetidine
Cocaine
Colchicine
Glucocorticoids
Ipecac
Penicillamine
Procainamide
Zidovudine (AZT)

Infections

Viral (influenza, Epstein-Barr virus, human immunodeficiency virus, coxsackie)
Bacterial (staphyloccoci, streptococci, clostridia, others)
Parasitic (toxoplasmosis, trichinosis, schistosomiasis, cysticercosis)
Envenomation by certain snakes

Endocrine Disorders

Hypothyroidism
Hyperthyroidism
Cushing's syndrome
Addison's disease
Hyperparathyroidism or hypoparathyroidism
Diabetes mellitus

Neuromuscular Disorders

Muscular dystrophies
Myotonic dystrophies
Spinal muscular atrophy
Myasthenia gravis and the Lambert-Eaton syndrome
Amyotrophic lateral sclerosis
Neuropathies: Guillain-Barré syndrome, prophyria, diabetes mellitus

Metabolic Myopathies

Mitochondrial myopathies
Disorders of carbohydrate metabolism: McArdle's disease
Adult acid maltase deficiency and others
Disorders of lipid metabolism: carnitine deficiency
Disorders of purine metabolism: myoadenylate deaminase deficiency

Electrolyte Disorders

Hypokalemia
Hypocalcemia
Hypercalcemia
Hypomagnesemia

Miscellaneous

Polymyalgia rheumatica
Sarcoidosis, Crohn's disease
Autoimmune diseases: systemic lupus crythematosus, Sjögren's syndrome, mixed connective tissue disease
Paraneoplastic neuromyopathy
Eosinophilia myalgia syndrome

muscular symptoms often persisted.[7] Colchicine, used for the treatment of gout, can cause myositis, particularly in patients with renal disease. Several lipid-lowering drugs, including the *statin* drugs (hydroxy methyl glutaryl–coenzyme A reductase inhibitors), gemfibrozil, nicotinic acid, and clofibrate, can induce a reversible myopathy characterized by proximal limb weakness, myalgia, elevated creatine kinase (CK), levels and myopathic changes on electromyogram (EMG). Zidovudine can cause a myopathy with ragged red fibers on muscle biopsy.[8]

An association of human immunodeficiency virus (HIV) infection with true polymyositis was first noted in 1983 and since has been confirmed by a number of reports.[9] HIV infection can also cause a heterogeneous group of noninflammatory destructive myopathies. HIV infection may predispose to other infections that might cause myositis, including infections with bacteria, protozoans, and mycobacteria. Pyomyositis is an increasingly recognized infection of the striated muscle in HIV-infected patients, especially with *Staphylococcus aureus*.

APPROACH TO THE PATIENT WITH MUSCLE WEAKNESS

Muscle pain and weakness are common complaints, but a careful history and physical examination can allow the clinician to obtain the necessary laboratory data and ancillary studies in the appropriate setting. Table 29–4 delineates some of the main features of the inflammatory myopathies (myositis), the metabolic myopathies, and muscular dystrophies, polymyalgia rheumatica, and fibromyalgia, as they may become apparent from an initial evaluation.

History

A careful and directed history is imperative. This history should include a family history; associated symptoms; and exposures to raw meat, toxins, or drugs. The age and gender of the patient are important: A younger man developing insidious muscle weakness with little or no pain may have an inherited disorder of muscle metabolism (metabolic myopathy or muscular dystrophy), in which case the family history can be revealing. The more sudden development in the younger patient of profound muscle weakness as well as pain, especially when associated with signs of systemic inflammatory illness, such as fever, weight loss, and general malaise, is much more suggestive of a form of myositis.

In women in their 20s and 30s, fibromyalgia is a common disorder characterized by widespread muscular pain; the weakness in this disease is mostly subjective due to the pain, rather than true muscle weakness. In patients older than age 50, myositis remains a possibility (in this age group, the association with malignancy must be considered), but another important diagnostic consideration is polymyalgia rheumatica. Associated features that should raise the suspicion of the latter are severe and disabling muscular pain, symptoms consistent with temporal arteritis, or symptoms suggestive of rheumatoid arthritis. Nevertheless, differentiating these two conditions may require nerve conduction studies, muscle biopsy, or both. An assessment of the degree to which the patient is impaired by symptoms is indicated, and the health assessment questionaire gives invaluable information as to current functional status. In particular, this questionnaire can help detect the impact of disease activity in terms of activities of daily living.

Table 29–4. CLINICAL AND LABORATORY FINDINGS IN COMMON MYOPATHIC SYNDROMES

	Pain	Weakness	CK Levels	ESR	EMG/NCS	Biopsy
Myositis	++	+++	↑↑	↑	Myopathic (sometimes diagnostic)	Diagnostic
Polymyalgia rheumatica	+++	+	—	↑	Normal	Normal
Muscular dystrophy and metabolic myopathy	+/−	+++	↑/—	—	Myopathic	Diagnostic
Fibromyalgia	+++	+/−	—	—	Normal	Normal

CK, creatine kinase; ESR, erythrocyte sedimentation rate; EMG/NCS, electromyography/nerve conduction studies.

Physical Examination

The affected muscle groups should be examined. Strength is difficult to quantify, but an impression of whether actual muscle weakness exists should be recorded. The degree to which proximal and distal muscles are affected should be compared. Muscle tone and bulk must be noted. Examination of the muscles should also include the tender points characteristic of fibromyalgia (see Chapters 3 and 18). The temporal arteries should be palpated to detect evidence for giant cell arteritis. The joints should be examined for concurrent arthritis, and a neurologic examination can provide evidence for a neurogenic cause by showing abnormal fasciculations, areflexia, or cogwheeling. Skin changes suggestive of dermatomyositis should be noted. If myositis is suspected, the lung examination may reveal fine dry crackles in the lower lobes indicating interstitial lung disease related to the autoimmune process.

Laboratory Tests

Laboratory tests play an important role in establishing a diagnosis in patients with muscle weakness. The initial evaluation should include an electrolyte panel, liver panel, a complete blood count, thyroid function tests, erythrocyte sedimentation rate (ESR), and CK. Total CK is most widely used to follow patients with myositis because of its high degree of sensitivity, relative muscle specificity, and good correlation with disease activity and muscle strength.[10] A small percent of patients have normal CK levels at the time of presentation, possibly related to the presence of inhibitors of CK enzyme activity in serum.[11] Serum aldolase concentration is elevated in myositis, but it is not a muscle-specific enzyme and may be elevated in other disorders, such as hepatic disease and hemolytic anemia. Aminotransferases may be elevated as an indication of muscle inflammation. These may be mistakenly attributed to hepatic disease rather than underlying muscle inflammation, and patients have been inappropriately subjected to a liver biopsy. Based on nature and severity of symptoms, an electrocardiogram, chest radiograph, pulmonary function tests, and fluoroscopic swallowing studies may need to be done.

Ninety percent of patients with myositis have autoantibodies to cellular antigens. Fluorescent antinuclear antibody test is the most frequent autoantibody test seen in inflammatory myopathy. It is usually a speckled pattern, although any other pattern can also be present. Rheumatoid factor is present in 20% of patients. Antibodies to extractable nuclear antigens (anti-RNP, anti-Smith, anti-Ro, anti-La) should also be sent; these may occur in myositis but have a primary association with other conditions and suggest an overlap syndrome. A group of antibodies directed against tRNA-related enzymes is found uniquely in myositis, and these are sometimes summarized as myositis-specific antibodies (MSA): they include antibodies such as anti-Jo, which can be ordered clinically, and a large number of antibodies that are available only in research laboratories. Each of the MSAs is found in only a small proportion of patients. An individual patient has only one MSA; therefore MSAs define subgroups of patients (Table 29–5). Although the MSAs are of considerable theoretical importance, their clinical utility remains limited at this time.

Nerve conduction studies and EMG are performed to distinguish neuropathies from myopathies. In myositis, a characteristic pattern of excessive spontaneous activity and polyphasic potentials of short duration and

Table 29–5. AUTOANTIBODIES IN POLYMYOSITIS AND DERMATOMYOSITIS

Antisynthetase (includes anti-Jo-1 antibody)	Seen in 20–25% of all myositis cases. High frequency of nonerosive arthritis, interstitial lung disease, fever, mechanic's hands, Raynaud's phenomenon; acute severe myositis with onset in spring. Moderate response to therapy
Anti-signal recognition particle (SRP)	Seen in <5% of myositis patients. Most often in African-American women. Cardiac involvement with palpitations and myalgias. Acute onset of polymyositis. Poor response to therapy
Anti-Mi-2	Classic dermatomyositis with V sign, shawl sign, and cuticular overgrowth; good response to therapy. Seen in 5%–10% of patients

low amplitude are seen in the acute stage and may in some instances be sufficiently diagnostic for myositis to obviate the need for a biopsy.[12] The use of magnetic resonance imaging (MRI) or magnetic resonance spectroscopy in the evaluation of muscular diseases is limited to research settings at this time.

Muscle biopsy remains the gold standard for the diagnosis of inflammatory myopathy. It is important that the biopsy site be distant from any site of the EMG testing because the needles for EMG testing may induce an inflammatory infiltrate. The biopsy specimen should be interpreted by an experienced neuropathologist.

Additional Work-up

In patients with myositis, the association between dermatomyositis and polymyositis and malignancy needs to be considered. In adults, approximately 25% of patients with dermatomyositis have been reported to have this association. There are no absolute guidelines as to when a search for occult malignancy should be undertaken. Some suggest a careful history and physical examination should be done, including pelvic, rectal, and breast examinations and a chest radiograph.[13] Women should have mammography and perhaps pelvic ultrasonography or serologic markers of malignancy, such as CA-125. Young men should have a careful testicular examination, and older men should be screened for prostate-specific antigen. A sensible rule to follow at the time of diagnosis is to pursue vigorously any abnormalities that turn up that cannot be ascribed to myositis. An unexplained finding, such as weight loss despite glucocorticoid therapy, should prompt a search for occult tumor. Table 29–4 summarizes the main laboratory findings in myopathic conditions.

Referral

Patients with muscular complaints that cannot easily be explained after an initial work-up as outlined should probably be referred to a specialist for a one-time consultation to pursue the diagnostic possibilities. Alternatively, if the diagnosis of myositis has been made or is strongly suspected, a consultation could help in designing the optimal treatment plan. Patients with a relapsing or refractory disease course should likewise be seen by an appropriate specialist.

TREATMENT OF IDIOPATHIC INFLAMMATORY MYOPATHY: POLYMYOSITIS AND DERMATOMYOSITIS

Early diagnosis and therapy offer the best chance for improvement in muscle strength and function, but assessing the effect of therapy may be difficult.[14] Before starting therapy, a patient's clinical status should be evaluated as objectively as possible, including testing strength of individual muscle groups. Stoll and colleagues[15] have attempted to quantify isometric muscle strength using handheld pull-gauge, but none of these methods are widely used. The CK level tends to correlate well with muscle inflammation and is the test recommended for following such patients.

Glucocorticoids

Glucocorticoids remain the agents of choice.[16] Three principles of glucocorticoid therapy predict a favorable biochemical and clinical outcome in the treatment of myositis: (1) administration of an adequate initial glucocorticoid dose, (2) continuation of the initial dose until the time that the serum CK has become normal, and (3) a slow glucocorticoid taper rate. Achievement of a CK level within the low-normal range predicts a prolonged biochemical remission, and a rise of CK, even within the normal range, signals a subsequent biochemical and clinical relapse.[17]

Standard practice is to begin daily oral divided dose therapy (equivalent to 60 mg prednisone) in the typical adult with active myositis. High divided dosing is continued until the serum CK levels fall into the normal range (generally 4 to 8 weeks). Thereafter, prednisone is consolidated to the same single morning dose (i.e., 60 mg) or a lower daily dose (i.e., 15 mg three times daily). Eventually, all patients should have their dose consolidated to once daily, or even every other day, to limit adrenal suppression, and glucocorticoid taper is continued on a monthly basis. Patients are seen monthly, and the serum CK is measured and manual muscle strength assessed. With disease relapse (i.e., worsening weakness and an increase in serum CK), prednisone dosage is increased or an immunosuppressive agent added. A critical factor in management of myositis patients is the recognition that clinical improvement in muscle strength lags behind CK by weeks or even months.[16]

When evaluating a patient whose condition is refractory to treatment, the differential diagnosis for myositis should be reconsidered in the context of the patient's history, including drug history. The most common problem in clinical practice is a superimposed myopathy resulting from the treatment with glucocorticoids. Steroid myopathy occurs unpredictably with longer-term glucocorticoid treatment and can range from mild to severe. Urinary creatine excretion is increased in steroid myopathy and can be used to distinguish this condition from reactivation of myositis.[17] In some difficult cases, a repeat biopsy is needed; steroid myopathy causes a typical pattern of type II muscle fiber atrophy. Whether MRI of the symptomatic muscles can be helpful and cost-effective in these difficult cases is unclear.[18]

Maintenance dosage of prednisone 5 to 10 mg daily is reached after about 6 to 8 months of therapy. Prolonged therapy may be necessary, and generally prednisone is continued until active disease has been suppressed for 1 year or more. Glucocorticoid-related morbidities—infection, osteoporotic compression fractures, and osteonecrosis, to name but a few—are common. All patients should be prescribed calcium and vitamin D supplements.

Pulse Methylprednisolone

The use of high-dose intravenous pulse methylprednisolone has not been studied extensively in adults with myositis but has been used in juvenile myositis.[17] One rationale for the treatment includes a decrease in daily glucocorticoid requirements, a shortened time to clinical response, and usefulness in life-threatening occurrences such as acute dysphagia. Doses range from 500 mg to 1 g/day for 3 days every 2 to 4 weeks.[19]

Immunosuppressive Therapy

Immunosuppressive agents (*second-line agents*) have traditionally been employed in patients with myositis who failed to respond to glucocorticoid therapy. It has been estimated that as many as 40% of patients have glucocorticoid-resistant disease.[20] More recently, it has been argued that those patients whose prognosis is poor (e.g., those who have had symptoms of weakness for more than 9 months before diagnosis or with autoantibodies to aminoacyl-tRNA synthetase) could benefit from addition of a second-line agent at the same time as starting glucocorticoid therapy. Taking this concept one step further, some have advocated addition of an immunosuppressive agent at the time of diagnosis in all patients unless a specific contraindication exists.[19] Because of the rapid rate at which these recommendations are evolving, the complexities of accurately prognosticating myositis, and the inherent challenges of using immunosuppressive medications, referral to a specialist for these patients is almost invariably indicated.

Methotrexate

Methotrexate is a commonly used second-line agent starting at a dose of 7.5 to 10 mg orally weekly. The dose may be increased weekly by 2.5-mg increments up to a maximal tolerated dose of 15 to 25 mg weekly. Higher dosages (>25 mg/week) can be administered as subcutaneous injections. Prednisone is often tapered as the methotrexate is increased, and this combination therapy is continued (at the lowest prednisone dose possible) until weakness and muscle enzymes improve or at least stabilize. At this point, the dosage of methotrexate may be continued for a few months and then slowly tapered watching for clinical and biochemical disease flares. In following a myositis patient on methotrexate, it is important to monitor liver function enzymes with the caveat that transaminases can be elevated because of the muscle disease rather than hepatic injury. For patients with severe or refractory myositis, other immunosuppressives are occasionally used, including *azathioprine, cyclophosphamide,* or *cyclosporin A.*

Intravenous Gamma Globulin

Some patients with refractory dermatomyositis appeared to benefit from intravenous gamma globulin in a placebo-controlled, randomized trial.[21] Effect size, however, was small, and concerns regarding the blinding of the study diminished its implications. Fever, headache, and aseptic meningitis are some of the side effects of intravenous gamma globulin. Costs are extremely high, and many insurance companies may not pay for this treatment.

Plasmapheresis

Although anecdotal reports of plasmapheresis alone or in combination with other treatments for myositis claimed benefit, a controlled trial by Miller and colleagues[22] showed no difference between treatment and control groups.

Physical Therapy

Physical therapy and rehabilitation should not be forgotten. The goal of any therapeutic program is to preserve existing muscle function, prevent disuse atrophy, and avoid the joint contractures resulting from limited joint mobility and fibrotic healing of inflamed muscles. Even in the face of active myositis, a more aggressive rehabilitation approach has not led to clinical or biochemical (CK) flares of disease.[23]

Skin Lesions

The skin lesions of dermatomyositis may be quite refractory to treatment with systemic glucocorticoids, or immunosuppressives, or both. If this is the case, the addition of an antimalarial, such as hydroxychloroquine 400 mg/day may be considered.

Calcinosis

Calcinosis, either cutaneous or within muscle itself, is common in juvenile dermatomyositis but can also occur in adults, although much less frequently. No satisfactory treatment exists for this problem, but colchicine, calcium channel blockers, and low-dose oral anticoagulants have all been tried with varying success.

INCLUSION BODY MYOSITIS

Inclusion body myositis[24] is now recognized as a common form of chronic myositis in the elderly, and it can be mistaken for treatment-resistant polymyositis. Inclusion body myositis occurs primarily in middle-aged to elderly individuals, with men predominating by a ratio of 2:1. Its onset is insidious, and consequently there may be a delay of several years before the diagnosis is made. There is progressive, painless muscle weakness affecting distal as well as proximal muscles, and involvement may be asymmetric. There appears to be a predilection to involve the quadriceps and iliopsoas muscle groups, resulting in severe atrophy of the upper legs. Laboratory findings are only mildly abnormal, with CK elevations of one to five times normal. Acute phase reactants are usually normal. Nerve conduction studies and EMG studies display a pattern similar to other forms of myositis (see Table 29–1). Muscle biopsy with electron microscopy is diagnostic in these cases (Fig. 29–3).

Although a trial of 40 to 60 mg of prednisone for 3 months is sometimes recommended for newly diagnosed inclusion body myositis, many patients do not report meaningful improvement in strength, and glucocorticoid-related toxicities are common, presenting a significant therapeutic dilemma for the clinician. In many instances, the better approach may be not to treat these patients medically, but to focus on quality-of-life issues and stress physical therapy, occupational therapy, and symptom relief.

CONCLUSION

Future developments relating to classification and prognostication of the various forms of myositis are likely to have profound effects on how physicians evaluate and care for such patients. Until that time, timely recognition of these syndromes and prompt referral to a rheumatologist, especially for patients with poor prognostic factors, such as severe myositis or pulmonary involvement, is essential. Oral glucocorticoids are the first line of therapy for the inflammatory myopathies. In the subset of patients with poorly responsive or progressive disease, the early use of second-line immunomodulating agents in a stepwise progression of therapies is recommended. All physicians who care for patients with myositis are soon humbled by the difficulty of achieving successful outcomes in the patients with the more seri-

ous forms of the disease. However it is clear that diligence in pursuing the correct diagnosis, timely institution of appropriate therapeutic measures, and care for the entire patient may greatly improve both short-term and long-term outcomes.

REFERENCES

1. Plotz PH: Not myositis: A series of chance encounters. JAMA 268:2074–2077; 1992.
2. Bohan A, Peter JB: Polymyositis and dermatomyositis (parts 1 and 2). N Engl J Med 292:344–347, 403–407, 1975.
3. Miller FW: Classification and prognosis of inflammatory muscle disease. Rheum Dis Clin North Am 20:811–826, 1994.
4. Kalovidouris AE: Mechanisms of inflammation and histopathology in inflammatory myopathy. Rheum Dis Clin North Am 20:881–897, 1994.
5. Mantegazza R, Bernasconi P, Confalonieri P, et al: Inflammatory myopathies and systemic disorders: A review of immunopathogenetic mechanisms and clinical features. J Neurol 244:277–287, 1997.
6. Zucker J: Drug-related myopathies. Rheum Dis Clin North Am 20:1017–1032, 1994.
7. Kaufman LD: The evolving spectrum of eosinophilia myalgia syndrome. Rheum Dis Clin North Am 20:973–994, 1994.
8. Dalakas MC, Illa I, Pezeshkpour GM, et al: Mitochondrial myopathy caused by long-term zidovudine therapy. N Engl J Med 322:1098–1105, 1990.
9. Espinoza LR, Aguilar JL, Espinoza CG, et al: Characteristics and pathogenesis of myositis in human immunodeficiency virus infection—distinction from azidothymidine-induced myopathy. Rheum Dis Clin North Am 17:117–129, 1991.
10. Bohlmeyer TJ, Wu AHB, Perryman BM: Evaluation of laboratory tests as a guide to diagnosis and therapy of myositis. Rheum Dis Clin North Am 20:845–856, 1994.
11. Kagen LJ, Aram S: Creatine kinase activity inhibitor in sera from patients with muscle diseases. Arthritis Rheum 30:213–217, 1987.
12. Szmidt-Salkowska E, Rowinska-Marcinska K, Lovelace RE: EMG dynamics in polymyositis and dermatomyositis in adults. Electromyogr Clin Neurophysiol 29:399–404, 1989.
13. Callen JP: Relationship of cancer to inflammatory muscle diseases: Dermatomyositis, polymyositis, and inclusion body myositis. Rheum Dis Clin North Am 20:943–953, 1994.
14. Mader R, Keystone EC: Inflammatory myopathy: Do we have adequate measures of the treatment response? J Rheumatol 20:1105–1107, 1993.

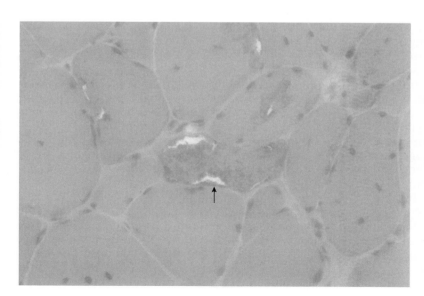

Figure 29–3. Transverse section of a fresh frozen muscle biopsy specimen from a patient with inclusion myositis (H&E, ×650). *Note* typical rimmed vacuoles (arrow).

15. Stoll T, Bruhlmann P, Stucki G, et al: Muscle strength assessment in polymyositis and dermatomyositis: Evaluation of the reliability and clinical use of a new, quantitative easily applicable method. J Rheumatol 22:473–477, 1995.

16. Oddis CV: Therapy of inflammatory myopathy. Rheum Dis Clin North Am 20:899–915, 1994.

17. Oddis CV, Medsger TA Jr: Relationship between serum creatine kinase level and corticosteroid therapy in polymyositis-dermatomyositis. J Rheumatol 15:807–811, 1988.

18. Fraser DD, Frank JA, Dalakas M, et al: Magnetic resonance imaging in the idiopathic inflammatory myopathies. J Rheumatol 18:1693–1700, 1991.

19. Villalba L, Adams EM: Update on therapy for refractory dermatomyositis and polymyositis. Curr Opin Rheumatol 8:544–551, 1996.

20. Joffe MM, Love LA, Leff RL, et al: Drug therapy of the idiopathic inflammatory myopathies: Predictors of response to prednisone, azathioprine, and methotrexate and a comparison of their efficacy. Am J Med 94:379–387, 1993.

21. Dalakas MC, Dambrosia JM, Soueidan SA, et al: A controlled trial of high-dose intravenous immune globulin infusion as treatment for dermatomyositis. N Engl J Med 329:1993–2000, 1993.

22. Miller FW, Leitman SF, Cronin ME, et al: Controlled trial of plasma exchange and leukapheresis in polymyositis and dermatomyositis. N Engl J Med 326:1380–1384, 1992.

23. Hicks JE, Miller FW, Plotz P, et al: Isometric exercises increases strength and does not produce sustained creatinine phosphokinase increases in a patient with polymyositis. J Rheumatol 20:1399–1401, 1993.

24. Calabrese LH, Chou SM: Inclusion body myositis. Rheum Dis Clin North Am 20:955–972, 1994.

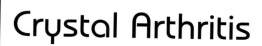

Chapter 30

Crystal Arthritis

Michael M. Ward

Crystal-induced arthritis comprises a group of acute and chronic conditions related to the tissue deposition of one of three types of crystals: monosodium urate crystals in gout, calcium pyrophosphate dihydrate crystals in pseudogout, and basic calcium phosphate crystals in calcific tendinitis and periarthritis. The crystal-induced arthritides are among the most common causes of inflammatory arthritis and can usually be well controlled with treatment. Correct diagnosis by identification of crystals in synovial fluid obtained from an inflamed joint is key to the proper management of these conditions and the prevention of recurrent attacks and chronic arthritis.

GOUT

Gout is best considered a chronic metabolic disease rather than an intermittent condition manifested by attacks of acute arthritis. When viewed in this way, there are four clinical stages in gout: asymptomatic hyperuricemia, acute arthritis, intercritical gout, and chronic gouty arthritis.

Normal Serum Urate

Normal serum levels of sodium urate are less than 7 mg/dL in men and less than 6 mg/dL in women. These limits, established in population studies, are close to the concentration of monosodium urate that results in supersaturation of serum (~7 mg/dL). This level is considered the best cut-off point for defining hyperuricemia because the probability that clinical gout will develop in patients with serum uric acid levels less than 7.0 mg/dL is extremely remote. In plasma, uric acid is in the ionized form of urate; it is only in acid pH in urine that uric acid is predominant. This level also defines the treatment goal for patients with clinical gout receiving allopurinol or uricosuric drugs and the serum level below which tophi resorb. Many clinical laboratories report *normal ranges* of serum uric acid to include levels up to 9 mg/dL. These limits should not be used to define hyperuricemia, but rather the physiologic level of 7.0 mg/dL should be used.

Serum uric acid levels are usually low in children but rise in boys at puberty, occasionally into the hyperuricemic range. This rise does not occur until menopause in women. In most cases, 20 to 30 years of sustained hyperuricemia are needed before tissue saturation occurs and clinical gout develops. This sequence accounts for the observation that men often have their first attack of gouty arthritis between ages 30 and 40 and women after age 65. Because women do not develop hyperuricemia until after menopause, with rare exceptions gouty arthritis should not be considered in the differential diagnosis of acute arthritis in premenopausal women.

Asymptomatic Hyperuricemia

Asymptomatic hyperuricemia is present in 5% to 10% of men. Hyperuricemia may be primary, in which it is not associated with medication use or other diseases, or secondary. Primary causes include uncommon genetic abnormalities in the enzymes involved in purine metabolism that lead to overproduction of uric acid and intrinsic defects in renal clearance that lead to underexcretion of uric acid. Secondary causes include conditions such as myeloproliferative and lymphoproliferative diseases, chronic hemolytic diseases, psoriasis, rhabdomyolysis, and other causes of extensive tissue breakdown, all of which lead to overproduction of uric acid. Renal insufficiency of any cause results in underexcretion of uric acid. Diuretics, low-dose aspirin (<1 g/d), niacin, cyclosporine, ethambutol, and pyrazinamide are among the commonly used medications that also decrease uric acid excretion. Excessive intake of purine-rich foods, including red meats, organ meats, shellfish, and alcohol, also contributes to hyperuricemia. Alcohol intake is often associated with hyperuricemia and acute gouty arthritis (Box 30–1), in part, because the metabolism of alcohol increases uric acid production by accelerating the breakdown of ATP and increases the concentration of lactic acid, which inhibits the renal excretion of uric acid. The accompanying box lists foods that may exacerbate hyperuricemia.

Acute Gout

The likelihood that persons with hyperuricemia will develop acute gouty arthritis depends somewhat on the degree and duration of hyperuricemia.[1] Factors that provoke acute attacks of gout are listed in Box 30–2.

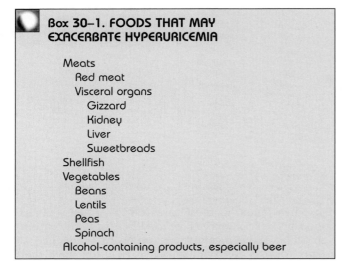

Box 30–1. FOODS THAT MAY EXACERBATE HYPERURICEMIA

Meats
  Red meat
  Visceral organs
    Gizzard
    Kidney
    Liver
    Sweetbreads
Shellfish
Vegetables
  Beans
  Lentils
  Peas
  Spinach
Alcohol-containing products, especially beer

Persons with serum uric acid levels greater than 9 mg/dL develop gouty arthritis at a rate of about 5% per year. Those with serum uric acid levels less than 9 mg/dL develop acute gouty arthritis at rates of less than 1% per year. Because some persons with hyperuricemia never develop clinical gout and because in many clinical gout develops only after decades of hyperuricemia, asymptomatic hyperuricemia should not be treated. Even though many patients with hyperuricemia develop urate deposits in the kidney, these deposits rarely interfere with kidney function, and treatment of hyperuricemia to preserve renal function is not indicated.

Acute gouty arthritis typically involves one joint, although up to 10% of attacks may be polyarticular.[2] Podagra, or inflammation at the first metatarsophalangeal joint, is the initial presentation of clinical gout in 50% of patients and is present at some time in the disease course in up to 90% of patients. Other joints commonly involved include the forefoot, knees, ankles, wrists, finger joints, and elbows. Gout may also cause acute bursitis, commonly in the olecranon or prepatellar bursa. Acute attacks of gouty arthritis often occur at night, with the patient aware of the arthritis only when attempting to get out of bed in the morning. Often, there are no premonitory symptoms, although occasionally patients may experience twinges of pain in the joint in the hours before development of a full-fledged attack. The affected joint is usually intensely painful, swollen, erythematous, and warm. Acute gouty arthritis may be accompanied by fever and chills. The peak in-

Box 30–2. FACTORS PROVOKING ACUTE ATTACKS OF GOUT

Trauma
Medication
  Raising urate levels; e.g., diuretics, low-dose aspirin
  Lowering urate levels; e.g., allopurinol, probenecid
High-purine diet
Dehydration
Surgery

tensity of the inflammation usually occurs in the first 24 hours, and patients with new onset of gouty arthritis often present for medical care within the first 12 hours. With treatment, symptoms usually decrease within 1 to 2 days, but complete resolution may take up to 7 days. Untreated attacks may last 3 to 4 weeks but eventually resolve.

Intercritical Gout

Patients are usually asymptomatic between attacks of acute gouty arthritis. This asymptomatic period is known as *intercritical gout,* emphasizing that the disease exists even in the absence of ongoing symptoms. Recurrent attacks of acute gouty arthritis are common. Attacks may be precipitated by trauma, surgery, dehydration, acute medical illness, alcohol consumption, and initiation of the drugs mentioned previously. Two thirds of patients have a second attack in the year after their first attack, three quarters have a second attack within 2 years of their first attack, and 90% have a second attack within 5 years of their first attack. Because some patients may have only one episode of acute gouty arthritis, and for many patients several years pass before they experience another attack, long-term treatment to lower serum uric acid levels is usually reserved for patients who have had at least two attacks of acute gouty arthritis. This threshold marks patients as being likely to go on to have repeated attacks, which may be reduced or eliminated by treatment. These patients are also the most likely to progress to chronic gouty arthritis.

Chronic Gout

Chronic gouty arthritis develops in up to 25% of patients with clinical gout who are not treated with hypouricemic medications. Patients with chronic gouty arthritis have a low-grade inflammatory synovitis in joints as a result of urate deposition in the synovium, cartilage, and underlying bone. The arthritis is polyarticular, with frequent involvement of the hands and feet. Although insidious in onset, chronic gouty arthritis is slowly progressive and often becomes severely deforming and disabling. Subcutaneous tophi may or may not be present. Rarely, patients with chronic gouty arthritis may present without a recalled history of acute gouty arthritis. This presentation is more likely in elderly patients with renal insufficiency who have taken anti-inflammatory medications for reasons other than gout.

Tophi are compact collections of urate. They form in skin, subcutaneous and soft tissue, tendons, and synovium (Fig. 30–1). Common locations include over the metatarsophalangeal joints or interphalangeal joints of the fingers, along the ulnar forearm and olecranon, over the Achille's tendon, and in the helix of the ear. Tophi over the finger joints are common in elderly women treated with diuretics. Most tophi are painless, asymmetric, firm masses that distend the skin, which may have a mottled hypopigmentation. Occasionally, small punctate tophi develop in the superficial layers of the skin of the finger pads. The skin over these tophi as well

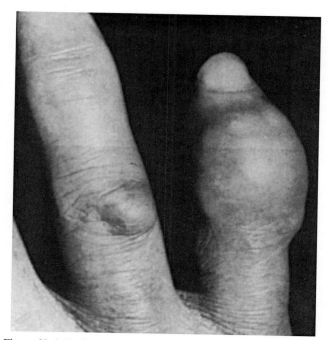

Figure 30–1. Tophus of fifth digit, with smaller tophus over fourth proximal interphalangeal joint. (From Kelley WN, Wortmann RL: Gout and hyperuricemia. In Kelley WN, Harris ED Jr, Ruddy S, Sledge CB, eds: Textbook of Rheumatology, 5th ed. Philadelphia, WB Saunders, 1997, p 1317.)

as larger ones may ulcerate and drain urate chalk. Chronic tophaceous gout is more likely to develop in patients with persistently high serum uric acid levels, and the likelihood is greatest in those with levels greater than 11 mg/dL. Chronic gouty arthritis and tophaceous gout are preventable with diligent hypouricemic treatment.

Diagnosis

The diagnosis of acute gouty arthritis depends on identification of monosodium urate crystals in the synovial fluid of an inflamed joint.[3] Urate crystals are usually easily found under polarizing microscopy as long, needle-shaped, and highly birefrigent (bright) crystals. These crystals demonstrate negative elongation, being yellow when aligned parallel to the direction of orientation of the red compensator and blue when aligned perpendicular to this direction. Urate crystals are often abundant in synovial fluid from acute inflamed joints, but the number of crystals observed has little relation to the intensity of inflammation seen clinically. Urate crystals should be seen within neutrophils to be confident that the inflammation is due to acute gout. Extracellular urate crystals are common even in noninflammatory synovial fluids from patients with a previous history of gouty arthritis. Crystals are most numerous on the first day of an attack and may be difficult to find in synovial fluid obtained more than 2 days after the onset of an attack. Urate crystals may also be demonstrated on microscopic examination of aspirates of tophi.

Synovial fluid leukocyte counts in acute gouty arthritis are usually greater than $20,000/mm^3$ and may be as high as $100,000/mm^3$, with a predominance of neutrophils. Peripheral leukocytosis may also be present, and other nonspecific indicators of inflammation, such as the erythrocyte sedimentation rate, are abnormal. These findings are usually not present in chronic gouty arthritis or tophaceous gout. During an episode of acute gouty arthritis, serum uric acid levels may be spuriously normal or even low. Therefore, serum uric acid levels at the time of an attack should not be used to support or refute a diagnosis of acute gouty arthritis. A search for prior laboratory studies demonstrating hyperuricemia is likely to provide much more useful and reliable information.

Radiographs of the joint affected by acute gouty arthritis usually show only soft tissue swelling or an effusion. Chronic gouty arthritis typically causes bone erosions, distinguished from those of rheumatoid arthritis by being large, often slightly removed from the margin of the joint, and surrounded by bone sclerosis (Fig. 30–2). Tophi may appear as cloudy soft tissue densities, but they do not calcify.

Acute gouty arthritis must be distinguished from infectious arthritis. Both usually present as an acute inflammatory monarthritis, and patients may have fever and laboratory markers of systemic inflammation. Synovial fluid leukocyte counts in these conditions of-

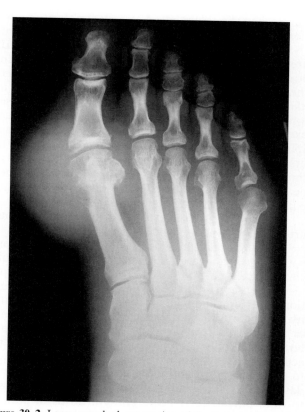

Figure 30–2. Large, punched-out erosion of the first metatarsal in a 63-year-old man with gout. The erosion underlies a large tophus, represented by the soft tissue density adjacent to the first metatarsophalangeal joint. Bone erosions in gouty arthritis need not be associated with tophi.

ten overlap. A prior history of similar attacks may provide some indication that gout is the cause of the acute arthritis, but the diagnosis depends on identification of intracellular urate crystals in synovial fluid and the absence of microorganisms on Gram stain and culture. Rarely, acute gouty arthritis and infectious arthritis may coexist. Acute gouty arthritis may also be confused with acute pseudogout, acute calcific periarthritis, or cellulitis. Any of the inflammatory polyarthritides, such as rheumatoid arthritis or psoriatic arthritis, may begin as a monarthritis and be confused with gouty arthritis. This may be more often the case in reactive arthritis, which is commonly acute in onset and typically involves the ankle or knee. The differential diagnosis of chronic gouty arthritis includes all conditions that cause inflammatory polyarthritis. Radiographs demonstrating changes typical of chronic gouty arthritis may be particularly helpful, as may a careful physical examination to detect subcutaneous tophi.

Treatment

ACUTE GOUT

The treatment of acute gouty arthritis includes rest of the affected joint and anti-inflammatory medication to reduce pain and swelling. Patients with acute gouty arthritis in lower extremity joints should avoid weight bearing and use crutches if possible. Wrists and finger joints may be splinted. Anti-inflammatory medications include nonsteroidal anti-inflammatory drugs (NSAIDs), glucocorticoids, and colchicine.[4] NSAIDs are the treatment of choice for most patients with acute gouty arthritis. Although indomethacin is often used for this indication, any NSAIDs at sufficiently high dose are likely to be effective. Salicylates should not be used, however, because in low doses they decrease uric acid excretion. High doses of NSAIDs (e.g., indomethacin 150 mg/day, naproxen 1000 mg/day) may be used for the first 1 or 2 days of an attack, with lower doses used thereafter until the attack has resolved. NSAIDs should be stopped once the attack has resolved, which in most patients occurs within 7 days (see Table 30A–1).

Glucocorticoids may be used to treat acute gouty arthritis in patients who have contraindications to NSAID treatment. Included in this group are patients with congestive heart failure, dehydration, renal insufficiency, recent gastrointestinal bleeding or recent peptic ulcer disease; patients receiving long-term anticoagulation treatment; and patients with NSAID hypersensitivity. Glucocorticoids may be given either intra-articularly or systemically. Intra-articular injections are often preferred when only one or two joints are involved in the acute attack. Inflammation usually responds quite well to these injections, and the attack abates within 3 or 4 days. Oral or intravenous glucocorticoids may be used to treat polyarticular acute gouty arthritis in patients who have contraindications to NSAID treatment. Prednisone, starting at a dose of 20 to 40 mg/day and tapered over one week, is usually well tolerated and successful. For hospitalized patients who are unable to take oral medications, intravenous methylprednisolone at a dose of 40 mg/day and tapered over one week may be used. Adrenocorticotrophic hormone (ACTH), in a dose of 40 to 80 IU parenterally, may also be used to treat acute gouty arthritis. Treatment with ACTH relies on the ability of the patient's adrenal glands to produce enough endogenous glucocorticoids to have an effect, and the clinical response may be less predictable, particularly in elderly patients. Rebound attacks of acute gouty arthritis may also be more common with this treatment.

Colchicine, long the traditional treatment for acute gouty arthritis, has been supplanted by NSAIDs because of their greater therapeutic-to-toxic ratios. When colchicine is given as one 0.6-mg tablet hourly until symptoms abate, side effects occur; a maximum of 10 tablets consumed almost invariably causes problems before symptoms resolve. The most common side effects are nausea, vomiting, diarrhea, and abdominal pain. Patients who are already in pain and who may have difficulty walking may not tolerate these side effects. This regimen of colchicine should not be used in patients with renal or hepatic failure. Colchicine treatment is most effective in the first day of an episode of acute gouty arthritis and tends to be less effective when used later in the course of an attack. Intravenous colchicine should never be used because of its toxicity, including bone marrow suppression, renal failure, liver necrosis, seizures, ventricular fibrillation, and death. Extravasation of the infusion may cause skin necrosis and sloughing. Safer alternatives exist.

CHRONIC GOUT

Long-term treatment to lower serum uric acid levels is indicated for patients who have had two or more attacks of acute gouty arthritis. The goals of this treatment are to decrease the frequency of acute attacks and to prevent chronic gouty arthritis and tophaceous gout. Treatment may be with either a uricosuric drug, such as probenecid or sulfinpyrazone, which lowers serum uric acid levels by increasing its renal excretion, or allopurinol, which lowers serum uric acid levels by decreasing its production. With either treatment, the dose is adjusted to achieve and maintain a serum uric acid level less than 6.5 mg/dL. Therefore, periodic monitoring of serum uric acid levels is necessary to gauge the effectiveness of treatment. Tophi may resorb faster if the serum uric acid level is reduced to less than 5 mg/dL. In most cases treatment should be lifelong.

It has been recommended that the choice of hypouricemic drug be determined by the underlying pathophysiologic defect responsible for the patient's gout. Patients whose gout is due to renal underexcretion of uric acid are best treated with uricosuric medications, and patients whose gout is due to overproduction of uric acid are best treated with allopurinol. Determination of underexcretion or overproduction is based on the 24-hour urinary excretion of urate. Patients excreting less than 600 mg/day of urate while on a purine-free diet are considered to be underexcretors, and those excreting more than 600 mg/dL are considered overproducers. The practical application of this scheme is difficult, however, because maintaining a purine-free diet is extremely difficult. Dietary indiscretion invalidates the test. Standards for urate underexcretion on unrestricted diets are less firmly established and are not available for groups other than white men. Because about 90% of patients with primary gout are underexcretors, there is also little risk in presuming most patients are underexcretors and treating them accordingly. Although correct in theory, measuring 24-hour urinary urate excretion and choosing the type of hypouricemic treatment based on this result has little clinical utility.

Probenecid is the uricosuric medication used most often. The initial dose is 250 mg twice daily, and the dose is slowly increased to a maximum of 2000 mg daily. The maintenance dose should be the lowest dose that maintains the serum uric acid level in the target range. Sulfinpyrazone is begun at a dose of 100 mg daily and increased slowly to a maximum of 200 mg four times daily. Probenecid and sulfinpyrazone are usually well tolerated but can decrease the excretion of other drugs. Low-dose aspirin inhibits the action of probenecid and sulfinpyrazone and should not be used in patients taking these medications. Patients needing hypouricemic treatment and who use aspirin for cardioprotective indications should be treated with allopurinol. A potential toxicity associated with uricosuric is acute uric acid nephropathy occurring when treatment is begun or the development of uric acid kidney stones with continued treatment. The likelihood of these complications can be reduced by beginning with low doses and ensuring patients are well hydrated when treatment is begun. Coadministration of sodium bicarbonate or sodium citrate to alkalinize the urine also promotes uric acid solubility and may decrease the likelihood of stone formation.

Allopurinol is indicated for patients with renal insufficiency (creatinine clearance <50 mL/min or serum creatinine >2.0 mg/dL) because uricosurics are ineffective for such patients. Allopurinol is also indicated for patients with a history of uric acid nephrolithiasis or tophi, for those known to be uric acid overproducers, and for those in whom uricosurics fail to control attacks or inadequately lower serum uric acid levels. For patients with normal renal function, the typical dose of allopurinol is 300 mg daily in a single dose. Many rheumatologists build up to 300 mg over several weeks from 100 mg/day in order to avoid precipitating acute attacks of gout. Some patients may require higher doses. The dose of allopurinol must be reduced in patients with renal insufficiency; a commonly used scheme is to use 250 mg/day in patients with a creatinine clearance of 80 mL/min, 200 mg/day in those with a creatinine clearance of 60 mL/min, 150 mg/day in those with a creatinine clearance of 40 mL/min, and 100 mg/day in those with a creatinine clearance of 20 mL/min. Those with creatinine clearances of less than 20 mL/min should be treated with 100 mg every other day or every third day. Diarrhea, headaches, or a pruritic rash can occur in up to 10% of patients who take allopurinol. Patients with a mild rash may be successfully desensitized.[5] Allopurinol hypersensitivity syndrome, with fever, urticaria, acute renal failure, hepatitis, or toxic epidermal necrolysis, develops in a small number of patients, can be severe, and can be fatal. Such patients should not be rechallenged. Allopurinol inhibits the metabolism of *azathioprine,* and the dose of azathioprine must be drastically reduced when allopurinol is started to avoid serious bone marrow toxicity.

Initiation of treatment with uricosurics or allopurinol can precipitate an attack of acute gouty arthritis. The likelihood of this event can be reduced if one delays the start of treatment with these medications for 4 to 6 weeks after resolution of an acute attack. Use of an NSAID or colchicine 0.6 mg/day during the time a uricosuric drug or allopurinol is started also reduces the likelihood that an acute attack will occur. Long-term treatment with colchicine 0.6 mg daily or twice daily or low doses of an NSAID daily can also be effective in reducing the frequency of attacks of acute gouty arthritis in patients who have recurrent attacks while receiving allopurinol or a uricosuric drug. Patients with frequent recurrences can benefit from an assessment of lifestyle factors that may be contributory, including diet and alcohol use. Rigid dietary restrictions are seldom necessary or practical, but moderation in the consumption of high-purine foods, avoidance of alcohol, and weight loss can be beneficial. Use of medications that can exacerbate gout, particularly diuretics, should be eliminated if possible.

Patients with chronic gouty arthritis or tophi should be treated with allopurinol. They will benefit from daily colchicine or NSAIDs to suppress inflammation and reduce the frequency of acute gouty attacks. NSAIDs or analgesics can also be helpful for pain control.

PSEUDOGOUT

Acute pseudogout is an episode of joint inflammation caused by crystals of calcium pyrophosphate dihydrate. As with gout, pseudogout is best viewed as a chronic metabolic disease, often referred to as *calcium pyrophosphate deposition disease* (CPDD). CPDD has four clinical stages that also parallel those seen in gout: asymptomatic chondrocalcinosis, acute arthritis, intercritical periods, and chronic arthritis. See Table 30–1 for differential characteristics of crystal-induced arthritis.

Asymptomatic Chondrocalcinosis

Chondrocalcinosis is a radiographic diagnosis that refers to the presence of fine, stippled or linear calcifications in cartilage (Fig. 30–3). Fibrocartilage is affected most often, and common sites of chondrocalcinosis include the menisci of the knees, the triangular cartilage at the wrist, the symphysis pubis, and the glenoid and acetabular labrum.[6] Chondrocalcinosis may also occur in hyaline cartilage, tendons, bursae, and ligaments. It is unclear if calcium pyrophosphate crystals deposit at sites of previously damaged cartilage or if crystal dep-

Table 30–1. CRYSTAL-INDUCED ARTHRITIS, DIFFERENTIAL CHARACTERISTICS

Characteristic		Gout	Pseudogout
Prevalence		• 1.5 to 2.6 cases per 1000 individuals • Increases with age in men and postmenopausal women • 15/1000 at age 58; men: 28/1000, women: 11/1000	• <1 case per 1000 individuals • Increases with age
Crystals	Chemistry	• Monosodium urate	• Calcium pyrophosphate dihydrate
	Appearance	• Negatively birefringent • Needle-shaped	• Weakly positively birefringent • Linear or rhomboidal
Articular Involvement		• Monarticular > oligoarticular • Polyarticular < 30%	• Monarticular > oligoarticular
Most Frequently Affected Joints		• 1st MTP joint initally 50% eventually 90% • Ankles, knees, other	• Knee, wrist, other
Associated Findings		• Tophi (in chronic disorder) • Hyperlipidemia	• Chondrocalcinosis (increases with age; most will not have pseudogout)
Predisposing Conditions/ Risk Factors		• Hyperuricemia,* obesity, hypertension, hyperlipidemia, alcohol ingestion, lead ingestion, hereditary enzyme defect (rare)	• Hemochromatosis, OA, chronic renal insufficiency, diabetes, hyperparathyroidism, hereditary (rare)
Therapeutic Options		• Acute attacks: NSAIDs, corticosteroids, colchicine • Chronic management: urate-lowering agents, colchicine	• Acute attacks: NSAIDs, corticosteroids, colchicine • Chronic management: NSAIDs ± colchicine

*Drugs associated with hyperuricemia include diuretics, low-dose salicylates, nicotinic acid, cyclosporine, ethanol, and ethambutol.

Modified from Roubenoff R: Gout and hyperuricemia. Rheum Dis Clin North Am 16:539, 1990 and Doherty M, Dieppe P: Clinical aspects of calcium pyrophosphate dihydrate crystal deposition. Rheum Dis Clin North Am 14:395, 1988. In Lipsky PE: Algorithms for the diagnosis and management of musculoskeletal complaints. Am J Med 103(6A):49S–85S, 1997.

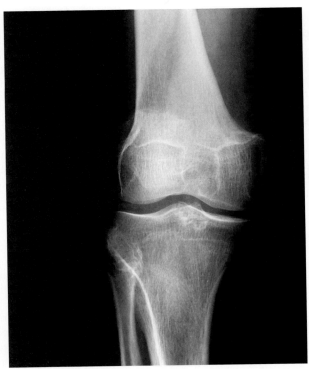

Figure 30–3. Chondrocalcinosis in the menisci of the knee in a 43-year-old man with acromegaly and several attacks of acute pseudogout.

osition is the primary event and cartilage damage follows. Chondrocalcinosis is rarely seen in patients younger than age 50, and its prevalence increases with age. Approximately one third of persons age 75 or older have chondrocalcinosis. Chondrocalcinosis per se is asymptomatic and requires no treatment.

Acute Pseudogout

Acute pseudogout has a prevalence of approximately 0.1% (1:1000 persons). From this prevalence, it is clear that the majority of patients with chondrocalcinosis never have an episode of acute arthritis associated with it. However, chondrocalcinosis is universally present in patients with acute pseudogout. In some cases, chondrocalcinosis may not be evident in the joint involved in acute pseudogout, but chondrocalcinosis is present in other joints. A radiologic survey of the knees, wrists, and pelvis is usually sufficient to detect at least one area of chondrocalcinosis in such patients. The likelihood that an episode of acute pseudogout will occur and the frequency of acute attacks are increased among patients with more extensive chondrocalcinosis. Because chondrocalcinosis is the precursor of acute pseudogout, most cases of acute pseudogout occur in elderly patients. Pseudogout occurring in patients younger than age 50 should alert the clinician to consider whether an associated disease is present (see later). Men and women are affected equally, and other than some rare hereditary subtypes, there are no differences in occurrence among ethnic groups.

Acute pseudogout usually presents as an inflammatory monarthritis. Polyarticular attacks can occur but are not common. Although chondrocalcinosis is recognized by calcification in cartilage, calcium pyrophosphate crystals also deposit in synovium. It is thought that crystal shedding from either the synovium or the cartilage surface is responsible for initiating inflammation in acute attacks. The joints typically involved include the knee, wrist, and ankle and less commonly the elbow, shoulder, and forefoot. Affected joints are swollen, warm, and tender, although the intensity of inflammation is often less than that in acute gouty arthritis. The arthritis often reaches its peak intensity on the second or even third day, rather than within the first 24 hours as is typical of acute gout. Acute pseudogout can last for days to weeks and may be accompanied by high fever and peripheral leukocytosis. The differential diagnosis, therefore, includes infectious arthritis as well as acute gouty arthritis.

The diagnosis of acute pseudogout depends on the demonstration of calcium pyrophosphate dihydrate crystals in the synovial fluid of an inflamed joint. These crystals can be identified by their typical appearance on polarized microscopy: linear or rhomboid crystals with blunt ends that are only weakly birefringent (dull).[3] These crystals also demonstrate positive elongation, being blue in color when aligned parallel to the direction of orientation of the red compensator and yellow when aligned perpendicular to this direction. Because they are dull in appearance and may be rare, calcium pyrophosphate crystals may be difficult to detect, and a diligent search is often needed to find them. Phase-contrast microscopy may also be helpful to detect crystals. Urate crystals can be differentiated by being thin, needle-shaped with pointed ends, bright, and negatively birefringent. Urate crystals may on occasion coexist with calcium pyrophosphate crystals. The synovial fluid in acute pseudogout also shows elevated leukocyte concentrations, although usually less than 50,000/mm^3, with a predominance of neutrophils.

An episode of acute pseudogout may occur without a preceding identifiable event or may be precipitated by trauma to the joint, intra-articular injection, surgery, or an acute medical illness, such as a myocardial infarction. Patients may have only one episode of acute pseudogout or may have multiple recurrences over years. Patients are usually asymptomatic between acute attacks.

Chronic Pseudogout

Chronic arthritis develops in about one half of patients with CPDD. Most of these patients develop a condition that mimics osteoarthritis, with chronic pain and joint deformity, that is termed the *pseudo-osteoarthritis variant of CPDD*. Patients with this variant may or may not have had previous episodes of acute pseu-

dogout, but most have chondrocalcinosis. The key to distinguishing pseudo-osteoarthritic CPDD from osteoarthritis is the distribution of involved joints. Pseudo-osteoarthritic CPDD often involves the metacarpophalangeal joints, intracarpal joints, wrist, elbow, and shoulder, whereas osteoarthritis does not typically affect these joints. Chronic CPDD should be considered among the possible diagnoses when radiographs demonstrate osteoarthritis at these sites. Pseudo-osteoarthritic CPDD can also involve the knees, hips, and spine, as does osteoarthritis, and these two conditions can coexist. Specific radiographic features help distinguish pseudo-osteoarthritic CPDD from osteoarthritis, including prominent subchondral cysts and variable osteophyte formation. Occasionally, patients with pseudo-osteoarthritic CPDD have severe joint destruction with features of a Charcot joint.

Five percent of patients with CPDD develop a chronic symmetric inflammatory polyarthritis that mimics rheumatoid arthritis and is known as the *pseudo-rheumatoid variant of CPDD*. These patients typically have low-grade inflammation, with swelling, tenderness, and warmth involving the knees, wrists, and small joints of the hands. Morning stiffness and fatigue are common, as in rheumatoid arthritis. One clinical indicator of pseudo-rheumatoid CPDD is that flares of arthritis tend to affect one or only a few joints, whereas in rheumatoid arthritis, flares are more typically polyarticular. Patients with pseudo-rheumatoid CPDD also have a history of episodes of acute pseudogout and have chondrocalcinosis on x-ray films. Radiographs show prominent osteoarthritic changes, rather than the erosions typical of rheumatoid arthritis. Because it is not uncommon for elderly persons to have low titer rheumatoid factor present in their serum, some patients with pseudo-rheumatoid CPDD can also be rheumatoid factor positive. Elevation of the erythrocyte sedimentation rate is common, adding to potential diagnostic confusion.

Several diseases have been reported to occur with increased frequency in patients with CPDD.[7] The strongest associations exist for hyperparathyroidism, hemochromatosis, and hypomagnesemia. Of the patients with hyperparathyroidism, 30% to 40% have chondrocalcinosis, and up to 15% may have clinical manifestations of CPDD. Similarly, 20% to 50% of patients with hemochromatosis have chondrocalcinosis, and one half of these patients have clinical CPDD. The presence of chondrocalcinosis or acute pseudogout should serve as an indication to evaluate the patient for these conditions. Associations have also been proposed between CPDD and familial hypocalciuric hypercalcemia, hypophosphatasia, amyloidosis, Bartter's syndrome, ochronosis, Wilson's disease, acromegaly, gout, diabetes mellitus, and hypothyroidism, but these have been less consistent.

The treatment of acute pseudogout is the same as that of acute gouty arthritis. The affected joints should be rested. NSAIDs, intra-articular or oral glucocorticoids, and colchicine can be used as anti-inflammatory agents and discontinued after resolution of the acute episode. Often, aspiration of the fluid from an affected joint is sufficient to relieve symptoms. There is no known treatment to deplete calcium pyrophosphate crystals from cartilage or synovium, and progression of chondrocalcinosis over time is common. Patients with frequent recurrences of acute pseudogout may benefit from prophylactic colchicine 0.6 mg daily or twice daily, or NSAIDs to reduce the frequency of attacks. Decisions to begin prophylactic treatment should be individualized but might be considered for patients who have two or more episodes of acute pseudogout yearly. Patients with chronic CPDD, either the pseudo-osteoarthritis or pseudorheumatoid variant, should be treated with analgesics or NSAIDs as needed. Daily colchicine may also help control symptoms, but there is no evidence that this treatment alters the long-term outcome of chronic CPDD. Patients with the pseudo-rheumatoid variant should not be treated with the second-line or immunosuppressive medications used to treat rheumatoid arthritis. A correct diagnosis is essential for appropriate treatment of this subgroup of patients.

CALCIFIC TENDINITIS, PERIARTHRITIS, AND ARTHRITIS

Tissue deposition of crystals of basic calcium phosphate may cause several different clinical conditions, including *calcific tendinitis, calcific periarthritis, acute inflammatory arthritis,* and *chronic destructive arthritis.*[8] Basic calcium phosphate crystals include a variety of different crystals, but the most common are calcium apatite crystals. These crystals deposit in tendons, bursae, and other soft tissue structures around joints as well as in cartilage, where they are asymptomatic. Shedding of crystals from these sites leads to acute inflammation and symptoms.

Calcific Tendinitis

Calcific tendinitis is an acute tendinitis, most often of the rotator cuff tendons, associated with periarticular calcification on radiographs (Fig. 30–4). Patients usually present with the acute onset of severe pain in the involved shoulder and often resist attempts at passive range of motion. Calcific tendinitis is most common among patients age 30 to 50. Patients with *diabetes mellitus* are at increased risk. There is often no history of antecedent trauma or chronic overuse. Radiographs commonly show a faint homogenous area of calcification that follows the contour of the involved tendon. The borders of this calcification may be more distinct when patients are asymptomatic and become blurred during an acute episode. The calcifications may resolve after several weeks and may recur later. Treatment of calcific tendinitis includes rest of the affected joint, local glucocorticoid injection, and early institution of range-of-motion exercises to prevent contracture. NSAIDs may be used but are often ineffective; failure to respond within 2 days of NSAID treatment is an indication for local glucocorticoid injection.

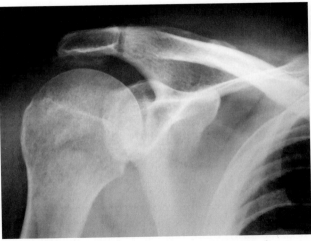

Figure 30–4. Calcific tendinitis in a 64-year-old man with recurrent shoulder pain. The density between the humeral head and the acromion represents a deposit of basic calcium phosphate.

Calcific Periarthritis

Calcific periarthritis is an acute inflammatory reaction near a joint, associated with local calcific deposits on roentgenograms. Patients with chronic renal failure are particularly prone to calcific periarthritis, but it may also be seen in patients without renal failure. Involved areas are painful and swollen and are often warm and erythematous, mimicking *cellulitis, acute gout,* or *pseudogout.* Episodes may last several weeks. Typical sites include areas around the shoulder, greater trochanters, elbow, wrist, and knee. Usually only one area is involved at a time, but it may recur at another site in the future. The diagnosis is based on finding typical calcifications in the soft tissue of the involved area. Treatment includes NSAIDs and colchicine, although some deposits may require aspiration or surgical removal.

Basic Calcium Phosphate Crystal Arthritis

Basic calcium phosphate crystals rarely cause an acute inflammatory arthritis with localized pain and swelling. This presentation has been most often noted in patients with osteoarthritis. Acute arthritis due to basic calcium phosphate crystals may occur more commonly than believed because these crystals are difficult to detect without specialized techniques, such as electron microscopy. These crystals cannot be identified by light microscopy or polarized microscopy, although clumps of basic calcium phosphate crystals may be detected when synovial fluid is stained with a special stain known as *alizarin red S.* Treatment options include NSAIDs, local glucocorticoid injection, and colchicine.

Rarely, basic calcium crystals are associated with a chronic destructive arthritis, most commonly known as the *Milwaukee shoulder syndrome.* This syndrome includes swelling and reduced range of motion at the shoulder, often with large effusions, and progressive destruction of the humeral head and glenoid. The arthritis usually develops gradually and may or may not be painful. More than half of affected patients have bilateral involvement. A similar process may occur at the knee. Most patients are elderly women. Synovial fluid examination often shows low leukocyte counts, but abundant basic calcium phosphate crystals are present when synovial fluid is examined by special methods. Analgesics, NSAIDs, and joint aspirations may help control symptoms, but many patients require shoulder replacement.

INDICATIONS FOR REFERRAL

Patients with possible crystal-induced arthritis should be referred to a rheumatologist if there is uncertainty about the diagnosis. Aspiration and crystal examination of synovial fluid is essential to establishment of the diagnosis, and consultation for this procedure may be necessary. Consultation may also be needed if an intra-articular injection is the preferred treatment for an acute attack. Although most patients with gout and CPDD can be managed effectively by primary care physicians, occasionally patients with frequent recurrences or symptoms that are difficult to control may benefit from the ongoing involvement of a rheumatologist in their care.

See Appendix to this chapter for algorithmic tables for the treatment of gout and pseudogout.

REFERENCES

1. Campion EW, Glynn RJ, DeLabry LO: Asymptomatic hyperuricemia: Risks and consequences in the the Normative Aging Study. Am J Med 82:421, 1987.
2. Lawry GV II, Fan PT, Bluestone R: Polyarticular versus monoarticular gout: A prospective, comparative analysis of clinical features. Medicine 67:335, 1988.
3. McCarty DJ: Crystal identification in human synovial fluids: Methods and interpretation. Rheum Dis Clin North Am 14:253, 1988.
4. Emmerson BT: The management of gout. N Engl J Med 334:445, 1996.
5. Fam AG, Lewtas J, Stein J, Paton TW: Desensitization to allopurinol in patients with gout and cutaneous reactions. Am J Med 93:299, 1992.
6. Resnick D: Calcium pyrophosphate dihydrate (CPPD) crystal deposition disease. In Resnick D, ed: Bone and Joint Imaging, 2nd ed. Philadelphia, WB Saunders, 1996, p. 409.
7. Jones AC, Chuck AJ, Arie EA, et al: Diseases associated with calcium pyrophosphate deposition disease. Semin Arthritis Rheum 22:188, 1992.
8. Halverson PB: Clinical aspects of basic calcium phosphate crystal deposition. Rheum Dis Clin North Am 14:427, 1988.

Recognition and Management of Patients with Specific Rheumatologic Problems

Table 30A–1. Managing Acute Gout

The patient has an established diagnosis of gout. A plan of treatment should be established for the acute attack.

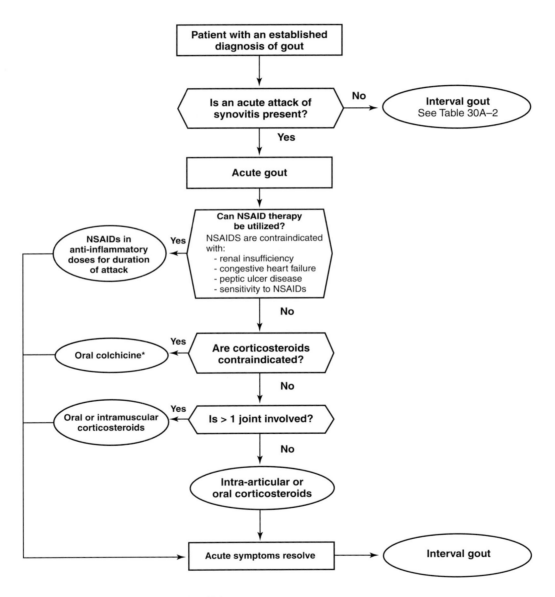

*Adjust dose in patients with renal insufficiency.
Modified from Lipsky PE: Algorithms for the diagnosis and management of musculoskeletal complaints.
Am J Med 103(6A); 69S, 1997.

Table 30A–2. Managing Interval Gout

The patient has an established diagnosis of gout. A plan of treatment should be established for the symptom-free interval between attacks.

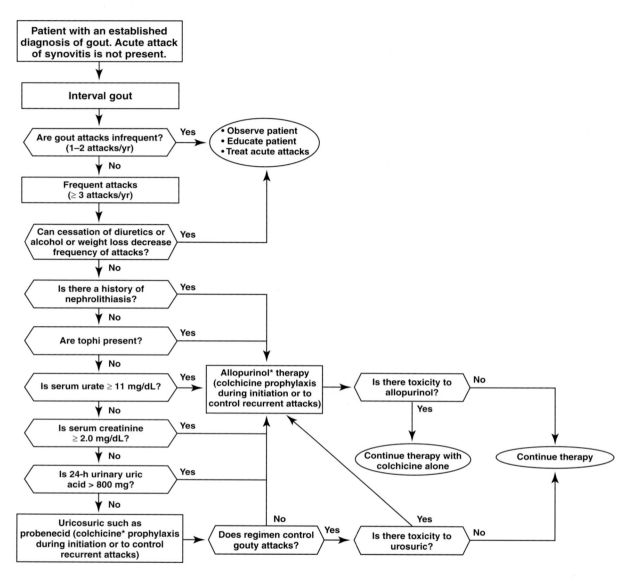

* Adjust dose with renal insufficiency.
Modified from Lipsky PE: Algorithms for the diagnosis and management of musculoskeletal complaints.
Am J Med 103(6A): 70S, 1997.

Table 30A–3. Treatment of Pseudogout

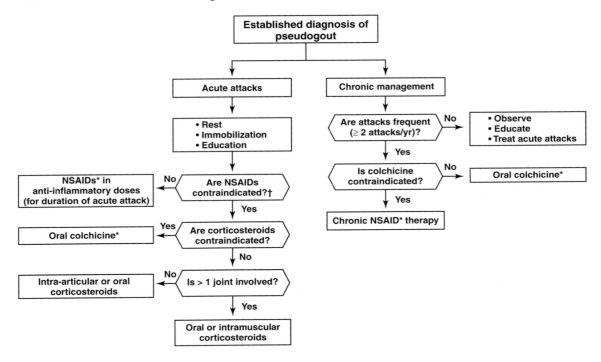

* Adjust dosage with renal insufficiency.
†NSAID contraindications: renal insufficiency, congestive heart failure, peptic ulcer disease, hypersensitivity.
Modified from Lipsky PE: Algorithms for the diagnosis and management of musculoskeletal complaints.
Am J Med 103(6A): 71S, 1997.

Chapter 31

Osteoarthritis of the Extremities

Boris Ratiner ■ Nancy E. Lane

Osteoarthritis (OA), also known as *degenerative joint disease,* is the most common form of arthritis in the United States[1] and a major cause of morbidity, especially in the elderly. Most likely, it is not a single disease but rather the end result of multiple diverse causes that produce degeneration and loss of the articular cartilage. It is often divided into either a secondary or an idiopathic form and can be localized or generalized, involving the knees, hands, spine, and, to a lesser extent, other joints in the body.[2]

The disease process is usually slow. Degeneration of articular cartilage leads to clinically evident joint stiffness and pain in the affected joints. With continued joint degradation and loss of function, local muscle weakness and atrophy become prominent and can lead to joint instability. In the later stages of OA, the diagnosis is easier; there are characteristic joint findings and radiographic appearance. Early in the disease process or in more inflammatory forms of the disease, OA can be difficult to distinguish from other forms of arthritis. Therefore, a thorough history and physical examination that includes risk factors for OA, such as past and present employment, history of serious joint injury, and exercise habits, is an essential diagnostic tool. This chapter includes a brief review of the structure of articular cartilage and pathogenesis of OA but focuses on diagnosis and treatment.

EPIDEMIOLOGY AND CLASSIFICATION

When one is considering the overall prevalence of OA, several factors need to be considered. Age, sex, and joint location are all important when trying to understand which patients are most susceptible to OA. When OA is diagnosed by thorough joint examination alone, the overall prevalence is approximately 9% to 12% in the general population of adults older than 25 years old. If only a history is used, 4.5% of men and 7.3% of women have symptoms consistent with OA. If radiographic criteria alone are used, as many as 32% of adults have mild and 8% of adults have moderate radiographic findings consistent with OA in at least one joint. Both the radiographic and the physical changes of OA are most commonly seen in the hand joints, followed by the foot, knee, and hip. These numbers, although impressive, are misleading because the prevalence of radiographic disease overestimates clinically

relevant OA. In fact, the prevalence of clinically symptomatic OA in adults between the ages of 25 and 75 years is highest in the hands and is approximately 2.4% for men and 3.8% for women.[1] The distribution of disease is shifted toward the elderly, and women seem to be affected more often than men. Although OA is seen all over the world, in westernized populations more than 70% of those older than age 65 have the disease by either radiologic or clinical criteria.[1, 3]

Since OA is the end result of multiple stimuli and can vary in clinical appearance, the American College of Rheumatology has proposed a classification scheme (Tables 31–1 to 31–3).[3, 4] The largest category is idiopathic OA, and it is divided into a localized (knee, hip, or hand) and generalized form (three or more joints affected). The distal interphalangeal and proximal interphalangeal joints of both the hands and the feet are often involved and are sometimes referred to as *Heberden's* and *Bouchard's* nodes. These are more common in women around the age of menopause and may have a hereditary predisposition.

Secondary Osteoarthritis

Secondary OA has numerous causes, the most common of which is secondary to trauma. Examples of affected patients include jackhammer operators who are more prone to hand OA, retired football players who have increased ankle and knee OA, linoleum floor layers who have increased knee OA, farmers who have increased hip OA, and individuals with other types of occupations or hobbies that require repetitive motions that stress particular joints.[5–7] In a retrospective study of middle-aged women, long-term weight-bearing exercises such as jogging and aerobics were associated with a twofold to threefold increase in the radiologic presence of hip and knee OA,[8] although other data suggest that vigorous sustained exercise of a joint that has not been previously injured does not produce OA.[4]

Other secondary causes of OA include congenital diseases, such as a type II procollagen defect that is linked to an early-onset familial OA,[9] and developmental abnormalities, such as hip dysplasias. Also, bone and joint diseases, such as *rheumatoid arthritis, crystal-induced arthropathies, Paget's disease, Charcot's arthropathy,* and *osteonecrosis,* can predispose to OA of both the affected joint and the joints proximal and distal to it.

Table 31–1. CLASSIFICATION CRITERIA FOR HAND OSTEOARTHRITIS

Hand pain, aching, or stiffness *and* at least 3 of the following:[*]
    Hard tissue enlargement of 2 or more of 10 selected joints[†]
    Hard tissue enlargement of 2 or more of DIP joints
    Deformity of at least 1 of 10 selected joints
    Fewer than 3 swollen MCP joints

[*]Sensitivity, 94%; specificity, 87%.
[†]These include the second and third DIP, the second and third PIP, and the first CMC joint on each hand.
    DIP, distal interphalangeal; MCP, metacarpophalangeal; CMC, carpometacarpal; PIP, proximal interphalangeal.
    Data from Altman R, Alarcon G, Appelrouth D, et al: The American College of Rheumatology criteria for the classification and reporting of osteoarthritis of the hand. Arthritis Rheum 33:1601–1610, 1990.

Finally, inherited metabolic diseases, such as *ochronosis* and *hemochromatosis,* and a number of endocrinologic diseases, which include *hyperparathyroidism, acromegaly, gout,* and *calcium pyrophosphate dihydrate disease,* can predispose the joints to OA.

There are good cross-sectional prospective data showing a strong link between obesity and OA of the knee.[4, 10] The evidence of its relationship to hip or hand OA is not as clear, but there is also a link here. Increased mechanical stress is the most plausible explanation for the weight-bearing joints being affected first, but systemic issues are also likely if obesity and hand OA are linked. Obesity in established OA patients can also increase the rate of disease progression and make treatment more difficult.

PATHOGENESIS

The primary disorder in OA involves degeneration of the articular cartilage. Hyaline cartilage is the smooth and slippery covering that coats the bony surfaces of all synovial joints in the human body. It is composed of 80% water and 20% organic material. The framework is a combination of type II collagen fibers, proteoglycans, and proteins secreted by chondrocyte cells. The proteoglycan monomers, composed of glycosaminoglycans, chondroitin-4-sulfate, chondroitin-6-sulfate, and keratin sulfate, are bound to hyaluronic acid to form the proteoglycan aggregates that are responsible for the compressive and elastic properties of cartilage. The tensile strength of cartilage is related to its collagen, whereas the load-bearing ability is determined by the proteoglycan content of the tissue.[2]

Table 31–2. CLASSIFICATION CRITERIA FOR HIP OSTEOARTHRITIS

Hip pain *and* at least 2 of the following:[*]
    Erythrocyte sedimentation rate <20 mm/h
    Radiographic femoral or acetabular osteophytes
    Radiographic joint space narrowing

[*]Sensitivity, 89%; specificity, 91%.
    Data from Altman R, Alarcon G, Appelrouth D, et al: The American College of Rheumatology criteria for the classification and reporting of osteoarthritis of the hip. Arthritis Rheum 34:505–514, 1991.

Table 31–3. CLASSIFICATION CRITERIA FOR KNEE OSTEOARTHRITIS

Knee pain *and* osteophytes *and* at least 1 of the following:[*]
    Age >50 y
    Crepitus on motion
    Stiffness <30 min

[*]Sensitivity, 91%; specificity, 86%.
    Data from Altman R, Asch E, Block G, et al: Development of criteria for the classification and reporting of osteoarthritis: Classification of osteoarthritis of the knee. Arthritis Rheum 29:1039–1049, 1986.

Hyaline cartilage itself is an avascular tissue and depends on the synovial fluid, circulated by joint movement, to bathe the chondrocytes and provide them with oxygen and nourishment. In healthy joints, an equilibrium exists between cartilage production and cartilage decay by the chondrocytes. In OA, this equilibrium is lost, which results in a net loss of cartilaginous mass. With progression of the disease, the ratio of water to proteoglycans increases, and the joint slowly loses its ability to rebound from a deforming load.[3] Also, the collagen network is disrupted, leading to blistering on the cartilaginous surface and exposure of the subchondral bone. Because cartilage lacks neural sensory fibers, there is usually no pain until a significant portion is gone and the joint capsule, underlying bone, or periosteum has been affected.[2] Loss of proprioception is also seen in OA. Whether it is a result or a causative factor is not known at this time, but it has been clearly demonstrated in several studies of knee OA.[11]

With progressive loss of both the gliding surfaces (i.e., articular cartilage) and the shock-absorbing capacity (i.e., proteoglycan molecules) of the joint, the resulting bone-on-bone trauma causes microfractures and increased joint vulnerability to stress. With time, local hypertrophic bone deposition and synovial hypertrophy can occur, and in some cases, bony cysts that indicate osteonecrosis and bony spurs can form. This joint destruction eventually leads to sclerosis, deformity, pain, and loss of function in the affected joint.

DIAGNOSIS AND CLINICAL FEATURES

Although the main clinical features of OA are pain, deformity, and progressive loss of motion, OA does not affect all joints in the same way. Therefore, both diagnostic and therapeutic measures must be tailored appropriately. In all patients, it is important to perform a thorough history and physical examination. The physician should

- Ask about any family or personal history of hemochromatosis or hyperparathyroidism.
- Ask about the patient's vocational, recreation, and weight history since early adulthood.
- Ask the patient if he or she has ever noticed joint swelling and how long it lasted.
- Note any lower back pain.
- Ask about any history of significant trauma.

- Ask about any septic or inflammatory arthropathies in the patient's past.
- Note the onset of pain, the joints involved, and any history suggesting ongoing inflammation, such as morning stiffness.[2]

Increased pain with joint activity or in the latter part of the day is more typical of OA than is morning stiffness or a gelling phenomenon, both of which are suggestive more of rheumatoid arthritis or other more inflammatory arthropathies.

Knee Joint

Knee pain that increases in severity when walking up or down stairs is more associated with patellofemoral disease than tibiofemoral joint OA. To test for patellofemoral disease, the physician places the patient supine, with knees in a neutral extended position, then pushes down on the proximal end of the patella while the patient contracts the quadriceps muscles (see Chapter 3). Pain or a sensation of crepitus with this procedure is a positive result. A radiograph of the knee can also be useful; typically, it shows bony spurring on the posterior surface of the patella or patellofemoral joint space narrowing.

On examination, any effusions or deformity in the knee joint and quadriceps wasting should be noted and are useful signs of OA. Local muscle weakness, particularly of the quadriceps group, is often seen with OA of the knee. Late-stage OA tends to cause a varus joint deformity with thickened synovium, crepitation and a limited range of motion.

Effusions, particularly in knee OA, are a common clinical finding and can be seen in about 20% of patients. The effusions range in size from a few milliliters to more than one liter. Occasionally a posterior synovial cyst (Baker's cyst) in an osteoarthritic knee ruptures, allowing the fluid to track down the posterior calf and cause lower extremity pitting edema with inflammation. This complication occurs more often in rheumatoid arthritis than in OA patients. A ruptured Baker's cyst can be misdiagnosed initially as cellulitis or a deep venous thrombosis. In general, a joint effusion in an osteoarthritic knee, especially if its onset correlates with exacerbation of pain or fever, should be aspirated. The studies that should be obtained from the synovial fluid include a Gram stain, culture, crystal examination, and cell count. The typical OA synovial fluid is straw colored and viscous, contains no crystals, and has a white blood cell count less than 2000/mm³. In many cases, removal of the fluid also helps with pain relief and mobility of the joint.

Radiographic findings suggestive of OA are joint space narrowing, osteophytes, sclerosis, malalignment, subchondral cysts, and deformities. The most helpful findings, especially in the knees and hips, are joint space narrowing and marginal osteophytes.[12] When writing the x-ray request to evaluate a patient for knee OA, the physician should request a weight-bearing radiograph with anteroposterior and lateral views. These views are the most helpful for evaluating the joint space and bony alignment of the knee. Although helpful for diagnosis, radiographic findings may not correlate with either the clinical progression of OA or the patient's symptoms. If the patient has locking of the knee on ambulation and physical examination suggests a meniscal tear, a magnetic resonance imaging (MRI) scan of the knee may be appropriate. MRI is much more sensitive for joint soft tissue injury, such as meniscal or tendon tears, than are ordinary radiographs and often is needed before any surgical intervention on the knee is undertaken.

Hip Joint

To examine the hip joint in OA, the physician should have the patient lie supine. Flexion, extension, and rotation are tested. The best clinical indicator of hip joint disease is pain, especially if exacerbated by external or internal rotation of the hip while the knee is in full extension. About 20% of patients have bilateral hip involvement with OA, so both hips need to be examined. Trochanteric bursitis, with tenderness over the greater trochanter, and sciatic nerve pain, with posterior hip and buttock pain, may both mimic the pain of hip OA. Anterior or inguinal pain and tenderness indicate true hip joint involvement. The x-ray findings of hip OA include joint space narrowing, osteophytes, femoral head migration, and bony sclerosis.[10]

Hand Joints

An examination of the hands often shows involvement of the distal interphalangeal and proximal interphalangeal joints. In fact, hand joint involvement has the highest prevalence rates of all clinically evident and symptomatic OA. The bony protrusions referred to as Heberden's and Bouchard's nodes are characteristic for the generalized primary form of the disease that also involves the knees and spine. Although subluxation and swelling of the distal interphalangeal and proximal interphalangeal joints can be marked, joint function is often preserved, and inflammation is minimal. These patients can suffer flares of the joint symptoms with swelling and inflammation, but the long-term prognosis for maintaining functional joint mobility is often good. In rare cases, a more erosive form of OA is seen with severe proximal interphalangeal and distal interphalangeal joint destruction and collapse of the subchondral bony plate on x-ray. More typical x-ray findings in hand OA, however, are subchondral sclerosis or cysts, joint deformity, and osteophytes. The first carpometacarpal joint is often symptomatic in OA. Pain or a decrease in the range of motion in this joint (particularly abduction) often demands more aggressive treatment because it may have a significant impact on overall functionality of the hand, limiting the patient's ability to grasp and hold objects.

TREATMENT

Once the diagnosis of OA has been established, there are two objectives of therapy: (1) to relieve pain and (2) to preserve function. Abnormal radiographic findings often do not correlate with clinical disease, and some amount of joint space narrowing can be seen with normal aging. Because, at this time, clinicians have no effective treatments that alter disease progression, therapy must focus on modifying the symptoms, including reduction of joint pain and functional disability. For this discussion, OA therapy is divided into pharmacologic, nonpharmacologic, and surgical treatments.

Nonpharmacologic Therapy

One of the most effective nonpharmacologic therapies for OA is patient education about joint protection. This education should be initiated by physicians, in the form of pamphlets and referral to a community arthritis support group, which are available through the Arthritis Foundation, and possibly a referral to a physical or occupational therapist. The support groups and the therapists can be helpful, both as educators and motivators of patients with OA. There is good evidence that health education for self-management of chronic arthritis can decrease pain, the number of physician office visits, and the patient's overall disability.[13]

As discussed previously, obesity and repetitive motion trauma are the most important and modifiable risk factors. Weight reduction may improve pain and progression of OA in the weight-bearing joints, such as the knee, for both the short-term and long-term.[14, 15] Weight loss can also significantly decrease a patient's pain medication requirement, so a weight reduction program should be recommended to all overweight OA patients.

Patients must begin to think in terms of using their affected joints sparingly, while keeping muscle strength and tone as good as possible. This is accomplished best by having the patient engage in a physical therapy or exercise program. The goals of physical therapy in OA are to decrease pain and to maintain joint functionality, endurance, and strength. Well-developed muscles are key to maintaining joint stability. Flexibility, aerobic conditioning, and muscle-strengthening exercises have been shown to be helpful in improving overall function and decreasing pain in patients with knee OA.[16, 17] This can include a low-impact aerobic regimen, such as walking or aquatics for 30 minutes, three times per week, and local muscle strengthening, such as quadriceps exercises for knee OA.[18] Other modalities that can be helpful include application of local heat or cold packs, isometric exercise programs, and splinting of affected joints to decrease pain and swelling and to protect the joint.[19] Improving body mechanics and posture training, often done by physical therapists, can also help to control pain and prevent further injury.

An occupational or physical therapist can also help with avoidance of repetitive motion injury during recreation or at work. They can provide a number of ergonomic and assistive devices that can decrease both joint load and repetitive motion. Examples of assistive devices include a cane for hip and knee problems, a knee brace for exercise, a tool to improve handgrip, and an elevated toilet seat. OA patients who walk for occupation or recreation may need special shoes with good shock absorption, extra depth, extra width, or metatarsal bars to improve toe alignment. In patients with already advanced OA, other simple measures can be taken to avoid further mechanical stress and decrease pain in affected joints. These include the use of lightweight utensils, use of electrical devices whenever possible, use of Velcro fasteners instead of zippers or buttons, installation of a single-lever faucet, avoidance of standing for long periods, and avoidance of lifting heavy objects.[2]

Pharmacologic Therapy

ANALGESICS

There are many medications that can assist with pain control (Table 31–4). Initially, patients with mild or moderate OA should be treated with a simple analgesic, such as acetaminophen. Treatment usually begins with 500 to 1000 mg twice per day, increasing up to 1000 mg three or four times per day as needed to control pain. The main side effect is liver toxicity; therefore, in alcoholics and patients with liver disease, this drug should be avoided or doses kept to less than 2 g/day, with periodic monitoring of liver enzymes. Studies suggest that in short-term trials (4-week duration), acetaminophen is as effective as ibuprofen.[20] In longer trials of 2 years' duration, however, acetaminophen was not as effective as naproxen for relieving the pain of knee OA.[21] Additionally, acetaminophen can be helpful as an adjunct to nonsteroidal anti-inflammatory drugs (NSAIDs) in more severe disease.

More potent analgesics, such as opiates, either

Table 31–4. COMMONLY USED ANALGESICS FOR OSTEOARTHRITIS

Drug Name	Usual Total Daily Dose for Osteoarthritis Patients (mg)	Short (S) or Long (L) Acting	Most Common Side Effects
Acetaminophen	650–3000	S	Liver toxicity
Codeine (alone or in combination with acetaminophen or aspirin)	30–180	S	Lightheadedness, dizziness, sedation, shortness of breath, nausea, respiratory distress
Tramadol	100–400	S	Dizziness/vertigo, nausea, constipation, headache, somnolence, pruritus, central nervous system stimulation, and rarely seizures

alone or in combination with acetaminophen or aspirin, have been shown to be helpful for acute painful flares of OA.[22] They can, however, mask symptoms of joint infection or ligamental damage and can be sedating in elderly patients, predisposing them to falls. Tramadol, a nonnarcotic analgesic, has been approved for use in OA. Preliminary studies show that it can also be effective for breakthrough pain in OA patients.[23] These agents are all best used in occasional short (2 to 4 weeks) bursts during times of severe pain, not responding to other medications.

NONSTEROIDAL ANTI-INFLAMMATORY DRUGS

NSAIDs are a large group of drugs that have analgesic effects at lower doses and anti-inflammatory effects at higher doses (see Chapter 9). They are all competitive inhibitors of the cyclooxygenase enzyme, which is a major branch point of the arachidonic acid pathway. They block the production of prostaglandins (particularly of the E series), lymphocyte function, neutrophil aggregation, and other proinflammatory mechanisms.[2] Their analgesic properties are thought to be due to inhibition of prostaglandin sensitization of peripheral pain receptors.[2] Although these agents vary in half-life, there is little evidence to suggest that they vary greatly in efficacy (Table 31–5). However, for unknown reasons, a different NSAID can help even though others have failed. It is best to begin with the drug that is likely to have the least side effects in a targeted patient and move to other NSAIDs if they fail to respond. In elderly patients with comorbid conditions, it is best to begin with an NSAID that has a short half-life. The patient should be started at the lowest available dose, which is increased slowly. A 2-year trial confirmed that NSAIDs were superior to placebo in relief of knee pain from OA.[24]

NSAIDs can precipitate acute renal insufficiency by decreasing glomerular filtration by inhibiting prostaglandin production. Less often, NSAIDs can cause interstitial nephritis with proteinuria. The shorter half-life preparations, such as ibuprofen, are preferred for older patients and those with poor renal function. NSAIDs inhibit platelet aggregation and can prolong bleeding time. For this reason, concurrent use of NSAIDs and warfarin (Coumadin) is relatively contraindicated and requires close monitoring of the prothrombin time. NSAIDs can occasionally cause tinnitus, headaches, confusion, depression, rashes, hypersensitivity reactions, and hepatic toxicity. The major side effect, however, and probably the most common cause of significant morbidity from NSAIDs is gastrointestinal toxicity. The inhibition of prostaglandins locally in the gastric mucosa can produce nausea, gastritis, esophagitis, ulcers, perforation, and gastroduodenal bleeding. It has been estimated that NSAIDs are responsible for 100,000 to 200,000 complicated ulcers each year in the United States, with 10,000 to 20,000 of those leading to death.[25] Obtaining any past history of positive *Helicobacter pylori* titer or biopsy and searching for history of gastric or duodenal ulcers help the physician decide if NSAIDs

are appropriate for use in individual patients. A baseline hematocrit and creatinine level should be obtained, and patients need to be educated about warning signs of gastrointestinal bleeding before NSAIDs are started. The advice not to take an NSAID on an empty stomach can help prevent gastrointestinal toxicity. For patients at high risk of gastrointestinal bleeding or with renal insufficiency, other therapeutic modalities should be used because NSAIDs relieve pain only and do not alter the course of OA.

To help patients tolerate NSAIDs, several groups of medications have been developed (see Chapter 9). The first is misoprostol (Cytotec). It is a prostaglandin E_1 analogue, which when taken at doses of 200 μg four times per day repletes the local gastric prostaglandin supply and can decrease the formation of gastric and duodenal ulcers.[22] Half this dose can be effective in many patients. Proton-pump inhibitors (omeprazole and lansoprazole) reduce gastric acid production and can also be useful to prevent gastrointestinal bleeding.[25] If a patient is found to have *H. pylori,* treatment to eradicate it from the gastric and duodenal mucosa before initiating NSAIDs has been shown to reduce the risk of developing NSAID-induced peptic ulcers.[23]

Work in the pathogenesis of inflammation has determined that cyclooxygenase (COX), the enzyme that catalyzes the production of prostaglandin, is two isoenzymes, COX-1 and COX-2. Most currently available NSAIDs inhibit both of the isoenzymes, and most are more potent COX-1 than COX-2 inhibitors. Studies suggest that COX-1 is the more nonspecific activator of the two and is the isoenzyme principally responsible for production of protective prostaglandins in the kidney and gastrointestinal tract. COX-2 is the form that is induced by inflammation.[26, 27] With this information in mind, a newer class of highly selective COX-2 inhibitors is available for use (see Chapter 9). Compared with traditional NSAIDs, these new agents have significantly less gastroduodenal toxicity (reduced endoscopically documented mucosal injury) and no impact on the coagulation system (no effect on platelet aggregation).[27, 28a–30] Currently, two selective COX-2 inhibitors are FDA approved for use in OA patients: celecoxib (Celebrex) and rofecoxib (Vioxx). Candidates for these new agents are patients with OA who either have complications from traditional NSAIDs (e.g., gastrointestinal or hematologic), or patients who are at an increased risk for NSAID complications (increased age, long duration of use, multiple concurrent medications, or concurrent use of prednisone, or warfarin).[28a–30]

TOPICAL THERAPY

Local application of capsaicin or salicylate cream over the affected joint has been shown to be effective over placebo in randomized, controlled trials. Other than local skin irritation, there are no side effects, and in some patients these agents seem to work quite well. Pain relief is local only, however, and the cream must be applied many times per day.[28] These medications can also be used for patients who are intolerant to NSAIDs.

Table 31–5. COMMONLY USED NONSTEROIDAL ANTI-INFLAMMATORY DRUGS

Drug Name	Usual Total Daily Dose for Osteoarthritis Patients (mg)	Short (S) or Long (L) Acting	Gastrointestinal Bleed Risk	Nausea or Dyspepsia	Risk of Dysuria, Renal Insufficiency, or Papillary Necrosis	Rash or Pruritus	Dizziness, Headache, or Tinnitus	Other
Aspirin	650–3000	S	++	+++	+	+++	++++	Enteric-coated available
Diclofenac	100–150	S	++	+++	+	++	++	Enteric-coated and long-acting (XL) available
Diflunisal	500–1000	L	+	+++	+	+++	+++	
Etodolac	600–1200	S	++	++++	++	++	++	Edema
Flurbiprofen	100–300	S	++	++++	+++	+++	+++	Edema
Ibuprofen	1200–2400	S	+	+++	+	++	++++	Long-acting (SR) available
Indomethacin	75–200	S	+	++++			+++	
Ketoprofen	75–300	S	+	++++	+++	+++	+++	Edema
Nabumetone	1000–2000	L	++	++++	+	+++	+++	Edema
Naproxen	500–1000	L	+	++++	++	+++	++	
Oxaprozin	600–1200	L	++	++++	++	++	++	Edema
Piroxicam	10–20	L	++	++++	+	+	++++	
Salsalate	750–3000	L	+	++++	+	+++	+++	Edema
Sulindac	300–400	L	++	++++	++	++	+++	Edema
Tolmetin	600–1800	S	++	++++				Edema

Incidence of adverse reaction:

+ = <1%
++ = 1–3%
+++ = 3–9%
++++ = >9%

INTRA-ARTICULAR INJECTIONS

GLUCOCORTICOIDS. Intra-articular preparations of glucocorticoids have a useful niche in the treatment of OA; their action is one of decreasing inflammation in the joint. Pain relief from such injections is generally good and lasts for an average of 7 to 10 days. There is some evidence that if used too frequently, glucocorticoid injections can induce damage to chondrocytes and, rarely, cause avascular necrosis, so most rheumatologists do not recommend more than four glucocorticoid injections in any one joint per year. The dose injected, type of glucocorticoid, and total volume depend on the joint being treated (Table 31–6). With time, the injections can lose efficacy, so patients begin to ask for injections more often. When injecting an acutely inflamed OA joint, it is important to aspirate as much of the synovial fluid as possible and send it for cell count, crystal examination, Gram stain, and culture. These tests rule out a crystal-induced arthropathy or joint infection. Oral glucocorticoids should be avoided because there is no evidence to support their use in OA.

HYALURONIC ACID. Two preparations of high-molecular-weight hyaluronic acid (Hyalgan and Synvisc) have been approved for use in knee OA. Hyaluronic acid (sodium hyaluronate) is the viscous macromolecule, a large repeating disaccharide molecule, that is a major constituent of synovial fluid and is responsible for soft tissue/cartilage and soft tissue/soft tissue lubrication within joints. Both of these agents require three to five joint injections to be administered over a period ranging from 2 to 5 weeks and can be given only twice per year. Although initial trials in animal models were promising, prospective controlled studies in humans have shown only mildly significant efficacy, with the difference in pain between the hyaluronate group and placebo being small (<10%).[31] However, older patients with functional disability had slightly more improvement in pain and function, after hyaluronate injections, than other groups of patients.[32] Other studies suggest that their efficacy is similar to NSAIDs and that the best use of these agents may be in patients who are unable to tolerate NSAIDs.

JOINT LAVAGE

Individuals with OA who do not respond to analgesics, NSAIDs, or intra-articular glucocorticoid injections may be candidates for joint lavage. There have been several published studies with favorable results of lavage of the knee for OA.[33, 34] This procedure is performed in an office setting using an arthroscope or a large-bore (14-gauge) needle and syringe. A total of about 1 liter of fluid is infused and removed after a few minutes from the joint. In one study, 58% of the 14 patients who underwent joint lavage reported clinical improvement after 1 year.[33] The mechanism for this effect is thought to be a washout of inflammatory mediators, debris, and loose bodies. This is just a hypothesis, however, and may be proven incorrect with further study.

ARTHROSCOPY

Although this procedure can be done on the wrist, hip, elbow, shoulder, and ankle, its use is most established in OA of the knee. It can be used in OA patients to detect chondral tears, loose bodies, ligamental tears, and some bony abnormalities. At the time of visualization, the arthroscopist can also repair meniscal tears, remove loose bodies, remove synovium, and, if needed, shave the articular cartilage. This procedure can improve knee locking, increase joint stability, and provide pain relief. Some investigators postulate that it can also be used as a *bridge* to joint surgery or replacement, but the population that would benefit most from such a procedure has yet to be established from randomized and controlled studies. The introduction of small arthroscopes and improved local anesthetic and sedation techniques can substantially reduce pain both during and after the procedure.[2]

SURGICAL APPROACHES

A large number of open surgical procedures can benefit OA patients. These include ligamental repairs, osteotomies, and total joint replacements. The most important reasons to undergo a surgical intervention include pain uncontrolled by other means, deformity that interferes with function, and severe disability. Timing for surgery and joint replacement is crucial because most prosthetic joints wear out with time. The average survival of a prosthetic hip joint, for example, is 10 to 15 years.[35] The patient's general medical condition and age are also important considerations. A patient younger than age 50 may require a second operation in future years. In this case, it may be better to delay sending the patient for replacement for as long as possible by maximizing their medical regimens and physical therapy. The longer patients are inactive, the more obese and deconditioned they become, and the more likely it is that they will have a worse outcome during surgery and immediately postoperatively. Predictors for early prosthesis failure include an imperfect fit, increased physical activity, and obesity.[2] Other important predictors of surgical outcome are the number of procedures that the surgeon has performed and the patient's cooperation with the prescribed rehabilitation regimen.[36]

OA of the weight-bearing joints, such as the knee and hip, tends to be the most disabling. Therefore, these joints are more commonly repaired and replaced than are the non–weight-bearing joints, such as the shoulder and small joints of the hands. The best postoperative re-

Table 31–6. RECOMMENDATIONS FOR GLUCOCORTICOID JOINT INJECTION	
Joint Size (Example)	Recommended Triamcinolone Hexacetonide Dose per Injection (mg)
Small (PIP, DIP)	5–10
Medium (wrist, elbow, ankle)	20–30
Large (knee, hip, shoulder)	30–40

PIP, proximal interphalangeal; DIP, distal interphalangeal.

sults occur with hip replacement, followed by knee replacement.

Osteotomy is a less commonly used procedure but in well-selected patients can be quite effective for pain relief, improved bone alignment, and stability. The technique is best for younger patients with knee deformities, such as genu valgum, and can delay knee replacement in these patients.[37] It can also be used for hip diseases, such as congenital hip dysplasia, nonunion after femoral neck fracture, slipped femoral epiphysis, Perthes' disease, and osteonecrosis.[38]

INVESTIGATIONAL THERAPIES

The oral supplements glucosamine and chondroitin sulfate, which are available in pharmacies and health food stores, are now under investigation for pain control. Both glucosamine and chondroitin are components of normal matrix in articular cartilage and are crucial to its stability. To date, the published trials on these supplements are few in number, have relatively small numbers of patients, and have short follow-up times. The data suggest that glucosamine was superior to placebo and similar to ibuprofen in improving pain and function in patients with OA within several weeks of beginning therapy.[39, 40] There appear to be few side effects from these agents, so that other than the cost of the supplements, there is little risk to trying them in patients who inquire about them.

In animal models, doxycycline has been shown to reduce breakdown of articular cartilage by inhibition of tissue metalloproteinases.[26] Clinical studies are currently underway to determine the ability of doxycycline or minocycline to decrease the progression of knee OA. Plaquenil and sulfasalazine, which are often used in rheumatoid arthritis and lupus, may also have a role in inflammatory OA; however, these agents are only now being studied in this group of patients. They have relatively few side effects and can be good adjunct medications in specific cases. At this time, however, their use in the primary care setting is not recommended. Other novel therapies, such as intra-articular NSAIDs and electromagnetic radiation, show some promising results in initial trials in OA but have yet to be used on large numbers of patients.[41, 42]

WHEN TO REFER TO A SPECIALIST

Although most OA patients can be managed by their primary care physician, in many cases, a referral is needed at some time. Initially, all patients should be provided with self-help materials, which can be obtained from local branches of the Arthritis Foundation. Patients can also contact the foundation directly, by phone (1-800-283-7800 or 1-404-872-7100), regular mail (1330 West Peachtree Street, Atlanta, Georgia 30309), or via the Internet (http://www.arthritis.org).

Most patients benefit from physical therapy. A therapist who has special training or experience with arthritis patients is of most help. The therapist can help relieve pain with modalities such as heat, ultrasound, and manual therapy. He or she can help identify joint dysfunction and teach patients how to strengthen appropriate muscle groups, how to use range-of-motion exercises, how to apply techniques of joint protection,

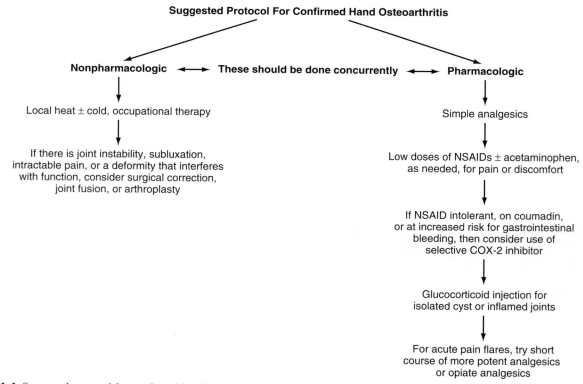

Figure 31–1. Suggested protocol for confirmed hand osteoarthritis. (Adapted from Ratner B, Gramas DA, Lane NE: Osteoarthritis. In Weisman MH, Weinblatt ME, eds: Treatment of the Rheumatic Diseases. Philadelphia, WB Saunders, 1995.)

and can instruct patients in home exercise programs. Physical therapists can also be helpful as motivators for more sedentary patients. They can help by evaluating gait and postural abnormalities and provide patients with assistive devices, such as canes, walkers, and splints. These goals can be accomplished in as few as three visits to the therapist, but most OA patients require more. Occupational therapists can also be helpful in increasing an OA patient's independence by providing equipment such as handrails, jar-opening devices, and special utensils.

Many OA patients benefit from an evaluation by a rheumatologist. The rheumatologist can assist with the diagnosis of OA; help rule out secondary causes; and provide a second opinion about therapy by *fine-tuning* ongoing medical management and providing advice on nonmedical management, joint injections, joint lavage, and in some cases diagnostic arthroscopy.[43, 44]

Orthopaedic surgeons offer a wide variety of procedures to benefit OA patients, ranging from arthroscopy to joint replacement. The main indications for joint replacement are intractable pain and inability to perform activities of daily living. These indications are patient dependent, so the timing of the procedure should involve collaboration between the patient, the medical physicians, and the orthopaedic surgeon. Good surgical outcome depends on a patient's overall health, type of surgery, the joint being repaired or replaced, the surgeon's experience with that particular procedure, and the patient's motivation for rehabilitation.[45]

Algorithms and additional guidelines for the treatment of osteoarthritis are in the Appendix to this chapter.

CONCLUSIONS

OA is a common disease that often presents more of a therapeutic than diagnostic problem for the primary care physician. It is usually an insidious, non–life-threatening disease that progresses over many years. For this reason, initial therapy should begin with simple measures, such as acetaminophen and physical therapy. As the disease progresses, however, more potent medications and, in some cases, surgery are required to control pain and preserve function in the involved joints. Recommendations for cost-effective and evidence-based management of OA for each joint can be found in Figures 31–1 to 31–3.

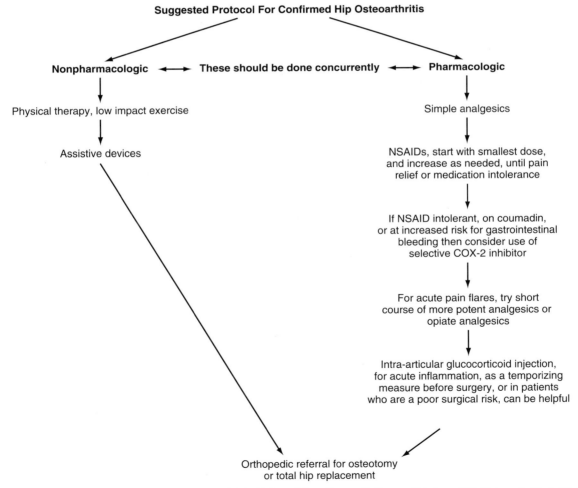

Figure 31–2. Suggested protocol for confirmed hip osteoarthritis. (Adapted from Ratner B, Gramas DA, Lane NE: Osteoarthritis. In Weisman MH, Weinblatt ME, eds: Treatment of the Rheumatic Diseases. Philadelphia, WB Saunders, 1995.)

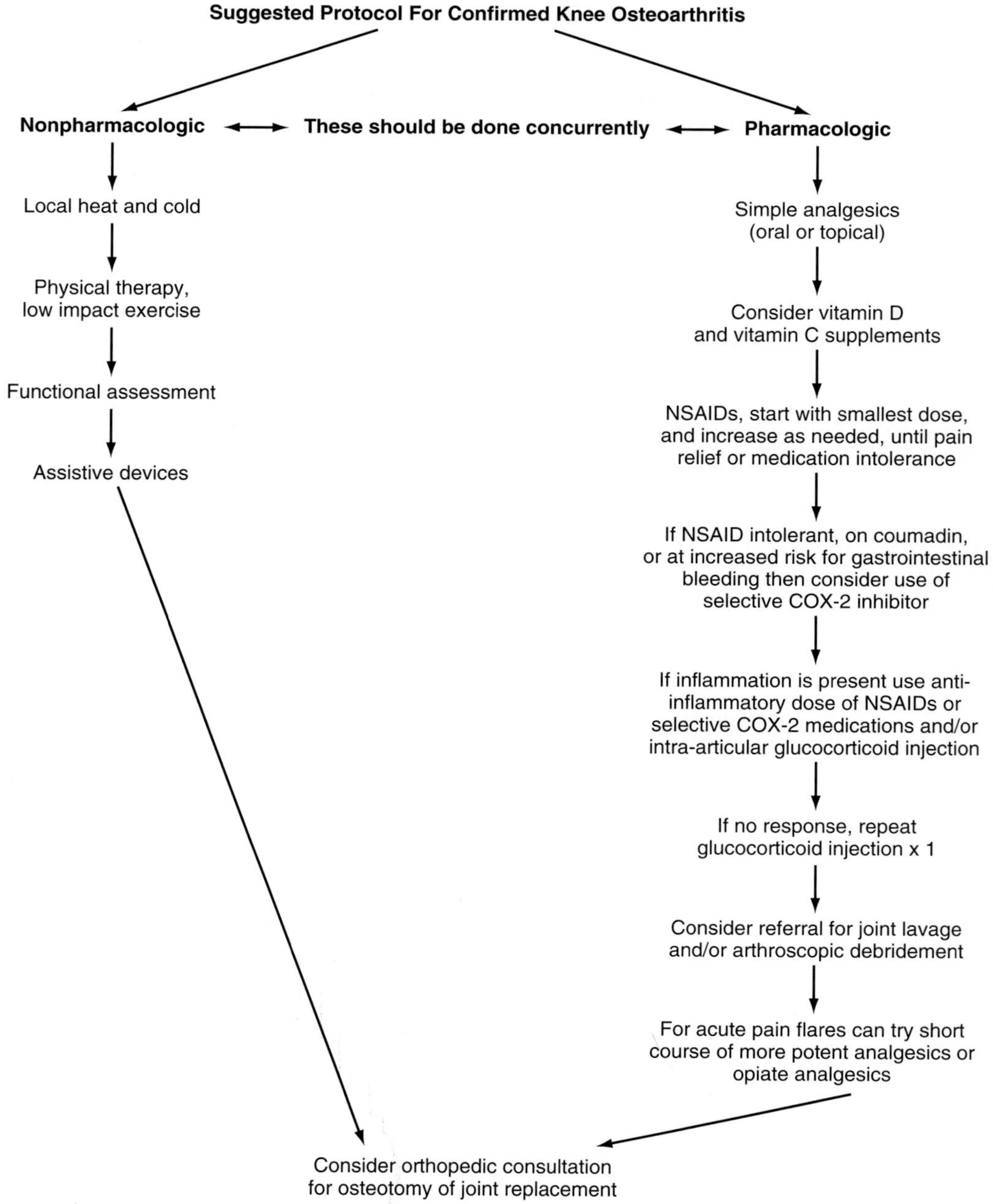

Suggested Protocol For Confirmed Knee Osteoarthritis

Nonpharmacologic ←→ These should be done concurrently ←→ Pharmacologic

Nonpharmacologic:
- Local heat and cold
- Physical therapy, low impact exercise
- Functional assessment
- Assistive devices

Pharmacologic:
- Simple analgesics (oral or topical)
- Consider vitamin D and vitamin C supplements
- NSAIDs, start with smallest dose, and increase as needed, until pain relief or medication intolerance
- If NSAID intolerant, on coumadin, or at increased risk for gastrointestinal bleeding then consider use of selective COX-2 inhibitor
- If inflammation is present use anti-inflammatory dose of NSAIDs or selective COX-2 medications and/or intra-articular glucocorticoid injection
- If no response, repeat glucocorticoid injection x 1
- Consider referral for joint lavage and/or arthroscopic debridement
- For acute pain flares can try short course of more potent analgesics or opiate analgesics

Consider orthopedic consultation for osteotomy of joint replacement

Figure 31–3. Suggested protocol for confirmed knee osteoarthritis. (Adapted from Ratner B, Gramas DA, Lane NE: Osteoarthritis. In Weisman MH, Weinblatt ME, eds: Treatment of the Rheumatic Diseases. Philadelphia, WB Saunders, 1995.)

Algorithms and guidelines for the treatment of chronic axial osteoarthritis are in the Appendix to this chapter.

REFERENCES

1. Lawrence RC, Hochberg MC, Kelsey JL, et al: Estimates of the prevalence of selected arthritic and musculoskeletal diseases in the United States. J Rheumatol 16:427–441, 1987.
2. Gramas DA, Lane NE: Osteoarthritis. In Weisman MH, Weinblatt ME, eds: Treatment of the Rheumatic Diseases. Philadelphia, WB Saunders, 1995, pp 286–311.
3. March LM: Osteoarthritis. Med J Aust 166:98–103, 1997.
4. Hochberg MC, Lethbridge-Cejku M: Epidemiologic consideration in the primary prevention of osteoarthritis. In Hamerman D, ed: Osteoarthritis: Public Health Implications for an Aging Population. Baltimore, Johns Hopkins University Press, 1997, pp 169–186.
5. Cooper C, Cambell L, Byng P, et al: Occupational activity and the risk of hip osteoarthritis. Ann Rheum Dis 55:680–682, 1996.
6. Vingard E: Osteoarthritis of the knee and physical load from occupation. Ann Rheum Dis 55:677–679, 1996.
7. Maetzel A, Makela M, Hawker G, et al: Osteoarthritis of the hip and knee and mechanical occupational exposure—a systematic overview of exposure. J Rheumatol 24:1599–1606, 1997.
8. Spector TD, Harris PA, Hart DJ, et al: Risk of osteoarthritis associated with long-term weight-bearing sports. Arthritis Rheum 39:988–995, 1996.
9. Bleasel JF, Cicuttini F, Baker J, et al: Genetic influences on osteoarthritis in women: A twin study. BMJ 312:940–943, 1996.

10. Creamer P, Hochberg MC: Osteoarthritis. Lancet 350:503–509, 1997.
11. Sharma L, Pai Y: Impaired proprioception and osteoarthritis. Curr Opin Rheumatol 9:253–258, 1997.
12. Mazzuca S: Plain radiography in the evaluation of knee osteoarthritis. Curr Opin Rheumatol 9:263–267, 1997.
13. Lorig KR, Mazonson PD, Halsted HR: Evidence suggesting that health education for self-management in patients with chronic arthritis has sustained health benefits while reducing health care costs. Arthritis Rheum 36:439–446, 1993.
14. Felson DT, Ahange Y, Anthony JM, et al: Weight loss reduces the risk for symptomatic knee osteoarthritis in women. Ann Intern Med 116:535–539, 1992.
15. Felson DT, et al: Obesity and knee osteoarthritis: The Framingham Study. Ann Intern Med 109:18–24, 1988.
16. O'Reilly S, Jones A, Doherty M: Muscle weakness in osteoarthritis. Curr Opin Rheumatol 9:259–262, 1997.
17. Fisher NM, Gresham GE, Abrams M, et al: Quantitative effects of physical therapy on muscular and functional performance in subjects with osteoarthritis of the knee. Arch Phys Med Rehabil 74:840–847, 1993.
18. Puett DW, Griffin MR: Published trials of nonsteroidal and noninvasive therapies for hip and knee osteoarthritis. Ann Intern Med 121:133–140, 1994.
19. O'Sullivan SB, Schmitz TJ: Physical Rehabilitation: Assessment and Treatment. Philadelphia, FA Davis, 1994.
20. Bradley JD, Brandt KD, Katz PB, et al: A comparison of an anti-inflammatory dose of ibuprofen and acetaminophen in the treatment of patients with osteoarthritis of the knee. N Engl J Med 325:87–91, 1991.
21. Williams HK, Ward JR, Egger MJ, et al: Comparison of naproxen and acetaminophen in a two year study of the treatment of osteoarthritis of the knee. Arthritis Rheum 36:1196–1206, 1993.
22. Graham DY, White RH, Moreland LW, et al: Duodenal and gastric ulcer prevention with misoprostol in arthritis patients taking NSAIDs. Ann Intern Med 119:257, 1993.
23. Chan F, Sung J, et al: Randomized trial of eradication of *Helicobacter pylori* before nonsteroidal anti-inflammatory drug therapy to prevent peptic ulcers. Lancet 350:975–979, 1997.
24. Dieppe P, Cushnaghan J, Jasani MK, et al: A two year placebo controlled trial of nonsteroidal anti-inflammatory therapy in osteoarthritis of the knee joint. Br J Rheumatol 32:595–600, 1993.
25. Bjorkman DJ, Kimmey MB: Nonsteroidal anti-inflammatory drugs and gastrointestinal disease: Pathophysiology, treatment, and prevention. Dig Dis 13:119–121, 1995.
26. Kuettner KE, Goldberg VM: Osteoarthritic disorders. Presented at American Academy of Orthopaedic Surgeons workshop, Monterey, CA, April 1994.
27. Lane N: Pain management in osteoarthritis: The role of COX-2 inhibitors. J Rheumatol 24(suppl 49):20–24, 1997.
28. Altman RD, Aven A, Holmburg CE, et al: Capsaicin cream 0.025% as monotherapy for osteoarthritis: A double blind study. Semin Arthritis Rheum 23(suppl 3):25–33, 1994.
28a. Simon LS, Lanza FL, Lipsky PE, et al: Preliminary study of the safety and efficacy of SC-58635, a novel cyclooxygenase 2 inhibitor: efficacy and safety in two placebo-controlled trials in osteoarthritis and rheumatoid arthritis, and studies of gastrointestinal and platelet effects. Arthritis Rheum 41:1591–1602, 1998.
29. Saag K, et al: A specific COX-2 inhibitor has clinical efficacy comparable to ibuprofen in the treatment of knee and hip osteoarthritis in a 6-week controlled clinical trial. Arthritis Rheum 41(9 Suppl):S196, 1998.
30. Karim A, et al: Celecoxib, a specific COX-2 inhibitor lacks significant drug-drug interactions with methotrexate or warfarin. Arthritis Rheum 41(9 Suppl):S315, 1998.
31. Dahlberg L, Lohmander S, Ryd L: Intra-articular injections of hyaluronan in patients with cartilage abnormalities and knee pain. Arthritis Rheum 37:521–528, 1994.
32. Lohmander S, Dalen N, et al: Intra-articular hyaluronan injections in the treatment of osteoarthritis of the knee: A randomized, double blind, placebo controlled multicenter trial. Ann Rheum Dis 55:424–431, 1996.
33. Chang RW, Falconer J, et al: A randomized, controlled trial of athroscopic surgery versus closed needle joint lavage for patients with osteoarthritis of the knee. Arthritis Rheum 36:289, 1993.
34. Ike RW, Arnold WJ, et al: Tidal irrigation versus conservative medical management in patients with osteoarthritis of the knee. J Rheumatol 19:772, 1992.
35. Emery DFG, Clarke HJ, Grover ML: Stanmore total hip replacement in younger patients. J Bone Joint Surg Br 79:240–246, 1997.
36. Peterson MG, Hollenberg JP, Szatrowski TP, et al: Geographic variations in the rates of elective total hip and knee arthroplasties among Medicare beneficiaries in the United States. J Bone Joint Surg Am 74:1530–1539, 1992.
37. Paley D, Maar DC, Herzenberg JE: New concepts in high tibial osteotomy for medial compartment osteoarthritis. Orthop Clin North Am 25:483–498, 1994.
38. Santore RF, Dabezies EJ: Femoral osteotomy for secondary arthritis of the hip joint in young adults. Can J Surg 38(suppl 1):33–48, 1995.
39. Lopez VA: Double blind clinical evaluation of the relative efficacy of ibuprofen and glucosamine sulfate in the management of osteoarthritis of the knee in outpatients. Curr Med Res Opin 8:145–149, 1982.
40. Potera C: Can supplements reduce arthritis symptoms? Physician Sportsmed 25:15–16, 1997.
41. Trock DH, Bollet AJ, Dyer RH, et al: A double-blind trial of the clinical effects of pulsed electromagnetic fields in osteoarthritis. J Rheumatol 20:456, 1993.
42. Pelletier JP, McMollum R, et al: Regulation of human normal and osteoarthritic chondrocyte interleukin-1 receptor by antirheumatic drugs. Arthritis Rheum 36:1517, 1993.
43. Mazzuca SA, Brandt KD, Katz BP, et al: Comparison of general internists, family physicians, and rheumatologists managing patients with symptoms of osteoarthritis of the knee. Arthritis Care Res 10:289–299, 1997.
44. Mazzuca SA, Brandt KD, Katz BP, et al: Therapeutic strategies distinguish community based primary care physicians from rheumatologists in the management of osteoarthritis. J Rheumatol 20:80–86, 1993.
45. Lavernia CJ, Guzman JF: Relationship of surgical volume to short-term mortality, morbidity, and hospital charges in arthroplasty. J Arthroplasty 10:133–140, 1995.

Algorithm G: Chronic Noninflammatory Articular Conditions
If the condition is chronic and noninflammatory, the provider should determine whether OA is likely or further evaluation is necessary.

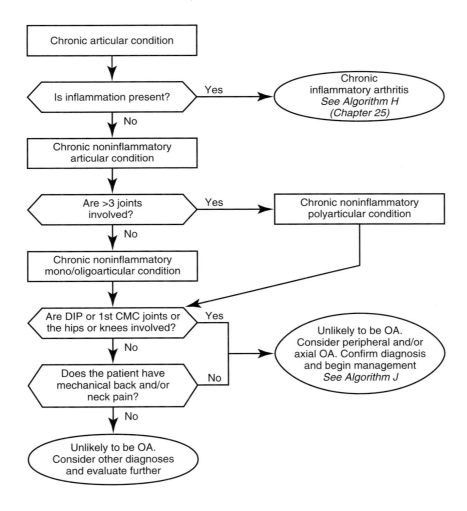

Recognition and Management of Patients with Specific Rheumatologic Problems

From Lipsky PE: Algorithms for the diagnosis and management of musculoskeletal complaints. Am J Med 103(6A):58S, 1997.

J Algorithm J: Management of Osteoarthritis

After the diagnosis of OA has been established, the provider should develop a plan of clinical management and assess outcomes.

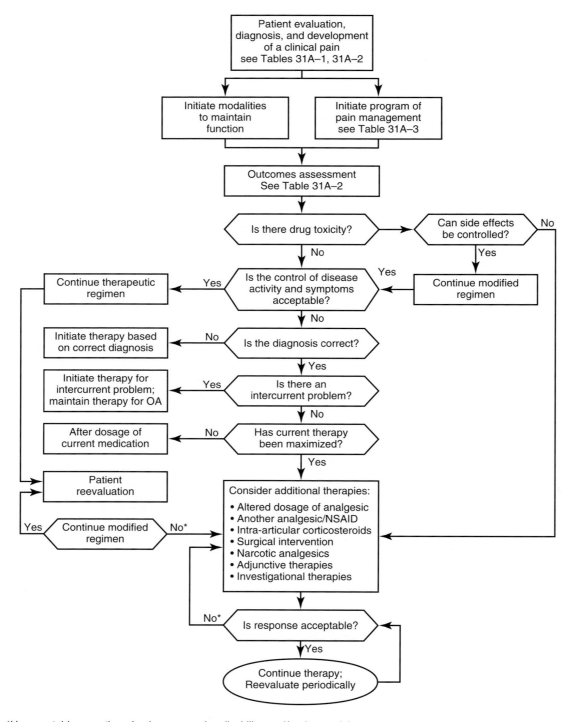

*Unacceptable = continued pain, progressive disability, and/or drug toxicity.

From Lipsky PE: Algorithms for the diagnosis and management of musculoskeletal complaints. Am J Med 103(6A): 61S, 1997.

**Table 31A–1. OSTEOARTHRITIS:
PATIENT EVALUATION**

Functional Status
- Joint function—limitation of movement/muscular atrophy
- Comorbid disease
- Psychological factors
- Socioeconomic factors/vocational factors
- Functional assessments (activities of daily living evaluations, functional questionnaires)
- Obesity

Peripheral Joint Pain
- Pain with activity or weight-bearing
- Pain at rest/night pain/sleep disturbance
- Small joint involvement
- Large joint involvement, damage, or instability
- Periarticular pain

Axial Pain

From Lipsky PE: Algorithms for the diagnosis and management of musculoskeletal complaints. Am J Med 103(6A): 79S, 1997.

**Table 31A–2. OSTEOARTHRITIS: GOALS
OF THERAPY**

- Relieve pain
- Maintain function
- Protect articular structures
- Educate patient, family

From Lipsky PE: Algorithms for the diagnosis and management of musculoskeletal complaints. Am J Med 103(6A): 79S, 1997.

**Table 31A–3. OSTEOARTHRITIS:
PAIN MANAGEMENT**

- OA of the hand usually responds adequately to analgesics and occupational therapy
- OA of the hip may require additional therapy, including NSAIDs at analgesic or anti-inflammatory doses, physical therapy, or surgical intervention
- OA of the knee may require additional therapy, including NSAIDs at analgesic or anti-inflammatory doses, intermittent intra-articular corticosteroids, physical therapy, or surgical intervention

Pharmacologic	Nonpharmacologic

• Primary therapy
  - non-narcotic analgesics
  - topical agents (eg, capsaicin)
  - nonacetylated salicylates
  - NSAIDs (consider analgesic dose initially)
  - intra-articular corticosteroids
	• Modification of activities
	• Exercise (bike, walk, swim)
	• Physical therapy
	• Heat/cold application
	• Psychosocial support
	• Pain management
	• Self-help programs

A survey of 440 practicing rheumatologists revealed the following preference for initial treatment of OA of the knee: non-narcotic analgesic, 37%; low-dose NSAIDs, 35%; high-dose NSAIDs, 13%; physical therapy, 10%; and intra-articular corticosteroids, 6%. If the initial treatment failed to curtail symptoms, the preferred second treatment was intra-articular corticosteroids, 33%; high-dose NSAIDs, 30%; low-dose NSAIDs, 23% physical therapy, 8%; and non-narcotic analgesics, 5%.

From Lipsky PE: Algorithms for the diagnosis and management of musculoskeletal complaints. Am J Med 103(6A): 80S, 1997.

Recognition and Management of Patients with Specific Rheumatologic Problems

Chapter 32

Osteoarthritis of the Spine

Glen S. O'Sullivan

DEGENERATIVE SPINE

Epidemiology

Spondylosis is the generalized degenerative process that affects all levels of the aging spine. If aging is a disease, degenerative discs are part of that disease state, especially when pain, disability, and dysfunction result. The morphologic, biochemical, and biomechanical changes that occur in spondylosis have been well documented. The greatest challenge in the evaluation of degenerative disc disease is to understand when normal maturation is transformed into abnormal degeneration and to determine which pathomorphologic changes may explain the clinical symptoms.

Correlations have been found between symptoms of pain and neurologic compromise resulting from spinal canal and foraminal encroachment with loss of intervertebral body height, herniated discs, enlarged facet joints, and thickened ligamentum flavum. Not all patients who have abnormal findings on radiographs and imaging studies are symptomatic. Most patients who have spondylotic changes occurring over time have no symptoms referable to the spine. In others, however, symptoms may become severe, possibly as a result of faster rates of degeneration or perhaps as a result of patients having smaller or less tolerant spinal canals.

Degenerative spinal conditions have inflicted a high cost to society in terms of patient pain and suffering, economic time lost from work, and permanent disability. Low back pain, for example, has resulted in estimated costs of $50 to $100 billion a year in North America alone. A small fraction of those affected, about 10%, account for the vast majority of the costs. There is a lack of clear definitions or well-controlled clinical studies to support much of the current treatment modalities used to treat these degenerative disorders. Most treating physicians believe that the predominant cause of persistent pain is incompetence of the disc. Others attribute symptoms to muscular strains or ligamentous sprains and facet arthritis. The Quebec Task Force achieved no consensus on the origin of low back or cervical pain and classified many of these disorders as activity-related spinal disorders based on presenting pain symptoms. There have been links to degenerative disc disease and occupations, especially when the spine is subjected to various vibrational and postural repetitive stresses. Psychological and socioeconomical factors, including personal problems and job dissatisfaction, also contribute to the disability associated with degenerative spinal disease.

General Evaluation

When evaluating a patient with spinal pain or neurologic symptoms and signs, it is important to distinguish the self-limited process of spondylosis from a more sinister underlying cause, such as trauma, infections, and neoplastic conditions. These may occur superimposed on the aging process. The clinician must maintain a high index of suspicion. Attention should be paid to the patient's age at onset of symptoms (spinal pain in patients younger than age 20 or older than age 50) and the quality of the pain, especially severe symptoms that occur at rest. A detailed history and physical examination that extract constitutional symptoms of fevers or weight loss, association with traumatic events, and past medical history of malignancy or immunosuppressant medications are important. Other conditions extrinsic to the spine can be confusing in the diagnostic work-up for a patient with a degenerative spinal disorder. It is not uncommon for patients to present with both neck pain and shoulder pathology, or lumbar pain and hip pathology, or peripheral nerve entrapment syndromes in the upper or lower extremities.

There appears to be a trend that in the early stages of the degenerative spinal process, patients present typically with radicular arm or leg pain as a result of herniated discs or axial spinal pain as a result of incompetent degenerative discs. Later on in life, as the spine becomes progressively stiffer, patients tend to have less axial neck or low back pain complaints but tend to present with evidence of neurocompromise (spinal claudication and myelopathy), resulting from central and foramenal spinal stenosis.

MORPHOLOGIC CHANGES IN SPINAL DEGENERATION

It is useful to consider each disc level as a three-joint complex or motion segment with the intervertebral disc and facet joints biomechanically linked to form a functional spinal unit. The intervertebral disc is a hydrostatic load-bearing structure between the vertebral bodies. The nucleus pulposus acts as a confined central fluid within the anulus fibrosis and is able to convert axial loads into tensile strain on the anulus fibers and the vertebral end-plates.

Beginning in the third to fifth decades of life, changes occur in the intervertebral discs with subsequent changes in the bones and articular processes. As the disc degenerates, it loses its hydrostatic properties. Changes occur in the molecular meshwork of proteoglycans and collagen, resulting in the reduced ability of the disc to imbibe water and eventually distribute load equally. With time, there is loss of clear distinction between the nucleus pulposus and outer fibrous anulus.

Pathophysiology of Disc Herniation

The annular wall is made up of type I collagen fibrils arranged in a lamellar configuration allowing the disc to accommodate complex stresses. As the disc ages, annular tears are seen and are associated with reduced proteoglycans and increase in larger collagen type III fibrils. There is reduced cellular activity, and the anulus possesses a poor ability to heal after these tears. Small annular tears can advance to a complete radial tear, which may result in herniation of the nuclear contents into the spinal canal. This disc herniation can be classified as a contained herniation if the herniating fragment is restricted by the posterior ligamentous structures, such as the outer annular fibers and posterior longitudinal ligament (Fig. 32–1). The herniation may be partially extruded if it breaks through the posterior ligamentous structures or completely extruded once this fragment is free in the spinal canal, in which case the fragment may migrate proximally or distally.

As the disc loses its hydrostatic properties, *increased creep* occurs, defined as time-dependent deformability resulting in diffuse bulging of the discs and loss of intervertebral body height. There is disc resorption with fibrocartilage replacement of nucleus pulposus, and as intervertebral height is lost, there is concomitant increased stress on the posterior element with synovial reactions occurring in the facet joint. Facet joint cartilage disruption and destruction occurs, and eventual enlargement and osteophyte formation occur within these joints. The functional spinal unit becomes increasingly lax with an uneven rolling motion occurring within the segment. The facet capsular laxity may result in *olisthesis,* which is slippage of one vertebral body on the other, and either anterior spondylolisthesis or retrolisthesis may occur. As the vertebral bodies and posterior elements come close together, there is buckling of hypertrophied ligamentum flavum and overriding of enlarged articular processes resulting in encroachment on the neuroforamen as well as central and lateral subarticular recess stenosis (Fig. 32–2).

DEGENERATIVE SPINAL SEGMENTAL INSTABILITY

Segmental instability is defined as a loss of motion segment stiffness such that force application to that motion segment produces greater displacement than would be seen in a normal structure. The condition usually causes pain and has the potential to result in progressive deformity placing neurologic structures at risk. Instability may declare itself on radiographs with an olisthy or a slip both forward and backward of one vertebral body on the other or development of osteophytes (either anterior or traction spurs or clasping, bridging osteophytes). Plain x-ray films confirming greater than 3 to 4 mm of anterior displacement or translation or 10 degrees of angular deformity may be considered evidence of segmental instability (Fig. 32–3).

Apart from translational and retrolisthetic instability occurring at one level, patients can present with axial rotation instability and progressive degenerative scoliosis over numerous levels (Fig. 32–4). The classic example of a one-level degenerative instability pattern is degenerative spondylolisthesis, usually occurring at L4–L5 (Fig. 32–5). Patients present with both back pain and lower extremity symptoms resulting from neurologic compromise. Should a surgical procedure be necessary when conservative efforts fail, a combined decompression and stabilization procedure is performed concomitantly.

As the spine ages, patients present with postural alterations. There is loss of lumbar lordosis in an attempt to unload the degenerating articular facet by maintaining a more flexed posture. There is a reduction of stature as a result of both loss of disc height and re-

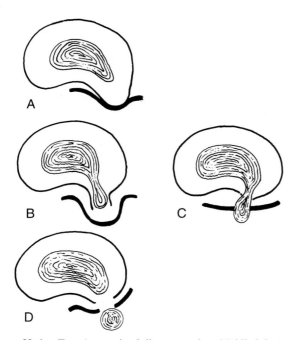

Figure 32–1. *Top,* A contained disc protrusion. *Middle left,* A noncontained subligamentous disc extrusion. *Middle right,* A noncontained transligamentous disc extrusion. *Bottom,* A noncontained disc sequestration. (From Hanley EN, et al: Surgical indications and techniques. In Wiesel SM, et al, the International Society for the Study of the Lumbar Spine, eds: The Lumbar Spine, 2nd ed, Vol 1. Philadelphia, WB Saunders, 1996, p 493.)

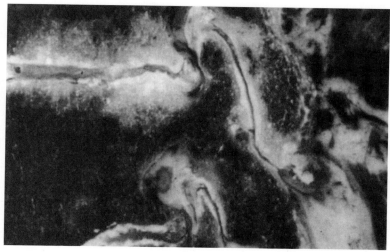

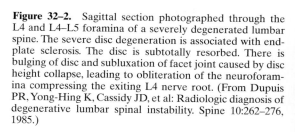

Figure 32–2. Sagittal section photographed through the L4 and L4–L5 foramina of a severely degenerated lumbar spine. The severe disc degeneration is associated with end-plate sclerosis. The disc is subtotally resorbed. There is bulging of disc and subluxation of facet joint caused by disc height collapse, leading to obliteration of the neuroforamina compressing the exiting L4 nerve root. (From Dupuis PR, Yong-Hing K, Cassidy JD, et al: Radiologic diagnosis of degenerative lumbar spinal instability. Spine 10:262–276, 1985.)

duced vertebral body height because of osteoporosis. Disorders of sagittal balance may result in patients who are quite markedly disabled because of this collapsing spine and present with both kyphosis and kyphoscoliosis (Fig. 32–6). It can be a difficult problem to manage because patients often do not tolerate bracing, and there are high risks involved in trying to balance the spine with surgical stabilization procedures.

CLINICAL PRESENTATION—SYMPTOMS AND SIGNS OF DEGENERATIVE SPINAL DISORDERS

Patients who have a degenerative spinal condition present with a number of symptoms and signs. The most common is pain, axial, referred, or radicular. Next most common is evidence of neurologic compromise: neuro-

logic signs of nerve root compromise, spinal cord compression (myelopathy), cauda equina compression, or spinal claudication.

Axial Pain

Pain is a complex perception and can occur in the absence of tissue damage. There are many potential sources of pain in the degenerative spine. The outer third of the anulus and posterior longitudinal ligament are richly innervated with nerve fibers, which may become sensitized by inflammatory agents such as phospholipase A_2. In addition, a degenerative spiral may occur as neuropeptides released from the dorsal root ganglion mediate a progressive degeneration of the functional spine unit by stimulating the synthesis of inflammatory agents and degradative enzymes.

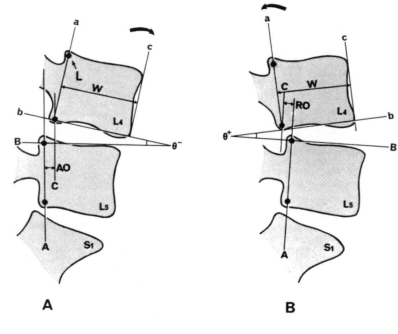

Figure 32–3. Measurement of angular displacement and translation in (A) flexion and (B) extension views. (From Frymoyer JW, et al: Segmental instability. In Wiesel SM, et al, International Society for the Study of the Lumbar Spine, eds: The Lumbar Spine, 2nd ed, Vol 2. Philadelphia, WB Saunders, 1996, p 789.)

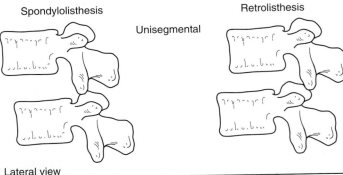

DEGENERATIVE INSTABILITY

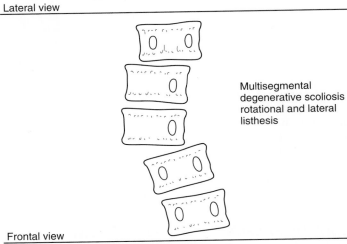

Figure 32–4. *Top*, Diagram demonstrating lateral view of typical unisegmental instability. *Bottom*, Diagram demonstrating multi-level, multisegmental instability pattern on frontal view.

It was hoped that magnetic resonance imaging would allow clinicians to follow the natural history of degenerating discs and help in the diagnosis of internal disc disruption, but this has not been the case. The only study available to establish the presence of a symptomatic disc is discography. This is a provocative study, which, although in widespread use, should be interpreted with caution.

MANAGEMENT OF SIMPLE NECK AND LOW BACK PAIN

Most patients with spinal degenerative mechanical pain in the neck and low back respond well to non-steroidal anti-inflammatory medications and physical therapy. Most acute episodes of pain respond to short

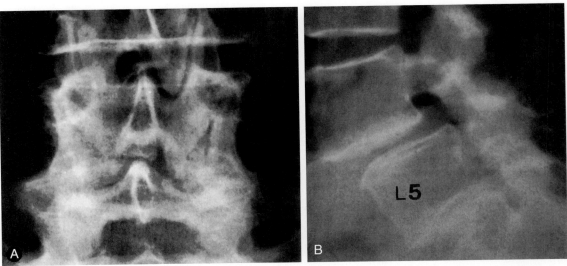

Figure 32–5. Anteroposterior (*A*) and lateral (*B*) radiographs of a 50-year-old woman with a degenerative spondylolisthesis at L4–L5. (From Postacchini F: Classification and treatment. Weinstein JN, Wiesel SW, International Society for the Study of the Lumbar Spine, eds: The Lumbar Spine. Philadelphia, WB Saunders, 1990, p 609.)

SAGITTAL BALANCE

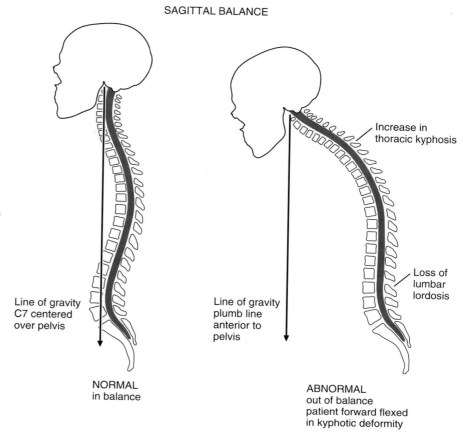

Figure 32–6. Alterations in body posture as a result of spinal degeneration.

Increase in thoracic kyphosis

Loss of lumbar lordosis

Line of gravity C7 centered over pelvis

Line of gravity plumb line anterior to pelvis

NORMAL
in balance

ABNORMAL
out of balance
patient forward flexed
in kyphotic deformity

periods of rest. Passive modalities, including spinal manipulation, have proved effective in the acute setting, as has the use of epidural glucocorticoid injections. Once the pain becomes chronic, and a sinister source of pain has been ruled out, passive treatments should be altered in favor of a more active program that includes isometric stabilization, strengthening, and posture programs as well as aerobic exercises. For mechanical degenerative disc disease or facet arthritis, spinal fusion techniques have been advocated. The results are mixed, averaging 60% clinical success rate. These techniques should be considered only in highly selected cases as a final resort.

Referred Pain

It was thought that extremity pain can result only from neurologic compromise, as in the traditional radicular-type pain mapped out with the standard dermatomal chart (Fig. 32–7). Typically, this pain, occurring in the proximal extremities originating from disc and facets, is usually more poorly localized, tends to be dull, and is less superficial than nerve root pain.

FACET SYNDROME

The facet syndrome was coined in 1933 and typically presents as back pain with additional referred pain in the posterolateral thigh. Back pain is related to activ-

ities such as extension and rotation of the lumbosacral spine. There has been controversy about the diagnosis and treatment of this syndrome. Although evidence exists that some patients benefit from facet injections, there are no good randomized clinical studies to confirm this.

Radicular Pain

Patients suffering radicular pain classically present with signs and symptoms of nerve root compression. The classic indications for treatment of this pathology have been the presence of the clinical triad of intractable extremity pain in a nerve root distribution; the presence of positive neurotensin signs, such as the straight leg raise test; and positive neurologic signs of nerve involvement (Table 32–1). Spinal nerves can also be compressed by encroachment in the spinal canal lateral recess or foramen, with a classic presentation of spinal stenosis, nerve root compression by posterior elements, hypertrophied ligamentum flavum, bony hypertrophy of the facet joints, and bulging of the disc anulus. The presence of an instability (e.g., spondylolisthesis) may lead to further nerve root irritation. Acute nerve root compression usually produces no pain but rather neurologic compromise, such as motor and sensory changes. The presence of inflammation, edema, and local demyelination generates the typical radicular pain of radiculopathy. A chronically injured

Pain Patterns in Lumbar Disease

Radicular pain due to nerve root compression

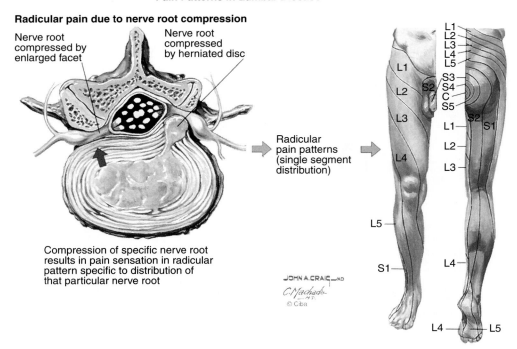

Nerve root compressed by enlarged facet

Nerve root compressed by herniated disc

Radicular pain patterns (single segment distribution)

Compression of specific nerve root results in pain sensation in radicular pattern specific to distribution of that particular nerve root

Figure 32–7. Radicular and referred pain patterns in the degenerative lumbar spine. (From Mooney V, Saal JA, Saal JS: Evaluation and treatment of low back pain. Clin Symp 48:4, 1996.)

Nonradicular, referred pain due to facet or disc disease

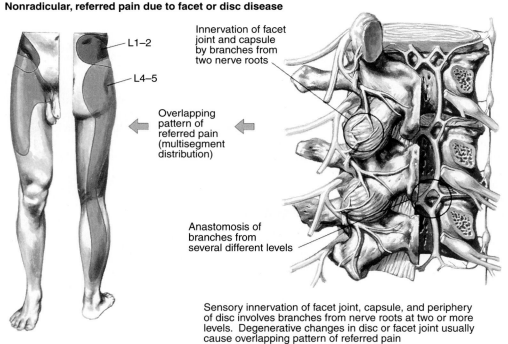

Innervation of facet joint and capsule by branches from two nerve roots

L1–2

L4–5

Overlapping pattern of referred pain (multisegment distribution)

Anastomosis of branches from several different levels

Sensory innervation of facet joint, capsule, and periphery of disc involves branches from nerve roots at two or more levels. Degenerative changes in disc or facet joint usually cause overlapping pattern of referred pain

dorsal root ganglion may be more sensitive and susceptible to mechanical compression than are peripheral nerve roots.

MANAGEMENT OF RADICULAR PAIN

Most patients with radicular disorders respond favorably to conservative efforts, 90% improve within 6 weeks if given nonsteroidal anti-inflammatory drugs and physical therapy. Occasionally, injections may be helpful, including epidural and selective nerve root blocks. These can be helpful both diagnostically and therapeutically. Indications for surgery include positive imaging studies consistent with clinical findings as well as the following:

1. Persistent or recurrent extremity pain unresponsive to a trial of nonsurgical treatment for at least 3 months

Table 32–1. RADICULAR SYMPTOMS AND SIGNS

Disc Space	C4–5	C5–6	C6–7	C7–T1
Root compressed	C5	C6	C7	C8
Motor weakness	Deltoid	Bicep	Tricep	Hand intrinsics
Sensory deficit	Shoulder	Arm and thumb	Fingers 2 and 3	Fingers 4 and 5
	L3–4	**L4–5**	**L5–S1**	
Root compressed	L4	L5	S1	
Reflex diminished	Knee jerk	No reflex	Ankle jerk	
Motor weakness	Knee extension	Great toe dorsiflexion	Ankle plantarflexion	
Sensory deficit	Medial ankle	Medial foot	Lateral foot	
Pain	Anterior thigh	Posterior leg	Posterior leg	

From Watts MC, Brem H: Neurosurgery. In Niederhuber JE (ed): Fundamentals of Surgery. Stamford, CT, Appleton & Lange, 1998, p 735.

2. Progressive neurologic deficit
3. Static neurologic deficit associated with significant radicular pain

Cauda equina syndrome is the rare presentation of low back pain and often bilateral lower extremity symptoms, including pain, weakness, numbness, and loss of reflexes. The presence of bladder or bowel dysfunction with loss of perianal sensation and rectal tone is considered a medical emergency, requiring rapid evaluation and consideration of acute surgical decompression.

Myelopathy

Myelopathy is common secondary to cervical spondylosis and is the most serious consequence of intervertebral disc degeneration. Spondylotic myelopathy is the most common cervical cord disorder during and after middle age. Patients often have long periods without the development of new or worsening signs and symptoms. Sixty-four percent of patients have no increasing symptoms, 36% of patients improve, and 26% of patients worsen. The typical presentations have been classified according to the anatomic portion of the spinal cord involved.

1. Central cord syndrome—disassociation in the degree of motor weakness, with the lower extremities being stronger than the upper extremities in the presence of sacral swelling
2. Brown-Séquard syndrome—modified hemisection of the spinal cord with hemilateral paralysis and contralateral sensor and temperature loss
3. Anterior cord syndrome—presence of motor paralysis with hypoesthesia and hypalgesia and preservation of the posterior column sensory function

It is important to differentiate cervical spondylosis from intrinsic degeneration of the central nervous system, such as motor neuron disease, particularly amyotrophic lateral sclerosis as well as multiple sclerosis. These intrinsic conditions may rarely coexist with cervical spondylosis.

The measurement of the canal size is important. The sagittal diameter of the adult cervical spine is 17 mm compared to the spinal cord at 10 mm. Various measurements have been made to assess the cervical spinal canal diameter. The most common method involves measuring the spinal cord from the midpoint of the posterior aspect of the vertebral body to the nearest point on the corresponding spinal laminal line (Fig. 32–8). This ratio compares the sagittal diameter of the spinal canal with the anterior-posterior width of the vertebral body measured through the midpoint of the body. This ratio method reduces the variability of mag-

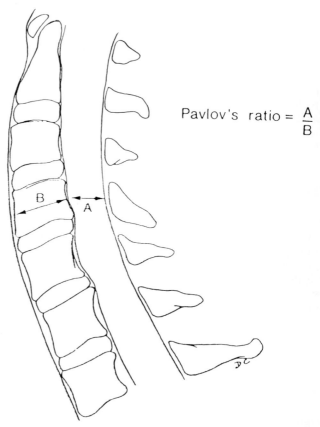

$$\text{Pavlov's ratio} = \frac{A}{B}$$

Figure 32–8. Diagram showing the measurements made on a plain lateral radiograph to determine Pavlov's ratio. Pavlov's ratio equals A over B. (From Frymoyer JW, Ducker TB, Hadler NM, et al, eds: Adult Spine: Principles and Practice, Vol 2. Philadelphia, Lippincott-Raven, 1991, p 1152.)

Table 32–2. DIFFERENTIAL DIAGNOSIS OF SPINAL CLAUDICATION

Diagnosis	Symptoms	Signs
Degenerative spine stenosis	Diffuse leg pain aggravated by standing and walking downhill	Limited lumbar range of motion, weakness only after exercise
Degenerative hip disease	Groin and/or anterior thigh pain	Limited hip rotation range, especially loss of internal rotation
Peripheral vascular disease	Distal leg pain relieved by standing	Bruits and diminished pulses
Diabetic neuropathy	Glove-and-stocking diffuse distal bilateral burning pain	Reflexes diminished or absent
Tumor or infection	Constant pain at rest, location of pain varying	Weight loss, elevated erythrocyte sedimentation rate, bone scan indicate malignancy or infection

From Mooney V: Lumbosacral Spine. Southwestern Orthopaedic Review Course, 1989, p 152.

nification, and in normal individuals, the Pavlov ratio should be 1 or greater. A ratio of less than 0.8 is associated with a statistically significant risk of developing spinal cord neuropraxia. Patients with stenotic spinal canals are usually asymptomatic; however, they are more vulnerable to encroaching lesions, such as herniated discs, protruding or bulging of the anulus fibrosis, osteophytes, and enfolding of the ligamentum flavum.

SURGICAL MANAGEMENT OF MYELOPATHY

Failing conservative efforts, including medications, bracing, physical therapy, and injections, surgical intervention may be necessary. Surgery involves decompression of the spinal cord, the extent of which depends on the number of levels and extent of stenosis and the underlying stability of the spine. Anterior cervical surgery includes discectomy or vertebrectomy with combined anterior column support, bone grafting, and fusion, whereas posterior surgery involves laminectomy or laminoplasty.

Spinal Claudication

The symptoms of claudication may involve one or multiple roots and are often described as a feeling of fatigue or weakness of the lower extremities with activity, particularly ambulation. This feeling may be relieved by sitting or squatting maneuvers that optimize lumbar spinal canal dimensions. These symptoms frequently may be vague. It is important not to overlook the possibility of claudication producing vascular disease, peripheral neuropathy, or an occult neoplasm as the source of pain or dysfunction. Physical findings may be minimal or reveal profound neurologic abnormalities. Spinal alignment may be normal, or a step-off deformity that goes with spondylolisthesis or scoliosis may be apparent. Lumbar lordosis is often diminished. Tension signs may be absent or present only to a mild degree. Neurologic examination may range from normal to the finding of profound sensorimotor and reflex abnormalities in one or both extremities, which may be referable

to one or more spinal levels. A complete physical evaluation of the patient should include an abdominal examination to exclude an abdominal aortic aneurysm or visceral abnormality, a rectal examination to rule out prostate and rectal pathology and to assess sphincter tone, and palpation of lower extremity pulses. Efforts should be made to distinguish between vascular and neurogenic provocation and to assess the possibility of peripheral neuropathy resulting from other disease processes (Table 32–2).

Typically the difference between neurogenic claudication symptoms and vascular claudication symptoms is that the pain in the former is severe in the leg after walking a short distance. The patient is forced to stop and bend forward or sit. Pain may occur at rest or in the standing position. This pain usually dissipates quickly. A noninvasive vascular work-up may be necessary.

SURGICAL MANAGEMENT OF SPINAL CLAUDICATION

If conservative efforts fail to alleviate the patient's symptoms, a decompressive procedure with preservation of the integrity of the facet joints by undercutting the medial facets and avoidance of excision of the disc leads to a 70% success rate. Spinal stenosis may occur at one level or involve multiple segments. The spinal segments involved may be either stable or unstble. If an instability pattern exists, a concomitant stabilization, instrumentation, and fusion may be considered.

BIBLIOGRAPHY

Bridwell K, DeWald R, eds.: Textbook of Spinal Surgery. Philadelphia, Lippincott-Raven, 1993.

Clark C: Degenerative conditions of the spine: Differential diagnosis and non-surgical treatment. In Frymoyer JW, Ducker TB, Hadler NM, et al, eds: The Adult Spine: Principles and Practice, vol II. New York, Raven Press, 1991, p 1152.

Mooney V, Saal JA, Saal JS: Evaluation and treatment of low back pain. Clin Symp 48:1–32, 1996.

Wiesel SM, Weinstein JN, Herkowitz HN, et al, edit com: The Lumbar Spine, 2nd ed. The International Society for the Study of the Lumbar Spine. Philadelphia, WB Saunders, 1996.

Chapter 33

Infections of the Joints and Spine

INFECTIONS OF PERIPHERAL JOINTS

James Posever

The infectious arthritides span a variety of clinical entities. At one end of the spectrum are the acute infections with nongonococcal and gonococcal bacteria. At the other are the more indolent, chronic, infections with mycobacteria and fungi. In the middle lie the viral-associated arthritides, which can result from joint infection or immune-mediated joint inflammation. Each of these topics is explored separately, with emphasis on understanding the risk factors, cause, presentation, diagnosis, therapy, and expected outcomes.

NONGONOCOCCAL BACTERIAL ARTHRITIS

Pathogenesis

Bacterial joint infections are responsible for one of the most rapidly destructive forms of arthritis. Such infections are often well established when patients present to a physician. These considerations require physicians to act quickly to confirm a diagnosis and initiate therapy. Septic arthritis originates from one of three mechanisms: hematogenous seeding, local extension, and direct inoculation. By estimates, 90% to 95% of cases result from blood-borne bacterial seeding of the synovium or subchondral bone, whereas the remaining 5% to 10% are caused by contiguous spread from a local infection or direct inoculation from a procedure.[1] Regardless of the mechanism, joint infections follow a similar course. Animal models have shown that the response to infection begins within 1 to 2 hours with proliferation of synovial cells, extravasation of perivascular mononuclear cells, and infiltration of the synovium with polymorphonuclear leukocytes. Synovial congestion ensues. In 24 to 48 hours, the synovium hypertrophies, and large numbers of inflammatory cells can form microabscesses. As inflammation intensifies over the first week, the synovium is filled with acute and chronic granulation tissue.[2] These synovial changes ultimately impede bacterial clearance from the joint.

Changes in joint fluid, articular cartilage, and subchondral bone progress simultaneously. By 24 to 48 hours, synovial fluid turns purulent and loses viscosity as hyaluronic acid is broken down. The intense inflammatory response is marked by release of cytokines and proteases, triggering damage to articular cartilage and subchondral bone. The insult to articular cartilage is reflected by the loss of proteoglycans, a major cartilage constituent, which can be depleted by 20% to 30% in 2 days, 50% to 60% in 10 days, and 65% to 80% in 3 weeks.[1,3] Irreversible joint damage includes loss of subchondral bone as early as the second day and cartilage loss by 7 to 10 days. This potentially destructive course emphasizes the importance of early identification of patients at risk of joint infection. *Articular cartilage once destroyed can never be replaced.*

Risk Factors

The incidence of septic arthritis among the general population is estimated to be 2 to 10 cases per 100,000 individuals per year, but the risk of infection is higher among specific groups.[4] The estimated incidence is 28 to 38 per 100,000 per year among patients with rheumatoid arthritis and 40 to 68 per 100,000 per year among patients with joint prostheses.[5] In general, risk factors for nongonococcal septic arthritis fall into three broad categories: history of prior joint damage, underlying systemic illness, and risk of bacteremia.

The risk of septic arthritis is increased among patients with prior joint damage regardless of whether it resulted from an inflammatory rheumatic disease, osteoarthritis, or joint trauma. What these conditions have in common are chronic synovial and bony changes that predispose a patient to bacterial seeding of a joint. Patients with inflammatory conditions at increased risk of joint infection include those with rheumatoid arthritis, systemic lupus erythematosus, and crystal-induced arthropathies. Of those patients with rheumatoid arthritis, at greatest risk are those who suffer from seropositive, aggressive disease usually of 10 or more years' duration on glucocorticoid therapy. Additional risks of infection among patients with joint disease include skin infection, hip or knee prostheses, joint surgery, age greater than 80 years, and diabetes mellitus.[5]

Further risk of joint infection is imparted by some chronic illnesses, medical therapies, and behaviors. Immunodeficiency syndromes may be the prototypic systemic illnesses with increased risk of joint infection. Among patients with humoral immunodeficiency, one study showed a 23% incidence over 20 years.[6] The risk with cellular immunodeficiency is less clear. For instance, in patients with human immunodeficiency virus (HIV), a risk of septic arthritis seems limited to individuals with acquired immunodeficiency syndrome (AIDS), unless they suffer from hemophilia or intravenous drug use, which carries concomitant risks of prior joint damage and bacteremia.[7] Decreased immunocompetence also is associated with cancer, diabetes mellitus, sickle cell anemia, and alcoholism; iatrogenic causes of immune dysfunction include cancer chemotherapy, immunosuppression for organ transplants, and systemic glucocorticoids. The risk of bacteremia accompanies burns, abrasions, catheters, hemodialysis, and intravenous drug use.

Presentation

Patients with septic arthritis usually present with complaints of severe joint pain. The history usually includes fever—although spiking temperatures are atypical—and patients commonly describe chills or malaise. Details of the onset and clinical course can vary with the infectious organism and host susceptibility factors. For instance, *Staphylococcus aureus* tends to have a rapid and intense onset leading to early presentation, whereas patients with infections with enteric organisms or compromised immune function may relate a more indolent clinical picture. Any joint can be affected, but the most common is the knee, which is involved in 50% of cases (Table 33–1). Although most patients present with symptoms limited to one joint, polyarticular infections occur in 10% to 20% of cases.

Patients should receive a complete physical exami-

Table 33–1. NONGONOCOCCAL BACTERIAL ARTHRITIS: PERCENTAGE OF CASES BY AFFECTED JOINT IN ADULTS AND CHILDREN

Region	Joint	Adults (%)	Children (%)
Upper extremity	Shoulder	8	4
	Elbow	6	11
	Wrist	7	3
Lower extremity	Hip	11	28
	Knee	55	40
	Ankle	8	14
Unspecified	Other	5	3
	Polyarticular infection	12	7

Adapted from Goldenberg DL: Bacterial arthritis. In Kelley WN, Harris ED, Ruddy S, Sledge CB, eds: Textbook of Rheumatology, 5th ed. Philadelphia, WB Saunders, 1996, pp 1435–1449.

nation with attention to identifying additional sites of infection, because 50% of patients have a source of infection involving the skin, lungs, or urinary tract.[4] Examination begins with observation of the patient. In septic arthritis, patients often hold the affected joint in a partially flexed position and limit voluntary movement or weight bearing. Infected peripheral joints may have obvious swelling or erythema. These features are often less conspicuous with involvement of the shoulder, hip, sacroiliac, or vertebral joints. Joint examination reveals significant discomfort with passive range of motion, and movement may also be limited by tense effusion. These findings should heighten a physician's clinical suspicion and prompt immediate joint aspiration. In the absence of a definitive history of trauma, an acutely inflamed joint should be presumed infected until proved otherwise.

Diagnosis

The diagnosis of septic arthritis requires joint aspiration and synovial fluid analysis. If adequate volume can be obtained, synovial fluid should be evaluated with a complete blood count (CBC) with differential, Gram stain, and aerobic and anaerobic cultures. Characteristic findings are an elevated white blood cell (WBC) count and predominance of neutrophils. A time-honored adage holds that the higher the synovial fluid WBC count, the greater the suspicion for infection, yet there is no lower limit that excludes the diagnosis of septic arthritis. In fact, recorded synovial fluid WBC counts at the time of presentation have decreased over the past 40 years. The current average is 36,000 WBC/mL, and 50% of cases now present with synovial fluid WBC counts less than 30,000.[8] If synovial fluid is of limited supply, bacterial cultures take first priority; the second priority is Gram stain, which is positive in one third of cases. All patients should have blood cultures performed, because 50% to 70% are positive.[4] Those suspected of harboring extra-articular infections should be evaluated accordingly with throat, sputum, or urine cultures when indicated.

A variety of additional tests can be useful in the initial assessment of a patient with acute monarticular arthritis. The presence of crystals in joint fluid does not rule out septic arthritis because bacterial infection can harvest existing crystal deposits from the synovium and produce a lower synovial pH causing precipitation of new crystals. Similarly the initial erythrocyte sedimentation rate (ESR) and blood WBC count can be deceptive when used to gauge suspicion for septic arthritis. The ESR and serum WBC counts are within normal range in 13% and 55% of patients with joint infections.[8] An ESR is most useful when assessing children with hip pain, in whom a value higher than 20 mm/h and fever greater than 37.5°C were 97% sensitive for pediatric hip infections.[9] If elevated, a WBC count can serve as an important adjunct in monitoring a patient's response to treatment. At one time, synovial fluid concentrations of protein, glucose, and lactate were thought to reflect infection; however, these tests have poor sensitivity and specificity and are no longer recommended for bacterial arthritis.

Imaging

Imaging studies have an important role in the evaluation of patients with septic arthritis, although they are rarely diagnostic. At the time of presentation, most plain radiographs of infected joints show only joint effusions and soft tissue swelling. If an infection has run a protracted course, characteristic findings include erosions with indistinct margins, random joint surface irregularities or bony destruction, and subchondral cysts. Independent of the duration of an infection, plain radiographs are indicated to establish a reference point for future evaluation of an affected joint. Under some circumstances, additional radiographic procedures can be helpful: Scintigraphy can be of value when trying to identify an infection at a deep site, such as the sacroiliac joint, and fluoroscopy or computed tomography (CT) can assist in arthrocentesis of the hip. When extension of an infection is suspected, further radiographic evaluation is necessary: CT scan is required to evaluate extension of infection at the sternomanubrial joint, whereas magnetic resonance imaging (MRI) is preferred to define deep, soft tissue, or bony involvement with infections of the extremities.

Microorganisms

Nongonococcal bacterial arthritis can be caused by a variety of organisms (Table 33–2). Gram-positive bacteria account for 50% to 90% of all cases. The single most common organism is *S. aureus,* which is responsible for 43% to 60% of infections in the elderly and 77% of infections in patients with rheumatoid arthritis. Staphylococcal species also should be suspected in postoperative joint infections, in which 75% to 90% of septic prosthetic joints are attributable to *S. aureus* or *Staphylococcus epidermidis.*[10] Streptococcal infections tend to follow a more indolent course when caused by the more frequent group A β-hemolytic streptococci, including *Streptococcus pyogenes,* and a complicated course when resulting from non-A serotypes. Group B infections are associated with diabetes mellitus, whereas group G infections are commonly preceded by cellulitis. Intravenous drug users commonly develop infec-

tions secondary to *Pseudomonas* and *Serratia* species. Although anaerobic infections are rare, they are relatively more frequent among patients with recent joint surgery or musculoskeletal trauma.[7, 11]

Treatment

DRAINAGE AND ANTIBIOTICS

The treatment of bacterial arthritis entails four steps: intravenous antibiotics, joint drainage, clinical monitoring, and rehabilitation. Initially, these patients should be hospitalized. Once joint fluid has been obtained, intravenous antibiotics should be started as quickly as possible. Gram stains are positive in one third of patients[12]; if this test proves unrevealing, empirical therapy should be started for both gram-positive and gram-negative organisms. Recommendations include a penicillinase-resistant synthetic penicillin or a first-generation cephalosporin and an aminoglycoside or ciprofloxacin; alternatively, ticarcillin/clavulanate, piperacillin/tazobactam, or ampicillin/sulbactam can be used alone. In patients with penicillin allergy, substitutes include vancomycin, or ciprofloxacin and rifampin.[13] In every case, the choice of antibiotics should be re-evaluated once culture results and bacterial susceptibilities are available. The duration of intravenous antibiotic therapy is usually 2 to 4 weeks; 2 weeks is often adequate for *Streptococcus* or *Haemophilus influenzae*; *Staphylococcus* and most gram-negative bacilli require at least 3 weeks of therapy.[11] Intra-articular antibiotics add no benefit and may exacerbate synovitis.

Drainage of a bacterial joint infection is essential. This requirement can be fulfilled with repeated joint aspiration, tidal irrigation, arthroscopy, and arthrotomy. The choice of drainage technique is an area of ongoing debate and may vary by institution. On one side, studies of serial joint aspiration have shown the potential for good results in approximately two thirds of cases.[14, 15] Not only does this technique avoid surgical risks, but also it provides a means of monitoring a clinical response to therapy. If joint cultures are persistently positive or if synovial fluid WBC counts fail to decline to less than 50,000/mm^3 by 5 to 7 days, patients should undergo more thorough joint exploration and débridement.[16] Joint aspiration and tidal irrigation can fail to drain adequately synovial abscesses or loculations within a joint. Critics add that joint aspiration is less successful at completely removing mediators of cartilage degradation, leading to poorer long-term outcome, and in some cases, it may even carry a higher risk of mortality.[17, 18] The middle ground may be held by arthroscopy, which can be an effective means of draining, débriding, and irrigating major joints, especially the knee.[19–21] Until pain and inflammation have subsided, the affected joint should be splinted except for passive full range of motion exercises twice daily by an experienced therapist.

Table 33–2. BACTERIAL ARTHRITIS: PERCENTAGE OF CASES BY INFECTIOUS ORGANISM IN ADULTS AND CHILDREN

Organisms	Adults (%)	Children (%)
Staphylococcus aureus	55	33
Streptococcus	27	13
Gram-negative bacilli	14	6
Anaerobes	<1	1
Unknown	3	34

Adapted from Smith JW, Piercy EA: Bacterial Arthritis. In Mandell GL, Bennett JE, Dolin R (eds): Principles and Practice of Infectious Disease, 4th ed. New York, Churchill Livingstone, 1995, p 1034.

Recognition and Management of Patients with Specific Rheumatologic Problems

SURGERY

It is generally accepted that some types of joint infections require surgical intervention. Because repeated aspiration of the hip is difficult and often inadequate, this joint should undergo surgical drainage either by arthrotomy or arthroscopy. Surgical intervention also may be required for deep infections at the sacroiliac, sternomanubrial, and shoulder joints. Further indications for surgical management are osteomyelitis, soft tissue extension of an infection, or thick purulent material that resists needle aspiration.[1, 8] One study suggests that knee arthrotomy should be performed when patients present with symptoms of more than 3 days' duration and when joint cultures grow either *S. aureus* or gram-negative organisms.[22] Less clear indications are host factors that carry a poor prognosis. Patients with rheumatoid arthritis, diabetes, and immunoincompetence are at risk of bacteremia and sepsis from a persistent joint infection. Under these circumstances, the possibility that aspiration could fail, leading to a delay in complete drainage, can weigh in favor of early surgical therapy providing complete drainage and removal of necrotic synovium.[18]

PROGNOSIS

Nongonococcal joint infections carry a significant risk of mortality and disability. The overall mortality is estimated between 10% and 16%.[4] This risk is enhanced by specific considerations, including the number and location of involved joints, the host's age and underlying medical condition, the infectious organism, and the duration of infection before therapy. Polyarticular infections lead to death in approximately one third of patients, and within this category the greatest risks are shared by patients with small joint involvement, bacteremia, or more than four infected joints.[8] Increased risk of mortality also accompanies infections in the elderly and patients with rheumatoid arthritis, prosthetic joints, and underlying immunocompromise resulting from illness or drugs.[1, 23] Within this latter group, gram-negative infections can be difficult to treat, resulting in an estimated mortality of 25%.[11] Among survivors, irreversible joint damage occurs in 50% of patients, with 16% developing dependency for activities of daily living.[4, 23] In otherwise healthy hosts, the most important prognostic factor is the amount of time that elapses before diagnosis and treatment. Patients treated within 5 to 7 days of their initial symptoms have good functional outcomes in up to two thirds of cases.[14] To optimize joint function, patients should have early mobilization and physical therapy once joint swelling begins to subside.[18]

Joint infections progress quickly, and some of the same considerations place a patient at increased risk for joint infection and poor prognosis. When an infection is suspected, physicians can best serve their patients by expediting the initial evaluation and therapy. Physical examination should include a search for possible extra-articular sites of infections, and laboratory assessment of synovial fluid is essential. Antibiotics should be started before laboratory results are available. As mentioned earlier, treatment also requires joint drainage and monitoring of the response to treatment. Once joint swelling begins to decrease, an infected joint should be mobilized with physical therapy. Despite the best efforts, nongonococcal bacterial arthritis continues to carry a significant risk of morbidity and mortality.

GONOCOCCAL ARTHRITIS

Gonococcal arthritis accounts for approximately 20% of all bacterial joint infections in the United States, and among patients younger than 30 years old, it is the most common form of septic arthritis, and most likely to present to primary care physicians. The overall incidence of gonococcal infection is approximately 150 cases per 100,000 individuals per year, but only 0.5% to 3% of mucosal infections progress to joint involvement, reducing the estimated yearly incidence of gonococcal arthritis to 2.8 per 100,000. Among patients with mucosal involvement, the development of gonococcal arthritis is influenced by both host susceptibility and bacterial virulence factors.

Although mucosal infections affect both genders equally, joint infections have a female predominance of 4:1. Women are most susceptible to disseminated gonococcal infection during menstruation and pregnancy when changes in vaginal pH, cervical mucus, genital flora, and endometrial vessels predispose patients to seeding of the blood. Once gonococci reach the bloodstream, the patient's first line of defense is complement-mediated bactericidal activity of host cells. Thus, patients with complement deficiencies are at increased risk of joint infection.

Gonococcal arthritis occurs mainly in young adults. The classic presentation includes the triad of dermatitis, tenosynovitis, and arthritis; however, disseminated gonococcal infections can assume two clinical pictures. The first is thought to correlate with a bacteremic phase when patients present with fever, rash, and tenosynovitis. Constitutional symptoms are usually mild, and fever rarely exceeds 39°C. Patients should be examined carefully for the characteristic rash because it spares the head and neck; it begins as a macule, painless and non-pruritic, and it progresses to be an erythematous base surrounding a vesicular, pustular, or necrotic papule. Lesions can be found in various stages as they erupt and resolve in a course of 4 to 5 days. Tenosynovitis commonly affects the fingers, hands, and wrists, but it also can involve the ankles and knees. This early clinical picture characterizes two thirds of patients at the time of hospitalization. A second phase involves progression of bacteremia to local infection of one or more joints. At the time of presentation, suppurative arthritis is found in only 25% to 50% of patients.

Independent of the phase of the infection, the most common presenting symptom is migratory or additive polyarthralgias. This presentation suggests a differential diagnosis for asymmetric polyarthritis that includes reactive arthritis, rheumatic fever, syphilis, hepatitis, and subacute bacterial endocarditis. Associated historical features and inspection of the rash may narrow this differential. For suspected gonococcal arthritis, patients should be evaluated with a CBC, ESR, joint aspiration as well as culture of blood and other possible mucosal sites of infection. These culture specimens require chocolate agar, often necessitating special instructions. Gonococcal arthritis causes a left shift and mild leukocytosis with mean serum values ranging between 10,500 and 12,500 WBC/mL. The ESR is typically elevated, with 50% of patients having values greater than 50 mm/h. Joint cultures are positive in only 50% of patients with suppurative arthritis, and, overall, only 25% to 30% of patients with gonococcal arthritis have positive synovial fluid cultures.

Because a majority of patients have negative joint cultures, three categories are used to describe the diagnostic certainty of disseminated gonococcal infections. Patients have *proven* infections when cultures are positive from a sterile source, such as synovial fluid (25% to 30%), blood (20% to 30%), and skin (< 5%). *Probable* infections describe patients with characteristic symptoms and positive mucosal cultures, including cervical (90%), urethral (50% to 75% in men), pharyngeal (20%), and rectal (15%) cultures. *Possible* infections have typical features, no culture growth, but a clear response to antibiotic therapy. Because of penicillin and tetracycline resistance of 5% and 12.5%, first-line therapy is a third-generation cephalosporine, such as ceftriaxone (1 g intramuscularly or intravenously every 24 hours). Additional options include cefotaxime or ceftizoxime (1 g intravenously every 8 hours). For beta-lactam sensitivity, the recommended alternative is spectinomycin (2 g intramuscular every 12 hours). Most gonococcal joint infections require no drainage, respond to antibiotics within 24 to 48 hours, and resolve without residual loss of joint function. Risk factors for poor outcome are an elevated ESR, positive joint cultures, and underlying systemic illness.[1, 4, 24]

MYCOBACTERIAL AND FUNGAL INFECTIONS

In contrast to the acute features of bacterial arthritis, mycobacterial and fungal joint infections often share a slowly progressive, indolent course. Common features include monarticular, nonspecific pain; stiffness; and occasionally only swelling. In the absence of obvious systemic disease, this presentation may disguise the diagnosis, leading to a protracted infection. The average delay in diagnosis is 8 months for mycobacterial involvement and 4.5 years for some fungal joint infections. This diagnostic challenge is compounded by potential requirements for special procedures and tests. Heightened clinical suspicion is essential to expedite diagnosis of joint infections caused by mycobacteria or fungi.

Mycobacterial Infections

Skeletal involvement accounts for 1% to 2% of all mycobacterial infections, 10% of extrapulmonary mycobacterial infections, and 20% of mycobacterial infections in AIDS patients. In addition to the immunocompromised state—whether from HIV, alcohol, or renal failure—risk factors include intravenous drug use, homelessness, age greater than 65 years, and debilitated health. Depending on patient age and infectious organism, the clinical presentation of mycobacterial joint infections can vary. *Mycobacterium tuberculosis* typically infects weight-bearing joints or the spine, although in elderly patients, non–weight-bearing joints are more commonly involved. Nontubercular species frequently affect the hand and wrist joints with accompanying symptoms of tenosynovitis and even carpal tunnel syndrome. For instance, *Mycobacterium kansasii* may present with monarticular synovitis, whereas *Mycobacterium leprosum* can produce symmetric polyarthritis of the wrist and small joints of the hands. *Mycobacterium marinum* is associated with fish or tropical aquariums, and this infection is characterized by lymphangitic spread.

Traditional methods of screening for mycobacteria are unreliable in the setting of joint involvement. In 50% of cases, a purified protein derivative (PPD) test is negative, and chest radiographs show no evidence of pulmonary involvement (in patients with documented mycobacterial joint infections, a positive chest x-ray typically reveals a miliary pattern). Joint fluid analysis shows an inflammatory cell count with a left shift; however, acid-fast stains are positive in only 20% of patients, and synovial fluid cultures are less than optimal, detecting 80% to 90% of cases. When a mycobacterial infection is strongly suspected, synovial tissue biopsy and culture may be required. In 90% of cases, synovial tissue reveals granulomas, and synovial tissue culture is diagnostic in 94% of patients. Because this procedure usually entails surgical intervention, an orthopaedic consultation is warranted. Similarly a positive diagnosis merits an infectious disease consultation for the choice of antimicrobial agents and duration of therapy.

Fungal Infections

Fungal joint infections can be caused by ubiquitous organisms or species that are endemic to certain geographical areas. The first group of organisms includes *Sporothrix, Candida, Cryptococcus, Aspergillus,* and *Scedosporium,* whereas the second category is limited to *Coccidioides, Blastomyces,* and *Histoplasma.* Joint involvement can result from local spread from a skin infection of sporotrichosis in patients who work in soil or from bone infections of cryptococcosis, aspergillosis, or blastomycosis. Hematogenous seeding of synovial tissue can occur in patients with pulmonary infections from coccidioidomycosis and histoplasmosis. Likewise, an immunocompromised state can lead to reactivation of prior infections or acute fungemia.

In all patients, joint evaluation should begin with aspiration and synovial fluid analysis, including fungal stains and cultures. Some infections require specific fungal screens and serologic tests; for instance, *Coccidioides* is isolated from joint cultures in less than 5% of cases, so alternative tests include serum latex agglutination or a skin test followed by a complement fixation titer. Diagnosis can also be confirmed with synovial tissue biopsy and culture; granulomas can be seen on synovial histology in all fungal processes except candidiasis, which tends to display only chronic inflammation. With bony involvement, plain radiographs may reveal periosteal elevation or, in chronic blastomycosis, characteristic punched-out lesions. Treatment often requires surgical débridement in addition to antifungal therapy. An infectious disease consultation can assist with the choice of optimal antifungal agents because they vary by organism and sometimes with the patient's underlying health.[11, 25]

VIRAL INFECTIONS

Many viruses are associated with arthralgias or arthritis, ranging from monarticular, oligoarticular, to symmetric, polyarticular processes. A list of common agents include parvovirus B-19, hepatitis B and C, HIV, herpes simplex virus-1, varicella zoster virus, Epstein-Barr virus, cytomegalovirus, rubella, mumps, coxsackieviruses, and echoviruses.[26] Joint symptoms can result from at least two pathogenic mechanisms. The first cause of viral arthritis is direct infection and viral replication within joint tissue. For example, parvovirus B-19 can trigger an acute or chronic arthropathy, with joint symptoms generally following a self-limited course that early on may mimic rheumatoid arthritis. The chronic form of parvovirus B-19 arthropathy illustrates the first pathogenic mechanism because viral DNA can persist within synovial tissue for years—long after serum clearance of viremia.[27] In the second setting, arthralgias or arthritis results from immune complex deposition in synovial tissues. This mechanism is illustrated by hepatitis B infection, in which joint symptoms occur in the prodromal phase of the illness, can be accompanied by a rash, and may correlate with complement consumption. In most syndromes, nonsteroidal anti-inflammatory drugs provide adequate relief of viral-related arthritic symptoms. If joint symptoms persist, a rheumatology or infectious disease consultation may be necessary; this rule of thumb is especially important when patients present with complicated rheumatic syndromes associated with hepatitis C or HIV infection.[28, 29]

REFERENCES

1. Goldenberg DL: Bacterial arthritis. In Kelley WN, Harris ED Jr, Ruddy S, Sledge CB, eds: Textbook of Rheumatology, 5th ed. Philadelphia, WB Saunders, 1996, pp 1435–1449.
2. Goldenberg DL: Pathophysiology—nongonococcal bacterial arthritis. In Espinoza L, Goldenberg D, Arnett F, Alaracon G, eds: Infections in the Rheumatic Diseases: A Comprehensive Review of Microbial Relations to Rheumatic Disorders. Orlando, Grune & Stratton, 1988, pp 3–8.
3. Smith LR, Merchant TC, Shurman DJ: In vitro cartilage degradation by *E. coli* and *S. aureus*. Arthritis Rheum. 25:441–446, 1982.
4. Goldenberg DL: Septic arthritis. Lancet 351:197–202, 1998.
5. Kaandorp CJE, van Schaardenburg D, Krijnen P, et al: Risk factors for septic arthritis in patients with joint disease: A prospective trial. Arthritis Rheum 38:1819–1825, 1995.
6. Furr PM, Taylor-Robinson D, Webster AD: Mycoplasmas and ureaplasmas in patients with hypogammaglobulinaemia and their role in arthritis: Microbiological observations over twenty years. Ann Rheum Dis 53:183–187, 1994.
7. Ike RW: Bacterial arthritis. In Koopman WJ, ed. Arthritis and Allied Conditions: A Textbook of Rheumatology, 13th ed. Baltimore, Williams & Wilkins, 1997, pp 2267–2295.
8. Javors J, Weisman MH: Principles of diagnosis and treatment of joint infections. In Koopman WJ, ed: Arthritis and Allied Conditions: A Textbook of Rheumatology, 13th ed. Baltimore, Williams & Wilkins, 1997, pp. 2253–2266.
9. Del Beccaro MA, Champuox AN, Bockers T, Mendelman PM: Septic arthritis versus transient synovitis of the hip: The value of screening laboratory tests. Ann Emerg Med 21:1418–1422, 1992.
10. Goldenberg DL, Reed JI: Bacterial arthritis. N Engl J Med 312:764–771, 1985.
11. Goldenberg DL, Brandt KD, Cathcart ES, Cohen AS: Acute arthritis caused by gram-negative bacilli: A clinical characterization. Medicine 53:197–208, 1974.
12. Smith JW, Piercy EA: Infectious arthritis. Clin Infec Dis 20:225–231, 1995.
13. Sanford JP, Gilbert DN, Sande MA: The Sanford Guide to Antimicrobial Therapy 1998. Dallas, Antimicrobial Therapy, 1998.
14. Goldenberg DL, Brandt KD, Cohen AS, Cathcart ES: Treatment of septic arthritis, treatment of needle aspiration and surgery as initial modes of joint drainage. Arthritis Rheum 18:83–90, 1975.
15. Broy SB, Schmid FR: A comparison of medical drainage (needle aspiration) and surgical drainage (arthrotomy or arthroscopy) in the initial treatment of infected joints. Clin Rheum Dis 12:501–522, 1986.
16. Rosenthal J, Bole GG, Robinson WD: Acute nongonococcal infectious arthritis. Arthritis Rheum 23:889–897, 1980.
17. Bynum DK, Nunley JA, Goldner JL, Martinez S: Pyogenic arthritis: Emphasis on the need for surgical drainage of the infected joint. South Med J 75:1232–1238, 1982.
18. Donatto KC: Orthopedic management of septic arthritis. Rheum Dis Clin North Am 24:275–286, 1998.
19. Ivey M, Clark R: Arthroscopic débridement of the knee for septic arthritis. Clin Orthop 199:201–206, 1985.
20. Smith MJ: Arthroscopic treatment of the septic knee. Arthroscopy 2:30–34, 1986.
21. Parisien JS, Shaffer B: Arthroscopic management of pyarthrosis. Clin Orthop 275:243–247, 1992.
22. Lane JG, Falahee MH, Wojtys EM, et al: Pyarthrosis of the knee, treatment considerations. Clin Orthop 252:198–204, 1990.
23. Kaandorp CJE, Krijnen P, Bernelot Moens HJ, et al: The outcome of bacterial arthritis: A prospective community-based study. Arthritis Rheum 40:884–892, 1997.
24. Cucurull E, Espinoza LR: Gonococcal arthritis. Rheum Dis Clin North Am 24:305–322, 1998.
25. Harrington JT Jr: Mycobacterial and fungal infections. In Kelley WN, Harris ED Jr, Ruddy S, Sledge CB, eds: Textbook of Rheumatology, 5th ed. Philadelphia, WB Saunders, 1996, pp 1450–1461.
26. Schnitzer TJ: Viral arthritis. In Kelley WN, Harris ED Jr, Ruddy S, Sledge CB, eds: Textbook of Rheumatology, 5th ed. Philadelphia, WB Saunders, 1996, pp 1473–1483.
27. Naides SJ: Rheumatic manifestations of parvovirus B-19 infection. Rheum Dis Clin North Amer 24:375–401, 1998.
28. McMurray RW: Hepatitis C-associated autoimmune disorders. Rheum Dis Clin North Am 24:353–374, 1998.
29. Cuellar ML: HIV infection-associated inflammatory musculoskeletal disorders. Rheum Dis Clin North Am 24:403–421, 1998.

INFECTIONS OF THE SPINE

Eugene J. Carragee

Spinal infections represent a particularly challenging problem to the clinician. In addition to all of the usual hazards of a deep-seated infection, the patient with a serious spinal infection is at risk for progressive spinal deformity, instability, and neurologic injury. The diagnosis of spinal infections is difficult. The main presenting symptom is spinal-type pain, and because back pain is nearly ubiquitous in the general population, early diagnosis has proven historically difficult.

The types of spinal infections have traditionally been divided between granulomatous and pyogenic infections. In the preantibiotic era, clinical experience led to a clear distinction between the more acute spinal inflammation seen with pyogenic infections and the chronic inflammatory condition typically associated with Pott's spondylitis (tuberculosis). The pyogenic form was characterized by an acute febrile illness, often progressing to paralysis and in many cases death in a short period of time. The granulomatous spinal infections were different. The patient had at some time in the past survived the acute pulmonary infection with tuberculosis, and the spinal infection was usually a process that progressed slowly, particularly in adults. The immunologic response was a granulomatous reaction about the infected areas.

The terms *pyogenic* and *granulomatous* have come to mean less over time as few cases are left to run their natural course. The influence of antibiotics has tempered the pyogenic response of bacterial infections, and the increased prevalence of less virulent infections in patients with compromised immune systems has led these infections to resemble chronic granulomatous infections. Similarly the emergence of antibiotic resistance in tuberculosis and the infection of immunocompromised patients have led to fulminant presentations of spinal tuberculosis more consistent with classic pyogenic infection. In reality, the presentation of spinal infections is quite variable. Distinctions are usually made according to the level of spinal involvement, involvement of the neural elements, and the mode of infection (hematogenous versus direct extension). Finally, spinal infections in children, adults, and the elderly appear to follow differing clinical patterns.

PYOGENIC INFECTIONS

Pyogenic vertebral osteomyelitis (PVO) is an uncommon infection but has been long recognized since first being described in 1897 by Lannelongue.[1] The clinical picture of this entity has changed over time to reflect medical and epidemiologic trends.[2-6] In the preantibiotic era, PVO infections were described as acute, subacute, and chronic syndromes. The organisms predominantly involved were *S. aureus* and *Streptococcus pyogenes;* these infections were associated with a 25% to 70% mortality and generally affected younger adults.[5, 7] It was common in that era for persons to be afflicted with the intractable suppurative conditions of the day: persistent furunculosis, ear infections, mastoid infections, and others, which although occasionally being drained, had no other effective treatment. The body was subject to intermittent bacterial showers, and in the presence of rheumatic valvular disease chronic endovascular infections were seen frequently. The individual who did not succumb in the early stages of the disease from sepsis or complications of paralysis could often clear the infection with time. Surgical measures risked further destabilizing the spine and were not effective in eradicating the infection.[8]

The course of the disease was noted to change with the introduction of effective antibiotic treatment in the 1940s and 1950s. Although acute cases frequently went undiagnosed, subacute and chronic infections were recognized by radiographic findings and treated with specific antibiotics. In modern times, PVO continues to be seen but often in the context of associated conditions, such as intravenous drug abuse, diabetes, and rheumatoid arthritis (Table 33–3).[2, 3, 6, 8–10]

Mechanism of Spinal Infections

The rise of low back disability and the aggressive treatment of degenerative conditions of the spine with surgery have increased the incidence of postoperative infections. Hematogenous spread, however; is the most frequently seen cause of spinal infection in most situations. Since the description of Batson's venous plexus in the pelvis in the 1930s, it has been assumed that a retrograde flow up these valveless veins accounted for the spread of bacteria to the spine from urogenital and rectal sources. Work, however, has shown that the pressure needed to cause this retrograde flow is probably not generated clinically. More likely is direct arterial delivery of pathogens to the spine. The metaphyseal area of the vertebral body is rich with end-arterial networks,

Table 33–3. IMMUNOLOGIC STATUS IN 111 CASES OF PYOGENIC VERTEBRAL OSTEOMYELITIS

Immunologic Status	No.	%
Apparently immunocompetent	67	61
Conditions associated with immunosuppression	44	40
Diabetes	28	
Glucocorticoid therapy	18	
Cancer chemotherapy	11	
Rheumatoid arthritis	9	
Renal failure	3	
Liver failure	3	
Malnutrition	1	
Myelodysplasia	1	
Intravenous drug abuse (current/confirmed)	15	13.5
Intravenous drug abuse (suspected or remote)	7	6.3

Data from Carragee E: Pyogenic vertebral osteomyelitis. J Bone Joint Surg Am 79:874–880, 1997.

and the blood flow is slow. Infections appear to start at these foci and spread quickly to the adjacent disc. The disc has no intrinsic blood supply and therefore is structurally ill equipped to control infection. The rapid spread through the disc and involvement of the next vertebral body give the classic pathologic and radiographic picture of PVO: a collapsed disc space with the end-plates on either side eroded.

The disc then becomes the center of bacterial proliferation and abscess formation. Purulent material may spread posteriorly to involve the spinal canal and neural element or anteriorly to track along the psoas or down the mediastinum.

Certain spinal levels may be predisposed to infection by co-existing arthritic conditions. The distribution of infections is greater in the lumbar region than the thoracic,[3] whereas the cervical region is the least frequently involved despite common arthritic changes with age. This distribution has important prognostic implications. Extension into the epidural space below the level of the spinal cord (i.e., below L1 vertebral body) does not frequently cause severe paralysis, and with treatment, recovery is the rule. Infections at the level of the cord more frequently lead to catastrophic neurologic injury that is largely irreversible. The neurologic risk of the area infected therefore dictates how aggressive surgical treatment may need to be. The distribution of infection by vertebral level in 111 cases is given in Figure 33–1; note that more than half of the infections in this series occurred below the cord terminus.

Bacteriology

The most common organism found in PVO infections is *S. aureus*. In older series, it was responsible for more than 50% of cases. More recently, less virulent organisms have been found, and the proportion of classic pyogenic species has decreased (Fig. 33–2).[3] Infections frequently arising from the urogenital tract are *E. coli*, *Proteus,* and *Pseudomonas* species. Mixed infections are seen, including aerobic and anaerobic organisms, and pyogenic and mycobacterial in the same abscesses. Some of these mixed infections may be due to iatrogenic contamination during biopsies.

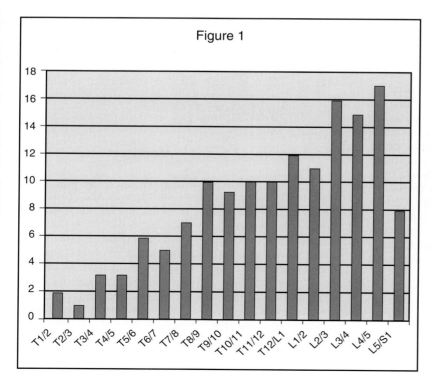

Figure 33–1. Distribution of pyogenic vertebral osteomyelitis in 111 patients. (Data from Carragee E: Pyogenic vertebral osteomyelitis. J Bone Joint Surg Am 79:874, 1997.)

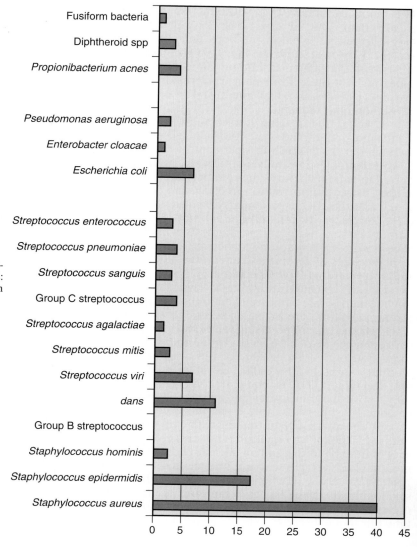

Figure 33–2. Organism cultured in 111 cases of pyogenic vertebral osteomyelitis. (Data from Carragee E: Pyogenic vertebral osteomyelitis. J Bone Joint Surg Am 79:874, 1997.)

Clinical Picture

Virtually all patients with PVO have back pain on presentation. Sixty percent to 80% of the adult population have back pain, however, and back pain is the second most common reason for patients to see a physician. Therefore, the presence of back pain alone is relatively unhelpful. The quality of the back pain may be important. Severe, disabling pain continuing over days or weeks, particularly if not associated with activity, is suggestive of infection. Pain that seems disproportionate to the physical findings is another clue. Fever and increased WBC counts are seen in a few cases. The ESR and C-reactive protein are almost invariably elevated.[3, 11]

Physical Examination

Subtle signs or symptoms of root or spinal cord irritation are present in most patients, but frank neuro-logic loss is much less common. Depending on the series, significant paralysis may be seen in 0% to 30% of cases. Spinal percussion may reproduce symptoms, but this is unreliable. Meningeal signs are rare and may not indicate cerebrospinal fluid infection.

Diagnosis

Until the advent of MRI, the diagnosis of spinal discitis and osteomyelitis was problematic. The classic radiographic finding of lysis in the vertebral metaphysis and disc height loss with end-plate changes is not seen until 2 to 3 weeks after infection. Technetium bone scans are nonspecific as are CT changes. Labeling WBCs with gallium is more specific but has largely been replaced with the MRI.[12–15]

MRI is sensitive and specific (see Chapter 4). It is the diagnostic study of choice. MRI is suggestive of infection within the first week of clinical infection. Along with blood culture, MRI is sufficient for diagnosis in greater than 30% of cases. The T1-weighted image shows decreased signal in the body and disc infected, and the T2-weighted image shows an increased signal intensity in the same distribution. This differs from the appearance of old compression fractures or degenerative disc changes, in which the signal intensity is decreased on both sequences.

Although the imaging studies and the ESR make the diagnosis likely, the bacteriologic diagnosis is a separate matter. In the rush to treatment of the diagnosis suggested on imaging studies, antibiotics are frequently started in patients before confirmatory cultures are obtained. This is not sound practice and should be avoided. Although the patient may be ill, it is unusual to see a patient so critically ill that antibiotics need to be started before a bacteriologic diagnosis is made. In the patient with sepsis requiring immediate antibiotic treatment, two sets of aerobic and anaerobic blood cultures and urine cultures should be taken.

In most instances, a thorough diagnostic approach can be taken before empirically initiating therapy. Blood and urine cultures are a starting point. If these are non-diagnostic, an experienced surgeon or radiologist should perform a needle or core biopsy of the spine. Blood cultures are positive about 25% of the time, and needle biopsies vary from 50% to 80% accuracy depending on the technique and thoroughness of the investigator.[3, 12, 16] If these measures fail, an open biopsy should be done. Most patients can tolerate this even if they are very ill. The alternative of treating with empirical antibiotics for an unknown organism is not attractive. The toxicity of multiple drugs and an unclear end point are significant disadvantages to this approach. In some centers, polymerase chain reaction techniques, which amplify small amounts of the bacteria, can directly identify the organism. This technique is not widely available at this time but should become so in the near future.

Treatment

The treatment of spinal infections is directed toward eradicating the infection while preserving or restoring neurologic function and spinal stability. Late progressive deformity and neurologic injury are still hazards even if the infection has been controlled. Antibiotics and immobilization of the involved spinal segments are the mainstays of treatment. In patients with no neurologic loss and an apparently stable spine, the success of this approach without surgery is related to the age and the immune status of the patient and the ESR response to treatment.[3, 11] Table 33–4 shows the relative probabilities of nonoperative success in patients without neurologic loss. In patients younger than 60 years old, with a normal immune status and a drop in ESR of more than 25% over the first month, treatment was successful greater than 90%. Only one third of older, immunosuppressed patients with a poor ESR response were successfully treated by antibiotics alone.

Experience has shown that most patients who improve are manifestly better within 2 weeks after antibiotic treatment and immobilization. The clearest indication of improvement is the subsidence of pain. The correct duration of antibiotic treatment in these cases is not known. Many authors recommend continuing antibiotics intravenously for about 6 weeks, then continuing oral treatment for another 6 weeks. The ESR may decline slowly over some months and would be a conservative measure to clinical cure. Immunosuppressed patients may need prolonged treatment. Patients with rheumatologic disease have an elevated ESR and C-reactive protein as part of their rheumatologic condition, and therefore antibiotic duration must be judged on other clinical grounds.

Over the first month or so, MRI is a poor indicator of clinical response.[12] The MRI study often appears to deteriorate despite obvious clinical improvement. It takes many months for MRI to reflect the successful eradication of the infection because the bone and disc continue to be metabolically active during that time.

Indications for Surgery

Because most patients can be adequately treated without surgery, surgical treatment should be reserved

Table 33–4. AGE, ERYTHROCYTE SEDIMENTATION RATE RESPONSE, AND IMMUNE STATUS AS PREDICTORS OF CLINICAL SUCCESS OF CONSERVATIVE TREATMENT IN 44 CASES WITH AT LEAST 1 MONTH OF NONOPERATIVE CARE					
Age	Immune Status	ESR response (+≥25% fall)	n	Success (%)	P Value
<60	Normal immune	+ ESR response	12	11 (92%)	—
>60	Normal immune	+ ESR response	7	6 (86%)	.68
<60	Immunosuppression	+ ESR response	3	3 (100%)	.60
>60	Immunosuppression	+ ESR response	4	3 (75%)	.38
<60	Normal immune	− ESR response	4	3 (75%)	.38
>60	Normal immune	− ESR response	4	2 (50%)	.06
<60	Immunosuppression	− ESR response	4	2 (50%)	.06
>60	Immunosuppression	− ESR response	6	2 (33%)	.009

ESR, erythrocyte sedimentation rate.
Adapted from Carragee E, Kim DD, Vlugt TVD, Vittum D: Erythrocyte sedimentation rate in pyogenic vertebral osteomyelitis. Spine 22:2089, 1997.

for specific circumstances. Indications for surgical treatment include:

1. Need for definitive diagnosis when noninvasive or percutaneous methods have failed
2. Profound or progressive sepsis from a spinal abscess
3. Neurologic loss because of instability or compression by epidural infection
4. Spinal instability
5. Failure to eliminate infection with an appropriate course of antibiotics

When indicated, operative treatment usually involves an anterior approach to the spine, cervical, thoracic, or lumbar, and it is important that the surgical team have experience in this approach. The anatomic landmarks in cases of infection may be obscure: The great vessels may be involved in phlegmon or abscess, and neural elements are at risk behind the abscess. The débridement of infected and necrotic tissue should be thorough. In most cases, the defect left after the débridement can be primarily grafted with autogenous bone for fusion. The surgery may be quite involved, but experience has shown that even these ill and often chronically debilitated patients can tolerate the operative trauma.[2, 3, 8, 17, 18] After surgery, a prolonged course of bed rest, immobilization in an orthosis, or both is usually required along with antibiotic therapy. The clinician should note that the ESR rises because of the surgery and does not reflect the status of the infection for several weeks.

Sometimes, simultaneous or delayed internal fixation with instrumentation should be considered. Although implantation of metal devices into an infected wound goes against common teaching, it has been found to be well tolerated and in some cases the only approach to salvaging a desperate situation.[17, 19] The special circumstances in which direct instrumentation of an infected spine may be prudent include:

1. Gross instability after débridement
2. Pulmonary or other medical disease precluding bed rest or bracing
3. Progressive deformity despite immobilization
4. Decubiti in the debilitated or insensate patient precluding bed rest or brace

Prognosis

Once cleared of infection, patients tend to do remarkably well. The recurrence rate of infection when a course of antibiotic has been completed is low. Chronic pain was found in fewer than 10% of patients and may be related to deformity or instability. Most patients despite considerable destruction of the spine do well and, in fact, have less ongoing symptoms than patients who undergo spinal fusion for degenerative conditions.

In many patients, neurologic recovery can be dramatic. In one series, nearly 50% of patients with complete loss at a spinal cord level at admission had full recovery. In the same series, about half of incomplete neurologic injuries also recovered completely. Neurologic injury, *S. aureus* infection, older age, and immune deficiency are all poor prognostic indicators.[3, 8]

GRANULOMATOUS INFECTION

A number of different organisms can cause spinal infections with primarily a granulomatous host reaction. In addition to *M. tuberculosis*, these include the atypical mycobacterium, atypical bacteria (*Actinomyces, Nocardia, Brucella* species), and fungi (*Coccidioides, Aspergillus, Cryptococcus,* and *Blastomyces*). Many of these are regionally specific around the world, and geography and travel must be considered. In addition, as stressed earlier, there is overlap with usually pyogenic organisms in presentation and pathologic appearance.

The most prominent of these infections historically had been *M. tuberculosis*. In modern times, the clinical picture has radically changed the patient demographics and clinical course. In the United States, the increase in immigration of many people from endemic areas, the emergence of drug-resistant strains, and the increase in individuals with serious cell-mediated immune deficiency (e.g., HIV, organ transplant) have all affected the nature of these infections.

Clinical Course

Pulmonary tuberculosis spreads to bone in about 10% of cases, and 50% of these involve the spine.[20, 21] This is usually a hematogenous spread, although direct erosion into the spine from intrathoracic foci has been seen. Neurologic progression depends on host resistance, treatment, and patient age. On admission, 10% to 50% of new spinal cases have some neurologic loss.[20–23]

The history is highly variable. Patients again almost invariably complain of back pain. Constitutional symptoms may not be volunteered but in retrospect are common. In some chronic cases, a pronounced deformity may be seen in patients with little pain. A history of pulmonary tuberculosis may be remote or nonexistant.

On examination, the spine can be tender, and a deformity may be apparent. Torticollis is often seen with cervical disease. The gibbus deformity of spinal tuberculosis (a sharp angulation) may be present and should not be confused with scoliosis or kyphosis. It may more closely resemble the curve of congenital spinal deformities or neurofibromatosis. The neurologic examination is also highly variable and may demonstrate meningeal signs.

Laboratory findings are usually nonspecific. Although in PVO the ESR is almost always elevated, in spinal tuberculosis, 25% of patients may have a normal ESR. The PPD is usually positive except in cases of severe metabolic or immunologic decline. Other possible sites of infection should be examined, such as the lung, chest, or kidney.

Radiographs are not sensitive or specific enough to make the diagnosis, although there are some characteristic features, including relative sparing of the disc space until late in the disease, multilevel involvement, and large paraspinal abscess shadows. The degree of destruction may be surprising given the patient's relatively comfortable presentation. Early granulomatous infection of the spine is more easily confused on radiographic examination with metastatic disease than PVO.[15, 24, 25] Technetium and gallium radionucleotide scans are less sensitive in granulomatous infections than in PVO (33% and 70% false-negative rates). CT scanning shows the bony anatomy well, particularly if planning surgery. MRI is again the imaging modality of choice. There may be confusion between granulomatous spinal disease and metastatic disease on MRI.

Treatment

The principles of treatment are the same as for PVO. Antibiotic treatment is dictated by the organism and drug sensitivities. Four-drug treatment is currently recommended in tuberculous infections, but regional variations in drug resistance make seeking consultation with local infectious disease and public health personnel important. Antibiotic treatment of the less common atypical granulomatous infections from bacteria and fungi warrants careful consideration and input from infectious disease specialists with an interest in these uncommon deep infections.

Urgent surgical intervention is considered when neurologic loss or acute instability is seen. The higher the lesion, the greater the neurologic risk. Cervical disease with any neurologic loss should be considered a surgical emergency because the results of delayed care are dismal.[26, 27] More commonly, however, patients needing surgery may be stabilized and the operation done on a semielective basis after some antibiotic treatment. The surgery usually involves a wide anterior débridement, primary bone grafting, and postoperative immobilization. The addition of instrumentation to eliminate the need for prolonged immobilization has been increasingly applied.

REFERENCES

1. Lannelongue O: *On Acute Osteomyelitis*. Paris, 1897.
2. Cahill D, Love L, Rechtine G: Pyogenic osteomyelitis of the spine in the elderly. J Neurosurg 74:878–886, 1991.
3. Carragee E: Pyogenic vertebral osteomyelitis. J Bone Joint Surg Am 79:874–880, 1997.
4. Garci A, Grantham S: Hematogenous pyogenic vertebral osteomyelitis. J Bone Joint Surg Am 42:429–436, 1960.
5. Guri J: Pyogenic osteomyelitis of the spine: Differential diagnosis through clinical and radiographic observations. J Bone Joint Surg 28:29–39, 1946.
6. Patzakis M, Rao S, Wilkins J, et al: Analysis of 61 cases of vertebral osteomyelitis. Clin Orthop 264:178–183, 1991.
7. Griffiths H, Jones D: Pyogenic infection of the spine: A review of 28 cases. J Bone Joint Surg 53:383–391, 1971.
8. Eismont F, Bohlman H, Soni P, et al: Pyogenic and fungal vertebral osteomyelitis with paralysis. J Bone Joint Surg Am 65:19–29, 1983.
9. Carragee EJ, Billys J, Sonu C: Pyogenic vertebral osteomyelitis in immunocompromised adults. Orthop Trans 84:1291, 1993.
10. Weissman G, Wood V, Kroll L: Pseudomonas vertebral osteomyelitis in heroin addicts. J Bone Joint Surg Am 55:1416–1424, 1973.
11. Carragee E, Kim DD, Vlugt TVD, Vittum D: Erythrocyte sedimentation rate in pyogenic vertebral osteomyelitis. Spine 22:2089–2094, 1997.
12. Carragee E: The clinical use of magnetic resonance imaging in pyogenic vertebral osteomyelitis. Spine 22:780–785, 1997.
13. Enzman D: Infection and inflammation. In Enzman D, Paz RDL, Rubin J, eds: Magnetic Resonance of the Spine. St Louis, Mosby, 1990, pp 260–300.
14. Modic M, Feilin D, Piraino D, et al: Vertebral osteomyelitis: Assessment using MR. Radiology 157:157–166, 1985.
15. Sharif HS: Role of MR in managing spine infections. Am J Radiol 158:133–145, 1992.
16. Fraser-Hill M, Renfrew D: Percutaneous biopsy of musculoskeletal lesions: 1. Effective accuracy and diagnostic utility. Am J Radiol 158:809–812, 1994.
17. Carragee E: Instrumentation of the infected and unstable spine: A review of 17 cases from the thoracic and lumbar spine with pyogenic infections. Spine 10:317–324, 1997.
18. Emery S, Chan, D, Woodward H: Treatment of hematogenous pyogenic osteomyelitis with anterior debridement and primary bone grafting. Spine 14:284–291, 1989.
19. Graziano G, Sidhu K: Salvage reconstruction in acute and late sequellae from pyogenic thoracolumbar infection. J Spinal Disord 6:199–207, 1993.
20. Boachie-Adje O, Squillante R: Tuberculosis of the spine. Orthop Clin North Am 27:95–103, 1996.
21. Ho E, Leong J: Tuberculosis of the spine. In Weinstein SL, ed: The Pediatric Spine: Principles and Practice. New York, Raven Press, 1994, pp 837–850.
22. Hodgson A, Skinsnes O, Leong CY: The pathogenesis of Pott's paraplegia. J Bone Joint Surg Am 49:1147–1156, 1967.
23. Hodgson A, Stock F: Anterior spine fusion for the treatment of tuberculosis of the spine. J Bone Joint Surg Am 42:295–310, 1960.
24. Smith A, Weinstein M, Mizushima A, et al: MR imaging characteristics of tuberculous spondylitis vs. vertebral osteomyelitis. AJR Am J Roentgenol 153:399–405, 1989.
25. Thrush A, Enzman D: MR imaging of infectious spondylitis. AJNR Am J Neuroradiol 11:1171–1180, 1990.
26. Hsu L, Cheng C, Leong J: Pott's paraplegia of late onset: The cause of compression and results after anterior decompression. J Bone Joint Surg Br 70:534–538, 1988.
27. Hsu L, Leong J: Tuberculosis of the lower cervical spine (C2 to C7): A report on 40 cases. J Bone Joint Surg B 66:1–5, 1984.

Chapter 34

Heritable Diseases Affecting the Immune and Musculoskeletal Systems

Edward D. Harris, Jr.

The primary care physician encounters patients with rheumatic problems that are caused by heritable defects in genetic material. This chapter focuses on underlying genetic abnormalities that cause musculoskeletal pain or deformity or predispose patients to commonly recognized rheumatic syndromes in adults. Some phenotypic expression of genetic defects in children is discussed as well. In each of these syndromes, there is potential for gene therapy.[1]

JOINT AND BONE PAIN WITHOUT INFLAMMATION

Genetic problems presenting as degenerative disease of bones and joints are often classified as heritable disorders of the structural proteins (collagen, elastin, and other proteins) and the glycoproteins and proteoglycans that make up the extracellular matrix. Before discussing the disorders, it is appropriate to review the characteristics of these molecules.[2]

COLLAGENS. Collagens are the most abundant proteins in the body. There are 19 distinct genetic types, representing 30 separate genes. For practical purposes, the function of these proteins can be considered as giving either compressive or tensile strength or an important barrier function. The most abundant collagens in the first group are as follows:

Type I collagen: This molecule is a collagen prototype, the first purified and characterized. It is the principal protein in bone, tendons, skin, fascia, and ligaments. As with the other collagens, its biosynthesis is complex. First, α chains of approximately 1000 amino acids are formed. These join in triads to form triple helical, rigid molecules that cross-link with other triple-helical molecules to form collagen fibrils and larger fibers. The *purest* examples of type I collagen are tendon and ligaments. Bone is primarily mineralized collagen type I. Skin is more complex: The dermis is principally type I collagen with more elastin and glycosaminoglycans than in tendon or ligament.

Type II collagen: This triple helical collagen is the principal protein of articular cartilage and fibrocartilage. Articular cartilage is one of the most highly differentiated tissues in the body. Although collagen provides tensile strength, the complex aggregates of proteoglycans and hyaluronic acid provide recoil and the ability of cartilage to rebound from the deforming loads that it experiences with each step taken or finger squeezed.

Type III collagen: Also triple helical, this molecule is more abundant in recently formed connective tissue but in highest concentrations never represents more than 2% or 3% of collagen in these tissues. It has an important role in the adventitia of blood vessels.

The important collagen that provides barrier function is *type IV collagen.* This is a complex molecule that has both triple helical and noncollagenous domains. It is a principal component of basement membrane of all tissues and blood vessels. Antibodies against an epitope on type IV collagen are found in Goodpasture's syndrome. The basement membrane is an extremely complex tissue, with type IV collagen, perlecan, sparc, laminin, entactin, and other extracellular molecules contributing to its structure and function.

ELASTIN. Just as collagens, structured as long thin rods, provide tensile strength, elastin molecules are linked to each other in aggregates that allow stretching of their domains with collapse to their original form when the force to deform them is gone. Thus, they are elastic. Elastin fibers are prominent in skin, the nuchal ligament, and arteries.[2]

MATRIX GLYCOPROTEINS AND PROTEOGLYCANS. Matrix glycoproteins and proteoglycans have a more amorphous structure than do the structural proteins, and the dominant characteristic of many of them is a strong anionic charge that enables them to recoil from a deforming load to their original configuration.[3] They are present in the solid phase (e.g., cartilage), fluid phase (e.g., hyaluronic acid in joint fluid), and cell surface phase. Along with some types of collagen (e.g., VI, VII, and IX), they are involved in attachment of cells to matrix. Examples of proteoglycans (glycosaminoglycans) prominent in connective tissue are as follows:

1. *Hyaluronan*—an enormous repeating disaccharide of glucuronic acid and *N*-acetylglucosamine that has no protein associated with it. Hyaluronan is produced by synovial cells, is responsible for the high viscosity of synovial fluid, and in high-molecular-weight form is used now for therapeutic injection into joints of patients with osteoarthritis. In cartilage, it combines by a link protein to aggregan to form a supermolecule responsible for the compressive characteristics of this tissue.

2. *Aggrecan*—a long core protein with glycosaminoglycan side chains (keratan sulfate and chondroitin sulfate) arranged in a formation similar to a bottle brush that link to hyaluronan.

3. *Fibronectin*—a major matrix glycoprotein with different forms. Fibronectin is involved in binding of cells to extracellular matrix, is found on the surface of cells, and in a fluid phase can serve as a chemoattractant. In cartilage, a similar molecule is named *chondronectin*. These *nectins* also have an important role in activation of various genes of cells leading to their expression of various proteins that can contribute to inflammatory or proliferative events.

Heritable Diseases of Connective Tissue

BONE PAIN, FRACTURES, AND DEFORMITIES

The prototype of disorders associated with bone pain, fractures, and deformities is *osteogenesis imperfecta*. The gene prevalence of osteogenesis imperfecta is 4 to 5 per 100,000. There are at least four types of this process, which has a dominant pattern of inheritance. It is associated with mutations in type I collagen genes so that insufficient amounts of collagen are synthesized for bone and other connective tissues.[4] One form is lethal, several others produce moderate osteopenia and fractures, and one form (Silence type I) can be undiagnosed for years and is characterized by excessive fractures without deformity, blue sclerae, and hearing loss during the second and third decades of life. Mild forms may be missed completely until they produce an obviously affected child, who, in turn, may be suspected of having been abused. Treatment awaits gene therapy; for now, the most important therapy is building muscle strength both before and after fractures.

HYPEREXTENSIBLE LIGAMENTS AND JOINT PAIN

The prototypes for this phenotype are the various forms of the Ehlers-Danlos syndrome (EDS) and Marfan's syndrome.

Ehlers-Danlos Syndrome

Types I and II of EDS often overlap. Type III is referred to as the *benign hypermobility syndrome* and merges with the normal population. These three types can make up to 5% of patients in a pediatric arthritis clinic.[5] Types I and II are characterized by joint hyperextensibility that may be widespread or limited to hands and feet (Fig. 34–1). Patients suffer from recurrent joint dislocations, periodic joint effusions from mild trauma, and the eventual appearance of osteoarthritis. The primary care physician who suspects the diagnosis should ask about the patient's birth: abnormally aggregated collagen in the placenta can lead to premature rupture of membranes and early birth. Skin of type I and II patients is velvety and distensible. When wounds heal, the edges oppose poorly, leading to a *fish-mouth* scar.

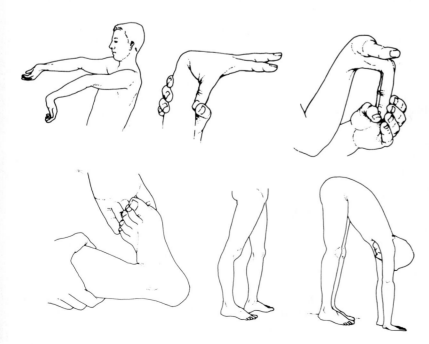

Figure 34–1. Maneuvers that may be used to establish the presence of clinically significant joint laxity. Examples of joint laxity found in the Ehlers-Danlos syndrome. It is not unusual to find extreme laxity of the small joints and less laxity in large joints. Laxity decreases with age, so that the dominant nature of most of these syndromes may not be appreciated when examining older family members. (Redrawn and modified from Wynne-Davies R: Acetabular dysplasia and familial joint laxity: two etiological factors in congenital dislocation of the hip. A review of 589 patients and their families. J Bone Joint Surg Br 52:704, 1970.)

The primary care physician is most likely to encounter type III EDS in the form of generalized joint pain, especially after exertion, and dislocation of joints (e.g., the patella). Progressive scoliosis can generate back pain. Frequent ankle sprains from instability can also be a problem. Lax joints may be assessed in a semiquantitative manner as follows:

- Passive approximation of the thumb to the forearm
- Passive hyperextension of fingers and toes
- Active hyperextension of the knee to greater than 10 degrees
- Excessive dorsiflexion of the ankle and eversion of the foot
 The ability to touch palms to the floor without bending the knees

The problem in diagnosis often arises in adolescent boys in the midst of a growth spurt who have some dissociation between bone and muscle and tendon growth. These are *growing pains* and can be disabling. Frequent sprains, some mild knee effusions, and moderate pain after sporting activities are the principal symptoms in this group. Unless there is a family history of EDS or characteristic malleable joints and velvety skin, a diagnosis of EDS should not be given until the growth spurts have ceased and the signs of hyperextensibility persist. Often, in adolescents with growing pains, emphasis on isometric exercise to build up muscle bundles without increasing flexibility is useful. In postadolescent athletes with well-developed musculature, the opposite situation may obtain: These young men may suffer from repetitive muscle tears because they lack flexibility.

Other forms of EDS are rare and have phenotypic changes in eyes (type VI) or skeletal dysplasias (type IX) and are diagnosed by pediatric specialists. In patients with type IV EDS, there is a heritable defect in type III collagen formation, and this leads to rupture of bowel diverticula or arterial rupture (e.g., iliac, splenic, or renal arteries) that can lead to massive hematomas or death. Patients have thin transparent skin revealing a prominent venous pattern, particularly on the abdomen, but do not have hyperextensible joints. Because vessels are friable, surgical repair is difficult. In most patients, mutations of the fibrillin gene (fibrillin is associated with elastin biosynthesis) are believed to be the cause.

Marfan's Syndrome

In its most recognized form, Marfan's syndrome is manifested as above-average height, arachnodactyly (long, thin fingers), dislocation of the lens of the eye, dilation of the ascending aorta with risk of dissection, mitral valve abnormalities, hernias, and skeletal abnormalities. This classic form can appear in up to 6 or 7 persons per 100,000. It is inherited as an autosomal dominant trait and is caused by mutations in the fibrillin gene that codes for proteins that form microfibrils close to basement membranes and in elastic fibers.[1] Patients may present with any one of the phenotypes listed previously as the signal for presence of the disease. Care must be taken not to confuse Marfan's syndrome with growing pains in a rapidly growing adolescent (see above). With awareness of the disease among laypersons, patients often arrive at a primary care physician's office asking whether or not they have Marfan's syndrome.

The first task for the physician is to do a careful family history, focusing on eye abnormalities and possible aortic aneurysms or aortic or mitral valve problems. In the patient, pointed questions about visual defects, chest pain, palpitations, hernias, joint dislocations, chest wall deformities (e.g., pectus excavatum or carinatum), and flat feet are suggestive elements of history. The following are an approximate prevalence of clinical abnormalities:

- *Arachnodactyly* (90%): Semiquantitative measures include a disproportionate excess of heel-to-pubis measurements to pubis-to-vertex of the skull and the ability to have the thumb protrude below the hypothenar eminence (Steinberg's test) (Fig. 34–2).
- *Ectopia lentis* (50% to 80%): This is usually bilateral and appears by 5 years of age.
- *Cardiovascular abnormalities* (approximately 80%): Auscultatory evidence for mitral or aortic valve involvement is common, with mitral valve prolapse, mitral regurgitation, and aneurysmal dilation of the ascending aorta being the primary lesions. Repeat echocardiograms are essential to measure the diameter of the ascending aorta. When it dilates to 6 cm or more in adults (or to >50% of normal for the body surface area), aortic graft surgery should be contemplated strongly. Antibiotic prophylaxis for dental visits and other invasive situations should be used in all Marfan's syndrome patients.
- *Skeletal abnormalities* (at least one in almost all patients): One or more of the following abnormalities are usually found in Marfan's syndrome patients:
  - A long narrow face with prognathism
  - A high arched palate
  - Loss of the normal curve of the cervical spine
  - Kyphoscoliosis
  - Pectus excavatum or carinatum
  - Spondylolistheses
  - Slipped epiphyses
  - Flat, unstable feet

Of these, kyphoscoliosis is the one that should be watched closely; it can progress rapidly during adolescence causing eventual compromise of pulmonary function.

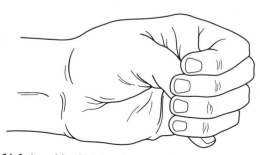

Figure 34–2. A positive Steinberg's test. When the thumb is flexed into the palm and held at an angle almost perpendicular to the radius, the distal tip, including most of the nail, protrudes on the ulnar side of the hand.

Pseudoxanthoma Elasticum

Pseudoxanthoma elasticum is much more rare than Marfan's syndrome and is characterized by degeneration and calcification of elastic fibers in the skin, retina, and blood vessels. In its autosomal dominant trait, it is recognized by the chamois-colored, slightly elevated papules and streaks on the skin of the neck and axilla. Breaks in Bruch's membrane of the retina can lead to blindness from hemorrhage into or around the retina. These *angioid streaks* can be seen with direct ophthalmoscopy. These patients should be referred to an ophthalmologist as soon as a diagnosis is made. Rupture of blood vessels in the gastrointestinal tract can cause severe bleeding. Mitral valve prolapse and symptoms suggestive of congestive heart failure may be found. Mutations in a gene responsible for this syndrome have not yet been identified.

GENETIC DEFECTS IN CARTILAGE

Mutations in chondrocyte genes affect the development of the entire skeleton because most bones arise from cartilaginous templates.[6] *Achondroplasia,* expressed as dwarfism, waddling gait, and a large head with normal intelligence, is an autosomal dominant trait. *Spondyloepiphyseal dysplasia* is characterized by a small trunk, short neck, barrel chest, and long extremities out of proportion to the trunk. Milder forms can be expressed in late adolescence and early adulthood as a particularly aggressive osteoarthritis. The type II collagen gene appears to have mutations in this syndrome.

Metaphyseal chondrodysplasia is the result of bone formation not progressing normally at the junction of bone and hypertrophic chondrocytes. Affected children are born with short limbs, enlarged joints, and shortened long bones that on radiographs slightly resembles rickets. Children with milder syndromes have a clinical picture of rickets (bowing of long bones of the legs) without the metabolic abnormalities. Children with another type with enlarged joints and short extremities have fine hair and susceptibility to viral and bacterial infections (McKusick's type). The possible genetic link between the skeletal and immune system has not been defined.

GENETIC DEFECTS IN BASEMENT MEMBRANE

Alport's syndrome (X-linked), characterized by renal failure and sensorineural hearing loss, is associated with a genetic abnormality of minor collagens.

PATIENTS WITH RECURRENT INFECTIONS OR DIFFUSE CONNECTIVE TISSUE DISEASES

Diagnosis

Awareness and understanding of human immunodeficiency virus (HIV) to associated infections and acquired immunodeficiency syndrome (AIDS) has increased the importance of recognizing heritable causes of immune deficiencies that can present as recurrent infections, often with the same or a related infectious agent. Of the various abnormalities, some of which present first in adulthood, B-cell defects far outnumber those affecting T cells, phagocytic cells, or complement proteins. Agammaglobulinemia occurs with a frequency of 1 in 50,000 live births and severe combined immunodeficiency with a frequency of 1 in 200,000 live births.[7]

When a patient is suspected of having an immune deficiency, is negative for HIV infection, and has abnormally high acute-phase reactants (erythrocyte sedimentation rate and C-reactive protein), the physician needs to measure immunoglobulin A levels; antibody titers against tetanus, penumococci, and diphtheria; and isohemagglutinins (i.e., antibodies against type A and B red blood cells). In the absence of antibodies to tetanus and diphtheria, levels can be measured again several weeks after vaccination. The absence of Howell-Jolly bodies in a smear of blood cells helps to exclude congenital asplenia, and the Wiskott-Aldrich syndrome (discussed later) is ruled out by a normal platelet count. A normal IgA virtually excludes permanent IgG deficiencies of all kinds because IgA is low in all of them. Measurements of subclasses of IgG should be done only if necessary in specialized clinics after the patient has been referred for consultation. T-cell function is assessed by absolute lymphocyte counts, CD4+ and CD8+ cell counts, and the *Candida albicans* intradermal skin test.

Killing defects in phagocytic cells, suspected when patients have recurrent staphylococcal, gram-negative bacterial, or fungal infections, can be assayed in specialized laboratories by measuring the respiratory burst in neutrophils during phagocytosis. A CH50 assay, which measures the function of all components of complement, is the most cost-effective assay to detect abnormalities of complement.

Immune Deficiencies That Are Relevant in Primary Care

Most severe immune deficiencies (e.g., X-linked agammaglobulinemia, thymic hypoplasia [DiGeorge's syndrome], cellular/immunodeficiency with intact immunoglobulins, and severe combined immunodeficiency) are diagnosed or detected early in life and manifested by severe and repeated infections. The Wiskott-Aldrich syndrome, usually diagnosed within the first year of life, is characterized by eczema, thrombocytopenia, and undue susceptibility to infections. There also is a 10% to 12% incidence of fatal malignancy. These patients rarely survive adolescence. Certain syndromes have a later onset and should be considered when an older child or young adult presents with a history of recurrent infections.

COMMON VARIABLE IMMUNODEFICIENCY

Patients with common variable immunodeficiency have a later onset of infections than do patients with X-linked agammaglobulinemia, and the two sexes are equally affected.[8] In addition to recurrent infections, they have autoantibodies; normal (or large) tonsils and lymph nodes; and, in about 25% of patients, splenomegaly. Associated syndromes have included sprue, lymphoid hyperplasia of the intestine, thymoma, alopecia, hemolytic anemia, gastric atrophy, pernicious anemia, thyroid dysfunction, vitiligo, and a symmetric moderately severe arthritis that is painful but not erosive. There is an almost 500-fold increase in the incidence of lymphomas in women in their 40s and 50s with common variable immunodeficiency. With the exception of those who develop polio, persistent enterovirus, rheumatoid arthritis, or a lymphoreticular malignancy (an incidence of approximately 6%), the overall prognosis for common variable immunodeficiency and X-linked agammaglobulinemia is good in patients who receive routine IgG replacement therapy.

SELECTIVE IGA DEFICIENCY

Selective IgA deficiency is defined as a deficiency of IgA but with normal other immunoglobulins. It is the most common immunoglobulin deficiency disorder, with perhaps 1 in 350 persons (blood donors) being affected. Because this immunoglobulin is the major immunoglobulin of external secretions, it is not surprising that these individuals have respiratory, gastrointestinal, and urogenital tract infections caused by bacteria but not viruses. Similar to common variable immunodeficiency, these patients have an excessive incidence of autoimmune diseases, including systemic lupus erythematosus, rheumatoid arthritis, dermatomyositis, pernicious anemia, thyroiditis, diabetes mellitus, chronic active hepatitis, idiopathic thrombocytopenic purpura, hemolytic anemia, and inflammatory bowel diseases. IgA deficiency appears to have an autosomal inheritance.

Most patients have normal IgG levels. Because a small amount of IgA may be present in intravenous immunoglobulin preparations, intravenous IgG should not be given for fear of causing anaphylactic reactions, as many patients have circulating IgE antibodies against IgA. Occasionally, selective IgA-deficient patients evolve into common variable immunodeficiency.

ANTIBODY DEFICIENCY WITH NEAR-NORMAL IMMUNOGLOBULIN

Patients with antibody deficiency with near-normal immunoglobulin are rare but perhaps overlooked in medical practices. They have normal T-cell function and near-normal or normal immunoglobulin concentrations but have deficient antibody responses to infectious agents. Accordingly, these patients have recurrent pyogenic infections, similar to those with agammaglobulinemia. Occasionally, they are observed to decline into a situation consistent with common variable immunodeficiency. Therefore, in a patient with recurrent infections but normal IgG levels, their ability to respond to antigenic challenge with pneumococci, diphtheria, or tetanus should be measured, and if subnormal, these individuals are candidates for monthly intravenous immunoglobulin infusions.

ATAXIA TELANGIECTASIA

Ataxia telangiectasia is a complex syndrome in which disease progresses through childhood until patients are wheelchair-bound. The process evolves from progressive cerebellar ataxia and cutaneous telangiectasia to chronic sinopulmonary infections, a high incidence of malignancy, and variable immune deficiency. Fifty percent to 80% of patients have a selective IgA absence and delayed cutaneous anergy.

COMPLEMENT DEFICIENCIES

Deficiencies of complement component proteins are inherited as codominant processes; a single *null* gene is expressed as half-normal levels of a complement protein, and with two null genes, the protein is completely absent.[9] As mentioned previously, the CH50, which measures function of all components of the classic pathway of complement, is the best screening test. Referral to a specialty laboratory is essential for sorting out the concentrations of complement proteins other than C3 and C4.

C1Q DEFICIENCY. Most patients have systemic lupus erythematosus or a mesangiocapillary glomerulonephritis.

C1R DEFICIENCY. These rare patients with this autosomal dominant disorder also have a lupus-like syndrome, nephritis, or both.

C1 INHIBITOR DEFICIENCY. Patients continually activate complement, have frequent attacks of hereditary angioedema, and have an increased frequency of systemic lupus erythematosus.

C4 DEFICIENCY. Homozygous C4-deficient patients typically present with acute and severe systemic lupus erythematosus. Diagnosis is difficult because the *typical* lupus patients have negative antinuclear antibody titers and DNA-binding activities.

C2 DEFICIENCY. This is, by far, the most frequent of complement deficiencies. The gene frequency is approximately 1%. Connective tissue diseases, such as systemic lupus erythematosus, polymyositis, glomerulonephritis, and vasculitis, or malignancy (Hodgkin's disease) occur in a third of patients.

MEMBRANE ATTACK PROTEIN DEFICIENCIES. These proteins are C5-/C9. Patients with deficiencies are particularly susceptible to *Neisseria* infections (some disseminated); some develop systemic lupus erythematosus.

CHRONIC GRANULOMATOUS DISEASE

Chronic granulomatous disease affects young patients, who have serious recurrent bacterial and fungal infections often associated with large granuloma formation related to an inability of neutrophils to kill adequately organisms that they have phagocytosed.

OTHER SYNDROMES

Increased skill and technology have enabled investigators to detect phenotypic subgroups of patients that have demonstrably similar genetic defects. They include syndromes such as (1) cartilage-hair hypoplasia, (2) immunodeficiency with thymoma; (3) hyperimmunoglobulinemia E syndrome; (4) leukocyte adhesion deficiencies; and (5) syndromes with defective T-cell receptors, cytokine (interleukin-2) production, and T-cell activation defects.

REFERENCES

1. Sakai LY, Burgeson, RE, Olson, BR, et al: Current knowledge and research directions in heritable disorders of connective tissue. Matrix Biol 15:211, 1996.
2. Williams CJ, Vandenberg P, Prockop DJ: Collagen and elastin. In Kelley WN, Harris ED Jr, Ruddy S, Sledge CB, eds: Textbook of Rheumatology, 5th ed. Philadelphia, WB Saunders, 1997, pp 23–36.
3. Trelstad RL: Matrix glycoproteins and proteoglycans. In Kelley WN, Harris ED Jr, Ruddy S, Sledge CB, eds: Textbook of Rheumatology, 5th ed. Philadelphia, WB Saunders, 1997, pp 37–54.
4. Cole WG: Osteogenesis imperfecta as a consequence of naturally occurring and induced mutations of type I collagen. Bone Min Res 8:167–204, 1994.
5. Yeowell HN, Pinell SR: The Ehlers-Danlos syndromes. Semin Dermatol 12:229, 1993.
6. Rowe DW, Shapiro JR: Heritable disorders of structural proteins. In Kelley WN, Harris ED Jr, Ruddy S, Sledge CB, eds: Textbook of Rheumatology, 5th ed Philadelphia, WB Saunders, 1997, pp 1535–1562.
7. Buckley RH: Specific immunodeficiency diseases, excluding acquired immunodeficiency syndrome. In Kelley WN, Harris ED Jr, Ruddy S, Sledge CB, eds: Textbook of Rheumatology, 5th ed. Philadelphia, WB Saunders, 1997, pp 1282–1304.
8. Cunningham-Rundles C: Clinical and immunologic analyses of 103 patients with common variable immunodeficiency. J Clin Immunol 9:22, 1989.
9. Ruddy S: Complement deficiencies and rheumatic diseases. In Kelley WN, Harris ED Jr, Ruddy S, Sledge CB, eds: Textbook of Rheumatology, 5th ed. Philadelphia, WB Saunders, 1997, pp 1305–1312.

Chapter 35

Osteoporosis

Robert A. Marcus

Osteoporosis is a condition of skeletal fragility resulting from reduced bone mass and disrupted skeletal microarchitecture. The consequence of porotic, or *spongy*, bone is fracture with low or even trivial degrees of trauma. A major public health problem in its own right, osteoporosis gains particular importance for patients with rheumatologic conditions. Some rheumatologic disorders are themselves conducive to accelerated bone loss (e.g., rheumatoid arthritis). The exercise tolerance of patients with rheumatic diseases may be limited, resulting in diminished habitual mechanical loading of the skeleton. Many such patients also receive drugs that profoundly disrupt skeletal maintenance, particularly glucocorticoids. Appropriate evaluation and management of skeletal risk is therefore essential to effective care. This chapter considers assessment of skeletal risk, prevention of bone loss, and treatment of osteoporosis in patients with rheumatologic conditions.

NORMAL ACQUISITION AND MAINTENANCE OF BONE

At any time in adult life, bone mass, the *amount* of bone that is present, reflects that which was gained during growth minus subsequent losses. Most discussions of osteoporosis have focused on conditions leading to accelerated bone *loss*, but it is now recognized that acquisition of robust bone mass in early adult life is critically important for skeletal health many years later. About 75% of peak bone mass reflects genetic endowment, but *environmental* factors contribute as well. Those factors that are best understood include physical activity, nutrient intake (particularly calcium), and reproductive hormone adequacy. About 60% of final adult bone mass is gained during a 3- to 5-year interval associated with the adolescent growth spurt. This *window of opportunity* can be jeopardized if illness, dietary or gonadal insufficiency, medications toxic to the skeleton, or prolonged immobilization limits bone acquisition. Once epiphyseal fusion brings an end to linear growth, opportunity for substantial bone gains ceases, and the adult phase of bone maintenance, followed by loss, ensues. For an individual with a substantial deficit in peak bone mass, even minimal additional loss constitutes an extreme risk for fractures. Several deleterious factors that constrain bone acquisition, such as restricted activity and glucocorticoid use, may plague young patients with *juvenile rheumatoid arthritis, ankylosing spondylitis, systemic lupus erythematosus,* and other rheumatic diseases.

Under normal circumstances, measurements of bone mineral density (BMD) after termination of bone acquisition are generally stable or decrease only slightly until about age 50 years, when BMD declines progressively from all skeletal regions in both men and women. The rate of loss is more rapid in women for several years, particularly in regions that are enriched in trabecular bone, such as the spine. This accelerated loss clearly reflects menopausal lack of estrogen.

BONE REMODELING

The basis for adult bone loss is bone remodeling, a continuous process of breakdown and renewal that takes place throughout life.[1] At least a passing familiarity with remodeling is essential to understand the mechanisms by which bone is lost normally or in disease states and by which bone is conserved or increased with therapy. During growth years, the impact of remodeling on skeletal economy is relatively meager and is overwhelmed by the effect of bone acquisition. Throughout adult life, remodeling is the final common pathway for various factors, whether they are dietary, mechanical, hormonal, or pharmacologic, to modulate the rate of bone loss. Remodeling is carried out by myriad independent *bone remodeling units* on bone surfaces. The surface density of trabecular bone far exceeds that of cortical bone, so the prevalence of remodeling activity and hence of remodeling-induced changes in bone mass is considerably greater in those same areas. About 90% of bone surfaces are normally quiescent, covered by a thin syncytium of lining cells. The remainder show evidence for a remodeling event in progress (Fig. 35–1).

The first event in a remodeling cycle is the appearance at a site on the bone surface of cells derived from macrophage-like precursors in the marrow. These cells fuse and develop characteristic features of the multinucleated giant cells known as *osteoclasts*. Osteoclasts remove, or resorb, a divot of bone from the surface, leaving a hole (osteoclast lacuna) that may reach a depth of 60 μ in a few weeks. Release of growth factors and cytokines embedded in the resorbed bone matrix attracts precursors of bone-forming cells (preosteoblasts) from the marrow stroma to the lacunar base, where they ma-

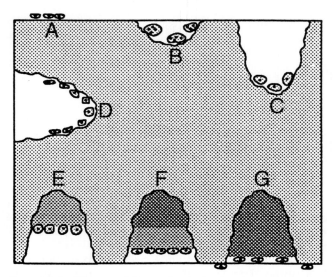

Figure 35–1. The remodeling cycle. *A,* Resting trabecular surface. *B,* Multinucleated osteoclasts dig a cavity of approximately 20 μm. *C,* Completion of resorption to 60 μm by mononuclear phagocytes. *D,* Recruitment of osteoblast precursors to the base of the resorption cavity. *E,* Secretion of new matrix by osteoblasts. *F,* Continued matrix secretion, with initiation of calcification. *G,* Completion of mineralization of new matrix. Bone has returned to quiescence, but a small deficit in bone mass persists. In addition, the black line represents a small filigree of woven collagen at the base of the resorption cavity. This cement line constitutes an area of weakened resistance to fracture. Accumulation of cement lines throughout adult life makes an important contribution to skeletal fragility at older ages.

ture into osteoblasts and produce new collagen and other components of bone matrix. Mineralization begins when newly synthesized matrix reaches a thickness of approximately 20 μ and continues on average about 6 months, until the resorbed bone is almost completely replaced by new mineralized bone. Similar to most biologic processes, bone remodeling is not completely efficient, so that on completion of each remodeling event, a small bone deficit remains. This *remodeling imbalance* underlies the process of age-related bone loss; that is, loss of bone should be viewed as a normal, predictable consequence of remodeling. Any stimulus that increases the rate of bone remodeling increases the rate of bone loss, and anything that suppresses remodeling lowers it.

Perturbations in remodeling can arise by distinct mechanisms, acting alone or in combination. Increased entry of new units into the active remodeling mode (i.e., in the birth rate of new remodeling units) accelerates bone loss simply because the number of remodeling-associated deficits per unit time also increases. Such perturbations are characteristic of patients with hyperthyroidism, hyperparathyroidism, and hypervitaminosis A and D. An exaggeration of remodeling inefficiency and therefore in the deficit remaining after each remodeling event is produced by agents that are toxic to osteoblasts; these include ethanol, glucocorticoids, and progressive age.

Another mechanism is observed with estrogen deprivation at menopause, when the efficiency of osteoclastic bone resorption may increase substantially, leading to trabecular perforation. Replacement of bone

requires a scaffold onto which osteoblastic cells can work. Trabecular perforation eliminates that scaffold, so that osteoblast proliferation is not possible, and the resorbed bone represents a permanent loss. Although these remodeling perturbations are presented as distinct entities, in most cases a mixture of dynamic alterations is present. Thus, in hyperparathyroidism, an increase in remodeling birth rate is accompanied by a decrease in the per cell activity of newly recruited osteoblasts. Estrogen-deficient bone may show evidence for osteoclastic hyperactivity as well as an increased remodeling birth rate.

ASSESSING SKELETAL RISK

History

A careful history to illuminate antecedent factors affecting the skeleton should be taken from every menopausal woman and man older than 60 years of age. The history should include exploration of events of early life. Important elements are fractures and immobilization; childhood illness and medications; previous and current diet and physical activity; chronology of pubertal development, menarcheal age, and regularity of menses; and tobacco and alcohol exposure. Eating disorders, pregnancy, and skeletally toxic medications should also be explored. Because the majority of peak bone mass is genetically determined, a family history of osteoporosis and fractures may also provide important information.

Bone Mass Measurement

Although osteoporosis is defined as a condition of low bone mass and disruption of normal skeletal microarchitecture, noninvasive tools currently available for clinical assessment provide estimates only of bone mass and do not address microarchitecture or other aspects of bone quality. Methods to estimate bone mineral density are generally based on the principles of densitometry (i.e., the attenuation of energy transmission through tissue by mineralized structures). Comprehensive discussion of bone densitometry is beyond the scope of this chapter, but a number of reviews are available for interested readers.[2] For most purposes, dual-energy x-ray absorptiometry (DXA) has emerged as a consensus optimal technique. DXA offers reasonable accuracy, precision, and a low exposure to ionizing radiation. It is less expensive than quantitative computed tomography (CT) and routinely permits measurements at sites other than the spine, such as hip, forearm, and whole body, whereas most CT facilities presently do not offer measurements beyond the lumbar spine.

Improvements in densitometry equipment have led to the introduction of several techniques to assess BMD at single peripheral sites, such as the forearm or calcaneus (single-energy and dual-energy peripheral x-ray absorptiometry, single-energy photon absorptiometry, peripheral CT). These devices offer reasonable accuracy and precision and are far less expensive than standard DXA. Although they cannot provide comprehensive assessment of skeletal status, they are useful for the primary application of bone densitometry, identifying patients at increased long-term risk of fracture.

Prospective studies clearly show that deficits in BMD are associated with increased fracture risk.[3, 4] For every 1 standard deviation (SD) below age-predicted mean values, fracture risk goes up twofold to threefold. By World Health Organization criteria, BMD values less than −2.5 SD from the mean value of a 25-year-old woman *define* the presence of osteoporosis, and values less than −1.0 SD are designated *osteopenia*. Although these criteria may be useful in selecting patients for intervention, they do not constitute a gold standard for diagnosis of an osteoporotic skeleton.[5] Proper uses of densitometry in patients with rheumatologic diseases include an initial ascertainment of fracture risk and subsequent monitoring of the effect of therapy. For initial determination of fracture risk, any of the available techniques gives reasonable information. For sequential monitoring, DXA of the spine, hip, and forearm remains superior, so patients who are identified to be osteopenic by peripheral methods and who may require multiple assessments over time should be referred for regular DXA assessment.

Biochemical and Other Assessments

In Northern latitudes and whenever exposure to sunlight is restricted, vitamin D sufficiency may be marginal or grossly deficient. Vitamin D nutritional status is determined by a measurement of circulating 25-hydroxyvitamin D (25-OHD), the major circulating form of vitamin D. Circulating concentrations of 25-OHD should approximate 30 ng/mL. Values less than 10 ng/mL are associated with florid osteomalacia, whereas values of 10 to 20 ng/mL may be associated with hypersecretion of parathyroid hormone (PTH) and increased bone loss. 25-OHD concentrations are not recommended as a routine screening test, but because vitamin D insufficiency may underlie poor responsiveness to therapy, its presence should be evaluated before starting patients on antiresorptive medications when there is reason to suspect that it may exist.

Laboratory Assessment

It is likely that most patients receiving treatment for rheumatic diseases already undergo periodic surveillance of blood counts and routine multiphasic chemistry profiles. Few additional tests are necessary for routine skeletal assessment, although physicians must remember that malignant diseases, particularly multiple myeloma, may be expressed initially as bone pain or fracture. Probably the most common metabolic abnormality that requires identification is vitamin D inadequacy. A fasting calcium × phosphorus product (mg/dL) less than 20 can indicate the presence of osteomalacia, a state of undermineralization of bone matrix.

Bone Turnover Markers

Assays are now available for determining the concentration in blood and excretion in urine of specific markers of bone turnover.[6] These may be useful in identifying patients with high turnover states, which are independently associated with increased fracture risk, and may also be useful in monitoring the response to therapy before a follow-up BMD measurement would give definitive results. For example, a change over time in BMD of approximately 4% may be required to conclude with 90% confidence that a real change has taken place. This magnitude of change might normally occur over 2 years or more. By contrast, suppression of bone turnover marker activity is generally detectable within a few weeks of initiating therapy. Thus, a biochemical check on patient compliance and dose adequacy can be made considerably earlier than BMD confirmation. Currently available bone turnover assays include urinary markers of resorption: deoxypyridinolines (D-PYD), and the telopeptides of type I collagen (NTx and Crosslaps). Markers of bone formation are measured in serum and include osteocalcin, bone-specific alkaline phosphatase, and the procollagen extension peptide of type I collagen. Although considerable evidence supports the utility of biochemical markers in assessing groups of patients in clinical trials, their utility in managing individual patients remains uncertain.

Radiographs

Standard radiographs are notoriously poor for assessing the amount of bone but provide definitive information regarding the presence of fracture and may be useful in demonstrating regional areas of bone loss. For assessing vertebral deformity, lateral thoracic and lumbar spine films are employed. Several approaches to quantifying vertebral deformities have been described, but for most clinical purposes, a 20% reduction in anterior, mid-, or posterior vertebral height compared with the other two measurements is taken as evidence for compression.

MANAGING SKELETAL RISK

For patients who are not prescribed glucocorticoids, the principles of skeletal management do not differ from those applied to the general population. These include both hygienic and pharmacologic approaches. Hygienic management involves attention to physical activity, diet, lifestyle behaviors, and safety.

Physical Activity

All patients should be encouraged to carry out regular and frequent physical activity to whatever degree is tolerated and acceptable. Most people are relatively sedentary and find it difficult to accomplish anything more than a program of walking. Therefore, assuming mobility is reasonable, initiating a schedule of brisk walking three to four times each week is a reasonable first start. Only after a successful activity pattern has been established can additional components be added to an exercise regimen. These could include more vigorous weight-bearing activity, such as dancing, running, and jumping, although in the patient with arthritis this may not be feasible. A supervised program of progressive resistance training (machine weights) can improve gait and balance and be of help in stabilizing bone mass. For older patients, reduction of falls is of far greater consequence to fracture risk than changes in bone density. Thus, an exercise regimen should give particular attention to strengthening the quadriceps group and other leg muscles.

Diet

From the skeletal perspective, adequate intake of calcium and avoidance of excess sodium are probably the most important considerations.[7,8] A dietary calcium intake of 1000 mg/day is recommended to meet skeletal requirements for young adult patients not taking glucocorticoids. After menopause, unless estrogen is taken, recommended intakes rise to about 1500 mg. One quart of milk contains about 1100 mg/day, so unless patients are able to drink the equivalent of 1 quart every day, it is highly likely that a supplement is necessary. Several reliable, reasonably inexpensive calcium supplements are available. The two major forms are carbonate and citrate salts. Evidence suggests that per tablet, the citrate salt may be better absorbed than carbonate, but this difference is minimal. A patient should be encouraged to sample two or three preparations to determine which is most palatable. Bioavailability is an important issue, particularly for some generic forms of calcium carbonate. Calcium preparations shown to be well absorbed include OsCal, Tums and Extra-Strength Tums, Caltrate, and Citracal.

Calcium homeostasis is determined not only by total calcium intake but also by other dietary constituents that affect calcium handling. Evidence suggests that dietary sodium constitutes an important modulator of calcium balance. Renal handling of sodium and calcium are tightly linked, so that a sustained reduction in sodium leads to substantial improvement in calcium balance.[8]

Attempts should be made to maintain vitamin D normalcy in all patients who may avoid sunlight, have reduced physical activity, have systemic diseases, and, particularly, may require glucocorticoid therapy. Daily doses of 400 to 800 units are appropriate and well-tolerated.

Lifestyle Habits

Epidemiologic evidence indicates that use of alcohol and tobacco creates an added risk for bone loss and fracture. Earlier reports that the added phosphorus in soft drinks led to bone loss are not correct. The primary issue related to soft drinks is that they are low in calcium. High-protein diets, particularly animal protein, have been implicated as a source of urinary calcium loss. Although a number of physiologic studies using liquid formula diets have successfully shown an effect of protein on urinary calcium, habitual protein intake does not appear to be an important risk factor for osteoporosis and associated fractures. In fact, patients with fracture are more likely to be deficient in multiple nutrients, including protein, and in-hospital intervention studies have shown that addition of a protein supplement improves outcomes for patients with hip fracture. There is no compelling evidence that caffeine makes an important contribution to bone loss or fracture risk.

Safety

Removing clutter and other factors around the home or workplace makes an important contribution to the goal of reducing falls. Patients should pay attention to adequate lighting, appropriate installation of safety rails in bathrooms and stairways, elimination of slippery throw rugs, and installation of carpet or other slip-proof materials on bathroom and kitchen floors. In many counties, public health nurses provide free or low-cost safety inspections to assist patients in this regard.

Pharmacologic Interventions

Although considerable work is being done to develop anabolic agents for bone, currently approved drugs for prevention and treatment of osteoporosis act by inhibiting bone resorption. The agent of first choice for women at menopause is estrogen. Hormone replacement therapy (HRT) conserves bone mass and when maintained long-term results in a decreased fracture incidence of about 60%. Other agents approved for prevention of bone loss at menopause include the selective estrogen response modifier raloxifene (Evista) and the potent amino-bisphosphonate, alendronate (Fosamax). Raloxifene is representative of a new class of estrogen-like drugs whose receptor interactions offer tissue specificity in response, so that some of the beneficial actions of HRT can be achieved without some of the less desirable effects. Whether every woman reaching menopause should undergo bone density testing before initiating HRT or its alternatives has been a topic of great controversy. Women with rheumatologic disease are clearly at added risk for bone loss, however, and assessment of such patients is appropriate. A comparison of HRT approaches is presented in Table 35–1.

Outside of the setting of menopause, such as for men of any age and premenopausal women, optimal therapy for low bone mass is uncertain and, in the absence of a rigorous clinical trial, highly individualized. In the absence of a prior fragility fracture and in cases in which glucocorticoids are not a factor, bisphosphonates are not routinely indicated for otherwise uncomplicated patients who simply have low bone mass. It seems more appropriate to assess by bone turnover

Table 35–1. CHARACTERISTICS OF CURRENT SELECTIVE ESTROGEN RECEPTOR MODULATORS

Agent	Actions				
	Bone	*Lipids*	*Uterus*	*Breast*	*Hypothalamus*
Estradiol-17β	4+ Agonist	4+ Agonist	4+ Agonist	4+ Agonist	4+ Agonist
Tamoxifen	2+ Agonist	2+ Agonist	3+ Agonist	Antagonist	Antagonist
Raloxifene	2+ Agonist	1+ Agonist	Null action	Antagonist	Antagonist

markers or by sequential densitometry whether the patient is in a high turnover state or is losing bone and to administer medication only under those circumstances. If fragility fractures have occurred, there is little choice but to use effective antiresorptive therapy. Alendronate 10 mg/day preserves and improves bone mass and, in a large 3-year clinical trial in women with osteoporosis, reduced fracture incidence by 50%.[9] Effective therapy with this agent requires fastidious attention to being in a fasted state, taking the medication with a full glass of water (and only water), and eating nothing and remaining upright for an additional 30 minutes after swallowing the pill. The primary adverse effect of alendronate is esophagitis, which occurred in fewer than 10% of patients in clinical trials but may be seen with greater frequency in clinical practice. Patients who already have gastric reflux may still take alendronate successfully, and use of H_2-blockers does not attenuate its affect.

GLUCOCORTICOID-INDUCED OSTEOPOROSIS

Characteristics

Treatment of glucocorticoid osteoporosis remains one of the most vexing challenges for rheumatologists and osteoporosis specialists.[10] Generally encountered when patients have been exposed to 15 mg/day of prednisone or its equivalent, bone loss proceeds at typical rates of 1% loss per month, then decreases after 6 to 12 months. Thus, interventions to prevent loss ideally would be initiated concomitant with, or shortly after, initiating glucocorticoid therapy. Glucocorticoid-induced bone deficits are greater in the axial skeleton than peripherally; trabecular deficits of 40% or greater are extremely common.

Mechanisms

A dominant model for glucocorticoid-induced bone loss has emerged over the past decade. By this model, the initial events take place at the intestine and kidney, where glucocorticoids directly inhibit the efficiency of gut calcium absorption and renal tubular calcium reabsorption, thereby slightly reducing blood-ionized calcium activity. In turn, compensatory hypersecretion of PTH develops. PTH action at the nephron improves reabsorption efficiency and also increases the production of 1,25-dihydroxyvitamin D, the primary active form of vitamin D, which ameliorates, albeit not completely, the impairment in intestinal calcium absorption. However, PTH also increases the birth rate of new remodeling units to increase the rate of bone loss, and, most important, in the presence of glucocorticoids, this increased bone remodeling activity is accompanied by marked inhibition of osteoblastic bone formation, so that not only are more remodeling units in action, but also the capacity of each to fill in with new bone is dramatically impaired, leading to substantial deficits in bone. For example, in some series of patients with polymyalgia rheumatica, glucocorticoid therapy resulted in 30% decreases in lumbar spine BMD within 1 year. Although this model is compatible with a broad range of experimental results, compelling demonstration of increased PTH concentrations has not been accomplished. Thus, a modification of the model holds that tissue responsiveness to PTH action is enhanced by glucocorticoids, permitting greater physiologic effect at usual circulating concentrations. Another action of glucocorticoids that carries adverse skeletal consequences is the suppression of the hypothalamic-gonadal axis, leading to hypogonadism, with its independent effects on remodeling rate and efficiency.[10]

Treatment

Treatment of established glucocorticoid osteoporosis, that is, patients with profoundly low bone mass and multiple fractures, remains highly unsatisfactory despite advances in osteoporosis therapeutics. The most satisfactory approach is to initiate early treatment to prevent the onset of glucocorticoid-related bone loss. The most effective strategy is for the physician to avoid glucocorticoids whenever possible and always to be alert for opportunities to minimize dosage and duration of therapy. If prolonged glucocorticoid treatment is unavoidable, a number of interventions appear rational and have been shown to be at least moderately useful. Identification and treatment of patients who are hypogonadal is an effective but often overlooked strategy. Prescribing supplemental calcium and vitamin D can overwhelm the intestinal block to calcium absorption and suppress the parathyroid axis, thus lowering remodeling rate. Where possible, regular, frequent exercise can promote mobility, limit muscular wasting, decrease the risk of falls, and help maintain bone mass.

Specific pharmacologic agents have also been shown to offer skeletal protection. In particular, beneficial effects of calcitriol and bisphosphonates have been confirmed in controlled clinical trials. In one study,[11] 1 year of treatment with calcitriol (0.5 to 1.0 μg/day) with or without intranasal salmon calcitonin (400 IU/day) substantially reduced bone loss from the spine, although no effect was apparent at the hip. In the next year of follow-up, patients who had received combined calcitriol/calcitonin continued to preserve spine BMD, although those who received calcitriol alone lost bone. The latter observation was complicated by the fact that patients in the calcitriol-alone group had also received more glucocorticoids during year 2.

In another study,[12] BMD was monitored in a large group of men and women shortly after initiation of high-dose glucocorticoids. This placebo-controlled trial assessed the effects of etidronate, a bisphosphonate, given cyclically as a 400-mg tablet for 14 days followed by 500 mg of supplemental calcium for 76 days. Patients receiving etidronate increased average spine and femoral trochanter BMD by 0.61% and 1.46%, whereas the calcium-only placebo group sustained losses of 3.2% and 2.7%. More importantly, postmenopausal women who received etidronate experienced substantially fewer vertebral fractures than those assigned to placebo. Although this study was the first of its kind to address the efficacy of bisphosphonates in the prevention of glucocorticoid osteoporosis, there is no reason to believe that etidronate is uniquely effective in this regard.

In a study of patients treated with glucocorticoids for variable periods of time, 48 weeks of daily alendronate (5 to 10 mg/day) significantly increased BMD of the spine and hip compared with a control group.[13] This response was independent of the duration of steroid use prior to initiating treatment. In a 2-year follow-up presentation at an international scientific meeting, the same authors reported that alendronate resulted in a 90% reduction in vertebral fracture, although an apparent reduction in nonvertebral fractures was not significant. Once again, these results indicate that the optimum time to initiate skeletal protection against glucocorticoids is early in the course of steroid treatment.

The development of anabolic therapies to restore glucocorticoid-induced bone deficits that already exist has been an attractive notion for several decades. Promising results have been occasionally reported in a few studies using fluoride, growth hormone, or PTH, but although some formal clinical trials have been conducted with encouraging results,[14] none of these agents is currently approved for this purpose.

Special Considerations in Rheumatic Diseases

For the most part, application of risk assessment, skeletal evaluation, hygienic measures, and therapeutics to patients with rheumatic diseases does not differ fundamentally from that appropriate for other individuals. In a few situations, the rheumatic process itself requires adjustment in diagnostic tests or recommended therapies to accommodate unique disease-specific features. For example, assessment of spine bone mass in patients with ankylosing spondylitis should not be undertaken with DXA but requires CT to obviate the artifactual elevation resulting from extraosseous calcification.[15] Patients with rheumatoid arthritis may have substantial osteopenia adjacent to involved joints, reflecting the rheumatic process itself, and the physician may wish to obtain densitometric measurements at these sites using special DXA regional software. Patients with photosensitivity may require additional supplementation with vitamin D to compensate for their habitual avoidance of sunlight.

Bone Loss After Joint Replacement

Although total hip replacement is extremely successful in alleviating pain, increasing mobility, and improving function for patients with end-stage arthritis, it is associated with severe loss of bone around the prosthesis. Specialized DXA software permitting estimation of BMD adjacent to the prosthesis has permitted studies indicating that loss of bone from the proximal femur is extremely common and may average about 20% within the first postoperative year.[16] This loss compromises fixation of the new prosthesis and leads to increased postoperative loosening, periprosthetic fracture, and surgical revision. Studies in animal models indicate that alendronate may be highly protective against prosthesis-induced bone loss, and clinical trials in humans are currently under way.

REFERENCES

1. Marcus R: Normal and abnormal bone remodeling in man. Ann Rev Med 38:129–141, 1987.
2. Wahner H: Use of densitometry in management of osteoporosis. In Marcus R, Feldman D, Kelsey J, eds: Osteoporosis. San Diego, Academic Press, 1996, pp 1055–1074.
3. Hui SL, Slemenda CS, Johnston CC Jr: Age and bone mass as predictors of fracture in a prospective study. J Clin Invest 81:1804–1809, 1988.
4. Melton LJ III, Atkinson EJ, O'Fallon WM, et al: Long-term fracture prediction by bone mineral assessed at different skeletal sites. J Bone Miner Res 8:1227–1234, 1993.
5. Marcus R: The nature of osteoporosis. In Marcus R, Feldman D, Kelsey J, eds: Osteoporosis. San Diego, Academic Press, 1996, pp 647–659.
6. Delmas PD, Garnero P: Utility of biochemical markers of bone turnover in osteoporosis. In Marcus R, Feldman D, Kelsey J, eds: Osteoporosis. San Diego, Academic Press, 1996, pp 1075–1088.
7. Marcus R: Calcium as a primary treatment and prevention modality for osteoporosis. In Rosen CJ, ed: Osteoporosis, Diagnostic and Therapeutic Principles. Totowa, NJ, Humana Press, 1996, pp 151–158.
8. Devine A, Criddle RA, Dick IM, et al: A longitudinal study of the effect of sodium and calcium intake on regional bone density in postmenopausal women. Am J Clin Nutr 62:740–745, 1995.
9. Black D, Cummings SR, Karpf DB, et al, for the Fracture Intervention Trial Research Group: Alendronate reduces the risk of fractures in women with existing vertebral fractures: Results of the Fracture Intervention Trial. Lancet 348:1535–1541, 1996.
10. Lukert B: Glucocorticoid-induced osteoporosis. In Marcus R, Feldman D, Kelsey J, eds: Osteoporosis. San Diego, Academic Press, 1996, pp 801–820.
11. Sambrook P, Birmingham J, Kelly P, et al: Prevention of cortico-

steroid osteoporosis: A comparison of calcium, calcitriol, and calcitonin. N Engl J Med 328:1747–1752, 1993.

12. Adachi JD, Bensen WG, Brown J, et al: Intermittent etidronate therapy to prevent corticosteroid-induced osteoporosis. N Engl J Med 337:382–387, 1997.

13. Saag KG, Emkey R, Schnitzer TJ, et al: Alendronate for the prevention and treatment of glucocorticoid-induced osteoporosis. Glucocorticoid-Induced Osteoporosis Intervention Study Group. N Engl J Med 339:292–299, 1998.

14. Lane NE, Sanchez S, Modin GW, et al: Parathyroid hormone treatment can reverse corticosteroid-induced osteoporosis: results of a randomized controlled trial. J Clin Invest 102:1627–1633, 1998.

15. Lee YSL, Schlotzhauer T, Ott S, et al: Skeletal status of men with early and late ankylosing spondylitis. Am J Med 103:233–241, 1997.

16. Marchetti ME, Steinberg GG, Greene JM, et al: A prospective study of proximal femur bone mass following cemented and uncemented hip arthroplasty. J Bone Miner Res 11:1033–1039, 1996.

APPENDIX

ICD-9 Codes for Diagnosis in Rheumatic Diseases

Mark C. Genovese

This appendix provides an easy-to-use listing of the most commonly used ICD-9 codes in the treatment of connective tissue diseases. Although not meant to be the definitive or all-inclusive source of codes, it is designed to make it easy to reference the codes a rheumatologist or a primary care physician would be most likely to encounter. Each table is devoted to a different aspect of musculoskeletal illness.

Table 1A–1. OSTEOARTHRITIS AND OSTEOPOROSIS

Osteoarthrosis, site unspecified	715.0
Osteoarthrosis, shoulder	715.1
Osteoarthrosis, upper arm	715.2
Osteoarthrosis, forearm	715.3
Osteoarthrosis, hand	715.4
Osteoarthrosis, pelvic region and thigh	715.5
Osteoarthrosis, lower leg	715.6
Osteoarthrosis, ankle and foot	715.7
Osteoarthrosis, other specified sites	715.8
Osteoarthrosis, multiple sites	715.9
Osteomalacia	268.2
Osteoporosis, symptomatic	733.00

Table A1–2. MUSCULOSKELETAL INJURY AND INFLAMMATION

Adhesive capsulitis, shoulder	726.0
Arthralgia	719.40
Articular cartilage disorder	718.0
Back syndrome (neuritis)	724.4
Backache, unspecified	724.5
Bunion	727.1
Bursitis	727.3
Bursitis, Achilles	726.71
Bursitis, anserine	726.61
Bursitis, olecranon	726.33
Bursitis, pes anserinus	726.61
Bursitis, prepatellar	726.65
Bursitis, shoulder	726.10
Bursitis, subacromial	726.19
Bursitis, trochanteric	726.5
Carpal tunnel syndrome	354.0
Chondromalacia of patella	717.7
Degenerative disc disease	722.6
Dupuytren's contracture	728.6
Effusion, joint	719.0
Effusion, ankle joint	719.07
Effusion, elbow joint	719.02
Effusion, foot joint	719.07
Effusion, hand joint	719.04
Effusion, hip joint	719.05

Table A1–2. MUSCULOSKELETAL INJURY AND INFLAMMATION (*continued*)

Effusion, knee joint	719.06	Sprain, lumbar (spine)	847.2
Effusion, multiple joints	719.09	Sprain, lumbosacral	846.0
Epicondylitis, lateral	726.32	Sprain, lumbosacral chronic or old	724.6
Epicondylitis, medial	726.31	Sprain, neck	847.0
Ganglion and cyst of synovium, tendon, and bursa	727.4	Sprain, rotator cuff (capsule)	840.4
		Sprain, toe phalanx	845.10
Hallux rigidus	735.2	Sprain, wrist (cuneiform) (scaphoid) (semilunar)	842.00
Hallux valgus	735.0		
Hemarthrosis	719.1	**Spur,** bone	726.91
Loose body in joint	718.1	Spur, calcaneal	726.73
Metatarsalgia	726.7	**Swelling,** ankle	719.07
Musculoskeletal pains, unknown cause	729.2	Swelling, finger	729.81
Myalgias	729.1	Swelling, foot	729.81
Rotator cuff sydrome of shoulder and related disorders	726.1	Swelling, hand	729.81
		Swelling, joint	719.0
Sciatica	724.3	Swelling, superficial, localized (skin)	782.2
Spasm of muscle	728.85	**Tendinitis** (tendonitis), unspecified	726.90
Sprain, strain (joint) (ligament) (muscle) (tendon)	848.9	Tendinitis, Achilles	726.71
		Tendinitis, adhesive	726.90
Sprain, ankle	845.00	Tendinitis, adhesive shoulder	726.0
Sprain, ankle and foot	845.00	Tendinitis, calcific	727.82
Sprain, cervical, cervicodorsal, cervicothoracic	847.0	Tendinitis, calcific shoulder	726.11
Sprain, collateral knee (medial) (tibial)	844.1	Tendinitis, elbow	727.09
Sprain, collateral lateral (fibular)	844.0	Tendinitis, patellar	726.64
Sprain, cruciate knee	844.2	Tendinitis, shoulder	726.11
Sprain, finger(s)	842.10	Tendinitis, wrist	727.05
Sprain, finger phalanx	842.10	**Tenosynovitis** and synovitis	727.0
Sprain, foot	845.10	Tenosynovitis, radial styloid	727.04
Sprain, hand	842.10	Trigger, finger (acquired)	727.03
Sprain, knee	844.9		
Sprain, low back	846.9		

Table A1–3. AUTOIMMUNE DISEASES OR CONNECTIVE TISSUE DISEASES

Ankylosing spondylitis	720.0	Lupus erythematosus, systemic	710.0
Arthropathy associated with other endocrine and metabolic disorders	713.0	Lyme disease	088.81
Arthropathy associated with gastrointestinal conditions	713.1	Myositis	729.1
		Paget's disease	731.0
Arthropathy associated with hematologic disorders	713.2	Panniculitis, unspecified	729.3
		Polyarteritis nodosa	446.0
Arthritis, unknown cause	716.90	Polyarthropathy, unspecified inflammatory	714.9
Arthritis, unspecified infective	711.9	Polychondritis, relapsing	733.99
Arthropathy associated with infections	711	Polymyositis	710.4
Arthropathy associated with Reiter's disease and nonspecific urethritis	711.1	Polymyalgia rheumatica	725
		Positive fluorescent antinuclear antibody	796.4
Arthropathy in Behçet's syndrome	711.2	Psoriatic arthritis	696.0
Arthropathy, postdysenteric	711.3	Raynaud's phenomenon	443.0
Arthropathy associated with other bacterial diseases	711.4	Reflex sympathetic dystrophy	337.20
		Reiter's syndrome	099.3
Arthropathy associated with other viral diseases	711.5	Rheumatic fever	390
Arthropathy, transient	716.4	Rheumatism, palindromic	719.3
Aseptic necrosis of bone	733.4	Rheumatism, psychogenic	306.0
Antiphospholipid syndrome	286.5	Rheumatoid arthritis	714.0
Chondrocalcinosis (pseudogout)	275.4	Sacroiliitis, not elsewhere classified	720.2
Chondrocalcinosis, unspecified	712.3	Sarcoidosis	135.0
Costochondritis	733.6	Scoliosis and kyphoscoliosis	737.3
Crystal arthropathies	712	Septic arthritis	711.00
Crystal arthropathy, unspecified	712.9	Sicca syndrome	710.2
Dermatomyositis	710.3	Sjögren's syndrome	710.2
Elevated erythrocyte sedimentation rate	790.1	Spondylopathy, unspecified inflammatory	720.9
Eosinophilia myalgia syndrome	710.5	Stiffness of joint, not elsewhere classified	719.5
Eosinophilic fasciitis	728.89	Symptoms, other, referable to joint	719.6
Erythema nodosum	695.2	Synovitis and tenosynovitis	727.0
Fatigue	780.7	Synovitis, villonodular	719.2
Fibromyalgia	729.1	Systemic lupus erythematosus	710.0
Giant cell arteritis	446.5	Systemic sclerosis	710.1
Gout	274.9	Unspecified diffuse connective tissue disease	710.9
Hypersensitivity vasculitis	446.20	Vasculitis, systemic arteritis	447.6
Juvenile rheumatoid arthritis	714.30	Wegener's granulomatosis	446.4
Lupus erythematosus, discoid	695.4		

Table A1–4. MISCELLANEOUS DIAGNOSES

Anxiety	300
Depression	311
Fever	780.6
Headache, migraine	346.9
Headache, tension	307.81
Lymphopenia	288.8
Neutropenia	288.0
Thrombocytopenia	287.5

Table A1–5. PROCEDURE CPT CODES

Injection, tendon sheath, ligament, trigger points, or ganglion cyst	20550
Arthrocentesis, aspiration and/or injection: small joint, bursa, or ganglion cyst (e.g., fingers, toes)	20600
Arthrocentesis, intermediate joint, bursa, or ganglion cyst (e.g., wrist, elbow, and ankle)	20605
Arthrocentesis, major joint or bursa (e.g., shoulder, hip, knee, subacromial bursa)	20610

Representative Case Studies

Mark C. Genovese

CASE NO. 1 ALL IS NOT WHAT IT APPEARS

Mrs. Motini is a 73-year-old woman who presented on referral from her primary care physician with a 6-year history of bilateral pain in her knees and wrists. She had been diagnosed with rheumatoid arthritis 4 years previously and was treated for 3 years with low doses of prednisone (5 mg/day) with sustained subjective improvement. In the past year, she was switched to a nonsteroidal anti-inflammatory drug (NSAID) with continued modest benefit. She had mild complaints of morning stiffness lasting 15 minutes or less, and had no significant impairments in her ability to function. She complained of occasional warmth and swelling in her wrists and knees but not in other small or large joints. Periodically, she used a right wrist splint to provide relief from pain. She used no other medications (e.g., acetaminophen) and had never been treated with a disease modifying antirheumatic drug (DMARD).

On examination, Mrs. Motini had bilateral volar subluxation of both wrists with mild soft tissue swelling and synovitis. Range of motion in both wrists was decreased to 45 degrees of flexion and 30 degrees of extension. There was mild tenderness of the right first carpometacarpal joint, but she had no involvement of any other joints. Laboratory test results are listed in Table A2–1.

Radiographs (Fig. A2–1) showed extensive bony erosions at the right first carpometacarpal joint as well as lytic lesions involving the carpal bones of the right wrist, distal ulna, and radius. The left wrist showed foreshortening of the left radius with osteophytes at the distal radioulnar joint.

Discussion

This patient presented with what might have initially appeared to be polyarticular, symmetric, inflammatory arthritis and was thus diagnosed with rheumatoid arthritis. The patient was treated with low-dose prednisone with good response, probably reassuring her physician that the diagnosis was the correct one. When the presentation is reviewed in a critical light, however, there are suggestions that this is not rheumatoid arthritis.

1. The patient complained of stiffness, but when questioned the stiffness rarely, if ever, lasted beyond 15 minutes in the morning. Typically, inflammatory arthritis is accompanied by morning stiffness lasting more than 30 minutes.
2. The distribution of joints involved is unusual for rheumatoid arthritis. Rheumatoid arthritis may initially present in an asymmetric fashion but usually within 6 months becomes symmetric.
3. In a patient with long-standing disease (e.g., 6 years), it is uncommon to find localization to only the wrists and the knees. Rheumatoid arthritis commonly involves the small joints of the fingers and toes with strong predilection for the metacarpophalangeal and proximal interphalangeal joints.
4. Inflammatory arthritis is usually accompanied by elevations in the acute-phase reactants, the nonspecific markers of inflammation. The erythrocyte sedimentation rate (ESR) and c-reactive protein were low in this patient.
5. The test for rheumatoid factor was negative. Eighty percent of patients with rheumatoid arthritis are seropositive for rheumatoid factor.
6. The most helpful radiographs are the anteroposterior film of the hands and the Norgaard view, also known as the *ball catcher's* view. In long-standing rheumatoid arthritis, one expects to see evidence of juxta-articular osteopenia, joint space narrowing, and erosion. The Norgaard view might aid in identification of early erosions. In a patient with a 6-year history of disease without the use of any disease-modifying medications, one would expect to find one or more of these abnormalities. The asymmetry and unilaterality of the lesions in the carpal bones, and the absence of erosions or periarticular osteopenia in the metacarpophalangeal and proximal interphalangeal joints speak against the diagnosis of rheumatoid arthritis. The pattern of destruction is more consistent with osteoarthritis, whereas the overall clinical story is suspicious for a crystalline arthropathy.

Table A2–1. LABORATORY STUDIES

White blood cell count	6.4 k/μL
Hematocrit	39.1%
Platelets	288 k/μL
Blood urea nitrogen	13 mg/dL
Serum creatinine	1.1 mg/dL
Thyroid-stimulating hormone	1.1 U/mB
Rheumatoid factor	Negative
Erythrocyte sedimentation rate	12 mm/hr
Uric acid	3.1 mg/dL

Although the radiographs do not show evidence of chondrocalcinosis, one could still presume that this patient is suffering from calcium pyrophosphate deposition disease (CPPD). Acute attacks of joint pain in such individuals are called *pseudogout.*

A full discussion of CPPD is found in Chapter 30. CPPD may present in various forms—acute, chronic, and asymptomatic. Most patients present with clinical findings and radiographs similar to those seen in osteoarthritis. Studies have suggested that 10% of patients with CPPD ultimately develop a chronic, symmetric inflammation resembling rheumatoid arthritis.[1] This variant has come to be called *pseudo–rheumatoid arthritis.*

The definite diagnosis of CPPD can be difficult. Although chondrocalcinosis is seen in a majority of patients with CPPD, it is not always present, especially when cartilage is lost from involved joints. Although the presence of crystals in the synovial fluid significantly aids in the diagnosis, it is not uncommon to be unable to visualize them. In this patient, no definitive diagnosis has been made yet; however, the clinical scenario suggests CPPD. Although the initial diagnosis of rheumatoid arthritis might have been premature, the therapy used (NSAIDs or low-dose glucocorticoids) works equally well for CPPD. Additional studies that might provide insight in this case include a weight-bearing anteroposterior radiograph of the knees looking for CPPD arthropathy and chondrocalcinosis, and an arthrocentesis of the knee or wrist when there are signs of inflammation.

REFERENCE

1. O'Duffy JD: Clinical studies of acute pseudogout attacks: Comments on prevalence, predispositions, and treatment. Arthritis Rheum 19(suppl):349–352, 1976.

CASE NO. 2   PAIN, BUT NO GAIN

Mrs. Valney is 60-year-old woman who was referred by her primary care provider for the complaint of bilateral shoulder pain. On presentation, she noted that her shoulder discomfort had begun gradually over a period of 3 months. She noted that the shoulder discomfort was accompanied by generalized fatigue. Over the past 4 weeks, she had developed mild discomfort in the hip girdle and lower extremities and was complaining of difficulty getting up from a chair and with dressing and undressing. When asked to describe further the discomfort, she characterized it as stiffness and as a dull ache. She had initially been treated for 4 weeks with NSAIDs without substantial benefit. When questioned, she also complained of a poor energy level, insomnia, and restless sleep. She noted feeling tearful and depressed since the onset of the symptoms, and she recently was started on fluoxetine (Prozac) for depression.

Her past medical history was remarkable for depression and hypercholesterolemia. She worked as an office manager and reported that this condition was interfering with her ability to function at her expected level at work. She denied fevers, headache, change of vision, or tiredness of her jaw when chewing (jaw claudication).

Physical examination revealed an obese woman with normal vital signs and no difficulty with walking. With the exception of the musculoskeletal examination, everything was normal. She had mild tenderness over the trapezius and the deltoid muscle groups bilaterally. Although she attained full range of motion in her shoulders and hip, both passive and active motion were painful. The location of the discomfort was the proximal extremities rather than the joints themselves. There was no pain over the areas of the subacromial bursa in the shoulder or over the greater trochanteric bursae of the hips. No weakness was found, and the neurologic examination was normal. No other tender points were identified, and there was no evidence of synovitis on examination of her joints. Laboratory findings are listed in Table A2–2.

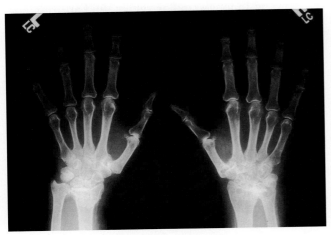

Figure A2–1. Case No. 1.

Table A2–2. LABORATORY STUDIES

Electrolytes	Normal
White blood cell count	Normal
Hematocrit	Normal
Platelets	Normal
Thyroid-stimulating hormone	Normal
Creatinine phosphokinase	Normal
Hepatitis C	Negative
Erythrocyte sedimentation rate	38 mm/hr

Discussion

Seldom do rheumatologic patients present in a textbook fashion with one clear diagnosis. The referring physician had initially diagnosed the patient with tendinitis/bursitis. The patient failed to improve, however, and the symptoms appeared more generalized; a referral was initiated. There was no pain to palpation over the bursae, and the persistent discomfort with both active and passive range of motion suggested this was not tendinitis/bursitis. The lack of synovitis and pain originating from the joints themselves made arthritis unlikely. The patient's difficulty getting out of a chair and with dressing might suggest myositis. Without objective weakness or evidence of muscle breakdown, however, myositis would be an incorrect diagnosis. Although the patient also had depressive symptoms, depression does not cause an elevation in the ESR. The elevation in ESR and lack of other tender points suggest that this is not fibromyalgia.

The constellation of symptoms—stiffness, location, symmetry as well as constitutional symptoms—all suggest that this patient is suffering from polymyalgia rheumatica. This suggestion is further confirmed by the elevation in ESR and the absence of other laboratory abnormalities. The reader should recognize this case as fairly classic for polymyalgia rheumatica (a more thorough discussion of polymyalgia rheumatica can be found in Chapter 27). This patient had no other symptoms suggestive of temporal arteritis, which always needs to be considered in the setting of polymyalgia rheumatica.

This patient was started on prednisone at 20 mg/day with rapid resolution of symptoms, then with a slow glucocorticoid taper as her symptoms permitted.

CASE NO. 3   MORE THAN MEETS THE EYE

Mr. Litner is a 53-year-old white man who presented with complaints of a painful, swollen right ankle. Mild warmth and erythema had started 24 hours before, and it progressed rapidly to severe swelling. He denied any prior history of arthritis. With the exception of hypertension, he was otherwise healthy. He worked intermittently as a manual laborer but denied recent physical exertion or trauma. He routinely consumed three or more cans of beer a day but denied drug use and recent sexual activity.

On physical examination, he was afebrile and normotensive. His foot and ankle were warm and pink from the dorsum of the right foot to an area 3 cm proximal to the ankle joint. The area was warm, diffusely swollen, and tender to palpation. Active and passive motion resulted in significant pain and discomfort. On detailed examination, dorsiflexion, plantar flexion, inversion, and eversion were severely reduced, indicating involvement of both the ankle and the subtalar joints.

Discussion

This patient presented with an acute monarticular arthritis. The cause of this event was not obvious. In Chapters 2 and 18, an approach to the evaluation of single-joint involvement is outlined. High on the differential diagnosis list must be trauma and infection. Crystalline arthritis (i.e., gout and pseudogout) must also be considered in the differential diagnosis, while other possibilities might include Reiter's syndrome (arthritis, urethritis, and iritis) or a reactive arthritis. Given the absence of ecchymoses and no history of trauma, acute injury was unlikely. The types of infection that might be involved include *Staphylococcus, Streptococcus, Pseudomonas,* and gonococcus. Gout and CPPD can develop in this fashion; however, the location is unusual. Reiter's syndrome or a reactive arthritis is also a possibility; however, the patient was without eye or urinary tract involvement, and he had denied any prodromal gastroenteritis.

Given the obvious joint effusion, an arthrocentesis was performed. Gram stain of the small amount of turbid yellow fluid aspirated from the ankle revealed gram-negative diplococci, suggesting the presence of *Neisseria gonorrhoeae.* With a directed sexual history, the patient admitted to unprotected sexual activity with a prostitute 4 days before presentation. The patient's throat and urethra were swabbed, the sample was sent for culture, the health department was informed, and the patient was treated for both gonorrhea and chlamydia. A more detailed discussion of infectious arthritis is found in Chapter 33.

Paramount in evaluation of any patient with acute monarticular arthritis is the detailed sexual history regardless of age, religion, or marital status. Although we were fortunate to see organisms on the Gram stain, more often than not Gram stain and cultures of synovial fluid are negative in gonococcal arthritis, highlighting the need for the clinical diagnosis. Had the Gram stain been negative, the patient would have been treated presumptively for gonococcal arthritis.

CASE NO. 4 YOU CAN RUN, BUT YOU CAN'T HIDE

Mr. Burke is a 37-year-old man who was referred by his primary care physician for evaluation of chronic hip pain. He was an active, otherwise healthy man. The patient ran 3 to 5 miles daily for the past 20 years, and he denied any injuries or trauma. He experienced 5 to 10 minutes of morning stiffness in the hips. Eight months ago, he noted the onset of mild hip pain that was worse on the left side. He noted it was exacerbated by weight bearing and exercise. Initially, the patient made alterations in his usual routine by cutting short his workouts when the hip pain was worse. Six months ago, he began taking NSAIDs and acetaminophen as analgesics to reduce the discomfort. When the discomfort began to limit his activities severely, he sought medical care.

On examination, he appeared fit and lean. When asked to jog in place, he complained of pain. There was no lower back pain on direct palpation or on straight leg raising to suggest lower back pathology as the underlying cause. Strength and neurologic examination were normal. Examination of his knees showed no evidence of malalignment, effusion, crepitus, or laxity, and there was little evidence to suggest that this was referred pain from the knee. Palpation of the hips revealed no suggestion of hernia and no tenderness over the groin or greater trochanteric bursa. In the supine position, passive range of motion revealed significant limitations to internal and external rotation of the hips secondary to pain. In addition, he had difficulty maintaining a straight leg raise against resistance because of groin and thigh pain.

Discussion

The constellation of symptoms and signs suggests that the process is intra-articular. The differential diagnosis includes osteoarthritis, stress fracture, avascular necrosis, septic arthritis, and labral tear (the labrum is a fibrocartilaginous structure lining the acetabulum).

The patient had plain radiographs taken (Fig. A2–2) that show narrowing of the joint space superolateral to both of the femoral heads. Sclerosis is seen at the acetabular margin, slightly more marked on the left. Subchondral cyst formation is seen in the lateral aspect of the left acetabulum. There is also hypertrophic spur formation at the inferior aspect of the femoral heads. The radiographs suggest significant bilateral osteoarthritis of the hips. Had the radiographs been less revealing and the pain persistent, magnetic resonance imaging (MRI) or a bone scan might have been useful to assess for early evidence of an insufficiency fracture or avascular necrosis.

This patient developed significant bilateral osteoarthritis of the hip for unclear reasons. Obviously the hip was subjected to repetitive stresses over the past 20 years of running. It is unknown to what degree strenuous weight-bearing activity predisposes to the develop-

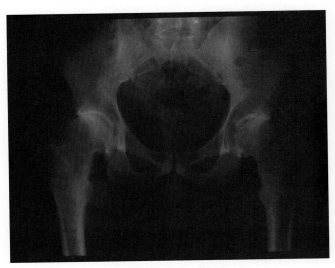

Figure A2–2. Case No. 4.

ment of osteoarthritis, but there is literature to suggest that running by itself does not predispose to increased risk of osteoarthritis of the hip or knees.[1, 2] It is more likely that this individual suffered from an unrecognized congenital hip disease. It has been reported that greater than 75% of hip osteoarthritis is a result of unrecognized childhood hip disease.[3, 4] Most often, however, early degenerative osteoarthritis of the hip results from mild dysplasia of the hips and incongruity on the articular surface between the femoral head and the acetabulum. Weight bearing and repetitive stress across the joint then leads to premature loss of cartilage.[5, 6]

The current degree of pain and arthritic change makes the patient's options somewhat limited. The continued use of acetaminophen, NSAIDs, or both may be useful from the standpoint of analgesia. Reduction in the degree of weight-bearing activity may delay his need for hip replacement surgery for a short period of time. Had the arthritis been identified earlier, there may not have been any difference in the outcome. Changing from weight-bearing to non–weight-bearing exercise, however, would have been recommended. As well, the patient would have been advised to maintain his ideal body weight because obesity is one of the modifiable risk factors for the development of osteoarthritis. In the future, agents (e.g., tetracycline-based antibiotics) that inhibit matrix metalloproteinases, enzymes known to degrade cartilage, might be used in an effort to slow the progression of osteoarthritis.

REFERENCES

1. Lane NE, Bjorkengren A, Oehlert J, et al: The risk of osteoarthritis with running and aging: A five-year longitudinal study. J Rheumatol 20:461–468, 1993.
2. Fries JF, Singh G, Morfeld D, et al: Relationship of running to musculoskeletal pain with age: A six-year longitudinal study. Arthritis Rheum 39:64–72, 1996.
3. Ranawat CS, Miyasaka KC, Umlas ME, Rodriguez JA: The hip. In Kelly WN, Harris ED Jr, Ruddy S, Sledge CB, eds: Textbook of Rheumatology, 5th ed. Philadelphia, WB Saunders, 1997, pp 1723–1738.

4. Stulberg SD, Cordell LD, Harris WH, et al: Unrecognized child-hood hip disease: A major cause of idiopathic osteoarthritis of the hip. In The Hip: Proceedings of the Third Open Scientific Meeting of the The Hip Society. St Louis, CV Mosby, 1975, p 212.
5. Stulberg SD, Harris WH: Acetabular dysplasia and development of osteoarthritis of the hip. In The Hip: Proceedings of the Second Open Scientific Meeting of the Hip Society. St Louis, CV Mosby, 1974, p 82.
6. Murphy SB, Kijewski PK, Millis MB, Harless A: Acetabular dysplasia in adolescent and young adult. Clin Orthop 261:214–223, 1990.

CASE NO. 5 SHE'S GOT HER HANDS INTO EVERYTHING

Ms. Willitts is a 55-year-old woman who was referred by her primary care physician for complaints of pain and swelling in the joints of her hands. Her symptoms started 3 years ago with swelling of her second proximal interphalangeal (PIP) joint of her left hand, accompanied by significant pain, warmth, and erythema. Approximately 2 years ago, she noted the involvement of the second PIP joint on the right side in a similar fashion to the left. In the last 4 months, she noted the progressive involvement of the third, fourth, and fifth PIP joints bilaterally. The chronic pain and swelling of those joints was also accompanied by morning stiffness of approximately 30 minutes in duration. She had initially sought care from her primary care physician, who had prescribed NSAIDs with only modest benefit. In general, she denied involvement of any joints outside the PIP joints already mentioned and denied any history of trauma.

On examination, she was a thin woman in good health. Examination of her hands revealed marked synovitis and swelling of the PIP joints bilaterally in virtually symmetric fashion. Most involved were the second and third PIP joints bilaterally, with both swelling and bony enlargement. There was also notable bony enlargement of the distal interphalangeal joints bilaterally consistent with Heberden's nodes. No other joints were involved, and the remainder of her examination was unrevealing. Her laboratory studies are listed in Table A2–3.

Radiographs of the hands (Fig. A2–3) show normal mineralization and an absence of involvement of the metacarpophalangeal joints. There is evidence of erosive changes in the right hand, particularly in the second and third PIP joints, with total destruction of the second PIP joint. There is joint space loss in the PIP joints of both hands. The distal interphalangeal joints show joint space narrowing of the third and fifth fingers of the right hand. There is evidence of soft tissue swelling in the right second and third PIP joints, with similar involvement on the left side. The metacarpophalangeal joints are normal. The findings are consistent with erosive osteoarthritis, worse in the right hand than the left hand.

Discussion

In this case, the radiographs are informative. This patient might mistakenly be clinically diagnosed with rheumatoid arthritis; after all, she is suffering from a

Table A2–3. LABORATORY STUDIES

White blood cell count	4.9 k/μL
Hematocrit	38%
Platelets	197 k/μL
Blood urea nitrogen	21 mg/dL
Serum creatinine	0.8 mg/dL
Aspartate transaminase	27 IU/L
Alanine transaminase	19 IU/L
Rheumatoid factor	Negative
Antinuclear antibodies	Negative
Erythrocyte sedimentation rate	8 mm/hr

polyarticular inflammatory arthritis in a symmetric distribution. Arthritis limited to the PIP and DIP joints, however, is classic for inflammatory/erosive osteoarthritis. This particular variant is most common in middle-aged women, and there may be a family history. In this setting, it was probably not necessary to obtain the rheumatoid factor and the antinuclear antibody test because the results would not have altered the diagnosis of this patient. The cell count and chemistry panel were helpful to assess baseline renal and liver function before initiating treatment.

The cause of the inflammatory variant of osteoarthritis is unknown. The treatment strategy usually revolves around the use of NSAIDs in an effort to reduce inflammation. There is no evidence that the use of NSAIDs affects the outcome of this disease, and the negative impact of NSAIDs on proteoglycan production within cartilage may, in fact, offset any anti-inflammatory benefits. Often, patients are cycled through numerous NSAIDs in an attempt to find the most effective agent. Acetaminophen may be added as an analgesic. As another adjunct, patients may undergo intra-articular glucocorticoid injections, which are usu-

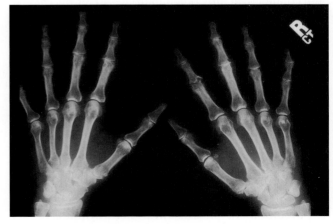

Figure A2–3. Case No. 5.

ally safe and quite effective, resulting in significant reductions in swelling and pain. Additional adjunctive therapies, such as hand therapy, paraffin wax treatments, capsaicin, and ergonomic modifications, can be quite helpful in reducing pain and improving the degree of function.

An alternative therapy that has shown some benefit in the treatment of inflammatory osteoarthritis is the use of hydroxychloroquine (Plaquenil). Hydroxychloroquine is an antimalarial and considered a DMARD because of its ability to slow the progression of disease in inflammatory arthritis. In a small series, investigators found hydroxychloroquine to be effective in six of eight patients with erosive osteoarthritis who had failed NSAIDs.[1] Although clearly not beneficial in the treatment of usual osteoarthritis, this agent might have a role in the inflammatory/erosive variant. Similarly, arguments could be made to initiate therapy with drugs that have been shown to inhibit matrix metalloproteinases (enzymes known to mediate the breakdown of cartilage), such as doxycycline or minocycline; however, these drugs are as yet unproven for this diagnosis.

REFERENCE

1. Bryant LR, des Rosier KF, Carpenter MT: Hydroxychloroquine in the treatment of erosive osteoarthritis. J Rheumatol 22:1527–1531, 1995.

CASE NO. 6 YOU'VE GOT THAT FIRE IN YOUR EYE

Mrs. Parker is a 47-year-old woman presenting for evaluation of dry eyes and dry mouth. She first noted scratchiness and burning in her eyes and the sense that she had sand in her eyes. Over the course of the next several months, she began feeling that her mouth was frequently dry and that she was consuming a lot of water. She simultaneously noted the development of mild swelling under her ears.

On examination, she appeared to be a healthy woman but had noticeable enlargement of her parotid glands (Fig. A2–4) Examination of her eyes revealed mild conjunctival infection and dryness. Her buccal mucosa was dry, and she had dental caries at the gum line. Her tongue was dry and smooth and had few papillae. The parotid glands were hard as well as being enlarged, but she had no evidence of adenopathy. The remainder of the examination was within normal limits.

Positive laboratory studies included Anti-SSA (Ro), Anti-SSB (La), and fluorescent antinuclear antibody. The constellation of symptoms, signs, and laboratory studies suggested that Mrs. Parker was suffering from Sjögren's syndrome.

Discussion

Traditionally, patients with sicca symptoms (dry eyes and mouth) are divided into primary Sjögren's syn-

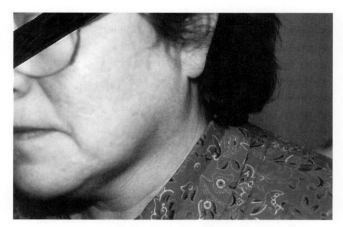

Figure A2–4. Case No. 6.

drome and secondary Sjögren's syndrome based on whether or not the sicca symptoms are related to another autoimmune or inflammatory disorder (rheumatoid arthritis, systemic lupus erythematosus [SLE], scleroderma, or mixed connective tissue disease [MCTD]). Primary symptoms include xerostomia (dry mouth) and keratoconjunctivitis. Although the involvement of the eye and mouth are well known, Sjögren's syndrome can cause symptoms in other organs, including the upper respiratory tract, gastrointestinal tract, thyroid, kidney, and vagina. The frequency of Sjögren's syndrome can vary significantly based on the criteria applied to make the diagnosis. In general, there should be symptoms of ocular dryness and xerostomia as well as some objective measures of dryness. Tests applied to assess ocular involvement have included Schirmer's test (measurement of tear flow by placing a strip of paper against the lower conjunctiva and measuring the distance of wetness after 5 minutes) or staining (fluorescein or rose bengal) of the cornea to visualize evidence of keratitis. Measures of salivary gland involvement have included a biopsy specimen of a minor salivary gland and measurement of parotid flow rates. In addition to the aforementioned features, there should be some evidence of an autoimmune process with an elevated antinuclear antibody, rheumatoid factor, anti-SS-A, or anti-SS-B.

The patient is suffering from primary Sjögren's syndrome because she has no evidence to suggest the presence of another inflammatory disorder and is taking no medications that could cause similar complaints. She had Schirmer's test performed and had less than 6 mm of tearing in 5 minutes. The only therapeutic options are symptomatic. No therapy is available to stop the lymphocytic infiltrate thought to be responsible for the salivary and lacrimal involvement. She was started on artificial tears, instructed on dental care, and given a dental referral. Should the traditional maneuvers prove inadequate, mouthwash and eyedrops with increased viscosity may be tried as can ophthalmologic occlusion of the lacrimal duct. Additional medications designed to stimulate tear and saliva production through muscarinic receptor stimulation have been developed but should not be tried without the guidance of the appropriate subspecialist. In the future, should there be any pain in or fluctuation in the size of the parotid or salivary glands, infection and malignancy should be considered. Infection occurs with increased frequency in Sjögren's syndrome related to decreased saliva flow. Patients with Sjögren's syndrome also have an increased risk of non-Hodgkin's lymphoma when compared with age-matched and sex-matched controls. If any questions exist that a lymphoma may be present, the glands should be imaged by MRI and possibly undergo biopsy.

CASE NO. 7   ALL TOO COMMON

Mr. Azul is a 60-year-old man referred for evaluation of arthritis in the knees. Over the past 6 years, he has noted a gradual worsening of the pain in his knees such that he was now having difficulty accomplishing ordinary tasks. The pain was worse with weight bearing, and he was having difficulty walking long distances or climbing stairs without significant pain. In the mornings, he had stiffness in his knees, but it never lasted longer than 5 to 10 minutes. His primary care physician diagnosed osteoarthritis, and he was seen once by an orthopaedic surgeon, who recommended total knee replacement. The patient chose not to undergo surgery. Instead, he was using large doses of NSAIDs until 3 weeks before presentation, when he vomited blood. He was hospitalized, and severe gastritis secondary to NSAID use was visualized by esophagogastric duodenoscopy. The NSAIDs were stopped, and he was placed on narcotic analgesics.

On physical examination, the patient was an obese man who had obvious knee pain while walking to the examining room. There was a mild varus deformity in his knees (bowlegged), and both knees were warm to the touch. He had a small effusion in his left knee (a positive bulge sign). The right knee had a larger effusion and a small Baker's cyst (synovial outpouching) in the popliteal fossa. There was no evidence of ligamentous laxity. He had mild pain on both active and passive range of motion.

Weight-bearing anteroposterior radiographs of both knees (Fig. A2–5) and a flexed lateral view (Fig. A2–6) were obtained. These two views allowed assessment of the three compartments of the knee: medial, lateral, and patellofemoral. The patient's radiographs showed narrowing of the medial compartment of the right knee with osteophyte formation in the medial, lateral, and patellofemoral compartments. A small calcific density was visible in the lateral compartment that may represent a loose body; additional calcific densities were noted on the lateral projection. The left knee also showed joint space narrowing of the medial and patellofemoral compartments with the development of osteophytes in all three compartments. Overall, the patient showed evidence of osteoarthritis of both knees slightly worse on the right.

Discussion

This case highlights the difficulty in treating patients with osteoarthritis, especially those that either

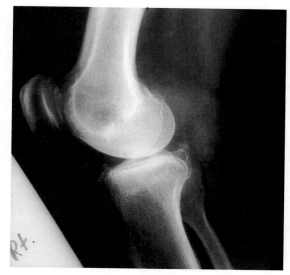

Figure A2–5. Case No. 7.

prefer to avoid surgery or are poor surgical candidates. Traditionally the risk factors for osteoarthritis include increased age, trauma, repetitive stress, obesity, race, genetic background, female gender, congenital or developmental defects, prior inflammatory joint disease, and metabolic or endocrine abnormalities.[1] Adaptations thought to be of use in delaying the progression of osteoarthritis include the avoidance of repetitive stress and the use of range-of-motion and strengthening exercises. The majority of therapy for osteoarthritis is directed toward pain relief. Traditionally, NSAIDs have been the agent of choice because of their anti-inflammatory and analgesic properties. NSAIDs, however, have been associated with significant side effects, including gastrointestinal bleeding. Some NSAIDs offer potentially less risk of gastrointestinal bleeding; these have traditionally included ibuprofen, nabumetone, and the nonacetylated salicylates choline magnesium trisalicylate (Trilisate) and salsalate (Disalcid). Now with the introduction of the new class of cyclooxgenase-2 (COX-2) inhibitors, patients taking selective NSAIDs may be at less of a risk for peptic ulcerations and bleeds

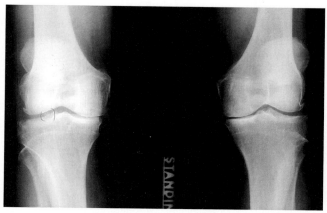

Figure A2–6. Case No. 7.

while taking these types of NSAIDs. Patients can alternatively be protected against the risks of NSAID gastropathy with proton-pump inhibitors or misoprostol (a prostaglandin E_1 analogue). In patients with a prior history of gastrointestinal bleeding, or in patients perceived to be at high risk for gastrointestinal bleeding, gastric prophylaxis or use of COX-2 selective agents should strongly be considered.

Alternatively, investigators have suggested that high doses of acetaminophen (up to 4000 mg/day) are effective in relieving the pain associated with osteoarthritis. When acetaminophen was compared to ibuprofen at both 1200 mg/day and 2400 mg/day, in a cohort of patients with chronic knee arthritis and moderate-to-severe osteoarthritis by radiograph, no significant difference in benefits could be found between the three groups at 4 weeks.[2] No medication is without side effects. An overdose of acetaminophen can lead to hepatic toxicity, and long-term use of acetaminophen has been shown to be associated with increased risk of renal failure.[3]

There are other therapies that might afford benefits in this patient. A glucocorticoid injection might be of use, although intra-articular glucocorticoids (in osteoarthritis) probably work best in patients with significant cartilage remaining, and they tend to be less effective when significant loss of joint space can be demonstrated. Injectable hyaluronic acid substances are available. Studies have suggested that a series of weekly injections (3 to 5 weeks) of hyaluronic acid into the knees of patients with osteoarthritis results in decreased pain. The mechanism of action of this therapy is unclear. The benefits over placebo and glucocorticoid injection are small, and this therapy is expensive (approximately $100 per injection at time of printing). Glucosamine and chondroitin sulfate have been touted as chondroprotective agents. There have been a number of small European studies looking at these agents compared to either placebo or NSAIDs, but all have been relatively short in duration (6 to 8 weeks). There might potentially be some mild clinical benefit, similar to that seen with modest NSAID use; however, claims of a cure for arthritis appear unfounded. Lastly, the application of topical medications such as capsaicin may provide benefit to some patients by working as counterirritants on the skin. Again, the studies suggesting efficacy are limited. Capsaicin, a topical application, works by the depletion of substance P (a chemical mediator responsible for the transmission of pain) from neurons and can give symptomatic relief.

REFERENCES

1. Hochberg M: Epidemiologic considerations in the primary prevention of osteoarthritis. J Rheumatol 18:1438–1140, 1991.
2. Bradley JD, Brandt KD, Kata BP, et al: Comparison of an anti-inflammatory dose of ibuprofen, an analgesic dose of ibuprofen, and acetaminophen in the treatment of patients with osteoarthritis of the knee. N Engl J Med 325:87–91, 1991.
3. Perneger TV, Whelton PK, Klag MJ: Risk of kidney failure associated with the use of acetaminophen, aspirin, and nonsteroidal anti-inflammatory drugs. N Engl J Med 331:1675–1679, 1994.
4. Constantz RB Jr: Hyaluronan, glucosamine, and chondroitin sulfate: Roles for therapy in arthritis? In Kelly WN, Harris ED Jr, Ruddy S, Sledge CB, eds: Textbook of Rheumatology, 5th ed. Update 27. Philadelphia, WB Saunders, 1998.

CASE NO. 8 A CASE FOR A CLOT, OR NOT

Mrs. Hingson is a 66-year-old white woman with a prior history of gout who was referred for the complaint of left leg pain of 6 months' duration. The pain started acutely while she was walking along the beach, then became dull and constant. The discomfort extended from the knee distally to the base of the calf, particularly posteriorly. Within a few hours of the development of pain, she noted swelling of the leg; and in a few days, she saw purple discoloration below the medial and lateral malleoli. The swelling and discomfort eased when she elevated her leg, but the pain returned when she stood or walked.

She was referred to physical therapy by her primary care physician, who also prescribed ibuprofen; neither physical therapy nor ibupofen helped. Because the pain and swelling persisted, a Doppler ultrasound was obtained. There was no evidence for a venous thrombosis or any other source of lower extremity swelling. The continued symptoms prompted a venogram; this also was normal. MRI of the lower extremities showed an effusion in the left knee, with an increased signal in the left calf muscles and posterior tibia. The cause of the increased signal remained unclear, and the patient was subsequently referred to the rheumatology clinic for evaluation.

On physical examination, the patient appeared healthy. There was no effusion, warmth, or erythema present in the left knee or ankle, and normal range of motion was present in both joints. There was no evidence of swelling, ecchymosis, or tenderness in the left thigh. The left calf did, however, have mild swelling and tenderness. There was a dark purple half-moon–shaped discoloration below the medial malleolus. Strength and neurologic examinations were normal.

Discussion

The difficulty in arriving at the correct diagnosis in this situation is that it must be part of the differential diagnosis from the beginning of symptoms. Based on the clinical story, it is relatively clear that this woman is suffering from a ruptured Baker's cyst, also known as pseudothrombophlebitis. A popliteal cyst (Baker's cyst) is an outpouching of synovium into the popliteal fossa. It is not an uncommon finding in rheumatoid arthritis but can also be found in other arthritides, including osteoarthritis. It usually presents with fullness in the medial aspect of the popliteal fossa. Occasionally, the popliteal cyst ruptures down into the calf. Rupture usually causes acute pain and the development of swelling in the lower part of the leg. The pain itself is related to the swelling, dissection, and possibly a mild compartment syndrome. The edema in the calf is worsened by impairment of venous or lymphatic flow. A *crescent sign*, a half-moon–shaped ecchymosis below the malleoli, is a telltale sign of hemorrhage into the calf. The presentation is commonly mistaken for thrombophlebitis. The worst outcome is that the patient is anticoagulated, a therapy that intensifies the hemorrhage.

Although the clinical presentation should have been adequate to make this diagnosis, an arthrogram was performed. The duration of the symptoms and the extent to which the patient had already been imaged made it necessary to establish the diagnosis clearly. The arthrogram (Fig. A2–7) shows evidence of a popliteal cyst enlarging with exercise. There is also evidence of a small amount of extravasation of contrast material from the joint into the popliteal fossa in Figure A2–8, establishing a ruptured Baker's cyst as the diagnosis. Doppler ultrasound usually reveals the diagnosis; in this case, however, neither a synovial outpouching nor contiguous extension of inflammation could be visualized. Although MRI provides outstanding visualization of the area involved, the intermittent nature of the swelling and the synovial rupture make it difficult to make the diagnosis. For this reason, MRI is usually not indicated. As well, the venogram was unnecessary because the clinical scenario and duration of symptoms made venous thrombosis highly unlikely.

The patient underwent glucocorticoid injection into the anterior compartment of the left knee, which resulted in a decrease in pain and swelling in the lower leg. The symptoms did not recur. Intra-articular glucocorticoid injection (triamcinolone hexacetonide

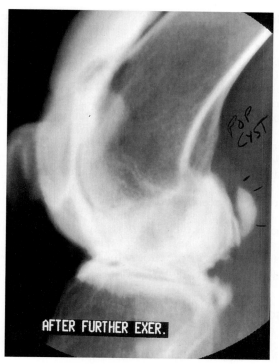

Figure A2–8. Case No. 8.

40 mg) usually results in a decrease in inflammation and synovial fluid. This decrease, in turn, reduces the force that pushes the fluid through the synovial herniation or outpouching and allows the tear in the synovium to heal. Should repeated injection fail to result in resolution, a referral to an orthopaedic surgeon should be made to have the synovial cyst resected.

CASE NO. 9 MAYBE JUST ANOTHER UPPER RESPIRATORY INFECTION

Mrs. Laguno is a 67-year-old woman who was seen in the hospital for consultation after developing palpable purpura on the lower extremities, hematuria, and hemoptysis. By her account, she was doing well until 3 weeks before admission, when she began to feel fatigued and developed a nonproductive cough. She was seen in an urgent care clinic 1 week before admission for the complaint of cough, nasal congestion, and mild epistaxis and was treated with amoxicillin for a possible bronchitis and sinusitis. She was taking no other medications and had no known drug allergies. Her symptoms continued to worsen. She developed a worsening cough, continued epistaxis, and blood-tinged sputum. Her family brought her to the emergency department because she continued to decline and had developed a fever to 101°F.

On examination, the patient had evidence of erythema and blood in the nasal mucosa. There were decreased breath sounds in her lungs and crackles in the lower two thirds of the lungs bilaterally. There were pal-

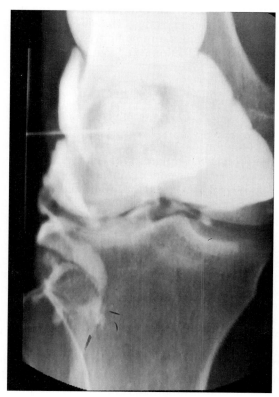

Figure A2–7. Case No. 8.

pable nonblanching purpuric lesions of varying size on the hands and lower extremities bilaterally. Chest radiographs showed diffuse interstitial and alveolar infiltrates bilaterally, and she was treated for presumptive infection.

Laboratory studies (Table A2–4) were markedly abnormal. At the time of admission, she had a vasculitic lesion on her foot; a biopsy sample later revealed leukocytoclastic vasculitis. On the second hospital day, she underwent a transthoracic echocardiogram looking for evidence of endocarditis, but the study was normal. Additionally, she had blood cultures and a purified protein derivative (PPD) test, which were negative. On the third day of hospitalization, she developed worsening hemoptysis and was subsequently started on intravenous glucocorticoids. The next day, she underwent an open lung biopsy of the right upper lobe and was started on oral cytoxan for the presumptive diagnosis of Wegener's granulomatosis.

Discussion

The patient presented with symptoms and signs suggestive of vasculitis. Wegener's granulomatosis classically presents with the triad of upper airway, pulmonary, and renal involvement (vasculitis is covered

Table A2–4. LABORATORY STUDIES

White blood cell count	22.1 k/μL
Hematocrit	27%
Platelets	172 k/μL
Blood urea nitrogen	34 mg/dL
Serum creatinine	1.7 mg/dL
Aspartate transaminase	45 IU/L
Alanine transaminase	38 IU/L
Serum albumin	3.1 g/dL
Erythrocyte sedimentation rate	82 mm/hr
24-hour creatinine clearance	35 mg/kg/day
Urinalysis	>100 RBC
Urinalysis	+++Protein
Antineutrophil cytoplasmic antibody titer	Positive cytoplasmic pattern 1 : 640
Anti–glomerular basement membrane antibody	Negative
Anti-streptolysin-O titer	Negative
Hepatitis B	Negative
Hepatitis C	Negative

more extensively in Chapter 27). Patients usually develop epistaxis, hemoptysis, and glomerulonephritis. There are limited forms with involvement confined to only one or two components of the triad. Other organ involvement can occur, including cutaneous vasculitis and otitis. The cause of the necrotizing granulomatous lesions is unknown, but activated neutrophils are thought to mediate the process.

The presence of antineutrophil cytoplasmic antibodies (ANCAs) has been useful as a marker of the disease, and it has been postulated that the antibody itself may be involved in the pathogenesis of the disease. There are two types of staining patterns associated with ANCAs: cytoplasmic and perinuclear. The cytoplasmic staining pattern (C-ANCA) is related to the proteinase-3 antigen and appears to be relatively sensitive and specific for Wegener's granulomatosis. The perinuclear staining pattern (P-ANCA) is related to the myeloperoxidase antigen and has been associated with other types of vasculitis but is much less sensitive and specific.

The patient manifested enough clinical and laboratory evidence of vasculitis to warrant empirical treatment. Formal diagnosis, however, requires pathologic evidence of necrotizing granulomas. It is important to be certain about the diagnosis before committing the patient to long-term therapy that has significant toxicity. The patient was empirically treated while awaiting biopsy results, which returned positive for granulomas with central necrosis and multinucleate giant cells, small arteries with lymphocytic and polymorphonuclear neutrophil infiltration, and perivascular inflammation. After 6 months of treatment, she remains on oral cytoxan but has been tapered to 5 mg/day of prednisone. Renal function has returned to normal, and the urinary sediment is no longer active. The nasal lesions have healed, and she denies any hemoptysis. The patient is back to work and functioning normally.

CASE NO. 10   A ROSE BY ANY OTHER NAME

Ms. Goulding, a 35-year-old woman with a history of hypothyroidism, is referred for complaints of fatigue and muscle pain. The patient states she was diagnosed with hypothyroidism 5 years ago and did well on thyroid replacement therapy. One year ago, she began to complain of increasing fatigue and the development of generalized musculoskeletal pain. She noted that the discomfort waxed and waned but became more progressive over the last year. She noted that exacerbating factors included stressful events at home and at work, physical exertion, and cold damp weather. She denied any relieving features but thought that her activity level had decreased significantly. She sought care from her primary care physician, who was unable to identify any significant physical findings but checked a number of laboratory studies. Her thyroid function appeared normal, as did her electrolytes, renal and liver function tests, and hematocrit. She had an antinuclear antibody (ANA) test performed which returned positive at a titer of 1:160, and she was subsequently referred to the rheumatologist for evaluation.

On presentation, she complained of generalized discomfort, but, when questioned, she was able to localize the areas of increased discomfort to her upper back and the lateral side of her hips. The complaints of fatigue and of stiffness were also paramount to this patient. When asked, she admitted to a great deal of difficulty with insomnia and to feeling depressed and anxious. She denied alopecia, rash, photosensitivity, aphthous ulceration, arthritis, serositis, renal disease, neurologic disorder, or immunologic/hematologic laboratory abnormalities.

On physical examination, she appeared depressed and irritable. Musculoskeletal examination revealed tenderness to palpation in relatively few areas, particularly across the occiput, upper back, epicondyles, upper and outer buttocks, greater trochanters, and at the medial fat pad of the knee. Examination of her joints showed no synovitis and normal active and passive range of motion. Strength was normal bilaterally, and neurologic examination was unremarkable.

Discussion

A number of issues need to be considered in the differential diagnosis of this patient. The patient has had a problem with her thyroid in the past; and although her symptoms are odd for thyroid disease, it is important to be confident that she is euthyroid, as her primary care provider was. Additionally, the positive ANA always generates the concern over possible systemic lupus erythematosus or other diffuse connective tissue diseases. The important question here is: Without the ANA, would there be any features suggestive of lupus? The patient does not have any significant features of systemic lupus erythematosus. The lack of synovitis based on normal joint examination virtually excludes an inflammatory arthritis. The lack of muscle weakness on examination indicates that she is not suffering from a myositis. Polymyalgia rheumatica, however, is a possibility. With polymyalgia rheumatica, the fundamental features are more of stiffness, particularly in the shoulder and hip girdles, and less of generalized pain, tenderness, and fatigue. There are a few additional laboratory studies that might ensure that one of the aforementioned diagnoses has not been missed. The ANA should be repeated, although it may be related to the history of thyroid disease. In addition, a small percentage of women in the population are ANA positive without any accompanying disease. Finally, the titer of 1:160 is probably not significant. Obtaining a urinalysis to look for additional evidence of renal disease is useful. This patient's urinalysis was negative. Obtaining a marker of muscle breakdown, such as a creatinine kinase, is important, and in this case it was normal. Lastly, the assessment of acute-phase reactants is justified in this patient because they are nonspecific markers of inflammation. The ESR and c-reactive protein were both within the normal range and suggested that this patient was not suffering from an inflammatory disorder.

In this light, it becomes clear that the patient is suffering from fibromyalgia. She has the typical features of musculoskeletal pain, tenderness, fatigue, poor sleep, and depression. Although a more thorough discussion is found in Chapter 18, some of the salient features are important. For the diagnosis of fibromyalgia, the 1990 American College of Rheumatology guidelines specify that the patient have a history of widespread pain for 3 months or longer.[1] The definition of *widespread* is above and below the diaphragm and on both the right and the left sides of the body. The pain is more often in an axial rather than a peripheral distribution. According to the criteria, the patient should manifest at least 11 out of the 18 possible tender points when 4 kg of force is applied. In practical reality, it is not that important to meet the exact quota of tender points. The more important issue is to consider the diagnosis, exclude legitimate other possibilities, and initiate a treatment plan. Fundamental to the treatment plan are the encouragement and support from the physician; an exercise regimen; a plan for improving insomnia; and muscle relaxants, NSAIDs, and acetaminophen to reduce pain and help the patient remain functional.

REFERENCE

1. Wolfe F, Smythe HA, Yunus MB, et al: The American College of Rheumatology 1990 criteria for the classification of fibromyalgia: Report of the Multicenter Criteria Committee. Arthritis Rheum 33:160–172, 1990.

CASE NO. 11 A DIAGNOSIS OF EXCLUSION

Mr. Sammon is a 34-year-old man referred to the rheumatologist with history of a rash, fevers, and arthritis. The patient was in normal health until 1 month before referral when he first developed an erythematous rash on the upper torso and upper extremities. Symptoms progressed over the next few days to include fevers to 102.5°F, myalgias, and arthritis. The arthritis involved the wrists and first carpometacarpal joints bilaterally. The patient was seen by his primary care physician and given an intramuscular glucocorticoid injection, which provided significant benefit, but symptoms returned within 2 days. The patient noted that the fevers and rash were worse in the evening and were often accompanied by a sore throat. He returned to his physician when the symptoms returned and was given a course of amoxicillin and prednisone (60 mg/day and a 2-week taper to 0). The patient experienced dramatic improvement initially; however, when the prednisone dose was tapered to 10 mg, the fevers, rash, and arthritis returned. He was subsequently admitted to the hospital for evaluation. He underwent a number of imaging studies, including chest radiograph (normal); computed tomography (CT) scans of the sinuses (normal), abdomen (hepatosplenomegaly), and pelvis (normal); and a ventilation/perfusion scan (normal). Many laboratory tests were performed (Table A2–5). A PPD (negative)

Table A2–5. LABORATORY STUDIES

Electrolytes	Normal
Creatinine	0.9 mg/dL
Aspartate transaminase	67 IU/L
Alanine transaminase	111 IU/L
Total protein	6.7 g/dL
Albumin	3.1 g/dL
Lactate dehydrogenase	538 IU/L
White blood cell count	30.1 k/μL
Differential	86% D to PMN
Platelets	490 k/μL
Hepatitis B	Negative
Urinalysis	Normal
Antinuclear antibodies	Negative
Rheumatoid factor	Negative
Creatinine phosphokinase	21 IU/L
Erythrocyte sedimentation rate	65 mm/hr
Rapid plasma reagin	Negative
Lyme titer	Negative
Complement	Normal
Thyroid function tests	Normal
Parvovirus	Normal
Epstein-Barr virus	Negative
Hepatitis C	Negative

Table A2–6. SYNOVIAL ASPIRATE

White blood cells	17 k/μL
Red blood cells	.820 k/μL
Differential	86% PMN
Gram stain	Negative
Tuberculosis smear and culture	Negative
Culture	Negative

PMN, Polymorphonuclear neutrophils.

Still's disease. This is the adult presentation of the systemic form of juvenile rheumatoid arthritis. Still's disease is a systemic inflammatory illness accompanied by the hallmark signs of spiking fever, rash, and polyarthritis. Commonly the clinical features include high spiking fevers (often accompanied by a sore throat); arthritis; and a subtle, fleeting erythematous salmon-colored rash typically referred to as *evanescent*. The rash is typically maculopapular and involves the torso and extremities. Arthritis commonly affects the knees, wrists, and PIP joints and less commonly the hips and shoulders. The accompanying synovitis is usually mild, but a minority of patients have radiographic progression of arthritis. Occasionally, carpal ankylosis (Fig. A2–9) may occur and has been described as a diagnostic sign in adult Still's disease.[1, 2] A waxing and waning sore throat, lymphadenopathy, and hepatosplenomegaly are among the more common symptoms and signs associated with Still's disease. Frequently, patients show elevations in the ESR, a leukocytosis with a predominance of neutrophils, and a transaminitis. More recently, serum ferritin values have been found to be markedly elevated in Still's disease, with values sometimes exceeding 20,000 μg/mL.[3]

The diagnosis of adult-onset Still's disease is based on a constellation of symptoms and signs and usually is a diagnosis of exclusion. The exclusion of infectious, in-

and bone marrow biopsy (negative) were also performed before rheumatology consultation.

On examination, the patient was febrile to 101.5°F with a prominent rash. The rash was maculopapular and nonconfluent. It was most prominent on the upper torso and upper extremities. The patient had mild adenopathy in the cervical chain. Lungs were clear, and there was no murmur. Abdominal examination revealed mild hepatosplenomegaly. Musculoskeletal examination revealed mild swelling, warmth, and decreased range of motion in the wrists and the left knee. The left knee was aspirated (Table A2–6).

Discussion

The patient underwent a substantial work-up, yet at the time of consultation it was unclear to all involved as to the illness. This case highlights one of the more enigmatic of the connective tissue diseases, adult-onset

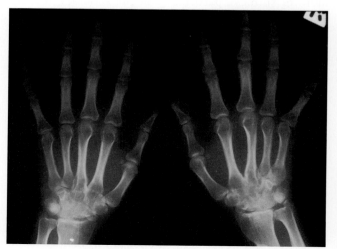

Figure A2–9. Case No. 11.

flammatory, and neoplastic diseases is crucial before making the diagnosis. For this patient, the exclusionary work-up had already been completed, and the constellation of symptoms made the diagnosis more straightforward.

Because the cause of Still's disease is unknown, the treatment is empirical. Patients are generally tried on NSAID therapy first, but for those with severe disease, glucocorticoid therapy is needed. Prednisone should be given in a dose of 1 to 2 mg/kg/day, although some patients may do well with smaller doses. For patients with severe disease and in those who cannot be successfully tapered off glucocorticoids, DMARDs are usually used. Methotrexate has been shown to be useful in adult-onset Still's disease and has been a useful glucocorticoid-sparing agent.[4]

The patient was started on prednisone, and low-dose methotrexate (7.5 mg/week) was added. He had a good response, and the prednisone was tapered off after 3 months; he has a good prognosis.

REFERENCES

1. Bywaters EGL: Still's disease in the adult. Ann Rheum Dis 30:121–133, 1971.
2. Medsger TA, Christy WC: Carpal arthritis with ankylosis in late onset Still's disease. Arthritis Rheum 19:232–242, 1976.
3. Ohta A, Yamaguchi M, Kaneoka H, et al: Adult Still's disease: Review of 228 cases from the literature. J Rheumatol 14:1139–1146, 1987.
4. Kraus A, Alarcon-Segovia D: Fever in adult onset Still's disease: Response to methotrexate. J Rheumatol 18:918–920, 1991.

CASE NO. 12   TIME WILL TELL

Mrs. Jimenez is a 34-year-old Hispanic woman referred for the complaint of bilateral hand pain of 5 months' duration. The patient noticed a gradual increase in pain and swelling bilaterally in the PIP, metacarpophalangeal, and wrist joints. She noticed a progressive increase in morning stiffness, now lasting up to 3 or 4 hours, and relieved somewhat by taking a warm shower and forcing herself to use her hands preparing breakfast. Later in the day, the pain is made worse by activity. She has worked as a housekeeper for 20 years but now is having difficulty doing her job. She has tried over-the-counter ibuprofen and acetaminophen; neither gave her significant relief. She has occasional discomfort and stiffness in her knees but substantially less than what she has been experiencing in her hands. When further questioned, she admitted to gradually worsening alopecia, and a mild persistent red rash on her cheek bones. She denies fever, aphthous ulcers, serositis, neurologic disorder, renal disease, and photosensitivity. She had no significant past medical history or family history.

On examination, the patient appeared healthy except for a subtle malar rash. She did not have any patchy alopecia, but she did have mild generalized thinning of the hair on her scalp. Examination of the hands revealed significant warmth and swelling in both wrists and a noticeable reduction in both flexion and exten-

Table A2–7. LABORATORY STUDIES

White blood cell count	6.5 k/μL
Hematocrit	38.3%
Platelets	275 k/μL
Differential	59% PMN, 31% lymphocytes
Blood urea nitrogen	11 mg/dL
Creatinine	0.7 mg/dL
Aspartate transaminase	22 IU/L
Alanine transaminase	16 IU/L
Urinalysis	Normal
Antinuclear antibodies	>1:640
Rheumatoid factor	Negative
Anti–double-stranded DNA	Negative
Extractable nuclear antigens	Negative
Complement (C3)	Normal
Complement (C4)	Normal
Thyroid-stimulating hormone	Normal
Creatinine phosphokinase	Normal
Erthyrocyte sedimentation rate	39 mm/hr

PMN, polymorphonuclear neutrophils.

sion. There was mild swelling of the PIP and metacarpophalangeal joints in bilateral and symmetric distribution.

Laboratory studies were obtained (Table A2–7). Radiographs of the hands (Fig. A2–10) showed areas that were suspicious for small bony erosions located in the left third distal metacarpal, right second distal

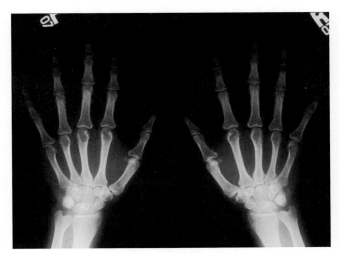

Figure A2–10. Case No. 12.

metacarpal, right third proximal phalanx, and right third distal metacarpal.

Discussion

The patient has symptoms, signs, and laboratory features of more than one illness. She is a good example of an overlap disorder or an undifferentiated connective tissue disease. The symptoms and signs of pain, stiffness, and swelling of hand and wrist joints and stiffness in a bilateral and symmetric distribution are diagnostic of an inflammatory arthritis. The ESR is elevated, providing nonspecific evidence of inflammation. The radiographs may have a subtle suggestion of early erosion, although the process has been going on only for 5 months, and it would be unusual to see erosion of bone. Against a diagnosis of rheumatoid arthritis, the rheumatoid factor is negative, and the antinuclear antibody is positive at a significant titer. She has a malar rash and alopecia suggestive of systemic lupus erythematosus. Arthritis is common in systemic lupus erythematosus but is not usually this prominent and almost never is erosive.

Other laboratory tests (see Table A2–7) were obtained. The urinalysis was normal reaffirming that there was no evidence for glomerulitis. Complement studies were also normal. Anti–double-stranded DNA (an insensitive but relatively specific marker for systemic lupus erythematosus) returned negative. Anti–extractable nuclear antigen (ENA) was sent; it also was negative. The extractable nuclear antigen is composed of an Sm antigen and ribonuclear protein, and, depending on the laboratory, may include SS-A (Ro) and SS-B (La). Thyroid studies were performed because there is a high association of thyroid disease and a positive antinuclear antibody, but these also were normal. Finally, a creatine kinase value was obtained to help insure that this was not a myositis associated with an overlap disorder. These tests failed to determine better whether this patient was suffering from systemic lupus erythematosus, rheumatoid arthritis, or another connective tissue disease.

For lack of better terms, this patient was given the diagnosis of an overlap syndrome with features of both systemic lupus erythematosus and rheumatoid arthritis. In the past, some authors have used the term *rupus* or *rhupus* to describe patients with these symptoms. Often, patients with this presentation go on to differentiate into one disease or the other after a number of years. This patient was treated with hydroxychloroquine (Plaquenil) because of its low toxicity, DMARD activity, and its efficacy in systemic lupus erythematosus. At 6 months, this patient had no evidence of arthritis or alopecia but continued to have a subtle malar rash. She requires periodic ophthalmalogic evaluation because of hydroxychloroquine use and vigilance on the part of her primary care physician and rheumatologist to help insure that she does not develop any significant joint or organ system damage in the future.

CASE NO. 13   WHEN JUST ONE WON'T DO

Mrs. Nguyen is a 30-year-old Vietnamese woman who was referred to a rheumatologist for Raynaud's phenomenon, fatigue, and progressive weakness. She was in good health until 6 months ago, when she noticed that her fingers began turning purple and white. Her symptoms were exacerbated by cold weather or by taking ice cream out of the freezer. During these last 6 months, Mrs. Nguyen began to develop significant fatigue; telangiectasias on her face, hands, and torso; alopecia; difficulty swallowing; and heartburn. Over the last 4 weeks, she has noticed progressive weakness and is now having difficulty continuing to function at her job as an electronics assembler.

On examination, she appeared fatigued and had numerous telangiectasias on her face. Her lungs were clear, and cardiac and abdominal examinations were normal. Examination of her hands showed a mild purple dusky tint across all her fingers, and they were cool. She had multiple telangiectasias, mild sclerodactyly, and some loss of digital pulp on the finger pads. There was mild puffiness in her hands and subtle synovitis. Her strength was notably decreased in the hip and shoulder girdles as well as in the muscles controlling flexion and extension of the neck. Laboratory studies were obtained and are listed in Table A2–8.

Discussion

At initial presentation, it is clear that this patient is suffering from Raynaud's phenomenon. The pres-

Table A2–8. LABORATORY STUDIES

White blood cell count	6.1 k/μL
Hematocrit	37.1%
Platelets	232 k/μL
Blood urea nitrogen	23 mg/dL
Serum creatinine	0.7 mg/dL
Aspartate transaminase	26 IU/L
Alanine transaminase	22 IU/L
ANA	1:320
Anticentromere	Negative
ENA	Anti-RNP 1:1,000,000
Anti-DS-DNA	Negative
Creatinine phosphokinase	1000 units
Urinalysis	Normal

ANA, antinuclear antibody; ENA, extractable nuclear antigen.

ence of many other features is suggestive of a more diffuse connective tissue disease. The constellation of symptoms is suspicious for the syndrome known as CREST (calcinosis, Raynaud's esophageal dysmotility, sclerodactyly, and telangiectasia). The term CREST is no longer used, in favor of the new term *limited systemic sclerosis*. In this patient, there was no evidence of calcinosis. Not all components of the syndrome need to be present to make the diagnosis, however. This syndrome has a high association with the presence of the anticentromere antibody, which serves as a sensitive marker for the process. In this patient, the anticentromere antibody was absent. More importantly, the patient was also suffering from fatigue and weakness, which is worrisome for myositis, a process not usually seen in CREST. The creatine kinase assay returned positive, confirming that muscle breakdown was taking place. Additionally, an extractable nuclear antigen was obtained. The extractable nuclear antigen is composed of an Sm antigen and a ribonuclear protein, and, depending on the laboratory, may include SS-A (Ro) and SS-B (La). In this patient, the anti–ribonuclear protein is positive at a substantial titer. This is indicative of mixed connective tissue disease.

Mixed connective tissue disease is an overlap disorder that has features of systemic lupus erythematosus, scleroderma, and polymyositis. The features of the disease include Raynaud's phenomenon, myositis, arthritis, and sclerodactyly. These symptoms do not have to appear concurrently but can appear sequentially over time. This patient's disease started with Raynaud's phenomenon, but probably she was developing subtle changes of sclerodactyly over a prolonged period of time. The patient underwent elecromyography/nerve conduction velocity studies that showed excessively abundant, low-amplitude, short-duration, polyphasic potential compatible with a myopathic process. She subsequently underwent muscle biopsy, which confirmed the presence of an inflammatory process in the muscles (myositis).

The treatment included high-dose glucocorticoids (1 mg/kg/day of prednisone) and the addition of methotrexate at 25 mg subcutaneously per week to control the myositis. The prednisone was tapered over a period of 8 weeks, and symptoms of weakness and muscle breakdown rapidly corrected. Additional therapies that proved beneficial included the use of calcium channel blockers for the Raynaud's phenomenon and proton-pump inhibitors for the esophageal discomfort. Although the original descriptions of mixed connective tissue disease suggested that the prognosis is good, there is no cure. Similar to systemic lupus erythematosus, scleroderma, and the other connective tissue diseases, the goal is to avoid organ damage and to keep the patient functional. Patients with this disorder are also at increased risk for the development of pulmonary hypertension, which is a major cause of mortality.

CASE NO. 14   IT'S NOT JUST SKIN DEEP

Mr. Spottes is a 48-year-old man who was in good health until 2 weeks ago, when he first began to notice fatigue, intermittent headache, and arthralgia. He also had pain, stiffness, and mild swelling in the hands. He did not seek medical care until he noticed the purplish discoloration of his lower legs. As the number of purple spots grew larger, he became concerned and presented to his primary care physician, who examined him and found discrete, purple papules that did not blanch on pressure. The lesions were seen in the feet and legs and appeared consistent with palpable purpura. Basic laboratory studies were obtained (Table A2–9), and the patient was referred to a rheumatologist for further evaluation.

The patient denied taking any prescription medications or herbal remedies and had no ill contacts. He did, however, admit to intermittent illicit drug use, including cocaine, amphetamines, and marijuana. As recently as 1 week prior, the patient had used amphetamines.

On examination, the patient appeared fatigued but in no distress. He was hypertensive with a blood pressure of 156/87 mmHg but afebrile. He had no adenopathy and had no oropharyngeal lesions. His lungs were clear, and he had no murmur. He had a mildly enlarged liver with the edge palpable 4 cm below the costal margin, and the spleen was also enlarged. He had trace-to-mild edema in the feet and ankles, but more striking were the purple lesions, predominantly on the extensor surface of the leg extending from the feet to just distal to the knee. As described previously, they were palpable, nonconfluent, nontender, nonblanching, and non-pruritic (Fig. A2–11). Examination of the hands revealed diminished grip strength and a trace of synovitis suggestive of arthritis.

Discussion

Vasculitis is often classified based on the size of the blood vessel involved: small, medium, or large. Vasculitis can be triggered by autoimmune disease, infection, and drug exposure. It is important to consider the possibilities in this situation (a more thorough discussion of vasculitis is in Chapter 27). Although this patient denied prescrip-

Table A2–9. INITIAL LABORATORY STUDIES

White blood cell count	4.1 k/μL
Hematocrit	38%
Platelets	135 k/μL
Blood urea nitrogen	18 mg/dL
Serum creatinine	1.6 mg/dL
Total protein	7.1 g/dL
Serum albumin	3.4 g/dL
AST	83 IU/L
ALT	78 IU/L

AST, aspartate aminotransferase; ALT, alanine aminotransferase.

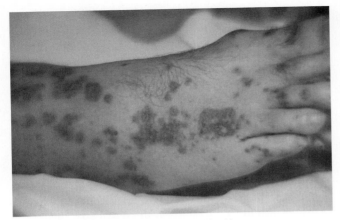

Figure A2–11. Case No. 14.

tion drug use, he admitted to recent amphetamine abuse. Amphetamines can lead to vasculitic syndromes and cause the development of palpable purpura; however, this diagnosis is probably insufficient to explain the enlargement of the liver and spleen as well as the arthritis.

Infections can precipitate vasculitic reactions. Streptococcal and staphylococcal infections can cause a leukocytoclastic vasculitis. Subacute bacterial endocarditis is one of the more common bacterial infections resulting in the development of a vasculitic syndrome. Human immunodeficiency virus has also been reported to cause a wide spectrum of vasculitic complications. Although parvovirus B19, the cause of erythema infectiosum (fifth disease) in children, can result in skin lesions and transient arthritis at initial presentation in adults, it would be unusual to result in palpable purpura or a true vasculitis.

Hepatitis C has been associated with a number of extrahepatic manifestations, with 36% to 54% of cases of hepatitis C having associated cryoglobulins. Cryoglobulins are immunoglobulins that reversibly pre-

Table A2–10. ADDITIONAL STUDIES

HIV	Negative
Hepatitis B	Negative
Anti–streptolysin O titer	Negative
Hepatitis C	Positive
Cryoglobulins	Positive

HIV, human immunodeficiency virus.

cipitate in the cold. Most cases of cryoglobulinemia associated with hepatitis C are mixed cryoglobulins of type II (monoclonal component) or type III (polyclonal component). This patient was subsequently checked for hepatitis C and cryoglobulins and was found to be positive for both. Additional laboratory tests were also performed (Table A2–10). Cryoglobulinemia is known to be responsible for a number of the features mentioned, including fatigue, arthralgia and arthritis, palpable purpura, and renal insufficiency and glomerulonephritis. In most cases, the hepatitis C virus is responsible for the cryoglobulin formation. Given this, therapy must be directed at the virus first. After the viral load and genotype of the hepatitis C virus were determined, therapy was instituted with interferon-α. Should the interferon-α fail to lead to a reduction in cryoglobulin formation and organ damage, the use of traditional agents, such as glucocorticoids, cytotoxics, and even plasmapheresis, would be considered.

REFERENCE

1. Pawlotsky JM, Roudot-Thoraval F, Simmonds P, et al: Extrahepatic immunologic manifestations in chronic hepatitis C and hepatitis C virus serotypes. Ann Intern Med 122:169–173, 1995.

Note: Page numbers in *italics* refer to illustrations; page numbers followed by b refer to boxed material, and those by t refer to tables.